Patient Derived Tumor Xenograft Models

Promise, Potential and Practice

Edited by

Rajesh Uthamanthil

Peggy Tinkey

Associate Editor

Elisa de Stanchina

ELSEVIER

AMSTERDAM • BOSTON • HEIDELBERG • LONDON
NEW YORK • OXFORD • PARIS • SAN DIEGO
SAN FRANCISCO • SINGAPORE • SYDNEY • TOKYO

Academic Press is an imprint of Elsevier

Academic Press is an imprint of Elsevier
125 London Wall, London EC2Y 5AS, United Kingdom
525 B Street, Suite 1800, San Diego, CA 92101-4495, United States
50 Hampshire Street, 5th Floor, Cambridge, MA 02139, United States
The Boulevard, Langford Lane, Kidlington, Oxford OX5 1GB, United Kingdom

Library of Congress Cataloging-in-Publication Data
A catalog record for this book is available from the Library of Congress

British Library Cataloguing-in-Publication Data
A catalogue record for this book is available from the British Library

ISBN: 978-0-12-804010-2

Publisher: Sara Tenney
Acquisition Editor: Sara Tenney
Editorial Project Manager: Halima Williams
Production Project Manager: Julia Haynes
Designer: Matt Limbert

Typeset by TNQ Books and Journals

Patient Derived Tumor Xenograft Models

Contents

Section III
PDX Models for Tumors of Various Organ Systems

Section IV
PDX Models in Cancer Research and Therapy Around the World

1. Global Practices in PDX Programs

G.Y. Ho, C.L. Scott and K. Pham

2. Role of Companies and Corporations in the Development and Utilization of PDX Models

J. Snyder, O. Duchamp, K. Paz and P. Sathyan

List of Contributors

O. Abdel-Wahab Memorial Sloan Kettering Cancer Center, New York, NY, United States

A. Akcakanat The University of Texas MD Anderson Cancer Center, Houston, TX, United States

S.F. Boyle Peter MacCallum Cancer Centre, East Melbourne, VIC, Australia; University of Melbourne, Parkville, VIC, Australia

T. Brabb University of Washington, Seattle, WA, United States

C. Brayton Johns Hopkins University School of Medicine, Baltimore, MD, United States

A. Bruna Cancer Research UK Cambridge Institute, Cambridge, United Kingdom; University of Cambridge, Cambridge, United Kingdom

D.M. Burgenske Center for Cancer and Cell Biology, Van Andel Research Institute, Grand Rapids, MI, United States

J.W. Cassidy Cancer Research UK Cambridge Institute, Cambridge, United Kingdom; University of Cambridge, Cambridge, United Kingdom

S. Chateau-Joubert Ecole Nationale Vétérinaire d'Alfort, Université Paris-Est, Maisons-Alfort, France

W. Cheng The First Affiliated Hospital of Nanjing Medical University, Nanjing, People's Republic of China

Y. Chen Memorial Sloan Kettering Cancer Center, New York, NY, United States; Weill Cornell Medical College, New York, NY, United States; New York-Presbyterian Hospital, New York, NY, United States

L.A. Colby University of Washington, Seattle, WA, United States

E. Corwin Seattle Genetics, Bothell, WA, United States

E. de Stanchina Memorial Sloan Kettering Cancer Center, New York, NY, United States

O. Duchamp Oncodesign, Dijon Cedex, France

J. Eswaraka Amgen Inc, Thousand Oaks, CA, United States

K.W. Evans The University of Texas MD Anderson Cancer Center, Houston, TX, United States

B. Fang The University of Texas MD Anderson Cancer Center, Houston, TX, United States

C.G. Fedele Peter MacCallum Cancer Centre, East Melbourne, VIC, Australia

J.B. Fleming The University of Texas MD Anderson Cancer Center, Houston, TX, United States

J.-J. Fontaine Ecole Nationale Vétérinaire d'Alfort, Université Paris-Est, Maisons-Alfort, France

A. Giddabasappa Pfizer Inc., San Diego, CA, United States

E. Girard Fred Hutchinson Cancer Research Center, Seattle, WA, United States

L.R. Hill The University of Texas MD Anderson Cancer Center, Houston, TX, United States

D.K. Hirenallur-Shanthappa University of Washington, Seattle, WA, United States; Amgen Inc., Thousand Oaks, CA, United States

G.Y. Ho The Walter and Eliza Hall Institute of Medical Research, Parkville, VIC, Australia; The University of Melbourne, Parkville, VIC, Australia; The Royal Women's Hospital, Parkville, VIC, Australia

G. Inghirami Weill Cornell Medical College, New York, NY, United States; University of Torino, Torino, Italy; New York University School of Medicine, New York, NY, United States

B.M. Iritani University of Washington, Seattle WA, United States

Y. Jiang The University of Texas MD Anderson Cancer Center, Houston, TX, United States; The First Affiliated Hospital of Nanjing Medical University, Nanjing, People's Republic of China

S.D. Kaffenberger Memorial Sloan Kettering Cancer Center, New York, NY, United States

A. Krivtsov Memorial Sloan Kettering Cancer Center, New York, NY, United States

M.G. Lawrence Monash University, Clayton, VIC, Australia

L. Liang The University of Texas MD Anderson Cancer Center, Houston, TX, United States

J. Liu The University of Texas MD Anderson Cancer Center, Houston, TX, United States; The First Affiliated Hospital of Nanjing Medical University, Nanjing, People's Republic of China

J.P. MacKeigan Center for Cancer and Cell Biology, Van Andel Research Institute, Grand Rapids, MI, United States

E. Marangoni Institut Curie, Paris, France

M. Mattar Memorial Sloan Kettering Cancer Center, New York, NY, United States

I. Mercado-Uribe The University of Texas MD Anderson Cancer Center, Houston, TX, United States

F. Meric-Bernstam The University of Texas MD Anderson Cancer Center, Houston, TX, United States

G.B. Mills The University of Texas MD Anderson Cancer Center, Houston, TX, United States

N. Niu The University of Texas MD Anderson Cancer Center, Houston, TX, United States

J.M. Olson Fred Hutchinson Cancer Research Center, Seattle, WA, United States; Seattle Children's Research Institute, Seattle, WA, United States; University of Washington, Seattle WA, United States

N. Paez-Arango The University of Texas MD Anderson Cancer Center, Houston, TX, United States

K. Paz Champions Oncology, Hackensack, NJ, United States

K. Pham The Walter and Eliza Hall Institute of Medical Research, Parkville, VIC, Australia; The University of Melbourne, Parkville, VIC, Australia

S.P.S. Pillai Fred Hutchinson Cancer Research Center Seattle, WA, United States

M. Pizzi University of Padova, Padova, Italy

J.T. Poirier Memorial Sloan Kettering Cancer Center, New York, NY, United States; Weill Cornell Medical College, New York, NY, United States

J.A. Ramírez University of Washington, Seattle, WA, United States

M.V. Rios Perez The University of Texas MD Anderson Cancer Center, Houston, TX, United States; University of Puerto Rico, San Juan, PR, United States

G. Risbridger Monash University, Clayton, VIC, Australia

P.J. Russell Queensland University of Technology at Translational Research Institute, Brisbane, QLD, Australia

P. Sathyan KEW Group Inc, Cambridge, MA, United States

M. Scaltriti Memorial Sloan Kettering Cancer Center, New York, NY, United States

S.C. Schmechel University of Washington, Seattle, WA, United States

C. Scott Walter and Eliza Hall Institute of Medical Research and Royal Melbourne Hospital, Parkville, VIC, Australia

C.L. Scott The Walter and Eliza Hall Institute of Medical Research, Parkville, VIC, Australia; The University of Melbourne, Parkville, VIC, Australia; Royal Melbourne Hospital, Parkville, VIC, Australia

J.-L. Servely INRA, Maisons-Alfort, France

M. Shackleton Peter MacCallum Cancer Centre, East Melbourne, VIC, Australia; University of Melbourne, Parkville, VIC, Australia

B.W. Simons Johns Hopkins University School of Medicine, Baltimore, MD, United States

J. Snyder University of Washington School of Medicine, Seattle, WA, United States

A.K. Sood The University of Texas MD Anderson Cancer Center, Houston, TX, United States

A.D. Strand Fred Hutchinson Cancer Research Center, Seattle, WA, United States

R. Taylor Monash University, Clayton, VIC, Australia

S. Thompson-Iritani University of Washington, Seattle, WA, United States

P.T. Tinkey The University of Texas MD Anderson Cancer Center, Houston, TX, United States

R. Uthamanthil Fred Hutchinson Cancer Research Center, Seattle, WA, United States

L. Wang The University of Texas MD Anderson Cancer Center, Houston, TX, United States

E.D. Williams Queensland University of Technology at Translational Research Institute, Brisbane, QLD, Australia

E. Yuca The University of Texas MD Anderson Cancer Center, Houston, TX, United States

J. Zhang Fourth Military Medical University, Xi'an, People's Republic of China

R. Zhang The University of Texas MD Anderson Cancer Center, Houston, TX, United States

Biographies

EDITORS

Dr. Rajesh Uthamanthil is the Director of Comparative Medicine Program at the Fred Hutchinson Cancer Research Center, Seattle, WA. He received a doctorate degree in veterinary medicine and veterinary sciences from the Kerala Agricultural University, a PhD degree in comparative biosciences from the University of Wisconsin–Madison, and completed a postdoctoral fellowship at the Rice University. Dr. Uthamanthil has more than 16 years of experience in animal models of human disease, most of it focused on cancer.

Dr. Uthamanthil also directs the patient-derived xenograft (PDX) core that supports studies using PDX models at the Fred Hutchinson Cancer Research Center. Dr. Uthamanthil has more than 20 peer-reviewed publications in the areas of translational research, has authored/coauthored two book chapters, and has made more than 30 presentations in national and international conference meetings.

Dr. Peggy Tinkey received degrees in veterinary science and veterinary medicine from the Texas A&M University, completed a postdoctoral fellowship in pathology at the Baylor College of Medicine, and is a Diplomate of the American College of Laboratory Animal Medicine. She is a Professor of comparative medicine and chairman of the Department of Veterinary Medicine and Surgery at the University of Texas M.D. Anderson Cancer Center (UTMDACC), where she directs the animal research program.

Dr. Tinkey has extensive experience in animal models of cancer, with an emphasis on mouse cancer models that includes genetically engineered and mutant mouse models, cell line xenograft models, and PDX models. She has published over 25 peer-reviewed manuscripts and book chapters on animal cancers and cancer models. She combines her expertise in animal models with extensive experience in regulatory medicine and has served on the UTMDACC Institutional Animal Care and Use Committee and Biosafety Committee for more than 20 years.

ASSOCIATE EDITOR

Dr. Elisa de Stanchina is the Director of the Memorial Sloan Kettering Cancer Center (MSKCC) Antitumor Assessment Core Facility, and over the past 8 years has overseen its evolution into a state-of-the-art "Mouse Hospital" that fosters preclinical drug development and coordinates efforts from basic scientists and clinicians to ensure that mouse trials effectively mimic treatment plans of human patients. She is an Associate Lab Member in the Molecular Pharmacology and Chemistry Program at the MSKCC. Her laboratory works closely with investigators to establish mouse models of cancer and has developed one of the largest academic PDX core support programs in the United States, with an extensive bank of clinically annotated models available to MSKCC investigators and their collaborators. Her work has resulted in over 65 publications in prestigious peer-reviewed journals, and she has recently authored one of the chapters in the new edition of the *Mouse Models of Cancer* book by the CSHL Press.

Foreword

One of the major challenges in cancer research has been the lack of models that faithfully mirror human cancer and that can be, therefore, used for research purposes. With limitations, xenograft models have been extensively used in preclinical cancer research. Over the past few years, models developed directly from patients have gained momentum and are now being widely used in academic and industry settings for preclinical studies and biomarker development and to personalize medicine.

This timely book by Uthamanthil, Tinkey, and de Stanchina provides a comprehensive and up-to-date summary of the state of the art in this field ranging from technical aspects on model development and maintenance to specific applications. Furthermore, it provides a comprehensive view of challenges and limitations in the field as well as strategies to overcome them. In addition, the book provides a road map for developments and areas of focus for the future. It is clear that this work will serve as a very valuable resource for trainees and groups starting to work in this field as well as a reference guide for current researchers.

Manuel Hidalgo M.D., Ph.D.
Harvard Medical School

Preface

Mouse models of cancer have been in use since the mid-1900s. Mouse models have evolved from the study of spontaneous and induced murine cancers in mice to transplanted syngeneic murine cancers in inbred mice to the paradigm-shifting discovery of the ability to transplant human tumors in immunodeficient mice. The hope that the study of human cancer xenografts in mice would yield the cure for human cancer has not yet been realized. Despite explosive increases in the use of all types of mouse models in cancer research over the past 70 years and great progress in treatments of some cancers, the worldwide burden of cancer morbidity and mortality remains high. Over the past 20 years, scientists have sought answers for the seeming failure of our current model systems to find cures for many types of cancers. A growing body of evidence has shown that the mouse cell line xenograft model, one of the primary model systems used for cancer drug discovery, has significant shortcomings in its ability to predict treatment responses in humans. Simultaneously, the advantages of patient-derived tumor xenograft (PDX) models to overcome these shortcomings is being recognized. The need to use new and innovative techniques to characterize the cell populations—cancer, stroma, immune system—and the complex intracellular interactions that occur in this milieu—genomic, epigenomic, proteomic, metabolomic, and others—are now being recognized as being absolutely critical to leverage PDX model systems to find cancer cures.

The history of PDX models is as old as the mouse xenograft models. However, setting up a new PDX program currently is an expensive and complex task that involves multiple challenges that extend far beyond the simple process of implanting a tumor fragment in a mouse. Considering the escalating costs and limited resources available for research, it is more imperative than ever for scientists to collaborate, share resources, avoid repetition, and work together to define strategic priorities. Many groups around the world are now working quickly to develop and refine PDX models to better predict patient response to treatment and identify biomarkers of drug resistance, metastasis, and recurrence. However, the literature on new techniques, standards, and discoveries is scattered in numerous sources and there has not yet been a single source that consolidated this information.

This book is an attempt to reduce the steep learning curve in understanding and setting up a PDX program. We attempt to consolidate and organize current literature on the topic of PDX and present details of technical and regulatory aspects that are keys to the success of such a program. In this book, we provide a brief review of several basic concepts including the history of mouse xenograft and PDX models and fundamentals of immunocompromised mice, recent developments and discoveries in tumor heterogeneity and humanized mouse models, current techniques in PDX models of several different cancer types, and practical information on the regulations, standards, infrastructure, processes, and programs involved in establishing and operating PDX programs. In Section IV, we gather information from global surveys of PDX programs in academia and industry to present an overview of PDX programs and resources around the world and we have included a brief catalog of companies that provide commercial PDX services. Finally, in Section V, present and future challenges and applications are discussed. We hope that this book will serve not only as a review and reference but also as a basis for stimulating discussion and decisions among the worldwide scientific community to develop a global, collaborative infrastructure to best leverage the use of PDX models for the benefit of cancer patients around the world.

We thought it fitting to dedicate this book to the laboratory mouse, the silent hero of research. These wonderful little animals have paved the way for tremendous progress in many areas of biomedical research, but their impact has been especially important in cancer research. These gentle creatures deserve our respect, care, and compassion in recognition of their important contributions to science.

Rajesh Uthamanthil
Peggy Tinkey

Section I

Mouse Xenograft Models of Cancer

Chapter 1

PDX Models: History and Development

S.P.S. Pillai, R.K. Uthamanthil
Fred Hutchinson Cancer Research Center Seattle, WA, United States

INTRODUCTION

This chapter aims to provide an overview of the rediscovery or resurgence of patient-derived xenografts (PDX) tumor models and their advantages. Different aspects of cancer (mouse) model development are discussed in other chapters in this section—including the history of mouse xenografts models (Section I, Chapter 2), limitations of conventional xenograft models (Section I, Chapter 3), advances in mouse models including immunocompromised mice (Section I, Chapter 5) and humanized mice (Section I, Chapter 6), and advances in scientific knowledge like tumor heterogeneity (Section I, Chapter 4). The scope of this chapter is limited to exploring the origin, development, resurgence, and utility of PDX mouse models and their increased relevance in translational research.

The major hurdle in oncology drug development include the lack of preclinical models that recapitulate the heterogeneity of patient tumors as well as the poor biologic and genetic reproducibility, and poor predictive value of the existing models.[1,2] To circumvent these limitations, preclinical models using PDX are being consistently characterized and applied in oncology research. These models, in which fresh human tumor tissue is directly transplanted, either subcutaneously or orthotopically, into immunodeficient mice or rats[3,4] have proven to be much better representative models of the human patient compared with other xenograft models or in vitro models.

HISTORY OF PDX MOUSE MODELS

It is interesting to note that the first reported mouse xenograft tumor model, reported in 1969, met the definition of what is considered a PDX model currently, even though the term "PDX" was developed only recently. Rygaard and Povlsen[5] minced primary colonic adenocarcinoma (collected within 15 min after removal of tumor) from a 74-year-old patient, and inoculated tumor

Patient Derived Tumor Xenograft Models. http://dx.doi.org/10.1016/B978-0-12-804010-2.00001-1

fragments subcutaneously in nude mice. The tumors in mice grew within weeks and were successfully transplanted to another cohort of mice. They reported that the tumors that grew in mice showed similarity to the initially implanted patient tumors. The authors also reported that of their four attempts to inoculate primary malignant human tumors in nude mice (two mammary carcinomas and two colon carcinomas), only one tumor showed successful take.[6]

Many of the fundamental questions that are currently addressed in the field of PDX tumors were asked in the early 1970s, despite the fact that a thorough understanding of tumor heterogeneity, its implications, and the powerful tool sets that current researchers have were lacking at the time. Many tried to answer questions of the potential changes that can happen to human tumors as they are passaged in mice and the relevance of such changes on the translational value of the model.[6,7] Observations were made on the gradual loss of properties of primary tumor after multiple passages in mice by the mid to late 1970s.[8] Multiple studies in the 1980s looked at the validity of PDX models comparing the response to chemotherapy in the mouse models to that in patients from whom the tumors originated,[9–11] and most of them found a high degree of correlation in the response to chemotherapy between the patients and the corresponding PDX models. The tumors collected from metastatic or recurrent sites were found to have better take rates.[12,13] A significant loss of tumor stroma after multiple transplantations was noted.[11,13] In fact, some researchers[9] wondered about the possibility of using "Avatar models" (even though the term "Avatar" was used much later) in the 1980s. For example, Shorthouse et al.[11] sum up the current discussion and challenges on the use of "avatar models in personalized therapy" in their 1980 article, which stated that "Although it has been claimed that xenografts may be potentially useful in a predictive capacity for the selection of appropriate chemotherapy in individual patients, it was found in the present series that the time required to establish xenografts and subsequently test drugs usually exceeded the survival of the patient. Therefore the major use of xenografts may be in the primary screening of new agents."

By the early 1970s, multiple human tumors were cultured in vitro, leading to collections of human tumor cell lines. This led to the emergence of mouse xenograft models that were derived from in vitro cultured tumor cell lines. The first mouse xenograft model derived from the injection of cultured tumor cells was reported in 1972.[14] By the late 1970s, the National Cancer Institute (NCI) led the development of extensive cell line–based assays for screening of cancer drugs, which continued through the 1980s and the 1990s. During the development of in vitro tumor cell line panel, it was envisioned that the cell lines in the panel would be used as mouse xenografts.[15] Nude mice models were initially used to confirm "tumorigenicity" of the cell line established in vitro from fresh human tumors. The establishment of a large number of tumor cell lines that could grow xenograft tumors in nude mice led to the popularity of these models. Compared with the xenograft (PDX) models that were developed in the 1960s and the early 1970s, which implanted primary human tumor tissues into mice, cell line–based xenograft models allowed simplicity, consistency (predictable growth rate based on which experiments can be scheduled), and cost-effectiveness.

RESURGENCE OF PDX MODELS

The resurgence of PDX models occurred in the early 2000s, driven by the significant limitations of cell line–based xenograft models that were used widely in translation research. For example, Johnson et al.[16] analyzed the activity of potential anticancer compounds in xenograft studies and Phase II preclinical trials. They found that the correlation between xenograft study results and the results from human patients in Phase II trials was very limited. The limitations of cell lines and cell line derived xenograft models compared with those of matching PDX models in recapitulating patient tumor characteristics were demonstrated in 2009 by Daniel et al.[17] It was also observed that colon cancer PDX and the cell lines derived from the cancer models significantly differed in their response to chemotherapeutic agents.[18] Cell line–based xenografts tend to lose the tumor heterogeneity and many key genetic signatures of the original tumor, whereas serially passaged PDXs typically maintain heterogeneity, the majority of key genes, as well as global pathway activity across multiple transplant generations.[17,19]

Since its resurgence in the early 2000s, PDX models have been gaining wide acceptance among cancer researchers. Large PDX tumor collections consisting of hundreds or thousands of tumor samples have been developed by academic and pharmaceutical organizations as well as consortiums and collaborations between government, academic, and commercial institutions.[20–23] In the past 5–10 years, results of using PDX tumors in various fields of cancer research, especially preclinical research, are very encouraging. A short description of the development and use of PDX tumors in various areas of cancer research is given below. Furthermore, although the requirement for immunocompromised mice currently precludes the use of PDX models for testing immunotherapies, PDX models may improve prediction of response to therapies that target cancer cell–intrinsic mechanisms of disease in patients.[24] The history and development of PDX models, as well as their varied applications, will be discussed in this chapter.

APPLICATIONS OF PDX MODELS

Tumor Biology

PDX models offer a powerful tool for studying tumor biology and evaluating oncologic therapy. Preclinical models often fail to capture the diverse heterogeneity of patient tumors. Intratumoral heterogeneity is governed by both cell-autonomous (genomic and epigenomic heterogeneity) and non–cell-autonomous (eg, stromal heterogeneity) factors. These factors are dealt in detail in Section I, Chapter 4. PDX models capture intra- and intertumor heterogeneity and have a clear advantage over traditional models in supporting their use in oncologic drug discovery and preclinical development. Mice xenografts of human breast cancers have been reported to represent the diversity of these cancers as well as maintain the essential features of the original tumors in terms of tumor histomorphology including fine histological features, such as gland formation and keratin deposition, imaging characteristics and gene expression profiles, metastases, clinical markers, hormone responsiveness, and drug sensitivity patterns.[1,25–28] Similarly, well-validated orthotopic and subcutaneous PDX models that evaluate tumor microenvironment, as well as metastases, have been developed for human pancreatic cancers,[29–31] non–small cell lung cancer,[32–34] melanoma,[35,36] colorectal cancers,[37,38] and ovarian and cervical cancers,[2,39–41] among others.

PDX models can be used to study tumor clonal dynamics and evolution. During tumor initiation and progression, cancer cells undergo repeated mutational events that may or may not increase survival and fitness. PDX models largely recapitulate the genomic clonal dynamics reminiscent of their originating tumor sample. The existence of variable subclones within a single tumor might explain variable responses to therapy and drug resistance. The integration of genomic and drug response data from breast cancer PDX models show that polygenomically engrafted tumors are more resistant to therapy than monogenomically engrafted tumors.[42] These genomic evolutions are also tools to study tumor metastasis. In a breast cancer study, the brain metastasis from a patient contained de novo mutations and deletions not present within the primary tumor. Following implantation in mice, the mouse xenograft retained the primary tumor mutations, but was genetically closer to the metastasis and displayed a mutation enrichment pattern resembling the metastasis.[43] Using a nude mouse PDX model of pancreatic ductal adenocarcinoma, the engrafted carcinomas were more often SMAD4 mutants, had a metastatic gene expression profile, and had worse prognosis. This suggested that the passage of tumor in mice selected a clonal population of cells with predilection to colonize new microenvironments and that the patients whose tumors showed higher rates of engraftment were more likely to have metastatic disease.[44] Other disease types also showed that engraftment success is a marker of poor prognosis.[45,46]

PDX models are a valuable source for studying tumor initiating cells (TICs) or cancer stem cells. Both solid and hematological malignancies harbor a distinct subpopulation of TICs that are capable of self-renewal and differentiation and remain largely quiescent in cancer tissues.[47,48] TICs make up only a small fraction of the total cancer cell population and there are no specific markers associated with these cells. Hence, it is difficult to consistently isolate sufficient amounts of TICs from primary tumor biopsies for further study. Expansion of tumor xenografts in mice can yield sufficient quantities of TICs from patient tissues to allow further analysis.[49] PDX models have been very useful in studying the role of TICs in primary tumor growth as well as metastasis.[50] Studies by Vingolu et al., have shown that human prostate TICs do not express the otherwise established markers of well-differentiated human prostate cancer cells like androgen receptor and prostate-specific antigen. Simultaneous targeting of TICs and differentiated tumor is necessary and expected to inhibit tumor initiation and burden.[51] PDX models of pancreatic cancers have been used to evaluate and validate hypoxia-activated drugs, such as TH-302 to increase treatment response of primary tumor as well as to prevent tumor recurrence and metastasis by reducing the number of TICs.[52]

Preclinical Research

PDX models have shown significant promise as an emerging platform for translational cancer research. An important component of validation of disease-specific PDX is determining the response to chemotherapeutic agents and correlating the response of the xenografts to that of the patient. Studies conducted as early as the 1980s have shown significant correlation in clinical response to cytotoxic drugs between patients with lung cancer and the mouse xenografts.[53] In a study using 15 colorectal cancer PDX models, involving treatment with three different agents, 5-fluorouracil, oxaliplatin, and/or irinotecan, the response to chemotherapy showed close correlation between the patient and the individual xenografts.[32] Combination treatment with a BRAF inhibitor and a small molecule MEK inhibitor showed a 100% response in BRAF-mutated melanoma PDX. This result is in concordance with the results seen in a combination Phase I/II clinical trial in BRAF(V600)-mutated melanoma patients that resulted in a 94% response rate.[54,55] Studies in colorectal cancer, non–small cell lung cancer, squamous cell carcinoma of the head and neck, breast cancer, renal cell cancer, and pancreatic cancers have reported that the response rates are comparable between PDX models and clinical data, for both targeted agents and cytotoxics.[49,56] Similarly, the lack of efficacy of chemotherapeutic agents in PDX models correlates with failure of treatment strategy in the clinic. Using pancreatic ductal adenocarcinoma PDX models, lack of efficacy of SRC inhibitor saracatinib and mTOR inhibitor sirolimus translated to negative clinical results.[57,58]

Cancer Drug Screening

Recently, PDX models are widely used as screening platforms for clinical drug trials. The NCI-sponsored pediatric preclinical testing program uses results from established mouse PDX models to screen drugs for pediatric clinical trials.[59] Successful clinical trials have been designed based on results from PDX models of pancreatic cancers[60] and rare tumors like adenoid cystic carcinoma of the salivary gland[61,62] among others. PDX models have been recently reported to be valuable in the development of Epstein-Barr virus–targeted treatment strategies for nasopharyngeal carcinoma.[63] Neutralizing antibodies targeting vascular endothelial growth factor (VEGF) were shown to be effective in inhibiting tumor growth in human PDX.[64] This led to the development of bevacizumab, a humanized monoclonal antibody that targets the VEGF-A. Bevacizumab was effective in Phase III clinical trials for colorectal and renal carcinoma and received US Food and Drug Administration approval in 2004.[65,66] In addition to solid tumors, preclinical PDX models of hematological malignancies including myeloma and myeloid leukemia have been established.[67,68] Results from PDX tumor models have been successfully adapted for the development of Phase I and II clinical trials for multiple myeloma.[69]

Personalized Cancer Therapy—Mouse Avatars

"Mouse avatars," that allow each patient's tumor to grow in an in vivo system, the mouse, allows for personalized drug efficacy and toxicity testing, leading to the identification and development of a personalized therapeutic regimen thereby eliminating the toxicities and cost of nontargeted therapy.[70] Avatar mice are used as a testing ground, with each patient having its own equivalent animal, with the premise that if the drug works in the avatar, it is highly likely to work in the patient. In addition, tumor profiling at different time points with different treatments using avatar models allows for understanding the molecular drivers, signaling pathways, and metabolic fluxes of tumor growth over time, as well as molecular changes driving metastasis and resistance to drugs.[71] In a recent study by Stebbing et al., 22 sarcoma PDX models were successfully established from 29 patients with a 76% take rate during a period of 3–6 months and screened for a panel of chemotherapeutic agents. Six patients died before test data were available. A correlation between PDX results and clinical outcome was observed in 81% of the tested cases.[72] Personalized therapy can be further tailored by integrating data obtained from full genomic analysis of the tumor DNA with using avatar models as an in vivo platform to test treatment strategies. Using exome sequencing and bioinformatics analyses, driver mutations are identified and the genetic signature is used to design effective treatments that are then tested in avatar models. Using this approach in patients with advanced cancers, such as pancreatic and colon cancers, treatments induced positive clinical responses in up to 77% of the patients.[73] Similar trials spearheaded by academic and biotechnology groups are ongoing. The research team at the Spanish National Cancer Research Center and the Comprehensive Cancer Center Clara Campal, Spain, have been undertaking clinical trials in patients with pancreatic cancer. The study includes assessment of mutations in a targeted panel of 409 cancer-relevant genes, selecting the most promising agents and testing their efficacy in the avatar model to determine patient treatment. Similar trials are being undertaken for ovarian cancer (Mayo Clinic, USA) and soft tissue sarcomas (Champions Oncology, USA).[19]

Biomarkers and Mechanisms of Drug Resistance

PDX models also enable the discovery of biomarkers predicting oncologic drug sensitivity and resistance. PDX models of colorectal cancer revealed that KRAS mutant tumors do not respond to the anti–epidermal growth factor receptor (EGFR) antibody, cetuximab.[56,74,75] KRAS wild-type status is now a well-documented clinical biomarker for this targeted therapy. An extensive analysis of cetuximab in 47 unselected colorectal cancer PDX models showed a 10.6% response rate, consistent with the response rate observed in patients with this disease.[75] Detailed analysis of the resistance mechanisms to EGFR inhibitors in these PDX models resulted in the identification of HER2 and MET amplification as a predictor of resistance leading to novel clinical trials.[75,76] Prolonged exposure to cisplatin in epithelial ovarian cancers led to the generation of platinum-resistant PDX models that are being evaluated for novel drug candidates, such as the DNA minor groove binder lurbinectedin.[77] PDX models of luminal breast cancer with acquired in vivo endocrine resistance have been recently generated and identified significant deregulation of estrogen receptor-mediated gene transcription, suggesting that endocrine resistance is tumor and treatment specific.[78] Similarly, melanoma PDX models treated with BRAF inhibitor vemurafenib identified a variety of resistance mechanisms to BRAF inhibition that were conserved in clinical cases. This led to testing of novel combination therapies involving vemurafenib with MEK inhibitor for treatment of melanoma.[79] An ongoing trial at the University of California, Davis [Serial Patient-Derived Xenograft Models to Eliminate Cancer Therapy Resistance (SPIDER)], aims to understand the molecular mechanisms underlying cancer therapy resistance. The study enrolls cancer patients with a known molecular driver, with biopsies taken at the time of initiation and at the time of resistance to targeted therapy. Biopsies are used to create pre- and posttreatment PDX models that receive that same targeted treatment that the patient received. The study anticipates similar treatment response, resistance, and genomic characters in patient and PDX tumors.[80] Coclinical trials utilizing parallel trials on patients and rodent PDXs have been useful in identifying biomarkers for pancreatic cancer.[57,81]

The PDX models thus serve as stable, renewable, quality-controlled resources for preclinical studies investigating treatment response and metastasis, analyze drug resistance pathways, and validate predictive biomarkers in oncology research. Over the past few years, there has been a growing interest in developing PDX collections and using them for different cancer research applications. Because of the significant expansion in the field, organized and collaborative efforts are needed to optimize the use of existing collections and generating new ones. In Section III of this book, the role of PDX models in different solid tumors including brain, prostate, pancreatic, breast, ovarian/gynecologic, lung, colorectal, as well as hematological malignancies will be covered.

REFERENCES

1. DeRose YS, Wang G, Lin YC, Bernard PS, Buys SS, Ebbert MT, et al. Tumor grafts derived from women with breast cancer authentically reflect tumor pathology, growth, metastasis and disease outcomes. *Nat Med* 2011;**17**(11):1514–20.
2. Tentler JJ, Tan AC, Weekes CD, Jimeno A, Leong S, Pitts TM, et al. Patient-derived tumour xenografts as models for oncology drug development. *Nat Rev Clin Oncol* 2012;**9**(6):338–50.
3. Morton CL, Houghton PJ. Establishment of human tumor xenografts in immunodeficient mice. *Nat Protoc* 2007;**2**(2):247–50.
4. Rubio-Viqueira B, Hidalgo M. Direct in vivo xenograft tumor model for predicting chemotherapeutic drug response in cancer patients. *Clin Pharmacol Ther* 2009;**85**(2):217–21.
5. Rygaard J, Povlsen CO. Heterotransplantation of a human malignant tumour to "Nude" mice. *Acta Pathol Microbiol Scand* 1969;**77**(4):758–60.
6. Cobb LM. The behaviour of carcinoma of the large bowel in man following transplantation into immune deprived mice. *Br J Cancer* 1973;**28**(5):400–11.
7. Pickard RG, Cobb LM, Steel GG. The growth kinetics of xenografts of human colorectal tumours in immune deprived mice. *Br J Cancer* 1975;**31**(1):36–45.
8. Selby PJ, Heyderman E, Gibbs J, Peckham MJ. A human testicular teratoma serially transplanted in immune-deprived mice. *Br J Cancer* 1979;**39**(5):578–83.
9. Fiebig HH, Schuchhardt C, Henss H, Fiedler L, Löhr GW. Comparison of tumor response in nude mice and in the patients. *Behring Inst Mitt* 1984;**74**:343–52.
10. Osieka R. Human malignant melanoma: preclinical and clinical drug evaluation. *Behring Inst Mitt* 1984;**74**:353–67.
11. Shorthouse AJ, Smyth JF, Steel GG, Ellison M, Mills J, Peckham MJ. The human tumour xenograft–a valid model in experimental chemotherapy? *Br J Surg* 1980;**67**(10):715–22.
12. Fogh J. *The nude mouse in experimental and clinical research.* Elsevier; 1978.
13. Shimosato Y, Kameya T, Nagai K, Hirohashi S, Koide T, Hayashi H, et al. Transplantation of human tumors in nude mice. *J Natl Cancer Inst* 1976;**56**(6):1251–60.
14. Giovanella BC, Yim SO, Stehlin JS, Williams LJ. Development of invasive tumors in the "nude" mouse after injection of cultured human melanoma cells. *J Natl Cancer Inst* 1972;**48**(5):1531–3.
15. Fogh J, Fogh JM, Orfeo T. One hundred and twenty-seven cultured human tumor cell lines producing tumors in nude mice. *J Natl Cancer Inst* 1977;**59**(1):221–6.
16. Johnson JI, Decker S, Zaharevitz D, Rubinstein LV, Venditti JM, Schepartz S, et al. Relationships between drug activity in NCI preclinical in vitro and in vivo models and early clinical trials. *Br J Cancer* 2001;**84**(10):1424–31.
17. Daniel VC, Marchionni L, Hierman JS, Rhodes JT, Devereux WL, Rudin CM, et al. A primary xenograft model of small-cell lung cancer reveals irreversible changes in gene expression imposed by culture in vitro. *Cancer Res* 2009;**69**(8):3364–73.
18. Dangles-Marie V, Pocard M, Richon S, Weiswald LB, Assayag F, Saulnier P, et al. Establishment of human colon cancer cell lines from fresh tumors versus xenografts: comparison of success rate and cell line features. *Cancer Res* 2007;**67**(1):398–407.
19. Aparicio S, Hidalgo M, Kung AL. Examining the utility of patient derived xenograft mouse models. *Nat Rev* 2015;**15**:311–6.
20. Novartis compiles mouse avatar "Encyclopedia". *Cancer Discov* 2015;**6**(1).
21. Gao H, Korn JM, Ferretti S, Monahan JE, Wang Y, Singh M, et al. High-throughput screening using patient-derived tumor xenografts to predict clinical trial drug response. *Nat Med* 2015;**21**(11):1318–25.

22. China plans large center for PDX models. *Cancer Discov* 2014;**4**(2):136–7.
23. Ledford H. US cancer institute to overhaul tumour cell lines. *Nature* 2016;**530**(7591):391.
24. Becker JC, Houben R, Schrama D, Voigt H, Ugurel S, Reisfeld RA. Mouse models for melanoma: a personal perspective. *Exp Dermatol* 2010;**19**(2):157–64.
25. Zhang X, Claerhout S, Prat A, Dobrolecki LE, Petrovic I, Lai Q, et al. A renewable tissue resource of phenotypically stable, biologically and ethnically diverse, patient-derived human breast cancer xenograft models. *Cancer Res* 2013;**73**(15):4885–97.
26. Marangoni EV-SA, Auger N, Degeorges A, Assayag F, de Cremoux P, de Plater L, Sigal Zafrani B, Delattre O, Dieras V, Poupon MF, et al. A new model of patient tumor-derived breast cancer xenografts for preclinical assays. *Clin Cancer Res* 2007;**13**(13):3989–98.
27. Kabos P, Finlay-Schultz J, Li C, Kline E, Finlayson C, Wisell J, et al. Patient-derived luminal breast cancer xenografts retain hormone receptor heterogeneity and help define unique estrogen-dependent gene signatures. *Breast Cancer Res Treat* 2012;**135**(2):415–32.
28. Reyal F, Guyader C, Decraene C, Lucchesi C, Auger N, Assayag F, et al. Molecular profiling of patient-derived breast cancer xenografts. *Breast Cancer Res* 2012;**14**(1):R11.
29. Walters DM, S JB, Adair SJ, Stelow EB, Borgman CA, Lowrey BT, et al. Clinical, molecular and genetic validation of a murine orthotopic xenograft model of pancreatic adenocarcinoma using fresh human specimens. *PLoS One* 2013;**8**(10):e77065. http://dx.doi.org/10.1371/journal.pone.0077065. eCollection 2013.
30. Loukopoulos P, Kanetaka K, Takamura M, Shibata T, Sakamoto M, Hirohashi S. Orthotopic transplantation models of pancreatic adenocarcinoma derived from cell lines and primary tumors and displaying varying metastatic activity. *Pancreas* 2004;**29**(3):193–203.
31. Delitto D, Pham K, Vlada AC, Sarosi GA, Thomas RM, Behrns KE, et al. Patient-derived xenograft models for pancreatic adenocarcinoma demonstrate retention of tumor morphology through incorporation of murine stromal elements. *Am J Pathol* 2015;**185**(5):1297–303.
32. Fichtner I, Rolff J, Soong R, Hoffmann J, Hammer S, Sommer A, et al. Establishment of patient-derived non–small cell lung cancer xenografts as models for the identification of predictive biomarkers. *Clin Cancer Res* 2008;**14**(20):6456–68.
33. Dong X, Guan J, English JC, Flint J, Yee J, Evans K, et al. Patient-derived first generation xenografts of non–small cell lung cancers: promising tools for predicting drug responses for personalized chemotherapy. *Clin Cancer Res* 2010;**16**(5):1442–51.
34. Nemati F, Bras-Goncalves R, Fontaine JJ, de Pinieux G, De Cremoux P, Chapelier A, et al. Preclinical assessment of cisplatin-based therapy versus docetaxel-based therapy on a panel of human non-small-cell lung cancer xenografts. *Anticancer Drugs* 2009;**20**(10):932–40.
35. Taetle R, Jones OW, Honeysett JM, Abramson I, Bradshaw C, Reid S. Use of nude mouse xenografts as preclinical screens: characterization of xenograft-derived melanoma cell lines. *Cancer* 1987;**60**(8):1836–41.
36. Fiebig H-H, Schüler J, Bausch N, Hofmann M, Metz T, Korrat A. Gene signatures developed from patient tumor explants grown in nude mice to predict tumor response to 11 cytotoxic drugs. *Cancer Genom Proteom* 2007;**4**(3):197–209.
37. Guenot D, Guérin E, Aguillon-Romain S, Pencreach E, Schneider A, Neuville A, et al. Primary tumour genetic alterations and intra-tumoral heterogeneity are maintained in xenografts of human colon cancers showing chromosome instability. *J Pathol* 2006;**208**(5):643–52.
38. Fichtner I, Slisow W, Gill J, Becker M, Elbe B, Hillebrand T, et al. Anticancer drug response and expression of molecular markers in early-passage xenotransplanted colon carcinomas. *Eur J Cancer* 2004;**40**(2):298–307.
39. Elkas JC, Baldwin RL, Pegram M, Tseng Y, Slamon D, Karlan BY. A human ovarian carcinoma murine xenograft model useful for preclinical trials. *Gynecol Oncol* 2002;**87**(2):200–6.

40. Scott CL, Becker MA, Haluska P, Samimi G. Patient-derived xenograft models to improve targeted therapy in epithelial ovarian cancer treatment. *Front Oncol* 2013;**3**:295.
41. Boone JD, Dobbin ZC, Straughn Jr JM, Buchsbaum DJ. Ovarian and cervical cancer patient derived xenografts: the past, present, and future. *Gynecol Oncol* 2015;**138**(2):486–91.
42. Cassidy JW, Caldas C, Bruna A. Maintaining tumor heterogeneity in patient-derived tumor xenografts. *Cancer Res* 2015;**75**(15).
43. Ding L, Ellis MJ, Li S, Larson DE, Chen K, Wallis JW, et al. Genome remodelling in a basal-like breast cancer metastasis and xenograft. *Nature* 2010;**464**(7291):999–1005.
44. Garrido-Laguna I, Uson M, Rajeshkumar NV, Tan AC, de Oliveira E, Karikari C, et al. Tumor engraftment in nude mice and enrichment in stroma-related gene pathways predict poor survival and resistance to gemcitabine in patients with pancreatic cancer. *Clin Cancer Res* 2011;**17**(17):5793–800.
45. Némati F, Sastre-Garau X, Laurent C, Couturier J, Mariani P, Desjardins L, et al. Establishment and characterization of a panel of human uveal melanoma xenografts derived from primary and/or metastatic tumors. *Clin Cancer Res* 2010;**16**(8):2352–62.
46. John T, Kohler D, Pintilie M, Yanagawa N, Pham N-A, Li M, et al. The ability to form primary tumor xenografts is predictive of increased risk of disease recurrence in early-stage non-small cell lung Cancer. *Clin Cancer Res* 2011;**17**(1):134–41.
47. Rosen JM, Jordan CT. The increasing complexity of the cancer stem cell paradigm. *Science* 2009;**324**(5935):1670–3.
48. Nguyen LV, Vanner R, Dirks P, Eaves CJ. Cancer stem cells: an evolving concept. *Nat Rev Cancer* 2012;**12**(2):133–43.
49. Rosfjord E, Lucas J, Li G, Gerber H-P. Advances in patient-derived tumor xenografts: from target identification to predicting clinical response rates in oncology. *Biochem Pharmacol* 2014;**91**(2):135–43.
50. Liu H, Patel MR, Prescher JA, Patsialou A, Qian D, Lin J, et al. Cancer stem cells from human breast tumors are involved in spontaneous metastases in orthotopic mouse models. *Proc Natl Acad Sci USA* 2010;**107**(42):18115–20.
51. Wang CY, Wei Q, Hu J, Zhang P, Wunder J, Alman B. Targeting tumor initiating cells in soft-tissue sarcoma. In: University of Toronto, ON, Canada, Hospital for Sick Children, ON, Canada, editors. 56th *Annual meeting of the orthopaedic research society* 2010, *Paper No. 4172005*.
52. Lohse I, Rasowski J, Ibrahimov E, Hill R, Tsao MS, Hedley DW. Abstract B46: targeting tumor initiating cells in patient-derived pancreatic xenograft models using the hypoxia-activated prodrug TH-302. *Cancer Res* 2012;**72**(14 Suppl.):B46.
53. Fiebig HH, Neumann HA, Henß H, Koch H, Kaiser D, Arnold H. Development of three human small cell lung Cancer models in nude mice. In: Seeber S, editor. *Small cell lung Cancer. Recent results in Cancer research*. vol. 97. Springer Berlin Heidelberg; 1985. p. 77–86.
54. Robert C, Karaszewska B, Schachter J, Rutkowski P, Mackiewicz A, Stroiakovski D, et al. Improved overall survival in melanoma with combined dabrafenib and trametinib. *N Engl J Med* 2015;**372**(1):30–9.
55. Flaherty KT, Infante JR, Daud A, Gonzalez R, Kefford RF, Sosman J, et al. Combined BRAF and MEK inhibition in melanoma with BRAF V600 mutations. *N Engl J Med* 2012;**367**(18):1694–703.
56. Hidalgo M, Amant F, Biankin AV, Budinská E, Byrne AT, Caldas C, et al. Patient-derived xenograft models: an emerging platform for translational cancer research. *Cancer Discov* 2014;**4**(9):998–1013.
57. Garrido-Laguna I, Tan AC, Uson M, Angenendt M, Ma WW, Villaroel MC, et al. Integrated preclinical and clinical development of mTOR inhibitors in pancreatic cancer. *Br J Cancer* 2010;**103**(5):649–55.

58. Rajeshkumar NV, Tan AC, De Oliveira E, Womack C, Wombwell H, Morgan S, et al. Antitumor effects and biomarkers of activity of AZD0530, a Src inhibitor, in pancreatic cancer. *Clin Cancer Res* 2009;**15**(12):4138–46.
59. Houghton PJ. The pediatric preclinical testing program: description of models and early testing results. *Pediatr Blood Cancer* 2007;**49**(7):928–40.
60. Hidalgo M, Bruckheimer E, Rajeshkumar NV, Garrido-Laguna I, De Oliveira E, Rubio-Viqueira B, et al. A pilot clinical study of treatment guided by personalized tumorgrafts in patients with advanced cancer. *Mol Cancer Ther* 2011;**10**(8):1311–6.
61. Morelli MP, Calvo E, Ordoñez E, Wick MJ, Viqueira B-R, Lopez-Casas PP, et al. Prioritizing phase I treatment options through preclinical testing on personalized tumorgraft. *J Clin Oncol* 2012;**30**(4):e45–8.
62. Siolas D, Hannon GJ. Patient-derived tumor xenografts: transforming clinical samples into mouse models. *Cancer Res* 2013;**73**(17):5315–9.
63. Hsu CL, Kuo YC, Huang Y, Huang YC, Lui KW, Chang KP, et al. Application of a patient-derived xenograft model in cytolytic viral activation therapy for nasopharyngeal carcinoma. *Oncotarget* 2015;**6**(31):31323–34.
64. Kim KJ, Li B, Winer J, Armanini M, Gillett N, Phillips HS, et al. Inhibition of vascular endothelial growth factor-induced angiogenesis suppresses tumour growth in vivo. *Nature* 1993;**362**(6423):841–4.
65. Yang JC, Haworth L, Sherry RM, Hwu P, Schwartzentruber DJ, Topalian SL, et al. A randomized trial of bevacizumab, an anti–vascular endothelial growth factor antibody, for metastatic renal cancer. *N Engl J Med* 2003;**349**(5):427–34.
66. Hurwitz H, Fehrenbacher L, Novotny W, Cartwright T, Hainsworth J, Heim W, et al. Bevacizumab plus irinotecan, fluorouracil, and leucovorin for metastatic colorectal cancer. *N Engl J Med* 2004;**350**(23):2335–42.
67. LeBlanc R, Catley LP, Hideshima T, Lentzsch S, Mitsiades CS, Mitsiades N, et al. Proteasome inhibitor PS-341 inhibits human myeloma cell growth in vivo and prolongs survival in a murine model. *Cancer Res* 2002;**62**(17):4996–5000.
68. Vick B, Rothenberg M, Sandhofer N, Carlet M, Finkenzeller C, Krupka C, et al. An advanced preclinical mouse model for acute myeloid leukemia using patients' cells of various genetic subgroups and in vivo bioluminescence imaging. *PLoS One* 2015;**10**(3):e0120925.
69. Field-Smith A, Morgan GJ, Davies FE. Bortezomib (Velcade™) in the treatment of multiple myeloma. *Ther Clin Risk Manag* 2006;**2**(3):271–9.
70. Malaney P, Nicosia SV, Dave V. One mouse, one patient paradigm: new avatars of personalized cancer therapy. *Cancer Lett* 2014;**344**(1):1–12.
71. Richmond A, Su Y. Mouse xenograft models vs GEM models for human cancer therapeutics. *Dis Models Mech* 2008;**1**(2–3):78–82.
72. Stebbing J, Paz K, Schwartz GK, Wexler LH, Maki R, Pollock RE, et al. Patient-derived xenografts for individualized care in advanced sarcoma. *Cancer* 2014;**120**(13):2006–15.
73. Garralda E, Paz K, López-Casas PP, Jones S, Katz A, Kann LM, et al. Integrated next-generation sequencing and avatar mouse models for personalized cancer treatment. *Clin Cancer Res* 2014;**20**(9):2476–84.
74. Julien S, Merino-Trigo A, Lacroix L, Pocard M, Goéré D, Mariani P, et al. Characterization of a large panel of patient-derived tumor xenografts representing the clinical heterogeneity of human colorectal cancer. *Clin Cancer Res* 2012;**18**(19):5314–28.
75. Bertotti A, Migliardi G, Galimi F, Sassi F, Torti D, Isella C, et al. A molecularly annotated platform of patient-derived xenografts ("xenopatients") identifies HER2 as an effective therapeutic target in cetuximab-resistant colorectal cancer. *Cancer Discov* 2011;**1**(6):508–23.

76. Bardelli A, Corso S, Bertotti A, Hobor S, Valtorta E, Siravegna G, et al. Amplification of the MET receptor drives resistance to anti-EGFR therapies in colorectal Cancer. *Cancer Discov* 2013;**3**(6):658–73.
77. Vidal A, Muñoz C, Guillén M-J, Moretó J, Puertas S, Martínez-Iniesta M, et al. Lurbinectedin (PM01183), a new DNA minor groove binder, inhibits growth of orthotopic primary graft of cisplatin-resistant epithelial ovarian cancer. *Clin Cancer Res* 2012;**18**(19):5399–411.
78. Cottu P, Bièche I, Assayag F, El Botty R, Chateau-Joubert S, Thuleau A, et al. Acquired resistance to endocrine treatments is associated with tumor-specific molecular changes in patient-derived luminal breast cancer xenografts. *Clin Cancer Res* 2014;**20**(16):4314–25.
79. Monsma DJ, Cherba DM, Eugster EE, Dylewski DL, Davidson PT, Peterson CA, et al. Melanoma patient derived xenografts acquire distinct Vemurafenib resistance mechanisms. *Am J Cancer Res* 2015;**5**(4):1507.
80. Gandara DR, Lara PN, Mack PC. Patient-derived xenografts for investigation of acquired resistance in oncogene-driven cancers: building a better mousetrap. *J Clin Oncol* 2015;**33**(26):2839–40.
81. Jimeno A, Amador ML, Kulesza P, Wang X, Rubio-Viqueira B, Zhang X, et al. Assessment of celecoxib pharmacodynamics in pancreatic cancer. *Mol Cancer Ther* 2006;**5**(12):3240–7.

Chapter 2

History of Mouse Cancer Models

L.R. Hill, P.T. Tinkey
The University of Texas MD Anderson Cancer Center, Houston, TX, United States

INTRODUCTION

For thousands of years, humans have selectively bred mice. As early as 1100 BC, the Chinese bred mice for specific somatic traits, such as body size and coat and eye color. Selective breeding spread throughout Europe in the 1700s, but the scientific use of mice did not begin until the 20th century. In 1900, William Castle at the Harvard University, Leo Loeb at the University of Pennsylvania, and Abbie Lathrop, a Massachusetts farmer, began to study the genetic determinants of inheritance of somatic traits and the correlation between spontaneous tumor incidence and mouse strain. Clarence Cook Little produced the first inbred mouse strains to minimize variation in his tumor transplantation work. In 1929, Little founded the Jackson Laboratory, a world-renowned institute for the study of genetics and genomics and the current home of the mouse genome database. Researchers eventually determined that 99% of mouse protein coding genes have human homologs, setting the stage for the mouse to become the predominant model for the study of human biology and disease.[1]

This chapter will focus on the history of murine tumor models in research, highlighting the models developed and used by the National Cancer Institute (NCI) for drug screening. We will briefly review the most commonly used immunodeficient mouse models and address some of the innovations in the use of xenograft models. Finally, we will discuss future directions of murine models in cancer research.

IMMUNODEFICIENT MOUSE MODELS

The growth of human tumors in a different animal species requires evasion of the normal immune response in the host animal to prevent rejection of the transplanted tissues (xenografts). Prior to 1960, many groups performed heterotransplantation of human cancer cells into immunoprivileged sites in other species, including the rabbit and guinea pig eye, the hamster cheek pouch, and via implanted diffusion chambers.[2,3] The possibility of inducing immunologic

Patient Derived Tumor Xenograft Models. http://dx.doi.org/10.1016/B978-0-12-804010-2.00002-3

tolerance to allow heterotransplantation of tissue was being explored in the 1960s.[4] This strategy set the stage for the scientific community to recognize the importance of the first report of successful human tumor xenograft in the then newly discovered mutant athymic nude mouse.[5] Since that time, many strains of immunodeficient mice have been developed for xenograft studies in cancer research.[6] Mice with single mutations [eg, nude mice, severe combined immunodeficiency (SCID) mice, beige mice, X-linked immunodeficiency (xid) mice, and mice with recombination activating gene 1 (*Rag1*) null or 2 (*Rag2*) null] were used extensively for xenograft studies. Over the past 50 years, nude mice followed by SCID mice have been used most frequently as hosts for human tumor xenografts.[7] The *nude* mutation results in a mouse that is T-cell deficient with maturational defects in B cells. The nude mouse retains innate immunity and tumoricidal macrophages and has an increase in natural killer (NK) cells.[8] This mutation has been introduced into many mouse strains.[9] The *Xid* mutation leads to B-cell defects in the offspring. Mice homozygous for the *Scid* mutation are severely deficient in B cells, T cells, and NK cells due to an arrest in the early development of B and T cells. Other hematopoietic cell types appear to function normally. The arrest in lymphocyte development is not absolute. Some young SCID mice are "leaky" and will generate a few clones of functional B and T cells.[10] Combining *Scid* with other background strains, such as the non-obese diabetic (NOD) strain and other mutations, such as the *Rag* mutation, produces mice that are no longer "leaky." Combination of the beige and *Scid* mutations results in blockage of the NK and myeloid-derived cell activity.[9] A pivotal achievement in the evolution of immunodeficient mouse models was the development of mice with an interleukin-2 (IL-2) receptor gamma chain deficiency. Combined with the *Scid* or *Rag* mutations, these models enabled the development of humanized mice through the improved engraftment of human hematopoietic cells.[7]

The unique characteristics, advantages, disadvantages, and utility of the ever-evolving varieties of immunocompromised and humanized mouse models are discussed in detail in Section I, Chapters 4 and 5.

HISTORY OF MOUSE MODELS IN CANCER RESEARCH

Early drug treatments for cancer evolved from three schools of thought. One concept was Ehrlich's "magic bullet," which envisioned that cancer drugs could be developed to aim at a specific target. This belief was fueled by the observation that different dyes had varying affinities for different parts of cells, which supported the idea that some compounds might preferentially affect cancer cells more than normal cells. A second theory was based on the observation of profound leukopenia in World War I soldiers following exposure to mustard gases, suggesting that these compounds might be effective against hematologic malignancies.[6] Regression of implanted lymphoid tumors in mice dosed with nitrogen mustard led to new treatments for patients with non-Hodgkin lymphoma in 1943, which stimulated interest in using alkylating compounds to treat cancer.[11] The third school of thought was based on the observations that hormonal manipulation could cause regression of some tumors derived from endocrine-responsive organs and that RNA content in tumor cells was higher than that in normal cells.[6]

As a result of these observations, scientists identified several new chemicals with antimetabolic activity that were candidates for anticancer efficacy testing; at that time, however, the pharmaceutical industry was not focused on cancer treatment.[6] Two major roadblocks to cancer drug development were the scarcity of effective models and the lack of clinical facilities to test agents.[11] Before 1955, analyses of various available screening methods indicated that nontumor systems (cell or bacterial cultures) were incapable of replacing tumor systems and that no single tumor system was capable of detecting all active antitumor compounds.[12] The need to develop common platforms for evaluating new compounds resulted in the development of panels of tumor models, generally using serially propagated tumor cells in syngeneic mouse hosts that were geared for high throughput. Initially, these screening efforts were used in academic research institutions, but as the demand for compound screening grew, Congress directed the NCI in 1955 to develop a publicly funded and accessible resource to provide preclinical evaluation and clinical testing of new compounds and therapies. This directive resulted in the formation of the Cancer Chemotherapy National Service Center, which was the predecessor for the present-day NCI Developmental Therapeutics Program. The NCI actively solicited test compounds from industry and academia, and results from NCI's screening tests were used to select promising compounds for development.[6]

NCI launched one of the first systems for systematic evaluation of new compounds and subsequently has played a predominant role in the development of anticancer drugs for 60 years. This is reflected in the fact that approximately half of the chemotherapeutic drugs currently in use were discovered and/or developed at the NCI.[11] From 1955 to 1975, testing relied on murine tumor screening systems.[12] The earliest in vivo systems were murine cell lines (L1210 and P388) derived from leukemias induced in DBA/2 mice by painting the skin with methylcholanthrene. Leukemia cell lines in mice were implanted intraperitoneally and provided a rapid and reproducible way to identify potential anticancer drugs.[7] Advantages of these mouse screening systems included speed, high throughput, and reproducibility. These models allowed the identification of important clinically relevant principles of cancer chemotherapy, and formed the basis of human chemotherapy regimens and practices. NCI focused on the in vivo P388 mouse leukemia model as the primary screening system between 1975 and 1985.[6] Compounds with anticancer activity were selected for testing in clinical trials, both in the United States and in other countries. However, many agents that appeared effective in murine models were not effective in humans.[13] Similar low success was reported by The European Organisation for Research and Treatment of Cancer Early Clinical Trials group, where more than 20 compounds identified for phase II studies over the course of 12 years yielded few effective drugs.[14] In addition, it became evident that only certain types of drugs, mostly alkylating agents and DNA-interacting drugs, were active in the mouse tumor models, and all of the drugs had similar toxicities to bone marrow and normal tissues.[7] The relevance of syngeneic mouse models to human cancer was also called into question because almost 30% of the compounds (eg, paclitaxel) that were deemed ineffective in syngeneic mouse models were active in some human tumors. It was also noted that some classes of compounds, eg, brefeldin and some DNA minor groove binders, seemed to have less activity in syngeneic mouse models than in patients.[6] A detailed evaluation of the sensitivities of individual tumor systems employed by the NCI from 1976 to 1982 revealed a wide range in sensitivity profiles as well as yield of active compounds. The data clearly indicated that rodent models were not capable of detecting all compounds with potential activity against human malignancies.[12] Other weaknesses of mouse models were the limited availability of tumor types, rapid growth of tumors, the lack of species-specific biological targeting of drugs, and intrinsic differences in drug metabolism and activity in mice compared with humans. Syngeneic murine solid tumors and human tumor xenografts eventually largely replaced murine leukemia cell lines in anticancer drug screening systems.[7]

The development of the nude mouse with its ability to sustain xenotransplant tumors signaled a pivotal change in many global drug testing programs.[5] In 1976, the NCI Division of Cancer Treatment started a new screening panel that used human transplantable solid tumors in nude mice. The panel was composed of matched animal and human tumors of the breast, colon, and lung as well as the L1210 leukemia and B16 melanoma models. Most of the early NCI testing conducted with human tumors used small tumor fragments grown under the renal capsule of nude mice. Although labor intensive, this assay provided a rapid means of evaluating new agents against human tumor xenografts at a time when testing large numbers of compounds against subcutaneous xenografts seemed infeasible.[12]

Retrospective studies performed during the mid-1980s showed no correlation between the preclinical and clinical efficacy of potential therapies on the basis of tumor type. It was thought that this finding might be due to the limited types of tumor models used, so different methods of increasing tumor types in panels were sought.[15] Groups in Europe and Japan began focusing on the use of human tumor xenografts combined with a disease-oriented rather than a compound-oriented approach to drug discovery. Beginning in the early 1980s, scientists began to see a strong correlation between the drug responses of direct patient xenografts in nude mice and the individual patient's response.[16,17] In 1988, a European multicenter collaboration (Netherlands, Germany, Belgium, Norway, Scotland) was created to study the feasibility and reliability of using a panel of human tumor cell line xenografts to predict the preclinical activity of new compounds. The results of this study, published in 1992, showed variable but overall promising results. The authors cautioned that it would be important to identify the mechanisms underlying the discrepancies between the responses in mouse models and cancer patients to be able to use the tumor panel more reliably.[18] During this same period, the NCI initiated a new project to assess the feasibility of using human tumor cell lines for large-scale drug screening. A concerted effort was made to establish a battery of subcutaneous mouse xenografts from human tumor cell lines from the NCI tumor repository. Seven cell lines representing common cancer types (brain, colon, lung, ovarian, and renal cancers; leukemia; and melanoma) were acquired from a variety of sources and subsequently subjected to a battery of in vitro and in vivo characterization testing, including drug sensitivity assays. Cell lines were preserved for future use via cryopreservation.[12] The relative technical simplicity of subcutaneous implantation and the ability to perform in vitro genetic modification of cancer cells before transplantation further enhanced the model's usefulness. As immunodeficient mice (eg, nude or SCID) became more widely available, the use of human tumor xenotransplants in cancer research increased. The approach was deemed suitable for large-scale drug screening in 1990.

During the 1990s, the NCI's strategy shifted from being compound oriented to being disease oriented.[15] In 1993, the composition of the NCI in vivo screening panel of 60cell lines (NCI-60), was modified to include various prostate and breast tumor lines.[7] Drug responses to the in vitro NCI-60 panel generated a characteristic profile or fingerprint, which was identified using COMPARE, a computer program. Studies showed that compounds with similar fingerprints often had related chemical structures or similar mechanisms of action. This observation highlighted the fact that a drug's efficacy is mediated by its interaction with a molecular target and underscored the need to molecularly characterize tumor models in order to match candidate drugs with models that have relevant targets.[15]

The hollow fiber assay was developed to combine multiple cell lines during in vivo pharmacodynamic/pharmacokinetic assessment. In this assay, fibers are seeded with 12 cell lines, which are implanted subcutaneously and intraperitoneally in mice that are then dosed with the test compound; later, tumor tissue is harvested and assessed. NCI started using the hollow fiber assay in 1995 as an in vivo prescreening assay, and active compounds were then selected for xenograft studies.[15] Because more than 85% of the screened compounds did not show activity, a highly sensitive three-cell-line prescreening system was adopted in 1999 to conserve time and resources.[7] This approach was validated by a study published by the NCI of Canada Clinical Trials group, which compared the predictive value of three of the most commonly used preclinical models at that time—in vitro cell lines, murine allografts, and human tumor xenografts. The study concluded that the in vitro cell line panel and the human xenograft model were more predictive of phase II performance than the murine allograft model and recommended continued use of the in vitro cell line complimented by use of appropriate panels of human xenograft models.[19]

Currently at the NCI, standard drug development of a candidate compound consists of demonstration of activity in the NCI-60 screening system and the hollow fiber assay followed by assessment of distal site antitumor activity in appropriate human tumor xenograft models in nude mice or, where relevant, in rodent tumor models.[20] This same basic strategy is used for most drug development programs around the world, with some variations. For instance, the Japanese Foundation for Cancer Research developed the JFCR39 cell line panel in 1990, which utilizes some of the same cells lines in the NCI-60 panel but includes cell lines of stomach and breast cancers that have a high incidence in Japan.[21] Orthotopic rodent xenograft models are not typically employed in the initial steps of in vivo drug evaluations. However, these models are used for subsequent, more detailed evaluations of compounds that exhibit activity in preliminary assays.[12] At the NCI, selection of compounds for antitumor efficacy testing and specific model conditions (tumor types, route of administration, dose, dosing schedule, etc.) are determined on a compound-by-compound basis after the compound has progressed through a series of prerequisite assays and the staff have evaluated the available data. Generally, previous identification of a novel mechanism of action and/or molecular target strengthens the case for initiating xenograft studies.[20]

XENOGRAFTS

The ability to grow human tumors in mice has revolutionized cancer research and set the stage for the quest for continual improvements in xenograft mouse models. The key element in xenograft mouse models is the immune impairments that allow implantation and prevent rejection of human tumors.[7] The development of mouse models with progressively sophisticated immune alterations has led to a rapidly increasing repertoire of models. While nude mouse models have been used most extensively for human tumor xenograft studies to date, the development of mice with combinations of severe immunodeficiencies (eg, SCID, beige, and xid) enabled the establishment of human xenograft tumors that were previously difficult to establish in nude mice, such as those of the hematopoietic system.[7] The development of mice with combined genetic mutations [NOD-SCID-IL-2g null (NSG), NOD-Rag-IL-2g null (NRG), and NOD-SCID-IL-2g null + human cytokine expression] has led to the creation of "humanized" mice via injection of human peripheral blood or bone marrow cells, which allows for an almost complete reconstitution of the immune response to the tumor.[22] Methods of tumor implantation and engraftment have also been refined to improve the relevance of mouse models to humans. Many investigators have moved away from subcutaneous implants and toward strategies, such as the use of orthotopic xenografts to mimic the human tumor microenvironment more completely.[22]

Despite these improvements, the value of xenograft models is still debated. Retrospective studies have shown that many compounds with promising activity in xenograft models did not have clinical success owing to limited efficacy or high toxicity.[15] Another complicating factor is that xenografts established from cell lines that have been maintained in in vitro culture for long periods often do not reflect the molecular characteristics of the original patient tumor,[15] therefore limiting the ability of established cancer cell lines to demonstrate how an individual cancer patient might respond to a particular treatment.[23] More and more, it is understood that xenograft models must be characterized molecularly and selected on the basis of rational matching of the drug to a model with a relevant target.

To address the shortcomings of cell line models, researchers are developing patient-derived xenograft models (PDX) as a promising tool for the development of anticancer drugs and predictive biomarkers.[23] Recent studies showed close correlation between the treatment response of human tumor xenografts developed directly from patient tumors and clinical response. Refinement of xenograft models to use samples directly from patients with no or limited culture has shown better predictive value of a drug's clinical activity and patient outcomes.[15] Future successful use of PDX models will require accurate genetic profiling of tumors and tumor-specific therapeutic targets.

The challenges, advantages, and limitations of xenograft mouse models and PDX models are discussed in detail in Section I, Chapters 1 and 3.

FUTURE DIRECTIONS OF MURINE MODELS IN BASIC RESEARCH

The holy grail of drug discovery methods continues to be a model that will reliably predict the clinical activity, response, and toxicity of candidate drugs in patients. The ideal preclinical animal tumor model could be evaluated objectively and quantitatively, and would be able to reproduce the biology of human cancer, predict clinical response and be reliable, available, and affordable. Over time, the ability of mouse models to predict clinical efficacy has improved, but the ultimate goal of identifying the ideal preclinical animal model has not yet been reached.

Current anticancer drug discovery is focused on proof of principle and target-oriented and tumor cell–specific approaches; however, there is still a need for a better understanding of tumor biology and to identify more target-defined models. As a consequence, scientists now recognize the need to define the molecular characteristics of both tumors and models. Xenograft tumor models can be utilized to analyze molecularly targeted therapeutics and to facilitate target validation via manipulation of potential targets in tumor cells. Scientists can then assess how that alteration affects the tumor's biological response to therapeutic agents.

The growing array of molecular tools that has become available to mouse geneticists and tumor biologists includes specifically designed genetically engineered mouse models (GEMs). GEMs have been developed to express specific genes, mutations, or deletions that are found in human tumors. Although these GEM models lack utility as a tool for large-scale drug discovery, they shed light on the cellular mechanisms that are vital to the progress of cancer research.[7]

There is continued promise to leverage the use of GEMs and PDX models by real-time integration of mouse data into co-clinical trials. Key aspects of such a program include a state-of-the art vivarium, animal care and veterinary staff with expertise in the care of GEMs and PDX models, a pharmacy where trial compounds are synthesized and optimized for mice, in vivo imaging capability, and centers for evaluating biomarkers, comparative pathology, bioinformatics, and mouse model development.[1]

With increasing molecular characterization of tumor lines and host organisms, continued development of increasingly specialized lines of immunodeficient and humanized mice, use of orthotopic methodology, and rational selection of model systems using knowledge of relevant molecular targets, mouse xenograft models will continue to make great contributions to targeted and disease-oriented cancer research and will remain useful in large-scale drug screening.[7]

REFERENCES

1. Lunardi A, Nardella C, Clohessy JG, Pandolfi PP. Of model pets and cancer models: an introduction to mouse models of cancer. In: Abate-Shen C, Politi K, Chodosh LA, Olive KP, editors. *Mouse models of cancer: a laboratory manual.* New York: Cold Spring Harbor Laboratory Press; 2014. p. 521.
2. Tanaka A, Imagi S, Mimura F, Nakatani S. Study of heterotransplantation of the human-cancer into rabbits and guinea pigs. *Jpn J Cancer Res* 1950;**41**:233–6.
3. Evgenjeva TP. Heterotransplantation of human cancers to animals by means of diffusion chambers. 1970 *Eur J Cancer* 1965;**6**:533. 4,IN21-IN26,5.
4. Southam CM. Immunologic tolerance to human cancer transplants in rats. *Cancer Res* 1966;**26**:2496–502.
5. Rygaard J, Povlsen CO. Heterotransplantation of a human malignant tumour to "Nude" mice. *Acta pathologica Microbiol Scand* 1969;**77**:758–60.
6. Decker S, Sausville E. Perspectives on the history and evolution of tumor models. In: Teicher BA, editor. *Tumor models in cancer research.* Springer Science & Business Media; 2010. p. 3–20.
7. Liu M, Hicklin D. Human tumor xenograft efficacy models. In: Teicher BA, editor. *Tumor models in cancer research.* Springer Science & Business Media; 2010. p. 99–124.
8. Committee on Immunologically Compromised Rodents. *Hereditary immunodeficiencies: mice with single mutations. Immunodeficient rodents: a guide to their immunobiology, husbandry, and use.* National Academies Press (US); 1989. p. 36–90.
9. Schuh JC. Trials, tribulations, and trends in tumor modeling in mice. *Toxicol Pathol* 2004;**32**:53–66.
10. Bosma MJ, Carroll AM. The SCID mouse mutant: definition, characterization, and potential uses. *Annu Rev Immunol* 1991;**9**:323–50.
11. DeVita VT, Chu EA. History of cancer chemotherapy. *Cancer Res* 2008;**68**:8643–53.
12. Plowman J, Dykes DJ, Hollingshead M, Simpson-Herren L, Alley MC. *Human tumor xenograft models in NCI drug development. Anticancer drug development guide.* Springer; 1997. p. 101–25.

13. Staquet M, Byar D, Green S, Rozencweig M. Clinical predictivity of transplantable tumor systems in the selection of new drugs for solid tumors: rationale for a three-stage strategy. *Cancer Treat Rep* 1983;**67**:753–65.
14. Winograd B, Boven E, Lobbezoo M, Pinedo H. Human tumor xenografts in the nude mouse and their value as test models in anticancer drug development (review). *In Vivo* 1986;**1**:1–13.
15. Suggitt M, Bibby MC. 50 years of preclinical anticancer drug screening: empirical to target-driven approaches. *Clin Cancer Res* 2005;**11**:971–81.
16. Fiebig H. *Comparison of tumor response in nude mice and in patients. Human tumour xenografts in anticancer drug development.* Springer; 1988. p. 25–30.
17. Inoue K, Fujimoto S, Ogawa M. Antitumor efficacy of seventeen anticancer drugs in human breast cancer xenograft (MX-1) transplanted in nude mice. *Cancer Chemother Pharmacol* 1983;**10**:182–6.
18. Boven E, Winograd B, Berger DP, et al. Phase II preclinical drug screening in human tumor xenografts: a first European multicenter collaborative study. *Cancer Res* 1992;**52**:5940–7.
19. Voskoglou-Nomikos T, Pater JL, Seymour L. Clinical predictive value of the in vitro cell line, human xenograft, and mouse allograft preclinical cancer models. *Clin Cancer Res* 2003;**9**:4227–39.
20. National Cancer Institute. *Developmental therapeutics program. Data retrieval and testing decisions*. 2015.
21. Kong D, Yamori T. JFCR39, a panel of 39 human cancer cell lines, and its application in the discovery and development of anticancer drugs. *Bioorg Med Chem* 2012;**20**:1947–51.
22. Richmond A, Su Y. Mouse xenograft models vs GEM models for human cancer therapeutics. *Dis Models Mech* 2008;**1**:78–82.
23. Jung J. Human tumor xenograft models for preclinical assessment of anticancer drug development. *Toxicol Res* 2014;**30**:1–5.

Chapter 3

Challenges and Limitations of Mouse Xenograft Models of Cancer

B.W. Simons, C. Brayton
Johns Hopkins University School of Medicine, Baltimore, MD, United States

INTRODUCTION

The successful development of effective anticancer drugs requires a preclinical model system that accurately predicts the safety and efficacy of promising compounds in clinical trials. The assessment of growth inhibition of immortalized cell lines in vitro and as subcutaneous xenografts in athymic nude mice remains the standard practice for preclinical drug evaluation. Despite enormous investments to translate these findings into clinically approved treatments, a majority of anticancer drugs that reach the Investigational New Drug stage fail in clinical trials. The discrepancy between preclinical promise and clinical disappointment raises concerns regarding the utility of the traditional subcutaneous xenograft model involving immortalized human cell lines and immunocompromised host mice.[1] Although their ability to predict clinical efficacy has fallen short of expectations, xenograft models have distinct advantages over in vitro assessments. Their primary advantage is the complex microenvironment that allows interaction between cancer cells and host vasculature and stroma. In addition, pharmacokinetic and safety studies can be done in the same species, and retrospective analyses of xenograft studies show good correlation between compounds with activity in multiple animal models and clinical efficacy in at least one human tumor type.[1] However, significant limitations to the use of cell line–based xenografts exist. This chapter discusses many of these limitations, emphasizing those related to the immortalized human cell lines and to the immunodeficient mouse hosts, and limitations in the design and interpretation of xenograft studies.

Patient Derived Tumor Xenograft Models. http://dx.doi.org/10.1016/B978-0-12-804010-2.00003-5

CONSIDER THE SOURCE: CELL LINES AS XENOGRAFTS

Typical xenograft studies involve subcutaneous injection of human cells taken from in vitro culture of an immortalized human cell line. Published, characterized, commercially available cell lines offer several advantages over alternatives, such as primary patient-derived xenografts (PDX) or genetically engineered mouse (GEM) models of cancer. Subcutaneous inocula of these cell lines often engraft and form rapidly growing, relatively synchronous tumors at very high rates, with a short latency until the tumors are palpable, and short doubling times of days to weeks.[2,3] In contrast, PDX models can show extended latency periods of months to a year and GEM models have similarly extended latency periods to cancer development ranging from several months to a year or more.[4,5] The shorter duration of xenograft studies can represent significant savings in time and costs. Well-characterized cell lines, in wide use for many years if not decades, offer the advantage of a wealth of published data concerning the expected behavior, genetic profile, and responses to treatments. Because most of these lines are available from public repositories, such as the American Type Culture Collection or their counterparts in Europe and Asia, studies can be replicated and confirmed by other laboratories using nearly identical populations of cells. The rapid growth rate and replicative potential of immortalized cancer cell lines allows them to be expanded to generate an essentially unlimited supply of cells to initiate xenografts. In contrast, tissue derived directly from patients often is of diagnostic importance, and very little can be diverted to initiate xenografts. Finally, the majority of established commercially available cell lines can be genetically modified to alter or induce the expression of genes, including vectors that facilitate quantitative imaging of luminescence or fluorescence. Labeled tumor cells facilitate the estimation of tumor burden in orthotopic xenografts and allow the identification of metastatic sites in a longitudinal, minimally invasive fashion.[6]

Xenografts derived from established cell lines have the advantage of homogeneous, readily available source material that can be passaged indefinitely, but these features may also contribute to their limited ability to generate xenografts that resemble the original human cancer. Cell lines have been established from most major histologic types of cancer, but many attempts to generate adherent cell lines directly from patient tumors are unsuccessful, and the peculiar cell lines that have this ability cannot reasonably be expected to reflect the spectrum of patient tumors. After passage in vitro, many cell lines no longer represent the native tumor. Many cell lines injected subcutaneously will form homogeneous sheets of cells with no recognizable architectural features of the primary tumor (Fig. 3.1). Intratumoral cellular and molecular heterogeneity is common in patient tumors, and contrasts with traditional xenograft cell lines, many of which were clonally derived.[7,8] Furthermore, the in vitro culture of cells has been shown to induce irreversible changes in gene expression compared to PDX models with primary tumor tissues.[9]

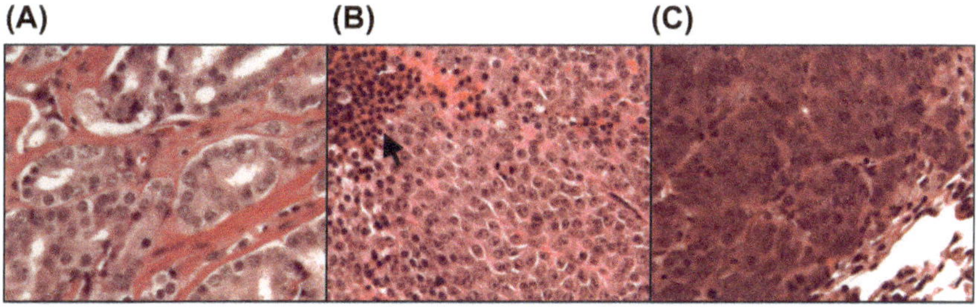

FIGURE 3.1 Morphologic differences between autochthonous tumors and cell line xenografts. A comparison of (A) human prostate adenocarcinoma showing cancer cells forming glands and surrounded by abundant stroma; (B) subcutaneous xenograft of prostate cancer cell line PC3 showing sheets of anaplastic cells with an area of necrosis (*arrow*); and (C) metastatic lung tumor formed after orthotopic prostate implantation of PC3 cells with similar anaplastic morphology.

Recent studies report numerous instances where cell lines were cross-contaminated by other cell lines or contaminated with microorganisms, especially mycoplasmas. Misidentified cell lines can occur through simple clerical error when maintaining cell lines, but can also occur through contamination by a faster growing line, such as HeLa cervical adenocarcinoma cells. Recognition of hundreds of cell lines as contaminated or inauthentic (ie, not the reported cell line) has invalidated the conclusions from numerous studies.[10] Although some cell lines were determined to be globally contaminated, inadvertent contamination of cell lines by a single laboratory can lead to confusing or contradictory publications. Long-term passage of cell lines has been shown to alter a variety of cellular parameters and results in the emergence of divergent sublines with very different properties.[11,12] Repeated passaging can result in xenograft studies on cells that differ by hundreds of generations, but which are reported as if they were performed with identical material.[13] Microbial contamination of cell cultures can affect survival and behavior of the cell lines, as well as survival and responses of the immunodeficient mouse host.[14] *Mycoplasma* contamination is well described to affect a wide variety of cellular parameters in vitro, and use of contaminated cell lines as xenograft models can affect tumor growth, immune response, and even metastatic potential.[15,16] Recognition of the role of xenotropic endogenous retroviruses as important genetic contaminants of cell lines is also emerging.[17] Many cell lines were contaminated with xenotropic rodent retroviruses during initial propagation as xenografts before passage in vitro. Cell lines can also be infected from coculture with a feeder layer of mouse fibroblasts. Many cell lines harbor replication-competent viruses, which can spread to other cell lines in laboratories. Multiple reports detail widespread contamination of nonxenograft cell lines by xenotropic retroviruses in laboratories that also culture xenograft-derived lines.[18] Infection of cell lines by xenotropic retroviruses has been shown to affect a variety of cellular parameters in vitro including growth, invasion, and cytokine expression.[19] These effects can translate to in vivo xenografts, where CWR22Rv1 prostate cancer cells, known to be infected by xenotropic murine leukemia virus–related virus, were treated with small hairpin RNA to reduce viral transcript expression and tumors derived from these lines grew more slowly and had more necrotic area than the parental lines.[19] A variety of other agents contaminate cell lines, via in vivo passaging in infected animals and by contact with contaminated reagents.[20] Microbial contaminations may be recognized by adverse effects on the cell line (loss of a cell line, cytolytic or cytopathic effects), or by adverse effects (morbidity, mortality) of inoculated hosts.[21,22] However, the effects may be fairly subtle, for example, parvoviruses remain prevalent in mouse colonies, target cells in S1, and have (potentially therapeutic) oncolytic effects that modulate xenograft growth.[23] Genetic and microbial contamination can be detected by routine quality assurance procedures that are not a standard of practice in many research programs, and prompt pathologic evaluation of unexpected morbidity and mortality of the rodent host may identify problems before a study is irretrievably compromised.[24]

The rapid growth of many traditional xenografts expedites evaluation of drug effect on the tumor, but may mask delayed toxicity that would not manifest until after the conclusion of the tumor assessment. In contrast to most human tumors, where only a small percentage of cells are dividing at a given time, a majority of xenograft cells can be actively replicating and contribute to the apparent effectiveness of cytotoxic drugs that target dividing cells in xenograft studies, followed by mixed success in clinical trials. Their rapid growth also predisposes the subcutaneous xenograft to large areas of necrosis, as the tumor growth outpaces the growth of vascular supply. The amount of necrosis varies among cell lines, but in some cases the majority of the xenograft becomes necrotic even without experimental intervention.[25] Necrotic areas in tumors complicate the measurement of tumor size, and influence drug distribution in the tumor.[26] Erratic or variable perfusion in xenografts can contribute to regional hypoxia and necrosis and affect the penetration and distribution of drugs.[27–29]

Considering the limitations of cell line–based xenografts described earlier, alternate approaches are clearly needed. PDX models can address some of these limitations, as they may reflect morphologic and genetic heterogeneity of patient tumors. Improvements in host models and engraftment techniques have increased the take rates and decreased the latency to logarithmic growth. Although these models have great potential for personalized medicine, they have not yet become the standard platform for preclinical drug development.

CONSIDER THE HOST: MOUSE XENOGRAFT MODELS

Compared with in vitro models, there are distinct advantages to studies using intact animal hosts. Cells grown in monoculture are typically exposed to a relatively homogeneous environment in liquid media unaffected by interaction with other cell types and with consistent distribution of oxygen, nutrients, and drugs or treatments. This contrasts with the microenvironment of a tumor in a human patient, where nutrient and oxygen gradients depend on the relative proximity to vasculature, and other direct and paracrine interactions among the tumor, stromal elements, immune system, and remote tissues through cytokine and hormone release. A xenograft mimics the complex tumor microenvironment better than in vitro cultures, including interactions with some portion of the innate immune system, even in immunodeficient mice.

Limitations inherent to the host (mouse) are similar for traditional xenografts and PDX models. Small size, short life span, and inbred genetics that make mice more readily available, less expensive, and more reliably consistent than larger animal models are also potential liabilities that limit the translational application of xenograft models. Genetic homogeneity of mice should not be expected to reflect the diversity in the human population. The size disparity between mice and humans is a practical limitation for some studies, as the maximum volume of drug that can be delivered to a mouse is limited, and imaging studies require access to high-resolution instruments. Mouse xenograft models are more relevant for pharmacodynamic studies of test compounds compared with in vitro systems. The small size and high metabolic rate of the mouse compared to humans requires adjusting the dose in mice to compensate for these differences, a process known as allometric scaling.[30] This principle is widely applied to translate pharmacodynamic studies from rodents to humans, but does not always accurately predict the clinical experience.[31] Camptothecin, an antitumor agent with excellent efficacy in mice, has shown relatively poor results in clinical trials. This failure was later determined to be due to the differential binding to serum proteins in mice and humans, rendering the drug inactive.[32] Metabolic clearance of drugs can also be estimated in mouse studies, but differences in specificity and activity of the CYP drug-metabolizing enzyme family can lead to pharmacokinetic data in mice that do not correlate with data from humans for drugs metabolized by this pathway. Models of hormone-dependent tumors, such as breast and prostate cancer, rely on estrogen or testosterone to support their growth. However, in prostate cancer, studies of adult male nude mice have shown that androgen levels vary dramatically among individuals, and that their mean serum testosterone concentration is well below the expected range for male humans.[33] Similarly, estrogen-responsive tumors are often grown in estrogen-supplemented mice. However, estrogen supplementation must be carefully controlled as hyperestrogenism can suppress bone marrow, and diet-derived phytoestrogens also may have effects.[34–36] Prolactin receptor–positive xenografts may be affected by species differences, as mouse prolactin does not activate the human prolactin receptor.[37] Therefore, hormone supplementation may be necessary to simulate the human hormonal microenvironment. Finally, species differences in susceptibility to toxic effects can lead to translational failure of some drugs. A major dose-limiting factor in clinical use of cytotoxic chemotherapeutic drugs is bone marrow toxicity. The toxic effect of these drugs can be underestimated in mice, as murine bone marrow progenitor cells are significantly more resistant to some cytotoxic therapies than their human counterparts are.[38] The reverse can in theory be true, with mice showing significant toxicity that may not apply to human patients due to differences in biology, resulting in the unnecessary abandonment of an otherwise promising drug. Even if the toxicity in mice and humans is comparable, the effects can be more severe in mice in the absence of intensive supportive care that is provided to human patients. For example, cisplatin is nephrotoxic, but is administered to patients along with aggressive fluid and supportive therapy to minimize renal damage.[39] In mice that do not receive similar supportive interventions and become dehydrated, the toxic effects can be enhanced. In practice, in vivo xenograft tests of any drug that causes dehydration in mice, whether through effects on the kidney or intestines, can appear to cause significant toxicity by inducing severe dehydration and the sequelae of reduced food intake, and potentially severe morbidity or mortality.[40] However, when recognized, these side effects can similarly be mitigated with supportive care of mice, and better represent drug efficacy and safety.[41]

Although much morbidity and mortality from many human tumors is related to metastatic disease, xenografts, especially subcutaneous xenografts, rarely metastasize, even when the tumors are large. Metastatic behavior may reflect inherent properties of the cell line, but also may reflect species differences between human and mouse microenvironment, and tumor–stromal interactions.[42–44] Table 3.1 summarizes examples of species differences that contribute to receptor–ligand mismatch between human tumors and mouse stroma. The

TABLE 3.1 Ligands With Limited or No Cross-Species Activity Between Mice and Humans

Ligands With Limited Cross-Species Reactivity
CD40L (partial)
CD47 (except NOD mice)
GITRL
GM-CSF
IFN-α
IFN-β
IFN-γ
IL-3
IL-4
Prolactin
TNF-α (partial)

These selected ligands are a few of the numerous cytokines, growth factors, and hormones that have limited cross-species activity between mice and humans. Nonfunctional ligand–receptor interactions are a critical limitation of mouse xenograft models. *GITRL*, glucocorticoid-induced tumor necrosis factor receptor-related protein ligand; *GM-CSF*, granulocyte-macrophage colony-stimulating factor; *IFN*, interferon; *IL*, interleukin; *NOD*, nonobese diabetic; *TNF*, tumor necrosis factor.

effect of stroma on tumor growth and behavior is amplified when implanted subcutaneously, as this microenvironment differs from the microenvironment of the tissue of origin. Orthotopic implantation can overcome this limitation somewhat. Species differences in stroma still exist, but the microenvironment in the orthotopic site is more relevant to the original tissue than is the subcutis. Studies have shown differences in drug sensitivity and higher metastatic potential for many cell lines when implanted orthotopically, as well as treatment responses that better reflect the clinical response in human tumors.[45–47] Recently, a major class of immunotherapy drugs was developed, designed to enhance antitumor immunity. This class of drugs works to increase the tumor-specific immune response by modulating the immune system. This precludes testing of these therapies in traditional xenograft models, which use immunodeficient hosts, and development is typically done in humanized mice engrafted with immune cells, or allograft and transgenic mouse models with a surrogate antibody targeting the homologous pathway. Although these drugs show clinical promise, preclinical safety testing is a challenge. In human patients, use of these drugs is often limited by autoimmune complications, an effect that was rare in mice treated with similar agents.[48] Testing immunotherapies in immune-sufficient mouse allograft models is an option, but interpretation of the results is limited by the strains in which this is feasible, and by the many differences between mouse and human immune systems.[49] Preconditioning or therapeutic interventions administered to xenograft host mice can affect host survival and research results. Variation in sensitivity of bone marrow to irradiation or estrogen effects is well recognized and myelosuppression contributes to adverse effects from opportunistic infections.[22,50–52] Antimicrobial agents may have unexpected effects on xenograft studies as well.[53] As in other studies involving mice, the housing environment can have a significant effect on the outcome of xenograft studies. Variables including diet, microflora or pathogen status, and ambient temperature have all been shown to impact xenograft studies and are reviewed elsewhere in this book.

Recent advances in PDX models have addressed some of these limitations, as these models typically contain mixed stromal elements derived from human patients and the mouse host. Furthermore, humanized models in which immunodeficient mice have been engrafted with human immune cells can recapitulate a portion of the immune microenvironment. The personalized "avatars" in which the immune system and tumor are both engrafted from the patient have great potential for interrogating the response to drug therapy and immunotherapy, and are discussed in other chapters.

CONSIDER THE METHOD: TECHNIQUE AND ANALYSIS OF XENOGRAFT MODELS

Variation in experimental design, even when using identical source material and host, can contribute to variable results and conclusions. Furthermore, the wide variation in analysis and reporting of data can make it difficult to compare experiments.

An early consideration is how and where to implant the xenograft. In general, more rostrally implanted subcutaneous xenografts are reported to grow faster than those implanted in the caudal flank.[54] Some orthotopic sites can be accessed in a relatively noninvasive fashion, whereas other sites, such as the prostate and pancreas may require major surgery to access the target organ, or require high-resolution ultrasound imaging for accurate percutaneous needle placement in the target organ. Although concern has been raised that surgical wounds release cytokines and growth factors that affect tumor growth, comparisons of invasive and noninvasive (direct or ultrasound guided) orthotopic injection did not find a difference in growth rate.[55,56] Surgical manipulation may have more impact on immunocompetent allograft models, where partial resection of established allografts has been shown to alter tumor immune cell infiltrates and antitumor immune responses, rendering them insensitive to immunotherapy that was effective in unresected tumors.[57] Implanting multiple tumors per mouse has been used to increase the experimental power, while decreasing animal number and cost, but there are significant limitations to this approach. Some statistical analyses assume that growth rates for all tumors are independent, but the potential for intra-animal correlation of tumors, or variation between rostral and caudal sites, may limit the additional power derived from these study designs.[58] Multiple tumors per mouse also would complicate the initiation of drug treatment when the tumors are not synchronous and the protocol requires initiation of treatment at a prescribed size. Finally, most studies have ethical limitations on the total volume or burden of tumors in an animal, and multiple tumors per animal significantly shortens the potential duration of studies and individual tumor size end points.

A second major variable in xenograft experiments is selecting a method to measure xenograft growth. For subcutaneous xenografts, a common method is to harvest all tumors at a given time point and measure their weights. Although this gives an accurate measurement of the excised mass, this method cannot longitudinally track tumor growth and fails to capture data concerning growth kinetics. For longitudinal assessment of growth, regular measurements of tumor size can be made with calipers to calculate an approximate tumor volume. Although many different formulas are described for this calculation, typically tumors are measured in two perpendicular dimensions and volume is calculated using formulas for ellipsoid volume.[59] This method assumes that the tumors grow in a symmetric, roughly ellipsoid mass, and measurement of irregular or multilobular tumors is difficult. Furthermore, this method cannot be applied to internal orthotopic xenografts. Micro computed tomography and ultrasound have been shown to be more accurate for assessing tumor volume, and can identify cystic or necrotic areas, but require specialized equipment and technical expertise.[60,61] To determine the relative number of viable cells, rather than tumor volume, cell lines can be engineered to express fluorescent or luminescent proteins. Optical imaging instruments detect light or fluorescence that is emitted only from living tumor cells, and can be used for orthotopic models.[62]

Finally, analysis and reporting of xenograft studies is critical. Although data analysis does not involve animals or cells per se, it can be one of the most challenging aspects of xenograft studies. End point analysis, where the final volumes or overall survival are compared, is useful, but it is the least powerful method of comparison.[63] Tumor doubling time is another option, but it is not applicable if the tumors fail to double in size, or if they shrink. Multivariate analyses and regression models may increase the statistical power and can identify subtle differences in experimental groups, but the complexity of this analysis puts it out of reach of most programs without dedicated support from experienced statisticians.[64]

CONCLUSION

Because agents selected for clinical trials have historically been, and continue to be, selected due to in vivo activity in xenografts, recognition of the limitations of these models is critical to maximizing their utility and validity in a humane and economical fashion. Despite the ongoing widespread use of these models, clinical translational success is the exception rather than the rule. New techniques, such as PDX and hollow fiber assays will provide additional tools for research and may improve the translational success of xenograft models. However, until these or other models become a standard in preclinical research, designing experiments with full awareness of the limitations inherent to cell lines, the mouse host, the environment, and the methodology can improve the reliability and predictability of data derived from cell line–based xenograft models. Review and retrospective analysis to determine where these models show the most success will also facilitate further refinement of experimental design.

REFERENCES

1. Johnson JI, Decker S, Zaharevitz D, et al. Relationships between drug activity in NCI preclinical in vitro and in vivo models and early clinical trials. *Br J Cancer* 2001;**84**:1424–31.
2. Perez-Soler R, Kemp B, Wu QP, et al. Response and determinants of sensitivity to paclitaxel in human non-small cell lung cancer tumors heterotransplanted in nude mice. *Clin Cancer Res* 2000;**6**:4932–8.
3. Giovanella BC, Vardeman DM, Williams LJ, et al. Heterotransplantation of human breast carcinomas in nude mice. Correlation between successful heterotransplants, poor prognosis and amplification of the HER-2/neu oncogene. *Int J Cancer* 1991;**47**:66–71.
4. Lin D, Wyatt AW, Xue H, et al. High fidelity patient-derived xenografts for accelerating prostate cancer discovery and drug development. *Cancer Res* 2014;**74**:1272–83.
5. Ittmann M, Huang J, Radaelli E, et al. Animal models of human prostate cancer: the consensus report of the New York meeting of the mouse models of human cancers consortium prostate pathology committee. *Cancer Res* 2013;**73**:2718–36.
6. Bhatnagar A, Wang Y, Mease RC, et al. AEG-1 promoter-mediated imaging of prostate cancer. *Cancer Res* 2014;**74**:5772–81.
7. Gerlinger M, Rowan AJ, Horswell S, et al. Intratumor heterogeneity and branched evolution revealed by multiregion sequencing. *N Engl J Med* 2012;**366**:883–92.

8. Zhang J, Fujimoto J, Zhang J, et al. Intratumor heterogeneity in localized lung adenocarcinomas delineated by multiregion sequencing. *Science* 2014;**346**:256–9.
9. Daniel VC, Marchionni L, Hierman JS, et al. A primary xenograft model of small-cell lung cancer reveals irreversible changes in gene expression imposed by culture in vitro. *Cancer Res* 2009;**69**:3364–73.
10. Capes-Davis A, Theodosopoulos G, Atkin I, et al. Check your cultures! A list of cross-contaminated or misidentified cell lines. *Int J Cancer* 2010;**127**:1–8.
11. Briske-Anderson MJ, Finley JW, Newman SM. The influence of culture time and passage number on the morphological and physiological development of Caco-2 cells. *Proc Soc Exp Biol Med* 1997;**214**:248–57.
12. Esquenet M, Swinnen JV, Heyns W, Verhoeven G. LNCaP prostatic adenocarcinoma cells derived from low and high passage numbers display divergent responses not only to androgens but also to retinoids. *J Steroid Biochem Mol Biol* 1997;**62**:391–9.
13. Hughes P, Marshall D, Reid Y, Parkes H, Gelber C. The costs of using unauthenticated, over-passaged cell lines: how much more data do we need?. *BioTechniques* 2007;**43**. 575, 577–578, 581-572 passim.
14. Drexler HG, Uphoff CC. Mycoplasma contamination of cell cultures: incidence, sources, effects, detection, elimination, prevention. *Cytotechnology* 2002;**39**:75–90.
15. Uno K, Takema M, Hidaka S, et al. Induction of antitumor activity in macrophages by mycoplasmas in concert with interferon. *Cancer Immunol Immunother* 1990;**32**:22–8.
16. Ushio S, Iwaki K, Taniai M, et al. Metastasis-promoting activity of a novel molecule, Ag 243-5, derived from mycoplasma, and the complete nucleotide sequence. *Microbiol Immunol* 1995;**39**:393–400.
17. Hempel HA, Burns KH, De Marzo AM, Sfanos KS. Infection of xenotransplanted human cell lines by murine retroviruses: a lesson brought back to light by XMRV. *Front Oncol* 2013;**3**:156.
18. Sfanos KS, Aloia AL, Hicks JL, et al. Identification of replication competent murine gammaretroviruses in commonly used prostate cancer cell lines. *PLoS One* 2011;**6**:e20874.
19. Stieler K, Schumacher U, Horst AK, Fischer N. XMRV induces cell migration, cytokine expression and tumor angiogenesis: are 22Rv1 cells a suitable prostate cancer model? *PLoS One* 2012;**7**:e42321.
20. Liu H, Bockhorn J, Dalton R, et al. Removal of lactate dehydrogenase-elevating virus from human-in-mouse breast tumor xenografts by cell-sorting. *J Virol Methods* 2011;**173**:266–70.
21. Lussier G. Potential detrimental effects of rodent viral infections on long-term experiments. *Vet Res Commun* 1988;**12**:199–217.
22. Baker DG. Natural pathogens of laboratory mice, rats, and rabbits and their effects on research. *Clin Microbiol Rev* 1998;**11**:231–66.
23. Marchini A, Bonifati S, Scott EM, Angelova AL, Rommelaere J. Oncolytic parvoviruses: from basic virology to clinical applications. *Virol J* 2015;**12**:6.
24. Peterson NC. From bench to cageside: risk assessment for rodent pathogen contamination of cells and biologics. *ILAR J* 2008;**49**:310–5.
25. Wexler EJ, Gravallese EM, Czerniak PM, et al. Tumor biology: use of tiled images in conjunction with measurements of cellular proliferation and death in response to drug treatments. *Clin Cancer Res* 2000;**6**:3361–70.
26. Minchinton AI, Tannock IF. Drug penetration in solid tumours. *Nat Rev Cancer* 2006;**6**:583–92.
27. Minchinton AI, Durand RE, Chaplin DJ. Intermittent blood flow in the KHT sarcoma–flow cytometry studies using Hoechst 33342. *Br J Cancer* 1990;**62**:195–200.
28. Chaplin DJ, Olive PL, Durand RE. Intermittent blood flow in a murine tumor: radiobiological effects. *Cancer Res* 1987;**47**:597–601.

29. Padera TP, Stoll BR, Tooredman JB, Capen D, di Tomaso E, Jain RK. Pathology: cancer cells compress intratumour vessels. *Nature* 2004;**427**:695.
30. Wajima T, Fukumura K, Yano Y, Oguma T. Prediction of human clearance from animal data and molecular structural parameters using multivariate regression analysis. *J Pharm Sci* 2002;**91**:2489–99.
31. Duconge J, Fernandez-Sanchez E, Alvarez D. Interspecies scaling of the monoclonal anti-EGF receptor ior EGF/r3 antibody disposition using allometric paradigm: is it really suitable? *Biopharm Drug Dispos* 2004;**25**:177–86.
32. Mi Z, Burke TG. Marked interspecies variations concerning the interactions of camptothecin with serum albumins: a frequency-domain fluorescence spectroscopic study. *Biochemistry* 1994;**33**:12540–5.
33. Michiel Sedelaar JP, Dalrymple SS, Isaacs JT. Of mice and men–warning: intact versus castrated adult male mice as xenograft hosts are equivalent to hypogonadal versus abiraterone treated aging human males, respectively. *Prostate* 2013;**73**:1316–25.
34. Heindel JJ, vom Saal FS. Meeting report: batch-to-batch variability in estrogenic activity in commercial animal diets–importance and approaches for laboratory animal research. *Environ Health Perspect* 2008;**116**:389–93.
35. Perry MJ, Samuels A, Bird D, Tobias JH. Effects of high-dose estrogen on murine hematopoietic bone marrow precede those on osteogenesis. *Am J Physiol Endocrinol Metab* 2000;**279**:E1159–65.
36. Simmons DJ. Collagen formation and endochondral ossification in estrogen treated mice. *Proc Soc Exp Biol Med* 1966;**121**:1165–8.
37. Utama FE, LeBaron MJ, Neilson LM, et al. Human prolactin receptors are insensitive to mouse prolactin: implications for xenotransplant modeling of human breast cancer in mice. *J Endocrinol* 2006;**188**:589–601.
38. Kurtzberg LS, Battle T, Rouleau C, et al. Bone marrow and tumor cell colony-forming units and human tumor xenograft efficacy of noncamptothecin and camptothecin topoisomerase I inhibitors. *Mol Cancer Ther* 2008;**7**:3212–22.
39. Pabla N, Dong Z. Cisplatin nephrotoxicity: mechanisms and renoprotective strategies. *Kidney Int* 2008;**73**:994–1007.
40. Jafri SH, Glass J, Shi R, Zhang S, Prince M, Kleiner-Hancock H. Thymoquinone and cisplatin as a therapeutic combination in lung cancer: in vitro and in vivo. *J Exp Clin Cancer Res* 2010;**29**:87.
41. Guindon J, Deng L, Fan B, Wager-Miller J, Hohmann AG. Optimization of a cisplatin model of chemotherapy-induced peripheral neuropathy in mice: use of vitamin C and sodium bicarbonate pretreatments to reduce nephrotoxicity and improve animal health status. *Mol Pain* 2014;**10**:56.
42. Cooper CR, Chay CH, Gendernalik JD, et al. Stromal factors involved in prostate carcinoma metastasis to bone. *Cancer* 2003;**97**:739–47.
43. Schmidt-Hansen B, Klingelhofer J, Grum-Schwensen B, et al. Functional significance of metastasis-inducing S100A4(Mts1) in tumor-stroma interplay. *J Biol Chem* 2004;**279**:24498–504.
44. De Wever O, Mareel M. Role of tissue stroma in cancer cell invasion. *J Pathol* 2003;**200**:429–47.
45. Francia G, Cruz-Munoz W, Man S, Xu P, Kerbel RS. Mouse models of advanced spontaneous metastasis for experimental therapeutics. *Nat Rev Cancer* 2011;**11**:135–41.
46. Wilmanns C, Fan D, O'Brian CA, Bucana CD, Fidler IJ. Orthotopic and ectopic organ environments differentially influence the sensitivity of murine colon carcinoma cells to doxorubicin and 5-fluorouracil. *Int J Cancer* 1992;**52**:98–104.
47. Zeineldin M, Jensen D, Paranjape SR, et al. Human cancer xenografts in outbred nude mice can be confounded by polymorphisms in a modifier of tumorigenesis. *Genetics* 2014;**197**:1365–76.

48. Liu J, Blake SJ, Smyth MJ, Teng MW. Improved mouse models to assess tumour immunity and irAEs after combination cancer immunotherapies. *Clin Transl Immunol* 2014;**3**:e22.
49. Mestas J, Hughes CC. Of mice and not men: differences between mouse and human immunology. *J Immunol* 2004;**172**:2731–8.
50. Pearson T, Shultz LD, Miller D, et al. Non-obese diabetic-recombination activating gene-1 (NOD-Rag1 null) interleukin (IL)-2 receptor common gamma chain (IL2r gamma null) null mice: a radioresistant model for human lymphohaematopoietic engraftment. *Clin Exp Immunol* 2008;**154**:270–84.
51. Duran-Struuck R, Dysko RC. Principles of bone marrow transplantation (BMT): providing optimal veterinary and husbandry care to irradiated mice in BMT studies. *J Am Assoc Lab Anim Sci* 2009;**48**:11–22.
52. Altholtz LY, La Perle KM, Quimby FW. Dose-dependant hypothyroidism in mice induced by commercial trimethoprim-sulfamethoxazole rodent feed. *Comp Med* 2006;**56**:395–401.
53. Gao P, Dang CV, Watson J. Unexpected antitumorigenic effect of fenbendazole when combined with supplementary vitamins. *J Am Assoc Lab Anim Sci* 2008;**47**:37–40.
54. Auerbach R, Morrissey LW, Sidky YA. Regional differences in the incidence and growth of mouse tumors following intradermal or subcutaneous inoculation. *Cancer Res* 1978;**38**:1739–44.
55. Huynh AS, Abrahams DF, Torres MS, Baldwin MK, Gillies RJ, Morse DL. Development of an orthotopic human pancreatic cancer xenograft model using ultrasound guided injection of cells. *PLoS One* 2011;**6**:e20330.
56. Fleming JM, Miller TC, Meyer MJ, Ginsburg E, Vonderhaar BK. Local regulation of human breast xenograft models. *J Cell Physiol* 2010;**224**:795–806.
57. Predina J, Eruslanov E, Judy B, et al. Changes in the local tumor microenvironment in recurrent cancers may explain the failure of vaccines after surgery. *Proc Natl Acad Sci USA* 2013;**110**:E415–24.
58. Heitjan DF, Derr JA, Satyaswaroop PG. The multi-site tumour transplantation model for human endometrial carcinoma: a statistical evaluation. *Cell Prolif* 1992;**25**:193–203.
59. Tomayko MM, Reynolds CP. Determination of subcutaneous tumor size in athymic (nude) mice. *Cancer Chemother Pharmacol* 1989;**24**:148–54.
60. Jensen MM, Jorgensen JT, Binderup T, Kjaer A. Tumor volume in subcutaneous mouse xenografts measured by microCT is more accurate and reproducible than determined by 18F-FDG-microPET or external caliper. *BMC Med Imaging* 2008;**8**:16.
61. Ayers GD, McKinley ET, Zhao P, et al. Volume of preclinical xenograft tumors is more accurately assessed by ultrasound imaging than manual caliper measurements. *J Ultrasound Med* 2010;**29**:891–901.
62. Caysa H, Hoffmann S, Luetzkendorf J, et al. Monitoring of xenograft tumor growth and response to chemotherapy by non-invasive in vivo multispectral fluorescence imaging. *PLoS One* 2012;**7**:e47927.
63. Heitjan DF, Manni A, Santen RJ. Statistical analysis of in vivo tumor growth experiments. *Cancer Res* 1993;**53**:6042–50.
64. Heitjan DF. Biology, models, and the analysis of tumor xenograft experiments. *Clin Cancer Res* 2011;**17**:949–51.

Chapter 4

Tumor Heterogeneity

J.W. Cassidy[1,2], A. Bruna[1,2]
[1]*Cancer Research UK Cambridge Institute, Cambridge, United Kingdom;* [2]*University of Cambridge, Cambridge, United Kingdom*

INTRODUCTION

Tumors have been known to be heterogeneous since their detailed study by experimental pathologists began at the start of the 19th century. As technologies improved, differences in cellular morphologies were described,[1] followed by heterogeneity across surface marker expression[2] and later differences in tumor growth rates[3] and response to therapy.[4] Following these early morphological and histological studies, large- and small-scale sequencing endeavors have helped elucidate the true scale of diversity across human neoplasms.[5] Early work in breast cancer, for example, allowed the stratification of patients based on the presence of estrogen receptor α (ER), which led to the successful therapeutic use of tamoxifen in ER+ patients.[6] The advent of high throughput sequencing technologies based on cancer genomics has enabled the comprehensive stratification of breast and other cancers into different subtypes.[5,7] Improving the taxonomy of cancer is the initial step toward a better understanding of the drivers of tumor growth and consequently toward improved precision medicines. It is hoped that this strategy may ultimately lead to the development of the next generation of targeted therapies.

Early evidence for functionally distinct cellular compartments within tumors came from Fidler and Kripke, who reported in 1977 that clonal population derived from mouse metastatic melanomas varied extensively in their ability to seed metastasis in syngeneic hosts.[8] Following on from this pioneering work, various studies around the late 1960s showed by in vivo radiolabeling that the morphologically distinguishable populations of human leukemic cells differed remarkably in their proliferative potential.[9–11] The observation that human cancers contain functionally different populations was echoed by Southam et al., who in 1962 showed that autologous engrafted human tumor cells differ in their ability to re-form tumors.[12] Evidence of this nature continues to be collected at present; John Dick's laboratory has generated revealing data in 2012 in colon cancer and hematological malignancies that cells sharing the same genotype can be functionally distinct.[13]

Patient Derived Tumor Xenograft Models. http://dx.doi.org/10.1016/B978-0-12-804010-2.00004-7

These early studies showed that tumors are not simply a growth of homogeneous cells with equal proliferative potential and tumor-forming ability, but rather a heterogeneous mixture of cellular populations. The observation that tumor cells differ in their ability to xeno- and autotransplant was added to seminal studies of teratocarcinomas,[14] small cell lung carcinomas,[15] and mammary adenocarcinomas,[16] to give rise to the cancer stem cell (CSC) model of tumor development and heterogeneity. Early evidence that genetic aberrations were the cause of a tumor's phenotypic traits[17] supported the idea that somatic evolution between genetic subclones could occur following darwinian selection in response to spatial and temporal selective pressures.[18] Together these theories have influenced a significant proportion of the cancer research occurring at present. Significantly, data derived from the use of statistical tools and sequencing data recently confirmed what was noted long ago.[1,18] Tumors are communities of cells with varying degrees of complexity and diversity with predefined evolutionary trajectories.[19–21] However, translation of this research into the clinical setting has been slower, hampered by the realization that traditional preclinical models lack the heterogeneity of human malignancies.[22] Currently, patient-derived tumor xenografts (PDXs) have emerged as powerful preclinical models capable of recapitulating most of the tumor heterogeneity.[23] As such, studies on PDXs are showing strong basic and translational impact in the field, which is crucial in order to avoid the unsustainable rates of attrition in oncological drug development.[24]

Although often considered disparate, the causes and consequences of intertumor heterogeneity (ie, different subclassifications of the same disease) and intratumor heterogeneity (ie, different subclonal architectures) are inherently linked (Fig 4.1). Moreover, compelling models of tumor heterogeneity, linking the theories of CSCs and somatic evolution have been proposed in 2014.[25] In this chapter, we will discuss these and other theories explaining tumor heterogeneity, before examining the clinical consequences. We will conclude by presenting the PDX as the model best reflecting the complex heterogeneity of human neoplasms. We argue for a greater reliance on the PDX in preclinical drug development but conclude by considering future improvements to the model. We stand at the brink of a new era of research into the causes and consequences of tumor heterogeneity. It is hoped that this new era of research will lead to new insights into the complex ecosystem, that is, cancer, and that these insights can be translated into the clinic to accurately stratify tumors and improve therapeutic strategies.

HERITABLE SOURCES OF HETEROGENEITY

Cancer is first and foremost a disease of the genome and it is through the acquisition of driver mutations (for example, *APC* loss in CRC) that initial clonal expansion of a transformed cell is fueled.[26,27] Far from being a static disease, however, cancers continue to acquire sequential (epi)genomic aberrations

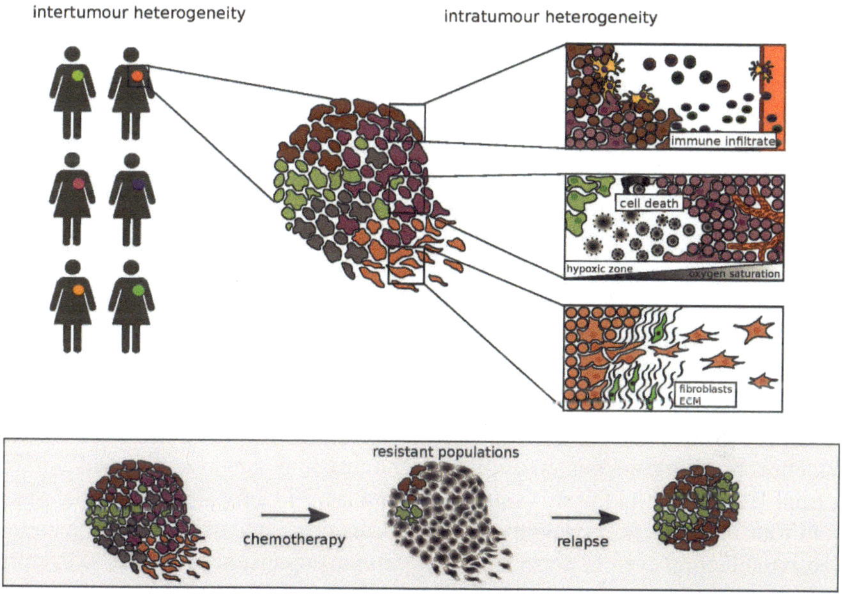

FIGURE 4.1 Overview of tumor heterogeneity. From left to right; intertumor heterogeneity ensures that no two malignancies are the same; genomic clonal populations exist within a tumor (colored) and functional heterogeneity (shape) exists within isogeneic populations. This nongenomic intratumor heterogeneity is due to intrinsic epigenetic differences (not shown), interaction with the immune infiltrate (top panel), differences in tumor metabolism (eg, hypoxia, middle panel), and interaction with the ECM/stromal component (bottom panel). Each of the depicted environments could have different effects on cellular phenotypes, and clearly these scenarios are not mutually exclusive. Intratumor heterogeneity has profound influence on both resistance to therapy and metastasis. In the lower half of the figure, two genomic clones are depicted as resistant to chemotherapy and able to repopulate the tumor after therapy. These resistant clones could be genomic or quiescent cellular.

throughout their development. Although genetic events (ie, copy number alterations and mutations) are by far the best characterized in this regard, the role of epigenetic modifications (eg, promoter methylation, histone modification) in tumor progression are beginning to become apparent.[28,29] It is through successive rounds of driver mutational events and subsequent clonal expansions that heterogeneity both between, and across, a tumor is achieved. This section will explore the role of these genomic and epigenomic events in tumor progression and the development of heterogeneity.

Genomic Influences on Tumor Heterogeneity

The earliest events in a tumor's evolution are fueled by specific genomic aberrations, which can have profound effects on intertumor heterogeneity. For example, *ESR1* and *ERBB2* amplification, leading, respectively, to ER[30] and human epidermal growth factor receptor 2 (HER2)[31] overexpression, can be early events in breast cancer initiation. *ESR1* and *ERBB2* amplification can also occur in the same tumors, with or without the presence of progesterone receptor (PR). These events are prognostic and predictive of drug responses, suggesting that they can be used to classify cancer into different subtypes. Indeed, the first molecular-based classification of breast cancers dramatically changed clinical practice and patient outcome and was based on ER, PR, and HER2 status.[32] With the advent of new technological advances it has become apparent that a wide range of (epi) genomic aberrations, beyond ER/PR/HER2, can drive the tumorigenic process in breast cancer. Indeed, as breast cancers are largely copy number driven,[33] a driver-based taxonomy has recently been defined based on copy number and gene expression data.[7,34] This study identified 10 subtypes with distinct prognosis and molecular drivers, reaffirming breast cancer heterogeneity.

Early disease-definitive driver events, such as *ERBB2* amplification in breast cancer are crucial for the classification and treatment of neoplasms. However, evidence is emerging that multiple driver mutations can coexist even within normal tissues. In addition, sequencing data on 234 biopsies of normal skin from four individuals showed that multiple cancer-associated genes were under positive selection even in normal tissue.[35] Clonal expansion of normal skin cells with early driver mutations were observed across patients. As this study focused on precancerous tissues, we cannot know if any of these early lesions would lead to tumor growth, although this study strongly suggests that clonal expansion occurs even in the earliest stages of a neoplasm's development and that not all cellular clones harboring single oncogenic drivers will develop a tumor.[35] Hence, driver mutations may not always be rare events that completely define a malignancy simply by their presence. It may be that the context in which the mutation is acquired is just as important in dictating the neoplasm's development. Indeed, the order in which cells acquire mutations can have profound effects on intertumor heterogeneity and disease progression. For example, in Philadelphia chromosome–negative myeloproliferative neoplasms (MPNs), recent work has demonstrated that within patients harboring both a *JAK2* and *TET2* mutation, those who acquired the *TET2* mutation first were less likely to present with polycythemia vera than essential thrombocythemia.[36] Thus, complete phenotypic heterogeneity is observed between patients with the same mutational burden depending on the order of mutational events.

Clearly, the presence of driver mutations is important for defining any malignancy. However, the observations that drivers coexist in normal skin and that the order in which these drivers are acquired can completely define the phenotype of MPN suggests that the processes involved in tumor progression are more complex. Indeed, the idea that clonal populations within a tumor coexist dynamically in space and time is well established in cancer biology.[18,21] Through the course of tumor initiation and progression, cancer cells undergo repeated mutational events,[17] which may or may not confer a survival advantage ("fitness") on their progeny. With time, this process generates a dominant clone that will expand and dominate the site where it was generated through darwinian selection in response to spatial and temporal selective pressures.[18] When clones arise with an increased fitness (or when selective pressures change), less-advantaged clones will either disappear or will be maintained as subclones alongside the dominant clone, acting as a reservoir from which evolution can continue.[37] It is through the dynamic evolution of these subclonal populations that genomic tumor heterogeneity is produced and maintained.

Numerous groups have been able to reconstruct the clonal hierarchy of individual tumors. For example, Nik-Zainal and colleagues were able to combine deep sequencing with new bioinformatics tools to reconstruct the clonal history of 21 breast cancers.[20] The authors showed that breast cancers evolve through the infrequent acquisition of driver mutations, each of which allows clonal expansion and eventual dominance. Interestingly, as the most recent common ancestor appeared relatively early, minor clones were able to coexist and diversify alongside the dominant clone.[20] This model of branched evolution allows for a genetic pool of minor clones able to fuel new stages of clonal evolution if selective pressures change. In agreement with this study, by reconstructing the clonal composition of 104 triple-negative breast cancers (TNBCs), we observed a complete spectrum of molecular and clonal compositions at patient diagnosis.[21]

Alongside this model of branched evolution, the survival of multiple subdominant clones can be explained by the spatial segregation of clones across the tumor as a whole. This pattern was hinted at in the precancerous clonal expansions of the normal skin[35] and fully considered in renal cell carcinoma[38] and lung cancers.[39] Furthermore, the notion that some clonal populations may cooperate through reciprocal signaling pathways can further contribute to tumor heterogeneity.[40] In this model, the survival of a minor clone can be assured if it contributes some degree of paracrine signaling to the dominant clone, ensuring expansion of the latter will never come at the expense of the former. Interestingly, this model does not require that cellular populations are genomically distinct; indeed, functional heterogeneity has been observed even in isogenic populations.[13]

Epigenomic Influences on Tumor Heterogeneity

As all cells in an adult organism are genomically identical (barring somatic mutations and immunoglobulin rearrangements in immune cells), the heterogeneity in cellular phenotypes found in normal tissues is predominantly defined by epigenetic mechanisms[41]. Epigenetic regulation of gene transcription, whether by promoter methylation, histone modification, or regulation of DNA-binding proteins, is the major mechanism by which a normal differentiated cell's phenotype is defined and maintained.[42] Perhaps unsurprisingly then, it is becoming apparent that aberrant DNA methylation patterns can be as essential for a cancer cell's survival as other genomic events.[28] For example, a recent study by Carvalho and colleagues identified promoter regions that require DNA methylation–mediated gene silencing for survival of cancer cell lines.[43] Novel experimental and bioinformatics methodologies have also recently uncovered epigenetic driver events required for the survival of breast cancer cells.[43] Moreover, coordinated epigenetic unmasking of multiple oncogenes has been reported in primary head and neck and lung cancers.[44]

One of the most important mediators of intertumor heterogeneity is the cell type from which the tumor arises.[45] Because of this, the underlying epigenetic state of a transformed cell is an important cause of intertumor heterogeneity. For example, breast cancer molecular subtypes have been linked to subpopulations of the normal epithelium by interrogation of specific gene expression signatures.[46] Challenging this argument is the recent finding that the acquisition of specific mutations (ie, oncogenic *PIK3CA*) can mediate switching between basal and luminal lineages as a tumor progresses.[47,48] Multiple examples link epigenetic alterations to genomic mutational events. Taking the most extreme example, hypermethylation of *MLH1* leads to a hypermutator phenotype in colorectal cancer (CRC).[49] This microsatellite instability phenotype both distinguishes *MLH1* mutant tumors from other CRCs and leads to widespread intratumor heterogeneity,[50] which has been linked to higher resistance to therapy.

The aforementioned studies demonstrated that DNA methylation and other epigenetic modifications are functionally important in cancer. Moreover, epigenomic regulation of lineage is important in normal tissues and tumors tend to retain some degree of functional relationship with their originating cell type.[41,42,46] Thus, epigenetic stratification of cancer could be a powerful technique to reveal novel biologically relevant subtypes. Indeed, early efforts are underway in this regard.[51] Stefansson and colleagues, in 2015, used DNA methylation–based arrays to describe distinct signatures associated with luminal B and basal-like breast cancer subtypes.[52] Although this classification was defined in only 40 samples, it was later validated in 212 tumors from the cancer genome atlas (TCGA) cohort. The epigenome thus contributes significantly to intertumor heterogeneity and large-scale studies, of the type performed by Molecular Taxonomy of Breast Cancer International Consortium and TCGA in genomics, should be encouraged.

CONTEXT-DEPENDENT SOURCES OF HETEROGENEITY

In addition to genomic and epigenomic diversity, cells within a tumor are characterized by functional heterogeneity related to their specific tumor microenvironment (TME). Indeed, components of the TME [encompassing immune infiltrate, stromal compartment, and extracellular matrix (ECM)] vary significantly between tumors and contribute to spatial heterogeneity in individual neoplasms. Moreover, localized signaling from stromal/immune components could lead to phenotypic plasticity within isogenic populations. For these reasons, we should consider a tumor as a complex ecosystem functioning at a level far exceeding the sum of its parts.[53]

Tumor Microenvironment

Tumor development depends on the coevolution of neoplastic cells along with the ECM stromal compartment, tumor vasculature, and immune cells. These tumor extrinsic factors collectively comprise the TME and are required for successful outgrowth of tumors and eventual metastasis.[54] As fitness is context dependent, we must consider tumors as complex organs and not simply as masses of transformed epithelial cells. The dynamic topology of the tumor, together with its microenvironment, varies drastically both between, and within the same lesions.[54] Thus, the individual compartments of the TME have profound influence on both inter- and intratumor heterogeneity.

Perhaps the most relevant facet of the TME for tumor stratification, given the success of immune checkpoint inhibitors, is the tumor's immune infiltrate.[55,56] For example, Th1 and cytotoxic (CD8+) T cells were recently found to be the strongest prognostic factor in the overall survival at all stages of CRC. Other studies have highlighted the vast heterogeneity seen in immune infiltrates of CRC patients.[57] As such, stratification of CRCs based on immune infiltrate could both provide more accurate prognosis information, and potentially identify patients who would benefit most from immune checkpoint inhibitors.

In breast cancer, efforts to develop immune-based subclasses are already underway. One study used immunohistochemical grading of CD8+ T cells, regulatory T cells, and natural killer cells to define three breast cancer subtypes.[58] Analysis of training ($n=440$) and validation ($n=382$) cohorts confirmed that these subtypes had significant prognostic value for relapse-free and overall survival.[58] Moreover, our own studies have shown that PD-L1 expression is correlated with infiltrating lymphocytes and highly enriched in basal-like breast tumors.[59] Anti–PD-L1 antibodies are currently in Phase 1A trials for metastatic breast cancer; it seems likely that stratification of breast cancers based on immune infiltrate or PD-L1 expression will aid in improving the efficacy of such agents.[60] Moreover, integration of immune and genomic-based classifications will further increase our resolution of intertumor heterogeneity and allow a more rational stratification of patients.

Phenotypic Plasticity

The epi(genomic) landscape can be conceptualized as containing "hills" (unstable states) and "valleys" (stable states). A pluripotent cell begins its differentiation process at the peak of a hill and progresses into a stable state (the valley) as it becomes restricted to a specific lineage.[61] Directing the cell down its lineage-restricted path are a multitude of environmental (eg, topology of the ECM[62]) and biochemical cues (autocrine and paracrine signaling) which directly stimulate the transition from one epigenetic state to the next.[63] During tumor development, the acquisition of numerous passenger mutations, coupled with irregular activation of signaling pathways, contributes to instability in these epigenetic "attractor states."[29] Thus, cancers are often described as caricatures of their normal tissue architecture, with phenotypic states that may be less stable and more susceptible to heterogeneity in the TME than the normal tissue equivalent.

As cancers develop, tight regulation of the ECM is lost and tissue architecture begins to degrade.[64] Solid-state ECM interactions are necessary for cells to maintain stem cell properties and regulated ECM helps maintain the stem cell niche.[65] As cancer is often associated with a blurring of the boundaries between stem and differentiated cells, it is possible that the loss of structured ECM is essential for the stability of multiple subdominant cellular clones within a tumor.[29] A study by Wang et al. in 2014 provides direct evidence that ECM-dependent signaling confers dynamic switching between expression signatures related to transforming growth factor β receptor 3 (TGFβR3) and jun D proto-oncogene.[66] Hence, depending on ECM stiffness and composition, heterogeneity in signaling pathways could be generated across a tumor.

The TME is further characterized by an influx of stromal cells. Infiltrating cancer-associated fibroblasts (CAFs) can confer resistance to cytotoxic and targeted therapies[67]; however, studies in 2014 confer on the fibroblasts a degree of plasticity, with antitumor properties observed in some populations.[68] Due to the high levels of CAF infiltrates seen in some tumor types, heterogeneity within their population would undoubtedly confer differential properties to the tumor bulk. For example, recent evidence suggests that CAFs may produce a variety of signaling molecules (TGFβ3, tenascin C, asporin, etc.) that initiate Wnt signaling in tumor cells.[69] As Wnt signaling is important for both tumor progression[40,70] and stem cell maintenance,[71] spatial heterogeneity in Wnt activation could also drive phenotypic heterogeneity in cancer cell populations.

Extensive spatial heterogeneity could also exist within a tumor in terms of immune infiltrate.[72] Areas close to blood vessels or lacking in normal lymphatic drainage, for example, may show increase buildup of immune cells. Different populations of leukocytes have been shown to harbor both pro- and antitumor properties depending on the tumor type. For example, CD8+ T-cell infiltration in breast cancer confers improved prognosis in ER− or ER+ HER2+ breast cancers but not in ER− HER2- cancers.[73] However, cytotoxic chemotherapeutics can induce colony-stimulating factor 1 (CSF1) expression in at least some breast tumor cells; CSF1 recruits macrophages to the tumor site and reduces CD8+ T-cell-mediated killing.[74] As such, localized tumor–immune cell interactions could reinforce intratumor heterogeneity and have profound effect on overall tumor development.

EVOLUTION OF THE CANCER STEM CELL MODEL

In summary, tumor heterogeneity is undoubtedly due, at least in part, to the stability of multiple genomic clonal populations within a neoplasm.[18] These arise from divergent evolution of the originating cells' progeny and may be sustained by geographical isolation within the tumor and cooperation between clones.[18] Changes in the nature and order of early driver mutations[36] can lead to highly divergent evolution between tumors and reinforce the profound intertumor heterogeneity seen in human tumors.[7,20] Passenger mutations in these populations may lead to altered epigenetic "attractor states" and a blurring of the boundaries between cellular phenotypes.[29] Tumor-extrinsic features of the ECM and TME lead to dynamic oscillations between epigenetically regulated phenotypes.[65,66] Spatial heterogeneity in TME components across a tumor may reinforce intratumor heterogeneity, whereas global changes in TME between patients influences intertumor heterogeneity.[56,58]

Recent research in the stem cell field identified various tissues with dormant or quiescent stem cell populations with the ability to regenerate tissues on damage.[75–77] The CSC theory of tumor initiation and progression posits that cancer follows the same principles as embryogenesis and normal tissue renewal. Thus, cancer "stem" cells produce all components of the tumor much as normal stem cells produce differentiated cells of the adult tissue.[25] These cells are resistant to normal genotoxic stress (of the type used in chemo- and radiotherapies) by virtue of their slow cycling nature. Kreso and Dick proposed in 2012 that certain cellular phenotypes within genomic clones may adopt a "dormant" (CSC-like) state but be able to reacquire malignancy in a context-specific manner. Such cellular populations have been described in CRC PDX models[13] in which quiescent cellular clones were linked to the acquisition of chemoresistance and later found to express the putative stem cell marker BMI1.[25,78]

Difficulties in robust isolation of CSCs from all malignancies have emerged challenging the CSC theory (leading to the term tumor-initiating cell for cells with CSC-like properties that cannot be prospectively purified). Interestingly, stem cell signatures do show prognostic features across multiple tumor types.[79–82] Moreover, studies in 2015 based on single-cell analysis have highlighted stem cell–like expression patterns in human metastatic breast cancer cells.[83]

Moreover, the realization that oncogenic driver mutations can lead to the reacquisition of mutlipotency has profound implications for this model.[47,48] Rather than resulting from oncogenic transformation of normal tissue stem cells,[84] a CSC-like phenotype could be the result of specific mutational events in a particular genomic clone. Moreover, as cells may transition between different epigenetic attractor states in cancer, cellular dedifferentiation, reacquisition of mutlipotency, and acquisition of a CSC-like phenotype could be driven by the epigenome.[41] Thus, the CSC and clonal evolution models of tumor development can be reconciled by considering that genomic clones may contain a heterogeneous mixture of cellular phenotypes. These cellular phenotypes could be maintained by the diversity in epigenetic state and TME-mediated (spatially heterogeneous) signaling pathways across a tumor. This unified model reinforces the need to study tumor growth and heterogeneity in complex model systems that are able to retain the complexity of human malignancies.

CLINICAL IMPLICATIONS OF TUMOR HETEROGENEITY

The typical attrition rate of new investigational drugs submitted for clinical trials is around 88%.[85] Consequently, the average cost of bringing a new therapeutic agent through to regulatory approval, a process that can take a decade, is over $2.56 billion.[85,86] Clearly as global life expectancy continues to rise, the cost of health care will become an even larger burden for our economies. Thus, the cost of new therapeutic agents is widely considered to be unsustainable. Moreover, even in cases in which a new agent is deemed "successful," the development of resistance is often seen as inevitable and clinical responses can often be fleeting at best.[87] In order to reduce the attrition of experimental cancer agents and improve the outcome of patients already treated with targeted agents, we must develop a more comprehensive picture of, and preclinical models able to capture, tumor heterogeneity.

Stratified Medicine

The first and most profound consequence of tumor heterogeneity for clinical practice is that chemotherapy and targeted agents do not have the same efficacy across malignancies of the same subtype or even across the same tumor.[88] The new generation of targeted therapeutics aim to selectively cause cell death in cancerous cells. Currently, two broad approaches are being explored in this regard. The first targets the oncogenic addiction process in which a tumor is defined by reliance on a single driver's process for growth (eg, ER antagonists or aromatase inhibitors in ER-addicted breast tumors). The second strategy, known as synthetic lethality, targets a different pathway, which when perturbed in the presence of a driver aberration will cause cell death (eg, poly ADP ribose polymerase inhibitors in *BRCA*-deficient cancers). Thus, successful targeted therapy can only be achieved when appropriate patient stratification based on molecular flags or biomarkers of drug response is attained.

Breast cancer provides an interesting example of how our understanding of heterogeneity has developed over time, how this has been translated to the clinic in terms of patient stratification, and how therapeutic strategies have ultimately been improved. Early studies into morphological heterogeneity across tumors formed the basis of a histological grading system and first identified the heterogeneity across tumors. Although multiple morphologies are observed, the vast majority are derived from the lining of the ducts or lobules, and are classified as such. Depending on whether cancerous cells proliferate within the epithelium or invade into the surrounding tissues, tumors can further be classified as carcinoma in situ or invasive carcinoma.[32] As our understanding of breast cancer developed, classifications were expanded to include the most relevant molecular features of breast cancer: presence or absence of hormone receptors (ER and PR) and HER2. This first molecular stratification had unprecedented clinical implications exemplified by the strong benefit of estrogen pathway inhibitors in ER+ and anti-HER2 therapy in HER2+ breast cancers. Later, with the advent of large-scale sequencing projects, our classification of subtypes across breast cancers moved from pathological analysis to genomic-based approaches.[89] Early genomic classifications based on single parameters (eg, PAM50 and gene expression) have evolved into complex integrative methodologies designed to capture heterogeneity across multiple levels, such as the 10 integrative clusters defined based on copy number and expression data by Curtis and colleagues in 2012.[7] Because breast cancer is defined mostly by copy number alterations,[33] this later classification is the most accurate one currently available and will likely allow the identification of subtype-specific therapeutic strategies.

The rational classification of breast cancers offers insight into the advances that can be made with large-scale sequencing endeavors. However, taxonomies must be identified in all areas of tumor biology. For example, efforts are underway to stratify both breast cancer[90] and CRC[91] based on immune infiltrates and immunogenomic signature. Such classification could allow more targeted use of novel immune checkpoint inhibitors.[55] It is only by integrating multiparametric layers of stratifying features that we will progress to treating cancers as truly stratified diseases. Thus, we must develop a deep understanding of the origins and molecular drivers of tumor heterogeneity and develop banks of preclinical models that capture the diversity of human malignancies.

Resistance and Progression

Clonal populations within the same tumor can have a profound influence on the response to therapy, the emergence of drug resistance, and disease progression. Currently, our ability to predict the emergence of drug resistance in tumors requires a priori knowledge of resistance mechanisms and the identification of resistance-associated clones within a tumor. However, there is some evidence that the development of resistance is an inevitable consequence of single agent–targeted therapies.[92]

Typically, resistance results from the outgrowth of specific preexisting populations within a tumor rather than from de novo evolution.[93] Indeed, the wider the diversity of minor clonal populations in a tumor, the more likely it is that resistance will arise. Such an association between tumor heterogeneity and drug resistance has been noted in ovarian[94] and esophageal[95] cancers. In addition, basal-like TNBCs tend to be associated with higher clonal diversity and have previously been linked with shorter disease-free survival compared with non–basal-like TNBCs.[21] Integration of genomic and drug response data from breast cancer PDX models generated in our laboratory show that polygenomically engrafted tumors are more resistant to therapy than monogenomically engrafted tumors (Bruna et al., 2016 under review). Thus, there may be multiple routes to the development of resistance within any single tumor.

Epidermal growth factor receptor (EGFR) is a well-established driver of CRC and anti-EGFR therapy shows clear benefit in a subset of the metastatic disease. However, a plethora of events have been shown to predict drug sensitivity (primary resistance) and acquired resistance to anti-EGFR therapy in this setting.[92] Interestingly, resistant populations have been shown with mutations in *RAS, BRAF*, and *PIK3CA* or amplifications in *KRAS, ERBB2*, and *MET*. Significantly, although the mechanisms of resistance are genetically heterogeneous, they functionally converge on key signaling pathways, which might aid the identification of biomarkers of disease progression.[96] Similarly, numerous avenues to PARP inhibitor resistance have been described in breast and ovarian cancers in either a BRCA1-dependent and BRCA1-independent (eg, 53BP1/REV7 loss) fashion.[97,98] Each mechanism of resistance results in a clone regaining the ability for homologous recombination activity, suggesting that functional biomarkers of resistance may be possible.

Thus, while the emergence of resistance may be an inevitable consequence of single agent–targeted therapy in a polyclonal neoplasm,[92] the use of combination therapies and functional biomarkers of resistance will allow rational therapy targeted to individual patients' malignancies.

Metastasis is the ultimate cause of 90% of all cancer deaths.[99] Heterogeneity among tumor populations widens the diversity available for the evolution of metastatic populations. The long-standing observation that some cells within a tumor were able to form secondary tumors at a higher frequency than others was one of the key arguments for the CSC hypothesis.[12] However, multiregion sequencing studies have found that multiple distinct genomic clones are able to form metastases in pancreatic cancer,[100] suggesting that a single "CSC clone" is not necessary responsible for cancer dissemination. In addition, new research suggests that metastatic sites must be "primed" before disseminating cells can form distant metastasis.[101,102] It is possible that clonal cooperation could contribute to this effect, with one cellular population releasing cytokines and the other disseminating into the circulation.

Both intra- and intertumor heterogeneity have profound clinical consequences in terms of differential response to therapy, development of drug resistance, and disease progression. The initial step in countering a lack of clinical efficacy and effectiveness of novel therapeutic agents is to stratify patients based on integrative clustering metrics, which capture both genomic and functional differences between tumors. Beyond stratified medicine, a better understanding of the causes and consequences of clonal heterogeneity within a tumor will allow a deeper understanding of the emergence of drug resistance. By studying the evolution of clonal populations we may be able to predict, and ultimately counter, the emergence of drug-resistant and metastatic clonal populations.

PDX MODELS TO PRESERVE TUMOR HETEROGENEITY

In order to capture intertumor heterogeneity, we must develop and characterize large banks of patient-derived experimental models. Clearly, such efforts may require substantial international collaborations, such as the EuroPDX consortium.[103] High-throughput drug screens on banks of patient-derived tumors has been possible using both organoid[104] and PDX models (Bruna et al., 2016 under review). However, the most suitable preclinical models must also be capable of preserving intratumor heterogeneity. As organoids are typically derived from single cells, they may not be suitable for preserving the heterogeneity seen in tumor subpopulations. Clonal heterogeneity across organoid pools has yet to be fully characterized; however, extensive efforts are underway to characterize clonal populations in PDX models.

Multiple groups have attempted to define clonal dynamics based on either lentiviral tagging (cellular clones) or mutational clustering (genomic clones) by population and single cell–based computational approaches.[13,19,105] For example, Eirew et al., reconstructed the genomic clonal dynamics of a panel of breast cancer PDX models using PyClone, a Bayesian clustering method for grouping somatic mutations.[19] In each of the 15 cases examined, clonal diversity was reduced by xenotransplantation. This varied from extreme engraftment bias, selecting minor clones present in the sample of origin, to only moderate clonal selection. Remarkably, similar clonal dynamics were observed in parallel xenografts established from the same sample. In a separate study, Ding et al., found that PDX models established from a basal-like breast cancer were more representative of the patient's metastatic lesion than the primary tumor.[106] Together, these observations suggest that deterministic, fitness-based mechanisms underline tumor-dependent clonal selection observed on engraftment. Eirew et al., further observed variable clonal dynamics between PDXs established from different molecular subtypes, underscoring the need for better representation of tumor molecular subtypes.[7,19] Seminal studies by both Kreso et al., (CRC)[13] and Nguyen et al., (breast cancer)[105] utilized lentiviral lineage tracing to mark the progeny of individual tumor cells in PDX models. Each group found a spectrum of clonal behaviors on serial xenograft passage, suggesting that complex clonal dynamics were present in PDX models.

In summary, PDX models can at least partially recapitulate the complex population dynamics of a human malignancy.[23] Reproducible patterns of clonal dynamics suggest that engraftment bias may represent a nonstochastic selection event, which defines a PDX model rather than limiting its utility. However, heterogeneity across a tumor is governed by both cell-autonomous (clonal heterogeneity) and non–cell-autonomous (ECM, immune infiltrate, stromal cells) factors.[23] Although PDX models appear to faithfully recapitulate the complex population structures of primary neoplasms, the current generation is notably lacking in these non–cell-autonomous drivers of heterogeneity. Future generations of PDX models should attempt to model the microenvironment of human neoplasms to a greater extent. The *Holy Grail* in this regard is to create a humanized PDX model through patient-matched coimplantation of stromal and immune components; we have discussed the advantages and technical challenges of this process at length previously.[23]

Ultimately the utility of PDX models will be confirmed in avatar trials, in which PDX models are treated with experimental therapeutics in parallel with their human counterparts. Although an experimental model system with clear limitations, the current generation of PDX models offer the best representation of the diverse heterogeneity seen in human neoplasms.

ACKNOWLEDGMENTS

Establishment of our patient-derived tumor xenograft models would not be possible without the dedicated work of the Cambridge Breast Unit at the Addenbrookes Hospital, the Cambridge Institute Biological Resources Unit, and our collaborators in EuroPDX consortium (http://www.EuroPDX.eu). The authors are grateful to Prof C Caldas, W Greenwood, A Sati, OM Rueda, Dr HR Ali, B Pereira, and OB Harris for valuable discussion. In addition, we are particularly grateful to the patients who donated tissues to further our research and cancer research, UK, for supporting both authors.

REFERENCES

1. Heppner GH. Tumor heterogeneity. *Cancer Res* 1984;**44**:2259–65.
2. Dexter D, Spremulli E, Fligiel Z. Heterogeneity of cancer cells from a single human colon carcinoma. *Am J Med* 1978;**71**(A40).
3. Danielson KG, Anderson LW, Hosick HL. Selection and characterization in culture of mammary tumor cells with distinctive growth properties in vivo selection and characterization in culture of mammary tumor cells with distinctive growth properties in Vivo1. *Cancer Res* 1980:1812–9.
4. Barranco SC, Ho DHW, Drewinko B, Romsdahl MM, Humphrey RM. Differential sensitivities of human melanoma cells grown in vitro to arabinosylcytosine differential sensitivities of human melanoma cells grown in vitro to arabinosylcytosine l. *Chart* 1972:2733–6.
5. Chang K, Creighton CJ, Davis C, Donehower L, Drummond J, Wheeler D, et al. The Cancer Genome Atlas Pan-Cancer analysis project. *Nat Genet* 2013;**45**:1113–20.
6. Cole MP, Jones CTA, Todd IDH. A new anti-oestrogenic agent in late breast cancer: an early clinical appraisal of ICI46474. *Br J Cancer* 1971;**25**:270–5.
7. Curtis C, Shah SP, Chin S-F, Turashvili G, Rueda OM, Dunning MJ, et al. The genomic and transcriptomic architecture of 2,000 breast tumours reveals novel subgroups. *Nature* 2012;**486**:346–52.
8. Fidler I, Kripke M. Metastasis results from preexisting variant cells within a malignant tumor. *Science* 1977;**197**:893–5.
9. Gavosto F, Pileri A, Gabutti V, Masera P. Non-self-maintaining kinetics of proliferating blasts in human acute leukaemia. *Nature* 1967;**216**:188–9.
10. Clarkson B, Fried J, Strife A, Sakai Y, Ota K, Ohkita T. Studies of cellular proliferation in human leukemia. III. Behavior of leukemic cells in three adults with acute leukemia given continuous infusions of 3H-thymidine for 8 or 10 days. *Cancer* 1970;**25**:1237–60.
11. Clarkson B, Ohkita T, Ota K, Fried J. Studies of cellular proliferation in human leukemia. I. Estimation of growth rates of leukemic and normal hematopoietic cells in two adults with acute leukemia given single injections of tritiated thymidine. *J Clin Invest* 1967;**46**:506–29.
12. Southam C, Brunschwig A, Dizon Q. Autologous and homologous transplantation of human cancer. In: Brennan MJ, Simpson WL, editors. *Biological interactions in normal and neoplastic growth: a contribution to the tumor-host problem*. Boston: Little, Brown; 1962. p. 723–38.
13. Kreso A, O'Brien CA, van Galen P, Gan OI, Notta F, Brown AM, et al. Variable clonal repopulation dynamics influence chemotherapy response in colorectal cancer. *Science* 2012;**339**:543–8.

14. Pierce G, Dixon F, Verney E. Teratocarcinogenic and tissue-forming potentials of the cell types comprising neoplastic embryoid bodies. *Lab Invest* 1960;**9**:583–602.
15. Baylin SB, Weisburger WR, Eggleston JC, Mendelsohn G, Beaven MA, Abeloff MD, et al. Variable content of histaminase, l-dopa decarboxylase and calcitonin in small-cell carcinoma of the lung. *N Engl J Med* 1978;**299**:105–10.
16. Bennett DC, Peachey LA, Durbin H, Rudland PS. A possible mammary stem cell line. *Cell* 1978;**15**:283–98.
17. Vogelstein B, Fearon ER, Hamilton SR, Kern SE, Preisinger AC, Leppert M, et al. Genetic alterations during colorectal-tumor development. *N Engl J Med* 1988;**319**:525–32.
18. Nowell PC. The clonal evolution of tumor cell populations. *Sci* 1976;**194**:23–8.
19. Eirew P, Steif A, Khattra J, Ha G, Yap D, Farahani H, et al. Dynamics of genomic clones in breast cancer patient xenografts at single-cell resolution. *Nature* 2015;**518**.
20. Nik-Zainal S, Van Loo P, Wedge DC, Alexandrov LB, Greenman CD, Lau KW, et al. The life history of 21 breast cancers. *Cell* 2012;**149**:994–1007.
21. Shah SP, Roth A, Goya R, Oloumi A, Ha G, Zhao Y, et al. The clonal and mutational evolution spectrum of primary triple-negative breast cancers. *Nature* 2012;**486**:395–9.
22. Auman JT, McLeod HL. Colorectal cancer cell lines lack the molecular heterogeneity of clinical colorectal tumors. *Clin Colorectal Cancer* 2015;**9**:40–7.
23. Cassidy JW, Caldas C, Bruna A. Maintaining heterogeneity in patient derived tumour xenografts. *Cancer Res* 2015;**75**:1–6.
24. Gao H, Korn JM, Ferretti S, Monahan JE, Wang Y, Singh M, et al. High-throughput screening using patient-derived tumor xenografts to predict clinical trial drug response. *Nat Med* 2015;**21**:1318–25.
25. Kreso A, Dick JE. Evolution of the cancer stem cell model. *Cell Stem Cell* 2014;**14**:275–91.
26. Sansom OJ, Reed KR, Hayes AJ, Ireland H, Brinkmann H, Newton IP, et al. Loss of Apc in vivo immediately perturbs Wnt signaling, differentiation, and migration. *Gene Dev* 2004;**18**(12):1385–90.
27. Barker N, Ridgway Ra, van Es JH, van de Wetering M, Begthel H, van den Born M, et al. Crypt stem cells as the cells-of-origin of intestinal cancer. *Nature* 2009;**457**:608–11.
28. Suvà ML, Riggi N, Bernstein BE. Epigenetic reprogramming in cancer. *Science* 2013;**339**:1567–70.
29. Marusyk A, Almendro V, Polyak K. Intra-tumour heterogeneity: a looking glass for cancer? *Nat Rev Cancer* 2012;**12**:323–34.
30. Holst F, Stahl PR, Ruiz C, Hellwinkel O, Jehan Z, Wendland M, et al. Estrogen receptor alpha (ESR1) gene amplification is frequent in breast cancer. *Nat Genet* 2007;**39**:655–60.
31. Kallioniemi OP, Kallioniemi a, Kurisu W, Thor a, Chen LC, Smith HS, et al. ERBB2 amplification in breast cancer analyzed by fluorescence in situ hybridization. *Proc Natl Acad Sci USA* 1992;**89**:5321–5.
32. Schnitt SJ. Classification and prognosis of invasive breast cancer: from morphology to molecular taxonomy. *Mod Pathol* 2010;**23**:S60–4.
33. Ciriello G, Miller ML, Aksoy BA, Senbabaoglu Y, Schultz N, Sander C. Emerging landscape of oncogenic signatures across human cancers. *Nat Genet* 2013;**45**:1127–33.
34. Ali HR, Rueda OM, Chin S-F, Curtis C, Dunning MJ, Aparicio S, et al. Genome-driven integrated classification of breast cancer validated in over 7,500 samples. *Genome Biol* 2014;**15**:431.
35. Martincorena I, Roshan A, Gerstung M, Ellis P, Van Loo P, McLaren S, et al. High burden and pervasive positive selection of somatic mutations in normal human skin. *Science* 2015;**348**:880–6.

36. Ortmann CA, Kent DG, Nangalia J, Silber Y, Wedge DC, Grinfeld J, et al. Effect of mutation order on myeloproliferative neoplasms. *N Engl J Med* 2015;**372**:601–12.
37. Cairns J. Mutation selection and the natural history of cancer. *Nature* 1975;**255**:197–200.
38. Gerlinger M, Horswell S, Larkin J, Rowan AJ, Salm MP, Varela I, et al. Genomic architecture and evolution of clear cell renal cell carcinomas defined by multiregion sequencing. *Nat Genet* 2014;**46**:225–33.
39. de Bruin EC, McGranahan N, Mitter R, Salm M, Wedge DC, Yates L, et al. Spatial and temporal diversity in genomic instability processes defines lung cancer evolution. *Science* 2014;**346**:251–6.
40. Cleary AS, Leonard TL, Gestl SA, Gunther EJ. Tumour cell heterogeneity maintained by cooperating subclones in Wnt-driven mammary cancers. *Nature* 2014;**508**:113–7.
41. Easwaran H, Tsai H-CC, Baylin SBB. Cancer epigenetics: tumor heterogeneity, plasticity of stem-like states, and drug resistance. *Mol Cell* 2014;**54**:716–27.
42. Lunyak VV, Rosenfeld MG. Epigenetic regulation of stem cell fate. *Hum Mol Genet* 2008;**17**:R28–36.
43. De Carvalho DD, Sharma S, You JSS, Su S-F, Taberlay PCC, Kelly TKK, et al. DNA methylation screening identifies driver epigenetic events of cancer cell survival. *Cancer Cell* 2012;**21**:655–67.
44. Smith IM, Glazer Ca, Mithani SK, Ochs MF, Sun W, Bhan S, et al. Coordinated activation of candidate proto-oncogenes and cancer testes antigens via promoter demethylation in head and neck cancer and lung cancer. *PLoS One* 2009;**4**:e4961.
45. Ince TA, Richardson AL, Bell GW, Saitoh M, Godar S, Karnoub AE, et al. Transformation of different human breast epithelial cell types leads to distinct tumor phenotypes. *Cancer Cell* 2007;**12**:160–70.
46. Lim E, Vaillant F, Wu D, Forrest NC, Pal B, Hart AH, et al. Aberrant luminal progenitors as the candidate target population for basal tumor development in BRCA1 mutation carriers. *Nat Med* 2009;**15**:907–13.
47. Koren S, Reavie L, Couto JP, De Silva D, Stadler MB, Roloff T, et al. PIK3CAH1047R induces multipotency and multi-lineage mammary tumours. *Nature* 2015;**525**:114–8.
48. Van Keymeulen A, Lee MY, Ousset M, Brohee S, Rorive S, Giraddi RR, et al. Reactivation of multipotency by oncogenic PIK3CA induces breast tumour heterogeneity. *Nature* 2015;**525**. [advance on].
49. Cancer T, Atlas G. Comprehensive molecular characterization of human colon and rectal cancer. *Nature* 2012;**487**:330–7.
50. Barnetson R, Jass J, Tse R, Eckstein R, Robinson B, Schnitzler M. Mutations associated with microsatellite unstable colorectal carcinomas exhibit widespread intratumoral heterogeneity. *Genes Chromosom Cancer* 2000;**29**:130–6.
51. Szyf M. DNA methylation signatures for breast cancer classification and prognosis. *Genome Med* 2012;**4**:26.
52. Stefansson Oa, Moran S, Gomez A, Sayols S, Arribas-Jorba C, Sandoval J, et al. A DNA methylation-based definition of biologically distinct breast cancer subtypes. *Mol Oncol* 2015;**9**:555–68.
53. Tabassum DP, Polyak K. Tumorigenesis: it takes a village. *Nat Rev Cancer* 2015:1–11.
54. Junttila MR, de Sauvage FJ. Influence of tumour micro-environment heterogeneity on therapeutic response. *Nature* 2013;**501**:346–54.
55. Gubin MM, Zhang X, Schuster H, Caron E, Ward JP, Noguchi T, et al. Checkpoint blockade cancer immunotherapy targets tumour-specific mutant antigens. *Nature* 2014;**515**:577–81.

56. Pagès F, Galon J, Dieu-Nosjean M-C, Tartour E, Sautès-Fridman C, Fridman W-H. Immune infiltration in human tumors: a prognostic factor that should not be ignored. *Oncogene* 2010;**29**:1093–102.
57. Mei Z, Liu Y, Liu C, Cui A, Liang Z, Wang G, et al. Tumour-infiltrating inflammation and prognosis in colorectal cancer: systematic review and meta-analysis. *Br J Cancer* 2014;**110**:1595–605.
58. de Kruijf E, Engels C, van de Water W, Bastiaannet E, Smit VHBM, van de Velde CH, et al. Tumor immune subtypes distinguish tumor subclasses with clinical implications in breast cancer patients. *Breast Cancer Res Treat* 2013;**142**:355–64.
59. Ali HR, Glont SS-E, Blows FM, Provenzano E, Dawson S-JS, Liu B, et al. PD-L1 protein expression in breast cancer is rare, enriched in basal-like tumours and associated with infiltrating lymphocytes. *Ann Oncol* 2015:1488–93.
60. Gibson J. Anti-PD-L1 for metastatic triple-negative breast cancer. *Lancet Oncol* 2015;**16**:e264.
61. Waddington CH. *The strategy of the genes. A discussion of some aspects of theoretical biology*. Taylor & Francis; 1957.
62. Cassidy JW, Roberts JN, Smith C-A, Robertson M, White K, Biggs MJ, et al. Osteogenic lineage restriction by osteoprogenitors cultured on nanometric grooved surfaces: the role of focal adhesion maturation. *Acta Biomater* 2014;**10**:651–60.
63. Mohn F, Schübeler D. Genetics and epigenetics: stability and plasticity during cellular differentiation. *Trends Genet* 2009;**25**:129–36.
64. Quail DF, Joyce JA. Microenvironmental regulation of tumor progression and metastasis. *Nat Med* 2013;**19**:1423–37.
65. Cassidy JW. Nanotechnology in the regeneration of complex tissues. *Bone Tissue Regen Insights* 2014;**5**:25.
66. Wang C-C, Bajikar SS, Jamal L, Atkins KA, Janes KA. A time- and matrix-dependent TGFBR3-JUND-KRT5 regulatory circuit in single breast epithelial cells and basal-like premalignancies. *Nat Cell Biol* 2014;**16**:345–56.
67. Straussman R, Morikawa T, Shee K, Barzily-Rokni M, Qian ZR, Du J, et al. Tumour micro-environment elicits innate resistance to RAF inhibitors through HGF secretion. *Nature* 2012;**487**:500–4.
68. Augsten M. Cancer-associated fibroblasts as another polarized cell type of the tumor microenvironment. *Front Oncol* 2014;**4**:62.
69. Kharaishvili G, Simkova D, Bouchalova K, Gachechiladze M, Narsia N, Bouchal J. The role of cancer-associated fibroblasts, solid stress and other microenvironmental factors in tumor progression and therapy resistance. *Cancer Cell Int* 2014;**14**:41.
70. Song J, McColl J, Camp E, Kennerley N, Mok GF, McCormick D, et al. Smad1 transcription factor integrates BMP2 and Wnt3a signals in migrating cardiac progenitor cells. *Proc Natl Acad Sci USA* 2014;**111**:7337–42.
71. Reya T, Clevers H. Wnt signalling in stem cells and cancer. *Nature* 2005;**434**:843–50.
72. Nawaz S, Heindl A, Koelble K, Yuan Y. Beyond immune density: critical role of spatial heterogeneity in estrogen receptor-negative breast cancer. *Mod Pathol* 2015;**28**:766–77.
73. Ali HR, Provenzano E, Dawson S-JS-J, Blows FM, Liu B, Shah M, et al. Association between CD8+ T-cell infiltration and breast cancer survival in 12,439 patients. *Ann Oncol* 2014;**25**:1536–43.
74. DeNardo DG, Brennan DJ, Rexhepaj E, Ruffell B, Shiao SL, Madden SF, et al. Leukocyte complexity predicts breast cancer survival and functionally regulates response to chemotherapy. *Cancer Discov* 2011;**1**:54–67.

75. Buczacki SJA, Zecchini HI, Nicholson AM, Russell R, Vermeulen L, Kemp R, et al. Intestinal label-retaining cells are secretory precursors expressing Lgr5. *Nature* 2013;**495**:65–9.
76. Huch M, Dorrell C, Boj SF, Van Es JH, Van De Wetering M, Li VSW, et al. In vitro expansion of single Lgr5+ liver stem cells induced by Wnt-driven regeneration. *Nature* 2013;**494**:247–50.
77. Cheung TH, Rando TA. Molecular regulation of stem cell quiescence. *Nat Rev Mol Cell Biol* 2013;**14**:329–40.
78. Kreso A, van Galen P, Pedley NM, Lima-Fernandes E, Frelin C, Davis T, et al. Self-renewal as a therapeutic target in human colorectal cancer. *Nat Med* 2014;**20**:29–36.
79. Schwede M, Spentzos D, Bentink S, Hofmann O, Haibe-Kains B, Harrington D, et al. Stem cell-like gene expression in ovarian cancer predicts type II subtype and prognosis. *PLoS One* 2013;**8**.
80. Soady KJ, Kendrick H, Gao Q, Tutt A, Zvelebil M, Ordonez LD, et al. Mouse mammary stem cells express prognostic markers for triple-negative breast cancer. *Breast Cancer Res* 2015;**17**:1–23.
81. Merlos-Suárez A, Barriga FM, Jung P, Iglesias M, Céspedes MV, Rossell D, et al. The intestinal stem cell signature identifies colorectal cancer stem cells and predicts disease relapse. *Cell Stem Cell* 2011;**8**:511–24.
82. Eppert K, Takenaka K, Lechman ER, Waldron L, Nilsson B, van Galen P, et al. Stem cell gene expression programs influence clinical outcome in human leukemia. *Nat Med* 2011;**17**:1086–93.
83. Lawson Da, Bhakta NR, Kessenbrock K, Prummel KD, Yu Y, Takai K, et al. Single-cell analysis reveals a stem-cell program in human metastatic breast cancer cells. *Nature* 2015;**526**.
84. Tomasetti C, Vogelstein B. Variation in cancer risk among tissues can be explained by the number of stem cell divisions. *Science* 2015;**347**:78–81.
85. Hutchinson L, Kirk R. High drug attrition rates–where are we going wrong? *Nat Rev Clin Oncol* 2011;**8**:189–90.
86. Moreno L, Pearson ADJ. How can attrition rates be reduced in cancer drug discovery? *Expert Opin Drug Discov* 2013;**8**:363–8.
87. Huang M, Shen A, Ding J, Geng M. Molecularly targeted cancer therapy: some lessons from the past decade. *Trends Pharmacol Sci* 2014;**35**:41–50.
88. Aparicio S, Caldas C. The implications of clonal genome evolution for cancer medicine. *N Engl J Med* 2013;**368**:842–51.
89. Weigelt B, Reis-Filho JS. Histological and molecular types of breast cancer: is there a unifying taxonomy? *Nat Rev Clin Oncol* 2009;**6**:718–30.
90. Engels CC, Fontein DBY, Kuppen PJK, de Kruijf EM, Smit VTHBM, Nortier JWR, et al. Immunological subtypes in breast cancer are prognostic for invasive ductal but not for invasive lobular breast carcinoma. *Br J Cancer* 2014;**111**:532–8.
91. Lal N. An immunogenomic stratification of colorectal cancer: implications for development of targeted immunotherapy. *Oncoimmunology* 2015;**4**.
92. Diaz La, Williams RT, Wu J, Kinde I, Hecht JR, Berlin J, et al. The molecular evolution of acquired resistance to targeted EGFR blockade in colorectal cancers. *Nature* 2012;**486**:537–40.
93. Bhang HC, Ruddy Da, Krishnamurthy Radhakrishna V, Caushi JX, Zhao R, Hims MM, et al. Studying clonal dynamics in response to cancer therapy using high-complexity barcoding. *Nat Med* 2015;**21**.
94. Bashashati A, Ha G, Tone A, Ding J, Prentice LM, Roth A, et al. Distinct evolutionary trajectories of primary high-grade serous ovarian cancers revealed through spatial mutational profiling. *J Pathol* 2013;**231**:21–34.

95. Maley CC, Galipeau PC, Finley JC, Wongsurawat VJ, Li X, Sanchez CA, et al. Genetic clonal diversity predicts progression to esophageal adenocarcinoma. *Nat Genet* 2006;**38**:468–73.
96. Misale S, Di Nicolantonio F, Sartore-Bianchi A, Siena S, Bardelli A. Resistance to anti-EGFR therapy in colorectal cancer: from heterogeneity to convergent evolution. *Cancer Discov* 2014;**4**:1269–80.
97. Lord CJ, Ashworth A. Mechanisms of resistance to therapies targeting BRCA-mutant cancers. *Nat Med* 2013;**19**:1381–8.
98. Xu G, Chapman JR, Brandsma I, Yuan J, Mistrik M, Bouwman P, et al. REV7 counteracts DNA double-strand break resection and affects PARP inhibition. *Nature* 2015;**521**:541–4.
99. Mehlen P, Puisieux A. Metastasis: a question of life or death. *Nat Rev Cancer* 2006;**6**:449–58.
100. Campbell PJ, Yachida S, Mudie LJ, Stephens PJ, Pleasance ED, Stebbings LA, et al. The patterns and dynamics of genomic instability in metastatic pancreatic cancer. *Nature* 2010;**467**:1109–13.
101. Padua D, Zhang XH-F, Wang Q, Nadal C, Gerald WL, Gomis RR, et al. TGFβ primes breast tumors for lung metastasis seeding through angiopoietin-like 4. *Cell* 2008;**133**:66–77.
102. Bruna A, Greenwood W, Le Quesne J, Teschendorff A, Miranda-Saavedra D, Rueda OM, et al. TGFβ induces the formation of tumour-initiating cells in claudin low breast cancer. *Nat Commun* 2012;**3**:1055.
103. Siolas D, Hannon GJ. Patient derived tumor xenografts: transforming clinical samples into mouse models. *Cancer Res* 2013;**73**:5315–9.
104. van de Wetering M, Francies HE, Francis JM, Bounova G, Iorio F, Pronk A, et al. Prospective derivation of a living organoid biobank of colorectal cancer patients. *Cell* 2015;**161**:933–45.
105. Nguyen LV, Cox CL, Eirew P, Knapp DJHF, Pellacani D, Kannan N, et al. DNA barcoding reveals diverse growth kinetics of human breast tumour subclones in serially passaged xenografts. *Nat Commun* 2014;**5**:5871.
106. Ding L, Ellis MJ, Li S, Larson DE, Chen K, Wallis JW, et al. Genome remodelling in a basal-like breast cancer metastasis and xenograft. *Nature* 2010;**464**:999–1005.

Chapter 5

Immunodeficient Mice: The Backbone of Patient-Derived Tumor Xenograft Models

D.K. Hirenallur-Shanthappa[1,2,a], J.A. Ramírez[1,a], B.M. Iritani[1]
[1]*University of Washington, Seattle, WA, United States;* [2]*Amgen Inc., Thousand Oaks, CA, United States*

INTRODUCTION

Mice have been extensively utilized as models for human diseases because of their small size, rapid propagation, and the availability of genetically identical inbred strains. However, preclinical studies in mice often do not predict therapeutic responses in humans, in part due to the relatively high genetic and phenotypic divergence of mice from humans. This is particularly true in oncology where the etiology of human cancers is complex, often arising from a wide array of genetic mutations and external factors that can differ extensively among similar tumor types, and are not easily recapitulated in murine models. As a result, the U.S. Food and Drug Administration approval rate for targeted therapies against cancer-driving proteins is only 5–7%. Given that the average time from discovery to therapy is 12 years with an average cost of US $0.5–2 billion, the price of failed drug development is immense.[1] Hence, there remains an enormous need to improve the abilities of current preclinical models to predict successful outcomes in humans.

Several strategies have been utilized to increase the incidence and breadth of cancer in murine models. For example, chemical carcinogens can be administered to induce cancer in mice. However, chemically induced cancers often behave differently than spontaneously occurring human cancers, in part because chemicals induce a different spectrum of genetic mutations than are found in naturally occurring cancers. An alternative strategy to generate cancer models in mice has been to utilize genetically engineered mouse (GEM) technology, which has significantly improved cancer modeling. GEM cancer models range from strains that overexpress human oncogenes, such as Myc or Ras in a

a. These authors contributed equally to this work.

Patient Derived Tumor Xenograft Models. http://dx.doi.org/10.1016/B978-0-12-804010-2.00005-9

tissue-specific manner (transgenic), to knock-in models whereby specific cancer-causing mutations are inserted into the corresponding mouse loci (gene targeting). GEM models have many advantages in that they have an intact immune system, represent the complete range of cancer development from tumor initiation through progression, and allow coevolution of tumors with tumor stroma. The major disadvantage of GEM models lies in the requirement for genetic engineering based on preconceived information regarding the pathogenesis of human tumors, which can vary from tumor to tumor and may result from multiple "driver" mutations. As the need became clearer for better animal models that recapitulated human tumor phenotypes and had better predictive value, transplantation of human tumors into mice (xenografts) became the gold standard in cancer modeling. The use of immunodeficient mice as hosts for human tumors is essential because xenografts of human tissue are ultimately rejected by the immune systems of normal mice.

The first major breakthrough in xenograft research began in 1966 when a Scottish farmer brought a hairless mouse found on his farm to a local university.[2,3] This mouse was the founder of the nude mouse strain, which was later discovered to have a spontaneous mutation in the *Foxn1* gene resulting in abnormal hair growth and the absence of a thymus,[4] the organ responsible for the development of T lymphocytes. Nude mice were found to more readily accept tissue grafts than wild-type mice and permit the growth of human tumor cell lines.[2] The discovery of nude mice revolutionized in vivo cancer modeling for therapeutic studies.

Although nude mice still play an important role in oncology research, the T-cell immunodeficiency associated with the *Foxn1* mutation is not sufficient to allow the growth of most primary human tumors, in part because of the presence of B and innate immune cells that contribute to antitumor immunity. Further advancements in GEM technologies have allowed the creation of many additional genetically engineered mouse and rat models that lack specific immune response genes. In this chapter, we review the immune system and anticancer immunity, introduce genetic and phenotypic characteristics of immunodeficient models commonly utilized in patient-derived xenograft (PDX) studies, and describe key factors and limitations to consider when choosing immunodeficient mouse hosts.

INTRODUCTION TO THE IMMUNE SYSTEM AND ANTITUMOR IMMUNITY

The mammalian immune system has evolved to recognize and eliminate foreign molecules produced by pathogens without attacking host (self) proteins. In the 1950s, Macfarlane Burnet[5] first proposed that the immune system also recognizes and destroys clones of pretransformed cells and kills tumor cells posttransformation. Over the past 60 years, numerous studies have provided support for Burnet's "immune surveillance" hypothesis.[6] Among the simplest observation was that immunodeficient animals and humans had increased incidence of many types of cancers. It is now known that multiple immune cell types contribute to recognizing and destroying transformed cells. How the immune system responds to tumors and foreign grafts, and methods of suppressing immunity to improve the acceptance of human tumor xenografts in murine models are discussed in the following.

The two main components of the vertebrate immune system, innate and adaptive immunity, cooperate to protect the host from exogenous and endogenous threats (see Abbas et al.[7] for review). The innate immune system is the earliest line of defense against microbes, and includes cellular and chemical barriers including skin, mucosal epithelia, and antimicrobial peptides; phagocytes, such as macrophages, neutrophils, and dendritic cells (DCs); natural killer (NK) cells; and circulating blood proteins including complement. Cells of the innate immune system express nonspecific pattern recognition receptors, such as the toll-like receptor (TLR) family that recognize pathogen-associated molecular patterns (PAMPs) common to pathogens but not found in higher plants and animals. Examples of PAMPs include lipopolysaccharides, flagellin, unmethylated CpG DNA motifs present in bacteria, and double-stranded RNA present in viruses. In response to infection, phagocytes engulf pathogens, digest proteins into small peptides, present peptide antigens bound to major histocompatibility complex (MHC) antigens to T lymphocytes, and produce proinflammatory cytokines that further activate immune cells. Macrophages have also been shown to kill tumor cells through the production of tumor necrosis factor alpha (TNF-α) and the release of lysosomal enzymes, reactive oxygen species, and nitric oxide. In addition, macrophages eliminate unrecognized cells through expression of signal regulatory protein alpha (SIRPα, also known as tyrosine-protein phosphatase nonreceptor type substrate 1), which binds to the CD47 ligand expressed on host cells. In the presence of host CD47, a "don't-eat-me" signal is sent to the macrophage.[8] This system is important in both graft rejection and antitumor immunity, in part because tumor cells can circumvent macrophage-mediated killing by upregulating the expression of CD47. Conversely, inhibiting macrophage function allows increased acceptance of tumor xenografts. For instance, naturally occurring polymorphisms in nonobese diabetic (NOD) locus results in alterations in the SIRPα gene and increased graft acceptance[8] (Table 5.2).

NK cells are very important in immunity to viruses and tumors. NK cells lyse virus-infected or transformed cells via a unique activating and inhibitory receptor system which recognizes stressed cells and decreased expression of MHC Class I, a strategy tumor cells utilize to avoid detection by T lymphocytes.[9] Inhibiting NK cell function is critical for maximizing tumor xenograft acceptance. For example, mice lacking expression of the interleukin (IL)-2 receptor common gamma chain ($IL2r\gamma_c^{-/-}$; IL2rg) completely lack NK cells and are commonly utilized in combination with other immunodeficient background stains [such as severe combined immunodeficiency (SCID)] to enhance tumor graft acceptance (Table 5.2).

The adaptive immune system consists of T and B lymphocytes, which contribute to cell-mediated (T-cell response–based) and humoral (antibody-based) immunity, respectively. In contrast to innate immune cells, adaptive immune cells have a highly diverse and constantly evolving repertoire of receptors [T-cell receptors (TCRs) and B-cell receptor (BCRs)], which adapt to changing conditions and newly encountered antigens.[7] T cells perform many essential functions in cell-mediated immunity. T cells bearing the CD8 coreceptors are known as cytotoxic T lymphocytes (CTLs). CTLs are activated by TCR recognition of peptide antigen derived from intracellular proteins (such as viral- or tumor-associated proteins) presented in association with MHC class I molecules present on all cells in the body. Activated CTLs kill cells by releasing enzymes including perforin and granzymes, which digest target cells. CTLs play an important role in antitumor immunity by recognizing and killing transformed cells that express peptide antigens derived from mutant cellular proteins, inappropriately expressed antigens, products of overexpressed genes, or oncogenic viruses in conjunction with MHC class I molecules.[7] In contrast to CD8 T cells, T cells bearing the CD4 coreceptor (called helper T cells) recognize extracellular antigens through interactions of the TCR with antigens presented by MHC class II molecules on the surface of antigen-presenting cells, such as macrophages, DCs, and B cells. CD4 helper T cells participate in antitumor immunity by promoting CD8 differentiation into antitumor CTLs, and by secreting TNF-α and interferon gamma (IFN-γ), which increase MHC class I expression on tumor cells and increase their sensitivity to lysis by CTLs and NK cells. In tissue transplantation, grafts between unrelated individuals (allografts) or unrelated species (xenografts) are rejected because host T cells are activated by foreign MHC molecules in the donor graft. Conversely, T cells present in the donor graft can also recognize foreign host antigens, resulting in graft-versus-host disease. In xenotransplantation, it is important that PDX recipient animals lack T cells (Table 5.1).

Humoral immunity, the other main arm of adaptive immunity, is dictated by B lymphocytes. In response to extracellular antigens binding to the BCR, B cells become activated and produce antibody molecules, which are released into the bloodstream and mucosal secretions. Circulating antibodies can target microbes and tumor cells for elimination by binding to and activating macrophages [via immunoglobulin Fc (fragment, crystallizable) receptors] and/or by activating the complement pathway, which kills cells through formation of pores in the membrane. B cells also present antigen in association with MHC class II molecules to CD4 T cells to further stimulate the immune response.

Regulatory (suppressor) subsets of B and T lymphocytes function to suppress inappropriate activation of lymphocytes and maintain tolerance, thus protecting from autoimmunity. Regulatory T cells and B cells function by producing suppressive cytokines, such as IL-10 and TGF-β, and by directly interacting with other immune cells. Regulatory lymphocytes also modulate antitumor and antigraft immunity by suppressing CTLs. Inhibition or removal of regulatory lymphocytes can enhance antitumor immunity[10] (Table 5.1).

TABLE 5.1 Adaptive Immune Compromised Mouse Strains

Strain	Genotype	Immune Cell Deficiency	Features	Leakiness (Serum Ig, B Cells, T Cells)	Thymic Lymphoma Incidence	Radiation Tolerance	References
Nude	*Foxn1*^{nu} Lacks the transcription factor Foxn1 Athymic	• T-cell deficient	• (+) Hairless-good tumor visualization • Cell line engraftment	(–) T cells leaky	(+) Low	(+) High	3
SCID	*Prkdc*^{scid} Lacks the DNA-dependent protein kinase required for V(D)J recombination and DNA repair	• T-cell deficient • B-cell deficient	• Cell line engraftment plus low level of primary human tumor engraftment	(–) T and B cells leaky	(–) High	(–) Low	10
Rag1 or Rag2 null	*Rag1*^{tm1Mom} *Rag2*^{tm1Fwa} Lacks recombinase activating genes 1 or 2	• T-cell deficient • B-cell deficient	• Cell line engraftment plus low, variable level of primary human tumor engraftment	(+) Absent	(+) Low	(+) High	11,12

+ Denotes advantages; – denotes disadvantages. Shown are three mouse strains with mutations resulting in adaptive immune dysfunction, which are commonly used for PDX studies. Immune features, leakiness, thymic lymphoma incidence, and radiation tolerance for each strain are shown.[3, 2,13,32]

Immunodeficient Mouse Models

Nude Mice

In order for human xenografts to grow in murine hosts, both antitumor immunity and T-cell-mediated antigraft immunity must be suppressed. The first immunodeficient mouse model utilized in PDX studies was the "nude" mouse, which accomplished a major portion of these goals. Nude mice have a mutation in the *Foxn1* gene (*Foxn1^{nu}*), which results in the absence of mature T cells.[3,4] Nude mice cannot mount CD8 CTL responses against xenograft MHC antigens or provide CD4 T-cell-mediated B-cell help, but they still retain functional B cells and a fully intact innate immune response (Table 5.1). Many human cell lines are able to grow in the absence of T cells only, and thus nude mice are still routinely utilized for cell line–derived xenograft research. Nude mice also lack hair, which facilitates tumor measurements following implantation. However, aged nude mice develop small populations of extrathymic T cells ("leaky") capable of rejecting tumor grafts, and female nude mice are poor breeders. In addition, most human primary tumor xenografts fail to grow because nude mice have intact humoral and innate immune responses.

Severe Combined Immunodeficiency Mice

In the 1980s a spontaneous mutation in the *Prkdc* gene (encoding for protein kinase DNA–activated catalytic polypeptide) was described in C.B17 mice.[11] This mutation (*Prkdc^{scid}*) causes a defect in DNA double-strand break repair, thus preventing rearrangements of the variable (V), diversity (D), and joining (J) gene segments of DNA encoding the T- and B-cell antigen receptors. In the absence of V(D)J gene rearrangements, both T- and B-cell development are arrested in the thymus and bone marrow, respectively, resulting in the absence of mature T and B cells. The combined absence of T and B lymphocytes is termed SCID. Following the development of gene targeting techniques in mice, additional targeted mutations were generated including deletions in the recombination-activating genes (*Rag*) (*Rag1^{null}* or *Rag2^{null}*), which also prevented V(D)J rearrangement and resulted in the absence of T and B cells.[12,13] Many other gene-targeted mutations have been generated that disrupt either B- or T-cell development. Mutations that arrest B- or T-cell development in mice can theoretically be combined together by intercrossing to generate new SCID strains.

Due to the deficiency of both T and B lymphocytes, *Prkdc^{scid}* mice can be engrafted with a larger range of primary human tumors than nude mice, and can support growth of low levels of human hematopoietic cells.[14] However, aged *Prkdc^{scid}* (but not *Rag* null) mice develop a low number of mature B and T cells with age (leaky), depending on their genetic background and environmental pathogen exposure (Table 5.1). In addition, *Prkdc^{scid}* mice, by virtue of the defect in DNA repair, spontaneously develop lymphoma. For the same reason, they are also more susceptible to chemical- or radiation-induced genotoxic stress than *Rag* null mice. All SCID mice retain an intact innate immune system, and thus do not permit the growth of many primary human tumors (Table 5.2).

TABLE 5.2 Combined Adaptive and Innate Immune Compromised Mouse Strains

Strain	Genotype	Immune Cell Deficiency	Features	Leakiness (Serum Ig, Functional B and T Cells)	Thymic Lymphoma Incidence	Radiation Tolerance	References
SCID Beige	*Prkdc*^{scid}*Lyst*^{bg} SCID plus mutated lysosomal trafficking regulator	• T-cell deficient • B-cell deficient • NK cell function low • Granulocyte functional deficits	(–) Very low level of primary human tumor engraftment (+) Better engraftment than SCID	(–) Low	(–) High	(–) Low	14
NOD-SCID	NOD-*Prkdc*^{scid}; *NOD-Rag1*^{tm1Mom} Sirpα polymorphism, SNP in *CTLA-4*, Lack MHC H-2^{g7}	• T-cell deficient • B-cell deficient • Macrophage, DC, and NK cell function impaired • Complement deficient	(–) Low level of primary human tumor engraftment (+) Better engraftment than SCID	(–) Very low	(–) High	(–) Low	42
NOD-SCID-gamma (NSG)	NOD.Cg-*Prkdc*^{scid} *IL2r*γ^{tm1wjl} NOD-SCID null plus complete null mutation of the IL-2 receptor common γ chain No signaling from IL-2, IL-4, IL-7, IL-9, IL-13, IL-15 cytokines.	• T-cell deficient • B-cell deficient • Macrophage, DC function severely impaired • Complement deficient • NK cells absent	(+) High level of primary human tumor engraftment relative to NOD-SCID (+) Long life span (+) Allows humanized immune system	(–) Very low to absent	(+) Low	(–) Low	21,22

Continued

TABLE 5.2 Combined Adaptive and Innate Immune Compromised Mouse Strains—cont'd

Strain	Genotype	Immune Cell Deficiency	Features	Leakiness (Serum Ig, Functional B and T Cells)	Thymic Lymphoma Incidence	Radiation Tolerance	References
NOG	NODShi.Cg-*Prkdc*^{scid} *IL2rγ*^{tm1Sug} NOD-SCID plus signaling-defective IL-2 receptor common γ chain	Similar to NOD-SCID, plus decreased macrophage, DC, and NK cell function	Similar to NSG	(–) Very low to absent	(+) Low	(–) Low	23,24
Rag-gamma and B alb-Rag-gamma (BRG)	C.Cg-*Rag2*^{tm1Fwa} *IL2rγ*^{tm1Sug} Rag null plus signaling-defective mutant of the IL-2 receptor common γ chain Can still bind cytokines	Similar to NOG	Similar to NOG	(+) Absent	(+) Low	(+) High	26
NOD-Rag-gamma (NRG)	*NOD. Cg-Rag1*^{tm1Mom} *IL2rγ*^{tm1Wjl} NOD-Rag null plus complete null mutation of the IL-2 receptor common γ chain	Similar to NSG	Similar to NSG	(+) Absent	(+) Low	(+) High	25

NOD-SCID-gamma HLA-A2.1 transgenic	NOD.Cg-*Prkdc*^{scid} *IL2rγ*^{tm1Wjl}Tg(HLA-A2.1)1Enge NSG plus transgenic expression of human MHC class I	Similar to NSG but will allow thymic development of humanized T cells	(+) Allows studies involving anticancer immune responses	(+) Absent	(+) Low	(−) Low	39
NOD-SCID-gamma IL-3, GM- CSF, SCF (NSG-SGM3) transgenic	NOD.Cg-*Prkdc*^{scid} *IL2rγ*^{tm1wjl} Tg(CMV-IL-3,CSF2,KITLG)1 Eav NSG plus transgenic expression of human IL-3, GM-CSF, and SCF	Similar to NSG, but has increased Treg cells, enhanced myelopoiesis	(+) Increased engraftment of hematopoietic cancers, especially AML (myeloid-derived) (−) Poor huHSC engraftment	(+) Absent	(+) Low	(−) Low	40,41

AML, acute myeloid leukemia; *HLA*, human leukocyte antigen; *SCF*, stem cell factor; + denotes advantages; − denotes disadvantages. Shown are selected mouse strains with combined adaptive and innate immune dysfunction, which are commonly used for PDX studies. Immune features, leakiness, thymic lymphoma incidence, and radiation tolerance for each strain are shown.[15,22–24,26,27,40,41,43]

Nonobese Diabetic (NOD)-SCID Mice

In order to develop immunodeficient mouse models which harbor innate as well as adaptive immune defects, several investigators crossed SCID mice onto the NOD genetic background.[14] NOD mice have innate immune system defects which include reduced activity of NK cells, macrophages, DCs, and an absent hemolytic complement response. NOD macrophages also feature a polymorphism in the *Sirpα* gene which results in a Sirpα protein that is more similar to human Sirpα, and reduces killing of engrafted human cells by mouse macrophages.[8] Results of these crosses (NOD-*Prkdc*^{scid} and NOD-*Rag1*^{tm1Mom}) produce mice with deficiencies in both adaptive and innate immune systems (Table 5.2). Another mutation was discovered that also produces mice with significant NK and CTL functional deficiencies, as well as abnormal chemotaxis and bactericidal activity of granulocytes. This mutation, known as the Beige (*Lyst*^{bg}) allele,[15] encodes a lysosomal trafficking regulator. The Beige mutation has been combined with *Prkdc*^{scid} (SCID Beige) to produce mice deficient in both the adaptive and innate immune responses. Other gene-targeted mutations in mice that attenuate NK cell function include alleles that target the beta-2 microglobulin (*B2m*) and perforin 1 (*Prf1*) genes.[16] These alleles have been introduced into various NOD-SCID and NOD-Rag strains. All these mouse strains offer significant advantages over SCID mice, including improved survival and growth of primary human solid tumors, hematopoietic cells, and hematologic malignancies. However, NOD-SCID and NOD-Rag mice still retain some innate immune cell activity, which prevents the growth of many human primary tumor cells, and have reduced life spans due to a high incidence of spontaneous thymic lymphoma.

SCID-INTERLEUKIN-2 RECEPTOR COMMON GAMMA CHAIN (IL2rg) NULL MICE

The development of mice carrying a targeted mutation in the IL-2 receptor common gamma chain (*IL2rg*^{null}) was a major advancement in the fields of xenotransplantation and cancer research.[17,18] The *IL2rg* gene encodes a shared component of the receptors for IL-2, IL-4, IL-7, IL-9, IL-15, and IL-21 important for innate and adaptive immune responses. In addition, *IL2rg*^{null} mice completely lack NK cells. When this mutation is combined with NOD-*Pkrd*^{scid} or NOD-*Rag1*^{null} the resulting mice completely lack adaptive immunity and have severely impaired innate immunity.[16,19,20] The development of these mice enabled engraftment of many human primary cells, tissues, and tumors.[21]

Two different mutations in the *IL2rg* gene have been bred to NOD-SCID mice and are commonly utilized today: the NOD-SCID-gamma (termed NSG, NOD.Cg-*Pkrd*^{scid} *IL2rg*^{tm1Wjl}), which do not express IL2rg[22,23], and the NOG (NOD-Shi.Cg-*Pkrd*^{scid} *IL2rg*^{tm1Sug}),[24,25] which express a signaling-defective IL2rg. Several strains have been developed which combine *Rag* and *IL2rg* mutations: NRG (NOD-Rag-gamma),[26] Rag-gamma,[27] and BRG (Balb-Rag-gamma), which have null mutations in either *Rag1* or *Rag2* in addition to one of the *IL2rg* alleles previously discussed. Importantly, these models are not all equivalent (Table 5.2). For example, NSG mice support higher levels of human stem cell engraftment than NOG mice.[28] Almost all types of human primary tumors have successfully been transplanted into NSG mice. Importantly, NSG PDX recipients are able to maintain some native stromal cell and tumor-infiltrating lymphocyte (TIL) populations after transplantation,[29] which can help support tumor growth.

Choosing Immunodeficient Mouse Models

As the number of immunodeficient mouse strains increase, so does the complexity of choosing the most appropriate model for specific research goals. In general, strains with the highest degree of combined innate and adaptive immunodeficiency enable the best engraftment of most primary human tumors. However, each model carries inherent advantages and disadvantages (Tables 5.1 and 5.2).

Research Goals and Tumor Type

Different types of tumors grow best in specific immunodeficient models, which are highlighted in detail in the following chapters and in several review articles.[14,30] In addition, some types of tumors require specific microenvironments and/or growth factors for engraftment. For example, human myeloma cells require human IL-6 for growth and thus fail to engraft in NSG mice. To better model human myeloid tumors and antitumor myeloid responses, mice have been developed that express human cytokines important for innate immune development and function.[31] Similarly, if the goal is to study immunotherapy and immune interactions with PDX tumors, then immunodeficient mice engrafted with functional human immune systems (termed humanized) are the best options.[19] Humanization of murine models is discussed in subsequent chapters.

Background Strain

It is well known that genetic background can have a significant effect on susceptibility to disease, behavior, immune function, phenotype, and engraftment rate. For example, *Jax* laboratories maintain three different strains of nude mice: NU/J inbred, B6-NU congenic, and J:NU outbred mice. Although NU/J, B6-NU, and J:NU mice are all homozygous for *Foxn1*^{nu}, their xenograft acceptance and growth rates vary significantly (https://www.jax.org/news-and-insights/jax-blog/2013/july/which-host-strain-should-i-use). Unlike NU/J and B6-NU, outbred J:NU mice exhibit variable and robust tumor growth, and are capable of handling more vigorous experimental manipulation. Mouse models that are on an albino background, NU/J and J:NU, are better for whole body imaging studies than the B6 background.

Leakiness

Some immunodeficient strains develop functional T and/or B cells with age, and are termed "leaky." For example, nude mice produce T cells as they age due to extrathymic T-cell development. Similarly, *Prkdc*^{scid} mice on certain backgrounds produce functional B and T cells and a varied range of circulating immunoglobins.[32] Leakiness in *Prkdc*^{scid} mice is higher when mice are housed under nonspecific pathogen-free conditions, are on C57BL/6 or BALB/cByJ backgrounds, and in older mice.[33] Leakiness can result in inconsistent tumor engraftment and growth between individual recipients, particularly with tumors that require longer growth periods.

Life Span

Long-term xenograft studies can be affected by the life span of immunodeficient mouse hosts. For example, SCID and NOD-SCID mice develop spontaneous lymphomas as they age, and so are less useful for long-term studies (Tables 5.1 and 5.2).

Sensitivity to Radiation and Genotoxic Agents

Some researchers irradiate immunodeficient mice to improve the engraftment and growth of human primary tumors. Irradiation further immunosuppresses the host and creates a niche for engraftment in the bone marrow. However, some strains such as SCID and NOD-SCID mice are susceptible to irradiation-induced DNA damage, since the SCID mutation results in a defect in DNA repair. Accordingly, SCID, NOD-SCID, and NSG mice are also highly susceptible to genotoxic agents, so alternative strains such as NRG should be considered if the study includes use of such agents. *Rag1*- or *Rag2*-null mice also lack B and T lymphocytes but are resistant to radiation and genotoxic agents (Tables 5.1 and 5.2).

Availability and Vendor

Immunodeficient strains from different vendors may have unique polymorphisms acquired through inbreeding that alter their phenotypes following xenotransplantation. Similarly, differences in husbandry practices, pathogen status, and normal microbiota between vendors may affect tumor engraftment or alter xenograft behavior.

Immunodeficient Mice: Limitations and Future Development

Despite advances in the development of immunodeficient mice as hosts for human tumors, many cancer therapies tested in PDX mice still fail to adequately predict clinical responses in humans. Specific limitations of using these models and potential strategies for improving PDX models are discussed in this section.

LIMITATIONS OF USING IMMUNODEFICIENT MICE AS PATIENT-DERIVED XENOGRAFT HOSTS

1. **The complexities of human tumor microenvironments are not recapitulated in immunodeficient mice.** Although human tumors can grow in immunodeficient mice, tumor-promoting cells within the tumor microenvironment, such as stromal cells, vascular cells, and tumor TILs are often replaced by mouse components, which may behave differently than human cells and may not be modulated by drugs that specifically target human cells. The use of NSG-eGFP mice, which constitutively express eGFP in all tissues, can help differentiate human versus mouse stroma in xenograft models (https://www.jax.org/strain/021937). Similarly drug metabolism may differ between human and murine hosts, resulting in differences in drug levels and activity. Drug doses may need to be modulated in mice to achieve blood levels found in humans. Recapitulation of human tumor microenvironments is required to test compounds that target the tumor environment including antiangiogenesis factors, hormone antagonists, and immune checkpoint inhibitors.
2. **Anticancer immunity and graft-versus-host immunity are not completely disrupted.** Some human tumor xenografts fail to optimally grow in current immunodeficient models because innate immunity (such as signaling from TLRs) is not completely disrupted.[34] In addition, human TILs present within grafts can recognize murine MHC antigens within host tissues, resulting in graft-versus-host disease.
3. **Limited utility for therapies that target the human immune system.** Some anticancer drugs function by blocking immune inhibitory receptors, whereas others function by directly activating the immune system.[35] Because most of these therapies target human proteins, it is often not possible to screen immune-modulating drugs or antitumor vaccines in standard immunodeficient mice (Table 5.1). This limitation has been partially overcome by the development of various types of humanized mice, which are discussed in more detail in subsequent chapters.
4. **Tumor growth and metastasis are regulated by the immune system.** Both macrophages[36] and B lymphocytes[37] can promote angiogenesis and lymphangiogenesis, which in turn can influence tumor growth and metastasis. Thus PDX tumors grown in immunodeficient mice may exhibit altered vascular and lymphatic infiltration, which could influence tumor growth.
5. **Trafficking or migration of human cancer cells may be altered.** The development of secondary lymphoid organs, such as lymph nodes are severely impaired in immunodeficient strains, such as *IL2rg*$^{-/-}$ mice, which have very small lymph nodes, and BRG mice, which lack all but mesenteric lymph nodes.[38] Thus, trafficking of hematopoietic cancers may be altered in these models. Differences between mouse and human adhesion molecules,

such as integrins and selectins may also prevent natural migration and retention of specific human cancer cells in murine hosts.

6. **Some human cancers are associated with infections by viruses, bacteria, and parasites.** Xenografts involving these tumors might respond differently in immunodeficient hosts, where microbial responses and microbiota are altered. For example, hepatocellular carcinomas caused by Epstein-Barr virus (EBV) have been reported to develop into EBV-induced lymphoblastoid cancers following transplantation into immunodeficient hosts.[39] This is presumably because immunodeficient murine hosts allow reactivation of latent EBV, which induces proliferation of B lymphocytes.
7. **Engraftment rates remain low for some tumors and establishment can be lengthy.** Ideally, PDX mice could be utilized to test therapies while cancer patients are undergoing initial treatment. However, some tumors require many months to establish and engraftment rates are inconsistent making it difficult to establish large cohorts of PDX mice for testing.
8. **PDX studies remain expensive.** Immunodeficient mice in particular are very expensive.

Approaches to Improving Modeling in Patient-Derived Xenograft Mice

To achieve optimal tumor engraftment, murine hosts must be completely tolerant of human tumor grafts, and TILs within the tumor graft must be tolerant of the mouse host in order to prevent graft-versus-host disease. Strategies for addressing these issues and improving PDX models include:

1. **Further decreasing antitumor immunity.** To achieve complete tolerance of human cells and allow engraftment of a higher percentage of human tumors, additional strategies to completely disrupt the adaptive and innate immune cells could be pursued. Although the NOD background confers phagocytic tolerance to human xenografts, other aspects of innate immunity remain intact. For example, TLR signaling may confer some antitumor immunity. Generation of NSG mice with additional innate immune defects (such as $Myd88^{-/-}$) or use of MISTRG mice (MITRG mice that also express human SIRPα), which lack alveolar macrophages[31] could further enhance tumor engraftment.[38]
2. **Humanizing the immune system.** Many limitations of using immunodeficient models can be partially overcome by humanization of the murine immune system, which is discussed in detail in a following chapter. In brief, NSG mice support the engraftment of functional human immune cells. Murine models can be further humanized by replacing the murine MHC locus with human MHC class I and class II genes, allowing the intrathymic development of a full repertoire of human T cells.[38,40] Humanization of the MHC locus allows human T cells to recognize antigen presented by human

MHC molecules present on mouse tissues. To further increase the survival of human immune cells in PDX mice, transgenic mice are being engineered to express human growth factors, cytokines, and adhesion molecules, which better support the proliferation, survival, and migration of human hematopoietic cells[19] (Table 5.2).

3. **Humanizing the tumor microenvironment.** Advancement in targeted genome editing technologies, such as (CRISPR/Cas9), zinc finger nucleases, and transcription activator-like effector nucleases have facilitated the creation of improved NSG mice, which express human cytokines and have additional innate immune defects.[38] For example, acute myeloid leukemia engraftment rates have been enhanced through use of NSG mice which express human granulocyte-macrophage colony-stimulating factor (GM-CSF), stem cell factor, and IL-3 transgenes (NSG-SGM3)[41,42] (Table 5.2), and by using modified Rag2-deficient, IL2rg-deficient mice that express human growth factors, including MITRG mice (*Rag2*-deficient, IL2rg-deficient mice which express human macrophage colony stimulating factor, IL-3, GM-CSF, thrombopoietin), and MISTRG mice.[31] Development of new models will continue as additional growth requirements for primary patient-derived tumors and stromal/immune cells are identified, enabling the use of better PDX tumor models that are more predictive of therapeutic response and patient survival.

REFERENCES

1. Day CP, Merlino G, Van Dyke T. Preclinical mouse cancer models: a maze of opportunities and challenges. *Cell* 2015;**163**:39–53.
2. Giovanella BC, Yim SO, Stehlin JS, Williams Jr LJ. Development of invasive tumors in the "nude" mouse after injection of cultured human melanoma cells. *J Natl Cancer Inst* 1972;**48**:1531–3.
3. Flanagan SP. 'Nude', a new hairless gene with pleiotropic effects in the mouse. *Genet Res* 1966;**8**:295–309.
4. Pantelouris EM. Absence of thymus in a mouse mutant. *Nature* 1968;**217**:370–1.
5. Burnet M. Cancer; a biological approach. I. The processes of control. *Br Med J* 1957;**1**:779–86.
6. Burnet FM. The concept of immunological surveillance. *Prog Exp Tumor Res* 1970;**13**:1–27.
7. Abbas AK, Lichtman AH, Pillai S. *Cellular and molecular immunology*. 6th ed. Philadelphia: Saunders/Elsevier; 2010.
8. Takenaka K, Prasolava TK, Wang JC, Mortin-Toth SM, Khalouei S, Gan OI, et al. Polymorphism in Sirpa modulates engraftment of human hematopoietic stem cells. *Nat Immunol* 2007;**8**:1313–23.
9. Yokoyama WM. Specific and non-specific natural killer cell responses to viral infection. *Adv Exp Med Biol* 2005;**560**:57–61.
10. Roychoudhuri R, Eil RL, Restifo NP. The interplay of effector and regulatory t cells in cancer. *Curr Opin Immunol* 2015;**33**:101–11.
11. Bosma GC, Custer RP, Bosma MJ. A severe combined immunodeficiency mutation in the mouse. *Nature* 1983;**301**:527–30.
12. Mombaerts P, Iacomini J, Johnson RS, Herrup K, Tonegawa S, Papaioannou VE. Rag-1-deficient mice have no mature b and t lymphocytes. *Cell* 1992;**68**:869–77.

13. Shinkai Y, Koyasu S, Nakayama K, Murphy KM, Loh DY, Reinherz EL, et al. Restoration of T cell development in rag-2-deficient mice by functional TCR transgenes. *Science* 1993;**259**:822–5.
14. Shultz LD, Goodwin N, Ishikawa F, Hosur V, Lyons BL, Greiner DL. Human cancer growth and therapy in immunodeficient mouse models. *Cold Spring Harb Protoc* 2014;**2014**:694–708.
15. Mosier DE, Stell KL, Gulizia RJ, Torbett BE, Gilmore GL. Homozygous scid/scid;beige/beige mice have low levels of spontaneous or neonatal T cell-induced B cell generation. *J Exp Med* 1993;**177**:191–4.
16. Shultz LD, Ishikawa F, Greiner DL. Humanized mice in translational biomedical research. *Nat Rev Immunol* 2007;**7**:118–30.
17. DiSanto JP, Muller W, Guy-Grand D, Fischer A, Rajewsky K. Lymphoid development in mice with a targeted deletion of the interleukin 2 receptor gamma chain. *Proc Natl Acad Sci USA* 1995;**92**:377–81.
18. Cao X, Shores EW, Hu-Li J, Anver MR, Kelsall BL, Russell SM, et al. Defective lymphoid development in mice lacking expression of the common cytokine receptor gamma chain. *Immunity* 1995;**2**:223–38.
19. Shultz LD, Brehm MA, Garcia-Martinez JV, Greiner DL. Humanized mice for immune system investigation: progress, promise and challenges. *Nat Rev Immunol* 2012;**12**:786–98.
20. Rongvaux A, Takizawa H, Strowig T, Willinger T, Eynon EE, Flavell RA, et al. Human hemato-lymphoid system mice: current use and future potential for medicine. *Annu Rev Immunol* 2013;**31**:635–74.
21. Agliano A, Martin-Padura I, Mancuso P, Marighetti P, Rabascio C, Pruneri G, et al. Human acute leukemia cells injected in NOD/LtSz-scid/IL-2R gamma null mice generate a faster and more efficient disease compared to other NOD/scid-related strains. *Int J Cancer* 2008;**123**:2222–7.
22. Ishikawa F, Yasukawa M, Lyons B, Yoshida S, Miyamoto T, Yoshimoto G, et al. Development of functional human blood and immune systems in NOD/SCID/IL2 receptor {gamma} chain(null) mice. *Blood* 2005;**106**:1565–73.
23. Shultz LD, Lyons BL, Burzenski LM, Gott B, Chen X, Chaleff S, et al. Human lymphoid and myeloid cell development in NOD/LtSz-scid IL2R gamma null mice engrafted with mobilized human hemopoietic stem cells. *J Immunol* 2005;**174**:6477–89.
24. Ito M, Hiramatsu H, Kobayashi K, Suzue K, Kawahata M, Hioki K, et al. NOD/SCID/gamma(c)(null) mouse: an excellent recipient mouse model for engraftment of human cells. *Blood* 2002;**100**:3175–82.
25. Yahata T, Ando K, Nakamura Y, Ueyama Y, Shimamura K, Tamaoki N, et al. Functional human T lymphocyte development from cord blood CD34+ cells in nonobese diabetic/Shi-scid, IL-2 receptor gamma null mice. *J Immunol* 2002;**169**:204–9.
26. Pearson T, Shultz LD, Miller D, King M, Laning J, Fodor W, et al. Non-obese diabetic-recombination activating gene-1 (NOD-Rag1 null) interleukin (IL)-2 receptor common gamma chain (il2r gamma null) null mice: a radioresistant model for human lymphohaematopoietic engraftment. *Clin Exp Immunol* 2008;**154**:270–84.
27. Goldman JP, Blundell MP, Lopes L, Kinnon C, Di Santo JP, Thrasher AJ. Enhanced human cell engraftment in mice deficient in rag2 and the common cytokine receptor gamma chain. *Br J Haematol* 1998;**103**:335–42.
28. McDermott SP, Eppert K, Lechman ER, Doedens M, Dick JE. Comparison of human cord blood engraftment between immunocompromised mouse strains. *Blood* 2010;**116**:193–200.
29. Simpson-Abelson MR, Sonnenberg GF, Takita H, Yokota SJ, Conway Jr TF, Kelleher Jr RJ, et al. Long-term engraftment and expansion of tumor-derived memory t cells following the implantation of non-disrupted pieces of human lung tumor into NOD-scid IL2Rgamma(null) mice. *J Immunol* 2008;**180**:7009–18.

30. Tentler JJ, Tan AC, Weekes CD, Jimeno A, Leong S, Pitts TM, et al. Patient-derived tumour xenografts as models for oncology drug development. *Nat Rev Clin Oncol* 2012;**9**:338–50.
31. Rongvaux A, Willinger T, Martinek J, Strowig T, Gearty SV, Teichmann LL, et al. Development and function of human innate immune cells in a humanized mouse model. *Nat Biotechnol* 2014;**32**:364–72.
32. Bosma GC, Fried M, Custer RP, Carroll A, Gibson DM, Bosma MJ. Evidence of functional lymphocytes in some (leaky) scid mice. *J Exp Med* 1988;**167**:1016–33.
33. Nonoyama S, Smith FO, Bernstein ID, Ochs HD. Strain-dependent leakiness of mice with severe combined immune deficiency. *J Immunol* 1993;**150**:3817–24.
34. Brehm MA, Cuthbert A, Yang C, Miller DM, DiIorio P, Laning J, et al. Parameters for establishing humanized mouse models to study human immunity: analysis of human hematopoietic stem cell engraftment in three immunodeficient strains of mice bearing the il2rgamma(null) mutation. *Clin Immunol* 2010;**135**:84–98.
35. Sharma P, Allison JP. The future of immune checkpoint therapy. *Science* 2015;**348**:56–61.
36. Qian BZ, Pollard JW. Macrophage diversity enhances tumor progression and metastasis. *Cell* 2010;**141**:39–51.
37. Ruddell A, Mezquita P, Brandvold KA, Farr A, Iritani BM. B lymphocyte-specific c-myc expression stimulates early and functional expansion of the vasculature and lymphatics during lymphomagenesis. *Am J Pathol* 2003;**163**:2233–45.
38. Brehm MA, Shultz LD, Luban J, Greiner DL. Overcoming current limitations in humanized mouse research. *J Infect Dis* 2013;**208**(Suppl. 2):S125–30.
39. Chen K, Ahmed S, Adeyi O, Dick JE, Ghanekar A. Human solid tumor xenografts in immunodeficient mice are vulnerable to lymphomagenesis associated with Epstein-Barr virus. *PLoS One* 2012;**7**:e39294.
40. Strowig T, Gurer C, Ploss A, Liu YF, Arrey F, Sashihara J, et al. Priming of protective t cell responses against virus-induced tumors in mice with human immune system components. *J Exp Med* 2009;**206**:1423–34.
41. Nicolini FE, Cashman JD, Hogge DE, Humphries RK, Eaves CJ. NOD/scid mice engineered to express human il-3, gm-csf and steel factor constitutively mobilize engrafted human progenitors and compromise human stem cell regeneration. *Leukemia* 2004;**18**:341–7.
42. Wunderlich M, Chou FS, Link KA, Mizukawa B, Perry RL, Carroll M, et al. AML xenograft efficiency is significantly improved in NOD/scid-IL2Rg mice constitutively expressing human SCF, GM-CSF and IL-3. *Leukemia* 2010;**24**:1785–8.
43. Shultz LD, Schweitzer PA, Christianson SW, Gott B, Schweitzer IB, Tennent B, et al. Multiple defects in innate and adaptive immunologic function in NOD/LtSz-scid mice. *J Immunol* 1995;**154**:180–91.

Chapter 6

Humanized Mice and PDX Models

J. Eswaraka[1], A. Giddabasappa[2]
[1]*Amgen Inc, Thousand Oaks, CA, United States,* [2]*Pfizer Inc., San Diego, CA, United States*

INTRODUCTION

Mouse models of cancer help preclinical researchers to confirm the biological relevance of drug targets, establish a therapeutic window between efficacy and toxicity for drugs, validate diagnostic hypothesis, and identify novel biomarkers.[1] Mouse xenograft models, either by xenotransplantation of cancer cell lines or patient-derived tumor xenografts (PDXs) in immune-deficient mice have been the most commonly used tool for in vivo researchers to understand the efficacy of cancer therapeutics. Despite the widespread use of these different mouse models, preclinical efficacy of drugs seen in mice has not always translated to efficacy in humans. Although the reasons may be many, one of the primary reasons is that mice despite having a similar genetic makeup as humans (>90% homology) cannot mimic the human immune system, especially T-cell signaling pathways, antigen (Ag)-presenting machinery, or immune receptor expression.[2,3]

The immune system contributes significantly to the eradication of tumor cells. Blockade of immune checkpoint inhibitors with targeted antibodies (Abs) has shown tremendous durable therapeutic responses to a variety of human cancers, such as melanoma,[4] renal cell carcinoma,[5] and non–small cell lung cancer.[6] Another significant advance within oncology is the adoptive transfer of antitumor lymphocytes to cancer patients. This approach has been successful in achieving durable responses or complete remission in melanoma patients.[7] Mouse models of cancer, such as GEMMs, xenograft, and PDX models that have helped to drive progress in oncology have very limited utility for exploring the mechanisms of immunotherapy for a variety of reasons, including the significant difference between the mouse and human immune system, inability to study human tumor–human stromal interactions, and lack of human origin tumor-infiltrating lymphocytes. In order to model and predict the efficacy of such novel immunotherapeutics and explore their potential against other

Patient Derived Tumor Xenograft Models. http://dx.doi.org/10.1016/B978-0-12-804010-2.00006-0

cancers, there is a pressing need to develop preclinical models that can recapitulate functional human immune responses in vivo. Humanized mice, that recapitulate the human system in mice to various degrees, have the potential to overcome the species differences between human and mice immune system and could become the main platform for modeling of immunotherapy targets and drugs. Humanized mice are highly immune-deficient mice that generate a functional human immune system through engraftment with human primary hematopoietic cells and human fetal tissues or engineered expression of human cytokine genes.[8] This chapter will focus on the development of these models as well as some of the challenges associated with their use in studying human tumor biology.

HISTORY OF HUMANIZED MICE

A key feature of developing humanized mice involves the selection of the right background strain of immunodeficient mice that allow transplantation of the human tissues or cells. Mice that have reduced to no xenograft rejection and that can support cellular differentiation and growth of human origin tissues are invaluable and significant efforts have been made to refine these models over the past 50 years since the first report in 1966 of a spontaneously hairless mice (nude mice).[9] Implantation of human tumor cell lines in these mice led to the development of tumors and provided an in vivo animal model for studying human tumors.[10] However, these mice have some components of the immune system, such as B cells, dendritic cells (DCs), granulocytes, and natural killer (NK) cells that reduce the engraftment rate of tumors and prevent the engraftment of human hematopoietic cells. In the 1980s, mice with severe combined immunodeficiency (SCID) caused by a spontaneous autosomal mutation in the *Pkrdc* gene (encoding for protein kinase DNA-activated catalytic polypeptide) were identified.[11] SCID mice support low levels of engraftment with mature human peripheral blood mononuclear cells (PBMCs) and hematopoietic stem cells (HSCs)[12,13] as well as a larger range of human tumors than nude mice.[14] However, the disadvantages of SCID mice include development of "leakiness" and sensitivity to radiation exposure (see Section I, Chapter 5 for more detailed information).[15,16] Mutation of Rag1/2 (recombination-activating gene 1 and 2) in these mice prevents the "leakiness" and formation of B and T cells.[17,18] But these mice still retain NK cell activity. Crossing the SCID mice into the nonobese diabetic (NOD) mouse background (NOD-SCID mice) results in mice that can efficiently engraft PBMCs and tumors as they had reduced levels of innate immunity; decreased NK cells, macrophages, and DCs; as well as absence of complement activity.[15,19] However, these mice have a limited life span (8 months) as they develop spontaneous lymphomas.[19] Development of NSG [NOD-SCID mice with null deletion of interlukin-2 receptor γ-chain locus (*Il2rg*)] or NOG mice [NOD-SCID mice with truncated mutation of the interleukin (IL)-2 receptor] were significant breakthroughs in the field. These strains of mice are more efficient in engraftment of HSCs, tissues, primary tumors, and PBMCs compared with the SCID and NOD-SCID mice (reviewed in Section I, Chapter 5 in detail). Currently, the NSG and the NOG mice are the main immunodeficient background strains of mice used for developing humanized mouse models.

RECONSTITUTION OF THE HUMAN IMMUNE SYSTEM IN IMMUNODEFICIENT MICE

To reconstitute a functional human immune system, investigators have developed various methods to engraft human hematopoietic cells derived from bone marrow or peripheral blood and tissues into immunodeficient mice, resulting in the establishment of different cell lineages required to reconstitute a functional human immune system. Based on the strain of mice used and the origin of the xenogeneic tissues a variety of different humanized immune system models have been developed. Table 6.1 provides an overview of the classical humanized mice models. For a more thorough review of these mice, readers are referred to other sources.[8,20–22] Each of the models has its own advantages and disadvantages for the study of the human immune system and is summarized in the following sections.

Hu-PBL-SCID

This model was established by intravenous (IV) or intraperitoneal (IP) injection of mature PBMCs into sublethally irradiated SCID mice.[13] The IP route resulted in a better human immune system than the IV route. Injected PBMCs are detectable in the peritoneal space for 3 weeks postinjection. By 1 month postinjection lymphocytes bearing human T (96–100%) and B (4%) cell markers are detectable in other organs (mainly lung, liver and spleen). A very minor fraction of the activated T cells are seen in the lymph nodes. No human macrophages or other immune cells are detectable.[13,23] The activated human T cells that are produced decline steadily with time and by about 5 months after implantation are virtually undetectable in the mice.[24] The human T cells in this model as with other SCID mice undergo thymic education and selection on mouse thymus and are mouse histocompatibility (H-2 Ag) restricted. As a result, the human T cells would not be able to recognize Ags presented by the human leukocyte antigen (HLA)–expressing human antigen-presenting cells (APCs) in peripheral tissues.[25] The APC compartment in SCID mice is functional and the H-2-restricted human T cells would encounter mouse APCs in the peripheral immune system. Therefore a functional H-2-restricted human T-cell response with a nonfunctional human B-cell system (due to lack of HLA-expressing B cells) is established in these mice.[24] The T cells in these mice are either CD4 or CD8 positive and show clonal heterogeneity.[26] Surprisingly, naive T cells which constitute 50% of the injected PBMC population seem to disappear over time and are not seen

TABLE 6.1 Characteristics of Classical Humanized Mice Models

Humanized Model	Human Tissue Implanted	Mouse Strain Used	Age of Mice for Implantation	Route of Implantation	Characteristics of Model	Key References
SCID-hu	Fetal liver/ thymus or bone marrow	CB-17-SCID	Adult	Kidney (renal capsule), bone marrow or SC	Thy/Liv model: Produce human T cells, B cells, macrophages, and dendritic cells; implants persist for long periods (6–12 months); presence of human thymus provides human HLA-restricted T cells; multilineage hematopoiesis observed; low levels in peripheral system. Bone marrow model: good for early hematopoiesis in hematolymphoid microenvironment; short window of 8–24 weeks for experimentation	12,33
Hu-SRC-SCID	HSCs	SCID	Adult or newborn	IV, IP	Implanted in newborn or adult mice; need exogenous cytokine administration; generates naive human immune cells; provides long-term engraftment; T cells are mouse MHC restricted	15,27
Hu-PBL-SCID	Peripheral blood lymphocytes (PBL)	CB-17-SCID	Adult	IP; IV	Implanted in adult mice; narrow window for naive T-cell response; T cells educated by mouse thymus; Mouse-activated T-cells response observed up to 5 months; T cells are mouse MHC restricted and can lead to GVHD	13,26
BLT	Bone marrow (HSCs), fetal liver, and thymus	NOD-SCID; NSG	Adult	Renal capsule and IV	Can produce a complete human system; human immune cells found in primary and secondary lymphoid system; no need of exogenous administration of cytokines; T cells are human HLA restricted (MHC I and II); able to mount a T-cell response to antigen; humoral response possible	39,40

3–4 weeks after engraftment suggesting that the mouse model does not provide the appropriate microenvironment for survival of naive human T cells.[24] Since the human T cells are H-2 restricted they are capable of stimulating the mouse immune system leading to the production of antimouse reactive T cells and can lead to graft versus host disease (GVHD). The narrow window of 3–4 weeks when the disseminated population of activated Ag-reactive T cells are produced in this model, provides an opportunity to study priming and effector functions of human T-cell responses to tumors.[24] Current versions of this model use the NSG or NRG [NOD mouse with Rag1 and Il2rg knockout (NOD.*Rag1*$^{-}$; γc^{null})] mice as background due to their higher engraftment rates for human cells and tissues.

Hu-SRC-SCID

This mouse model was established by injecting newborn or adult immune-deficient mice with human CD34^{+} HSCs [also called as SCID-repopulating cells (SRCs)] derived from fetal liver, cord blood or bone marrow, or granulocyte colony-stimulating factor–mobilized peripheral blood cells. Since the human stem cells cannot utilize the murine hematopoietic factors, exogenous administration of cytokines was necessary. Coadministration of erythropoietin, Hu-mast cell growth factor, and granulocyte-macrophage colony stimulating factor (GM-CSF) along with bone marrow–derived HSCs in SCID mice resulted in the repopulation of murine bone marrow with human progenitors, mature cells of myeloid, lymphoid and erythroid lineages.[27] The primary advantage of this model is that T cells, B cells, myeloid cells, NK cells, and APCs are engrafted thereby generating a naive human immune response. By injection of human umbilical cord blood cells in these mice engraftment was seen without exogenous cytokine expression possibly due to the presence of immature T cells in the inoculum.[28] The SRC model provides for long-term engraftment (over 6 months), and serial transfer of human CD34^{+} CD38^{-} cells into irradiated secondary *nod-scid* recipients generates multiple lineages of human cells[29] suggesting that these mice can regenerate a population of human stem cells (SRC). SRC cell frequency has been determined to be 1 per 1×10^6 cord blood cells, 1 per 3×10^6 bone marrow cells, and 1 per 6×10^6 mobilized PBMCs obtained from human donors.[15,30] Although multiple lineages of cells were repopulated, SCID mice had lower overall percentage of human cells (~0.5–5%) in the SCID recipient bone marrow compared with murine cells. Similar to the Hu-PBL-SCID model the human T cells in this model are also murine H-2 restricted and do not respond to human HLA-positive APCs. In addition, the T-cell development in general is very poor. The engraftment and the diversity of immune cell development in the Hu-SRC-SCID depends on the background strain of the immune-deficient host. When engrafted into CB17.SCID mice, there is poor engraftment of the HSCs and very few human T cells are generated.[20] Ablation of NK cell activity using NK-depleted C57BL/6J mice, loss of hemolytic complement using the DBA/2J-scid mice, or reduced macrophage activity using C3H/HeJ-*scid* mice do not increase human cell engraftment in the model.[15] NOD/LtSz-scid mice have an enhanced engraftment of HSCs compared with the other strains of SCID.[31] When HSCs were transplanted into NSG and NOG mice (defective IL2rg), de novo lymphopoiesis and T-cell development was seen. However, even within these strains differences exist. When irradiated NOD-SCID mice with $IL2rg^{-/-}$ or macrophage-depleted (by clodronate administration) BALB/c-$Rag2^{-/-}$ are used for engraftment, both B and T cells are generated. However C57BL/6-$Rag2^{-/-}$ $Il2rg^{-/-}$ do not successfully engraft with HSCs. The intrahepatic injection of HSCs into conditioned newborn NRG, NSG, or NOG mice results in better HSC engraftment and formation of human T cells, B cells, macrophages, NK cells, and DCs.[8,32] The Hu-SRC-NOD-SCID mice model has been widely used for studying the human hematopoiesis in *scid* mice and is the host strain of choice for most laboratories.[15] Similar to the other *scid* models, thymic lymphomas which limit the life span to ~8 months, low NK cell activity, mouse major histocompatibility complex (MHC) priming, and extreme radiosensitivity are significant limitations for the use of this model.

SCID-Human

In this model tissue fragments from human organs are transplanted instead of isolated cells. These models were initially created to study the immunological responses to human immunodeficiency virus infection in humans. These models were established by the coimplantation of human fetal liver and/or thymus under the renal capsule (SCID-hu Thy/Liv) or fetal bone into SCID mice (SCID-hu Bone).[12,33] Human thymus fragments provide an autologous thymic epithelium that helps in education of the human T cells and HLA restriction of the T cells. Under these conditions the T cells also become tolerant to murine histocompatibility Ag $H\text{-}2^d$. When thymus fragments alone are implanted followed by intrathymic injection of HSCs, the HSCs grow and differentiate into T and myeloid cells. However, only low and transient levels of human $CD4^+$ and $CD8^+$ T cells are seen in the periphery. To overcome this effect researchers then engrafted fragments of fetal liver (~10^7–10^8 cells). The implants persisted for over 6–12 months and produced detectable levels of circulating human T cells. It is hypothesized that the liver as a source for multilineage hematopoiesis provides the microenvironment necessary for the HSCs' maintenance and differentiation. The T-cell compartment of the Thy/Liv implant is similar to that of the fetal thymus and has $CD3^{+/-}$ $CD4^+$ $CD8^+$ "cortical thymocytes" and $CD3^+$ $CD4^+$ $CD8^-$ or $CD3^+$ $CD4^-$ $CD8^+$ "medullary thymocytes."[12] The $CD4^+$ and $CD8^+$ T-cell clones from these mice are phenotypically normal, functional,[34] exist in normal CD4/CD8 ratios, and produce cytokines in similar quantities as normal human peripheral blood cells.[35] A limitation of the model is that the mature T cells are predominantly confined to the *Thy/Liv* organoids and very few of them are seen in the peripheral circulation. Lymph nodes in these mice are very small. The T cells are functional in in vitro tests but do not seem to mount a normal immune response in vivo.

The SCID-hu Bone model was created by subcutaneously implanting human fetal bone. After 4–6 weeks of implantation the bone was vascularized and histologically similar to human bone marrow.[36] Proliferation and differentiation of multilineage HSCs were maintained up to 20 weeks postimplant. The levels of erythropoiesis and myelopoiesis were relatively low. Exogenous administration of erythropoietin increased erythropoiesis. These mice provide the opportunity to do studies on human hematopoietic cells in the context of human hematolymphoid microenvironment (eg, effects of lethal irradiation followed by adoptive transfer) that can help characterize long-lived, self-renewing, human HSCs that are not possible in the in vitro setting.[33,37,38] These self-renewing HSCs can be serially passaged from one human bone to another in the SCID-hu mice without affecting the multilineage potential.

BLT Model

This model is established by subrenal capsule implantation of human fetal liver and thymus fragments followed by sublethal irradiation and IV injection of autologous $CD34^+$ HSCs derived from the same fetal liver donor into NOD-SCID or NSG mice.[39–41] HSCs engraft at higher rates than the other models. This method allows for the engraftment of a complete human system with the generation of T cells, B cells, NK cells, macrophages, and DCs, without exogenous human cytokine supplementation. Human T cells are educated on the human thymus and are human MHC class I and II restricted[42] and can thereby offer T-cell help to Ag-stimulated B cells. Unlike other humanized models strong in vivo immune responses that can lead to rejection of skin xenografts are seen in these mice.[39] The multilineage lymphoid cells are seen in the secondary lymphoid tissues, such as the bone marrow, spleen, liver, and lymph nodes. Unlike SCID-human (*Thy/Liv*) mice the BLT mice show enlarged lymph nodes that are populated by $CD45^+$ human cells ($^+$~90% of the population) originating from T cells ($CD4^+$ and $CD8^+$), B cells ($CD19^+$), and DCs.[39] These mice are able to mount a T-cell response that can recognize the APCs and recruit Ag-specific T cells at the target organs as evidenced by the delayed-type hypersensitivity (DTH) response to both Th1 (tetanus toxoid induction) or Th17 (collagen V–induced) Ags.[43] DTH responses are elicited when an Ag is presented by APCs to sensitized memory T cells in the draining lymph node and at the challenge site. BLT-NSG mice develop a B-cell-induced immunoglobulin response to Ag; however, the Ab isotype response is an IgM and not an IgG response. This could be due to the inability of these mice to form germinal centers in lymph nodes and facilitate immunoglobulin class switching.[43]

LIMITATIONS OF HUMANIZED MICE MODELS FOR CANCER BIOLOGY

To a certain extent development of the humanized mice, such as NSG or NOG which have severe impairment in their innate and adaptive immunities have allowed for a significant increase in tumor engraftment of patient-derived tumors of ovarian,[44,45] lung,[45] gastrointestinal,[46] and leukemic[47] origin. Despite these advances as with any xenogeneic implantation, there are several limitations with the use of these models. These include the following:

1. **GVHD**: Humanized mice that have received xenogeneic bone marrow or PBMC or cancer cell transplantation develop fatal GVHD at later points postengraftment. GVHD symptoms, such as dermatitis, poor tumor implantation, emaciation, and wasting are correlated with the activation of human T cells that attack recipient mouse tissue and increased levels of human immunoglobulins (IgG and IgM) in the serum. These results suggest activation and loss of self-tolerance that allows the human immune system to respond to the mouse immune system.[41] Another cause of this rejection could be mismatching of HLA Ags between the tumor cells and hematopoietic cells of the host. Onset of GVHD is not delayed even in mice that lack mouse MHC 1 and 2 Ags indicating that the human $CD4^+$ and $CD8^+$ T cells probably mediate GVHD.[41]
2. **Poor engraftment**: Endogenous mouse immunity can limit the rate of xenogeneic cell implantation. NSG mice have innate immune cells, such as macrophages, DCs, and neutrophils that can impede engraftment.[48] Although mouse proteins do not cross-react with human cells, some of the human proteins can cross-react with mouse immune system that can affect the engraftment rates. Some tumors, such as prostate carcinoma do not engraft well in NSG mice and this could be a function of the tumor type as the same problems are encountered with engraftment of these tumors in other immunodeficient mice, such as nude and SCID mice. Human origin cells also require species-specific growth factors and cytokines to improve engraftment. This has been partly overcome by the expression of human genes, such as growth factors and cytokines by a variety of genetic engineering technologies, such as transgenic expression of complementary DNA constructs driven by tissue-specific or ubiquitous promoters, transgenic expression of bacterial artificial chromosomes (BACs), and knock-in-technology.[49] Various strains of NSG or BRG [Balb/c mouse with Rag1 and Il2rg KO (NOD.$Rag1^{-}$; γc^{null})] mice (such as NSG-HLA-A2/HHD that expresses human HLA class I heavy and light chains and BRG CSF-1 that expresses macrophage colony-stimulating factor) have been used for the transgenic expression of human genes. These strategies allow enhancement of specific populations of immune cells directed by the transgene in the humanized mice. Despite these advances, various issues exist, such as improper levels of transgene expression, poorly controlled temporal kinetics, and lack of expression in the target organ.

3. **Incomplete human immune system:** In the Hu-PBL-SCID and Hu-SRC-SCID models, human T cells are restricted on the murine H-2d Ags. Therefore the human T cells lack the ability to recognize Ags in an HLA-restricted manner. Due to this defect, tumor metastasis studies can be affected due to the inability of the mice to develop human origin cytotoxic T-lymphocyte (CTL) responses. The development of the humanized NSG-HLA-A2/HHD overcomes this limitation by producing CTL responses.[8] Humanized mice in general do not develop all the key characteristics of a functional human immune system even with the transplantation of HSCs derived from the human thymus, liver, or bone marrow. Development of peripheral lymph nodes is very limited except in the BLT model, as described previously. Even in the BLT mouse, lymph nodes do not develop a germinal center and so no class switching of Ig responses is seen. The lymphoid structures are poorly organized in the liver, spleen, thymus, etc., and very few mature human T cells are seen in the peripheral circulation.
4. **Reactivation of endogenous infectious agents**: Tumors (PDX) and human tissue can harbor some endogenous viruses, such as the Epstein-Barr virus or retroviruses that when implanted into mice can reactivate. Reactivation of such agents can induce tumors which are different in character and morphology from the original tumor biopsy.[50–52]
5. **Divergence of human tumor**: When human tumors are passaged or transplanted from one mouse to the other the tumors undergo significant changes to their structure. The human stromal cells in the primary graft are replaced by mouse fibroblasts during subsequent passages. Mouse immune cells infiltrate the tumors and disrupt the architecture of the tumor thereby altering the local microenvironment. All these factors can severely impair the reproducibility of the data between different experiments.
6. **Ethics and logistics**: A key limitation to the utilization of the humanized models is the ethics of utilizing human fetal origin liver or thymus. Depending on the country, use of human fetal tissue is either restricted or banned, limiting the use of these models. The ability to acquire human bone marrow is also limited. Another key factor is that the cost of developing these models is high and technically challenging.

UTILITY OF HUMANIZED MICE IN CANCER

Cancer researchers have expanded the range of humanized mouse models by cotransplantation of human stem cells with human tumor cells. These models have a functional human system that gets activated by the presence of human tumor cells which mimics the situation in cancer patients. These models show promise for studying human tumor–stromal interactions, opportunity to investigate cancer immunotherapy, and tumor resistance. A variety of models that utilize these cotransplantation methods are available through commercial (Champions Oncology's TumorGraft models) and academic sources. Two examples of well-described models are listed in the following sections.

Humanized Xenochimeric Mice (XactMice)

These mice are established by bone marrow injection of an ex vivo expanded HSC and human stem cell progenitor cells (HSPCs) into sublethally irradiated NSG mice.[53] Following the establishment of these humanized mice, tumors derived from head and neck cancer patients were subsequently implanted in the flank of these mice to study the interaction of the HSPCs and the grafted tumors. In these mice even 6 months after engraftment, human origin CD3/CD45^{+} cell population remain stable in peripheral blood. In addition, human origin T and B cells are seen in bone marrow and spleen for over 12 months, demonstrating that these HSPCs continue to proliferate after engraftment. The human cell population was about 2–5% of the total bone marrow cells. These human bone marrow cells infiltrate the subcutaneously implanted tumors and produce alpha-smooth muscle actin-positive cells that are interspersed with mouse stromal cells. In addition, the HSPCs can produce human cytokines that helps the tumors maintain the native characteristics of the original patient-derived tumor and avoid the genetic drift that is seen with xenograft models. The re-created native tumor microenvironment is an improvement over the other animal models and could provide a tool for studying stroma- and immune-directed drug development.

Humanized Tumor Mice

This model was established by concurrent transplantation of HSCs and human breast cancer cells into the liver of irradiated neonatal NSG mice.[54] In this model, mice developed a functional immune response that was detectable by 5 weeks posttransplantation. Tumor cells disseminate into the lymphoid and nonlymphoid organs with the formation of macroscopic tumors in liver and spleen by 3 months posttransplantation. Humanized tumor mice (HTM) mice can reconstitute a complete T cell receptor repertoire in spleen, lymph node, and liver. Tumor growth was accompanied by T-cell maturation (from naive CD4^{+} toward a memory phenotype) and tumor cell–specific T-cell activation [CD4^{+} T cell, NK cell proliferation, interferon γ (IFNγ), and perforin production]. These results indicate that the HTM mice can be a useful tool to study human immune cell modulation, such as immune therapeutics based on Ab-dependent cellular cytotoxicity.

An elegant extension of this model was developed for studying the efficacy of Abs against immune check point inhibitors hCD137 (urelumab) and hPD-1 (nivolumab).[55] In this study, 3–4-week-old NSG mice were implanted with human PBMCs (IP). Following IP injection, the hPBMCs engrafted well with both CD4^{+} and CD8^{+} T cells seen in the peritoneal lavages by 5–6 days. These T cells also showed an induction in the immune checkpoint receptors CD137 and programmed cell death protein-1 (PD-1) on their surface. As expected a xenogeneic GVHD against the engrafted cells by 4–5 weeks posttransplantation was seen. When these mice were treated with urelumab or nivolumab either as single agent or combination therapy, the GVHD was exacerbated by the checkpoint inhibitor Abs and the response was primarily driven by human IFNγ-producing $CD4^+$ T cells. In these mice, subcutaneous administration of HT29 cells or human gastric carcinoma biopsy resulted in slower tumor growth rate than controls. This model provides an elegant method to assess the efficacy of human monoclonal Abs against immune checkpoint inhibitors. The potential to create "human avatars" with patient-derived tumor xenografts in this model is very exciting. New treatment strategies as well as novel Ab therapeutics could be designed and tested in these models which could then help inform clinical trial design.

FUTURE DIRECTIONS

Although the humanized mice models described in this chapter can produce some of the human immune responses, they still cannot replicate the entire diversity of human in vivo immune responses to tumors and tumor Ags. The inability to form peripheral lymph nodes is especially a challenge. Humanized mice have defects in their ability to support development and function of several human immune cells, such as monocytes, macrophages, and NK cells. Several strategies to overcome this defect by exogenous cytokine delivery, transduction of cytokine-encoding plasmids, and introduction of human transgenes expressing cytokines have been developed. There are ongoing efforts within the field to overcome this limitation by the exogenous administration of human IL-17 and other cellular factors. However, the supraphysiological concentration of the cytokines in the peripheral blood of these mice leads to mobilization and exhaustion of the HSCs. An alternate strategy that has also been employed is to knock-in genes expressing these human cytokine genes into the mouse genome. Some of the gene knock-ins that have been created by this method include thrombopoietin (*Tpo*), *IL-3, GMCSF (Csf-2),* and *MCSF(Csf-1)* into NSG mice. Tpo knock-in results in enhanced maintenance of HSC engraftment that can undergo mulitlineage differentiation and sustain high rates of engraftment and serial passage into other animals.[56] Csf-1 expression results in increased number of human monocytes and macrophages in the recipient mouse tissues.[42] New humanized mouse models have been described where multiple of these genes are knocked into the respective loci of the NSG mice—MITRG (knock-in of M-CSF, IL3/GMCSF, and TPO)[57] and MISTRG (knock-in of BAC transgene encoding human signal regulatory protein alpha).[58] These mice which express these human cytokines that are essential for innate immune cell development are highly permissive to human hematopoiesis and development of monocytes, macrophages, and NK cells from the engrafted HSCs are seen. These models could support primary hematopoietic malignancies, such as myeloproliferative neoplasia or myelodysplastic syndrome that are plagued by low proliferative ability. However, a drawback of the MIRTG or MISTRG mice is that the development of mouse red blood cells is suboptimal and the mice die of severe anemia. In addition, the adaptive immune responses in these mice are weak with low cytotoxic and humoral responses seen. NSG mice that are deficient in MHC class I and II expression,[59] HLA class I (A-2) transgenic,[60] have also been developed. These models have the potential to increase HSC and human tumor engraftment, delay xenogeneic GVHD, and generate human CTL responses. These models will allow us to understand the mechanism of tumor resistance to the human immune system and also provide us with an opportunity to develop novel therapeutics that can overcome these resistance pathways. An alternative to these genetically modified mouse model approaches is to create peripheral humanized lymphoid organs using a tissue engineering approach. Several investigators have examined the possibility of implanting polymers or bioengineered bone containing HSCs or human growth factors subcutaneously into NSG mice. Early results are encouraging in that these implanted materials can attract transplanted human progenitor cells and can form a local HSC niche. It would be interesting in the future to see if these niches allow transplanted cells to differentiate into different lineages of cells and can result in bone and bone marrow formation.[61] A combination of humanized mice with this tissue engineered niches could be useful to study tumor metastasis, bone formation, or hematological malignancies in their native microenvironment.

REFERENCES

1. Gould SE, Junttila MR, de Sauvage FJ. Translational value of mouse models in oncology drug development. *Nat Med* 2015;**21**:431–9.
2. Mestas J, Hughes CC. Of mice and not men: differences between mouse and human immunology. *J Immunol* 2004;**172**:2731–8.
3. Platzer B, Stout M, Fiebiger E. Antigen cross-presentation of immune complexes. *Front Immunol* 2014;**5**:140.
4. Eggermont AM, Maio M, Robert C. Immune checkpoint inhibitors in melanoma provide the cornerstones for curative therapies. *Seminars Oncol* 2015;**42**:429–35.
5. Weinstock M, McDermott D. Targeting PD-1/PD-L1 in the treatment of metastatic renal cell carcinoma. *Ther Adv Urol* 2015;**7**:365–77.
6. Garon EB, Rizvi NA, Hui R, et al. Pembrolizumab for the treatment of non-small-cell lung cancer. *N. Engl J Med* 2015;**372**:2018–28.
7. Besser MJ, Shapira-Frommer R, Treves AJ, et al. Clinical responses in a phase II study using adoptive transfer of short-term cultured tumor infiltration lymphocytes in metastatic melanoma patients. *Clin Cancer Res Off J Am Assoc Cancer Res* 2010;**16**:2646–55.
8. Shultz LD, Brehm MA, Garcia-Martinez JV, Greiner DL. Humanized mice for immune system investigation: progress, promise and challenges. *Nat Rev Immunol* 2012;**12**:786–98.
9. Flanagan SP. 'Nude', a new hairless gene with pleiotropic effects in the mouse. *Genet Res* 1966;**8**:295–309.
10. Fogh J, Fogh JM, Orfeo T. One hundred and twenty-seven cultured human tumor cell lines producing tumors in nude mice. *J Natl Cancer Inst* 1977;**59**:221–6.
11. Bosma MJ, Carroll AM. The SCID mouse mutant: definition, characterization, and potential uses. *Annu Rev Immunol* 1991;**9**:323–50.
12. McCune JM, Namikawa R, Kaneshima H, Shultz LD, Lieberman M, Weissman IL. The SCID-hu mouse: murine model for the analysis of human hematolymphoid differentiation and function. *Science* 1988;**241**:1632–9.

13. Mosier DE, Gulizia RJ, Baird SM, Wilson DB. Transfer of a functional human immune system to mice with severe combined immunodeficiency. *Nature* 1988;**335**:256–9.
14. Phillips RA, Jewett MA, Gallie BL. Growth of human tumors in immune-deficient scid mice and nude mice. *Curr Top Microbiol Immunol* 1989;**152**:259–63.
15. Greiner DL, Hesselton RA, Shultz LD. SCID mouse models of human stem cell engraftment. *Stem Cells* 1998;**16**:166–77.
16. Tian X, Woll PS, Morris JK, Linehan JL, Kaufman DS. Hematopoietic engraftment of human embryonic stem cell-derived cells is regulated by recipient innate immunity. *Stem Cells* 2006;**24**:1370–80.
17. Mombaerts P, Iacomini J, Johnson RS, Herrup K, Tonegawa S, Papaioannou VE. RAG-1-deficient mice have no mature B and T lymphocytes. *Cell* 1992;**68**:869–77.
18. Shinkai Y, Rathbun G, Lam KP, et al. RAG-2-deficient mice lack mature lymphocytes owing to inability to initiate V(D)J rearrangement. *Cell* 1992;**68**:855–67.
19. Christianson SW, Greiner DL, Hesselton RA, et al. Enhanced human CD4+ T cell engraftment in beta2-microglobulin-deficient NOD-scid mice. *J Immunol* 1997;**158**:3578–86.
20. Shultz LD, Ishikawa F, Greiner DL. Humanized mice in translational biomedical research. *Nat Rev Immunol* 2007;**7**:118–30.
21. La H, Ralph G. *An overview of humanized mouse models for experimental medicine*. 2015. [p. Taconic Webpage].
22. Akkina R. New generation humanized mice for virus research: comparative aspects and future prospects. *Virology* 2013;**435**:14–28.
23. Ito M, Hiramatsu H, Kobayashi K, et al. NOD/SCID/gamma(c)(null) mouse: an excellent recipient mouse model for engraftment of human cells. *Blood* 2002;**100**:3175–82.
24. Tary-Lehmann M, Saxon A, Lehmann PV. The human immune system in hu-PBL-SCID mice. *Immunol Today* 1995;**16**:529–33.
25. Watanabe Y, Takahashi T, Okajima A, et al. The analysis of the functions of human B and T cells in humanized NOD/shi-scid/gammac(null) (NOG) mice (hu-HSC NOG mice). *Int Immunol* 2009;**21**:843–58.
26. Tary-Lehmann M, Lehmann PV, Schols D, Roncarolo MG, Saxon A. Anti-SCID mouse reactivity shapes the human CD4+ T cell repertoire in hu-PBL-SCID chimeras. *J Exp Med* 1994;**180**:1817–27.
27. Lapidot T, Pflumio F, Doedens M, Murdoch B, Williams DE, Dick JE. Cytokine stimulation of multilineage hematopoiesis from immature human cells engrafted in SCID mice. *Science* 1992;**255**:1137–41.
28. Vormoor J, Lapidot T, Pflumio F, et al. SCID mice as an in vivo model of human cord blood hematopoiesis. *Blood Cells* 1994;**20**:316–20. Discussion 20–2.
29. Hogan CJ, Shpall EJ, McNiece I, Keller G. Multilineage engraftment in NOD/LtSz-scid/scid mice from mobilized human CD34+ peripheral blood progenitor cells. *Biology Blood Marrow Transplant: J Am Soc Blood Marrow Transplant* 1997;**3**:236–46.
30. Wang JC, Doedens M, Dick JE. Primitive human hematopoietic cells are enriched in cord blood compared with adult bone marrow or mobilized peripheral blood as measured by the quantitative in vivo SCID-repopulating cell assay. *Blood* 1997;**89**:3919–24.
31. Lowry PA, Shultz LD, Greiner DL, et al. Improved engraftment of human cord blood stem cells in NOD/LtSz-scid/scid mice after irradiation or multiple-day injections into unirradiated recipients. *Biology Blood Marrow Transplant: J Am Soc Blood Marrow Transplant* 1996;**2**:15–23.
32. Berges BK, Rowan MR. The utility of the new generation of humanized mice to study HIV-1 infection: transmission, prevention, pathogenesis, and treatment. *Retrovirology* 2011;**8**:65.

33. McCune JM. Development and applications of the SCID-hu mouse model. *Seminars Immunol* 1996;**8**:187–96.
34. Krowka JF, Sarin S, Namikawa R, McCune JM, Kaneshima H. Human T cells in the SCID-hu mouse are phenotypically normal and functionally competent. *J Immunol* 1991;**146**:3751–6.
35. Vandekerckhove BA, Krowka JF, McCune JM, de Vries JE, Spits H, Roncarolo MG. Clonal analysis of the peripheral T cell compartment of the SCID-hu mouse. *J Immunol* 1991;**146**:4173–9.
36. Kyoizumi S, Baum CM, Kaneshima H, McCune JM, Yee EJ, Namikawa R. Implantation and maintenance of functional human bone marrow in SCID-hu mice. *Blood* 1992;**79**:1704–11.
37. McCune J, Kaneshima H, Krowka J, et al. The SCID-hu mouse: a small animal model for HIV infection and pathogenesis. *Annu Rev Immunol* 1991;**9**:399–429.
38. Chen BP, Fraser C, Reading C, et al. Cytokine-mobilized peripheral blood CD34+Thy-1+Lin-human hematopoietic stem cells as target cells for transplantation-based gene therapy. *Leukemia* 1995;**9**(Suppl. 1):S17–25.
39. Lan P, Tonomura N, Shimizu A, Wang S, Yang YG. Reconstitution of a functional human immune system in immunodeficient mice through combined human fetal thymus/liver and CD34+ cell transplantation. *Blood* 2006;**108**:487–92.
40. Melkus MW, Estes JD, Padgett-Thomas A, et al. Humanized mice mount specific adaptive and innate immune responses to EBV and TSST-1. *Nat Med* 2006;**12**:1316–22.
41. Covassin L, Jangalwe S, Jouvet N, et al. Human immune system development and survival of non-obese diabetic (NOD)-scid IL2rgamma(null) (NSG) mice engrafted with human thymus and autologous haematopoietic stem cells. *Clin Exp Immunol* 2013;**174**:372–88.
42. Rathinam C, Poueymirou WT, Rojas J, et al. Efficient differentiation and function of human macrophages in humanized CSF-1 mice. *Blood* 2011;**118**:3119–28.
43. Rajesh D, Zhou Y, Jankowska-Gan E, et al. Th1 and Th17 immunocompetence in humanized NOD/SCID/IL2rgammanull mice. *Hum Immunol* 2010;**71**:551–9.
44. Bankert RB, Balu-Iyer SV, Odunsi K, et al. Humanized mouse model of ovarian cancer recapitulates patient solid tumor progression, ascites formation, and metastasis. *PloS one* 2011;**6**:e24420.
45. Simpson-Abelson MR, Sonnenberg GF, Takita H, et al. Long-term engraftment and expansion of tumor-derived memory T cells following the implantation of non-disrupted pieces of human lung tumor into NOD-scid IL2Rgamma(null) mice. *J Immunol* 2008;**180**:7009–18.
46. Maykel J, Liu JH, Li H, Shultz LD, Greiner DL, Houghton J. NOD-scidIl2rg (tm1Wjl) and NOD-Rag1 (null) Il2rg (tm1Wjl): a model for stromal cell-tumor cell interaction for human colon cancer. *Dig Dis Sci* 2014;**59**:1169–79.
47. Agliano A, Martin-Padura I, Mancuso P, et al. Human acute leukemia cells injected in NOD/LtSz-scid/IL-2Rgamma null mice generate a faster and more efficient disease compared to other NOD/scid-related strains. *Int J Cancer* 2008;**123**:2222–7.
48. Zhou Q, Facciponte J, Jin M, Shen Q, Lin Q. Humanized NOD-SCID IL2rg-/- mice as a preclinical model for cancer research and its potential use for individualized cancer therapies. *Cancer Lett* 2014;**344**:13–9.
49. Drake AC, Chen Q, Chen J. Engineering humanized mice for improved hematopoietic reconstitution. *Cell Mol Immunol* 2012;**9**:215–24.
50. Radaelli E, Hermans E, Omodho L, et al. Spontaneous post-transplant disorders in NOD.Cg-Prkdcscid Il2rgtm1Sug/JicTac (NOG) mice engrafted with patient-derived metastatic melanomas. *PLoS One* 2015;**10**:e0124974.
51. Fujii E, Kato A, Chen YJ, Matsubara K, Ohnishi Y, Suzuki M. Characterization of EBV-related lymphoproliferative lesions arising in donor lymphocytes of transplanted human tumor tissues in the NOG mouse. *Exp Anim/Jpn Assoc Lab Anim Sci* 2014;**63**:289–96.

52. Wetterauer C, Vlajnic T, Schuler J, et al. Early development of human lymphomas in a prostate cancer xenograft program using triple knock-out immunocompromised mice. *Prostate* 2015;**75**:585–92.
53. Morton JJ, Bird G, Keysar SB, et al. XactMice: humanizing mouse bone marrow enables microenvironment reconstitution in a patient-derived xenograft model of head and neck cancer. *Oncogene* 2015;1–11.
54. Wege AK, Ernst W, Eckl J, et al. Humanized tumor mice–a new model to study and manipulate the immune response in advanced cancer therapy. *Int J Cancer* 2011;**129**:2194–206.
55. Sanmamed MF, Rodriguez I, Schalper KA, et al. Nivolumab and urelumab enhance antitumor activity of human T lymphocytes engrafted in Rag2-/-IL2Rgammanull immunodeficient mice. *Cancer Res* 2015;**75**:3466–78.
56. Rongvaux A, Willinger T, Takizawa H, et al. Human thrombopoietin knockin mice efficiently support human hematopoiesis in vivo. *Proc Natl Acad Sci USA* 2011;**108**:2378–83.
57. Willinger T, Rongvaux A, Strowig T, Manz MG, Flavell RA. Improving human hemato lymphoid-system mice by cytokine knock-in gene replacement. *Trends Immunol* 2011;**32**:321–7.
58. Strowig T, Rongvaux A, Rathinam C, et al. Transgenic expression of human signal regulatory protein alpha in Rag2-/-gamma(c)-/- mice improves engraftment of human hematopoietic cells in humanized mice. *Proc Natl Acad Sci USA* 2011;**108**:13218–23.
59. Pino S, Brehm MA, Covassin-Barberis L, et al. Development of novel major histocompatibility complex class I and class II-deficient NOD-SCID IL2R gamma chain knockout mice for modeling human xenogeneic graft-versus-host disease. *Methods Mol Biol* 2010;**602**:105–17.
60. Shultz LD, Saito Y, Najima Y, et al. Generation of functional human T-cell subsets with HLA-restricted immune responses in HLA class I expressing NOD/SCID/IL2r gamma(null) humanized mice. *Proc Natl Acad Sci USA* 2010;**107**:13022–7.
61. Holzapfel BM, Wagner F, Thibaudeau L, Levesque JP, Hutmacher DW. Concise review: humanized models of tumor immunology in the 21st century: convergence of cancer research and tissue engineering. *Stem Cells* 2015;**33**:1696–704.

Section II

Components of a PDX Program

Chapter 1

Regulations of Patient-Derived Xenografts

S. Thompson-Iritani, S.C. Schmechel
University of Washington, Seattle, WA, United States

REGULATIONS SURROUNDING THE PROCUREMENT OF HUMAN TISSUES FOR RESEARCH

The regulations described are for the use of human biospecimens and associated data in the United States. Many countries have differing regulatory standards, and awareness of standards that may differ from the US regulations is required prior to initiating patient-derived xenograft (PDX) programs in other countries.

The procurement and distribution for research of human biospecimens annotated with health information is subject to complex US regulations. Biospecimens obtained solely for research (pathway labeled "research biospecimen pathway 1" in Fig. 1.1) are subject to (1) standards of medical practice—for example, limiting the volume of phlebotomized blood to safeguard against inappropriately low patient hematocrit levels; (2) protocol and consent approval from an Institutional Review Board (IRB); (3) proper handling of individually identifiable health information as mandated by the federal Health Insurance Portability and Accountability Act of 1996 (HIPAA)[1] and; (4) in some cases, state laws that may be more stringent than federal requirements.

Research biospecimens obtained as residual portions of clinical specimens are subject to more extensive regulations. A clinical specimen is defined as one removed primarily for diagnostic, prognostic, or theragnostic testing, and/or removed for therapy. In addition to the standards of medical practice, IRB approval, HIPAA compliance, and state law compliance, use of biospecimens derived from clinical specimens may be subject to (1) hospital accreditation requirements such as those of The Joint Commission (TJC), (2) the federal Clinical Laboratory Improvement Amendments of 1988 (CLIA) as implemented by accreditation organizations such as the College of American Pathologists (CAP), and (3) relevant individual hospital policies.

Patient Derived Tumor Xenograft Models. http://dx.doi.org/10.1016/B978-0-12-804010-2.00007-2

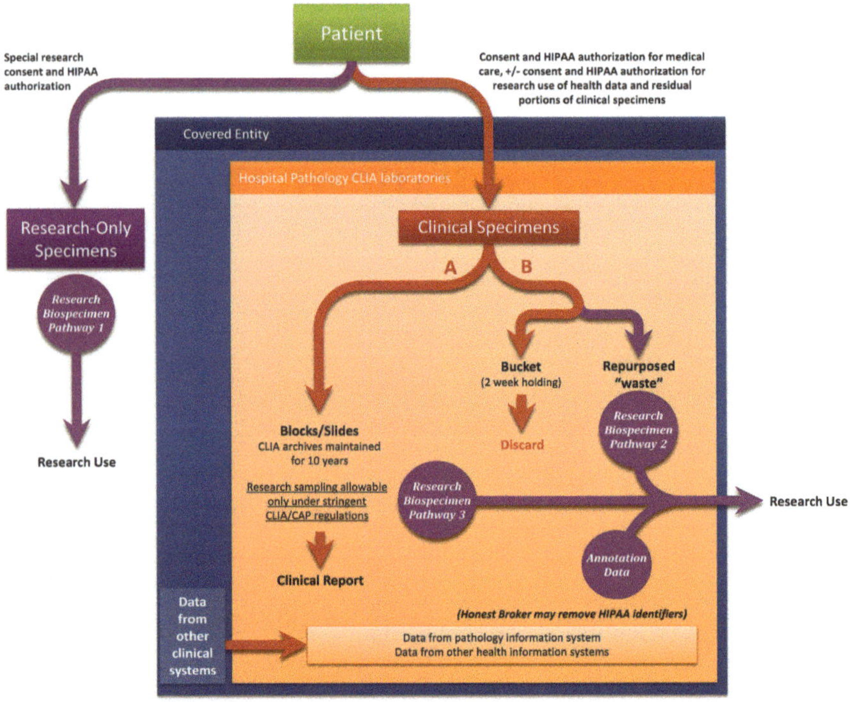

FIGURE 1.1 Potential specimen flows from a human research subject. Research biospecimen and data flows are indicated by *purple arrows*; clinical biospecimen and data flows are indicated by *red arrows*. With special consent, research-only biospecimens, such as peripheral blood or tissue obtained solely for research, may be obtained specifically for a research protocol ("research biospecimen pathway 1"). These specimens may or may not be processed or analyzed in a clinical laboratory. Research biospecimens derived from residual portions of clinical specimens are processed and analyzed in the clinical laboratory and are subject to requirements imposed by federal law called the CLIA. Under CLIA, many laboratories are accredited by the CAP. Those portions of clinical specimens that are submitted to prepare tissue blocks and slides used in generating the pathology clinical report (*arrow A*) are subject to CLIA/CAP-mandated holding requirements, although research sampling from these materials is permitted under stringent conditions ("research biospecimen pathway 3"). Those portions of clinical specimens that are not needed for clinical purposes (*arrow B*) may either be discarded/incinerated as medical "waste" or, alternatively, repurposed for research protocols ("research biospecimen pathway 2"). Collection and release of materials and data by the laboratory for research, including with respect to patient identifiers, may be subject to additional regulations imposed under IRBs and the federal HIPAA. For many projects, IRB and other regulations favor the use of unidentified, anonymized, or coded/deidentified specimens and data, particularly if the research protocol does not require patient identifiers. In these circumstances, an individual serving an honest broker role may remove identifiers from specimens and data prior to their release for research.

Institutional Review Boards

The Federal National Research Act of 1974 established the formation of IRBs to oversee most forms of human subjects research. The work of IRBs is guided by Federal Policy for the Protection of Human Subjects, published as Title 45, Part 46 of the Code of Federal Regulations (45 CFR 46; the "Common Rule").

[For drug, biologic, and medical device work involving human specimens to be submitted to the US Food and Drug Administration (FDA), distinct guidance is available as Title 21 CFR Parts 50, 56, and 812.[2]] The Common Rule incorporates principles published as the Belmont Report.[3] This report defined the boundary between practice and research: "the term 'practice' refers to interventions that are designed solely to enhance the well-being of an individual patient or client and that have a reasonable expectation of success," whereas research was defined as "an activity designed to test an hypothesis, permit conclusions to be drawn, and thereby to develop or contribute to generalizable knowledge."[3] This distinction is important, since practice and research may occur concurrently in health care settings. For example, a clinical specimen removed for therapy (eg, removal of a patient's tumor and the surrounding marginal tissue) may simultaneously undergo examination in the pathology laboratory for clinical purposes including removing portions of the specimen to prepare paraffin blocks and microscopic slides used to generate a pathology report, and for research purposes including removing for research portions of the specimen not needed for clinical purposes. It is important for pathologists and others to recognize when their role is part of practice versus research.

The Belmont Report importantly defined three ethical principles relevant to research involving human subjects: (1) respect for persons, (2) beneficence, and (3) justice. Respect for persons includes the concept that individuals are autonomous and entitled to protections, including making judgments and choices about whether to voluntarily take part in a research protocol. The concept of beneficence includes minimizing potential harms associated with research and maximizing potential benefits. The concept of justice incorporates that, to the degree possible, there should be equitability in who bears the burdens versus who reaps the benefits of research. For example, where appropriate, attempts should be made to include individuals of various racial and ethnic backgrounds and socioeconomic groups in research, rather than to rely on more homogeneous populations simply because they may be more readily available to the research team. Further, the justice principle compels researchers to consider additional factors, such as whether an international setting providing a convenient population may be appropriate for a drug clinical trial if the population in that setting may not be able to benefit from the drug whose approval is a consequence of the research. These ethical principles are reflected in the Common Rule guidance and HIPAA requirements for the use of individually identifiable health information.

Common Rule

The Common Rule guides IRBs in their oversight of research involving human subjects. It defines research as a systematic investigation that may lead to generalizable knowledge. A process for obtaining informed consent is generally required, and must include sufficient information to allow potential subjects to make an informed decision to participate in the research, including ensuring that potential subjects understand the nature of the research, its duration, benefits, and potential risks including risks associated with genetic sequencing. Research involving human biospecimens or data identifiable to individuals is considered human subjects research, even if the researcher/research team does not interact with subjects themselves, but rather interacts only with identifiers from subjects. Importantly, under the current Common Rule guidance, research using unidentified, anonymized, or study-coded/deidentified biospecimens which lack individually identifiable information [because individually identifiable patient protected health information (PHI) has been removed from specimens and data by an individual serving an honest broker role], and for which the researcher/research team cannot relink the biospecimen study codes back to individually identifiable information, may not constitute human subjects research. For projects determined to be not human subjects research, no member of the research team—those obtaining, interpreting, or analyzing research information, or serving as an author on subsequent research reports—can be involved in the study coding or have access to patient-identifiable information or a code key. Under these circumstances, a determination often provided by a relevant IRB or other mechanisms permitted by the institution, such as allowing researchers to self-determine that the research does not constitute human subjects research, and a signed "gatekeeper" agreement between the honest broker and the research team ensuring that researchers will not attempt to relink codes back to patient identifiers, may be sufficient authorization to obtain human unidentified, anonymized, or study-coded/deidentified biospecimens and data for research. [However, for study results to be submitted to the FDA, the FDA generally considers all work with human biospecimens (whether identifiable or not identifiable) to be human subjects research and recommends IRB review of such study protocols.[4]] The Common Rule allows IRBs to waive the requirement for consent if all of the following conditions are met: (1) the research involves no more than minimal risk to participants, (2) the waiver will not adversely affect the rights and welfare of participants, (3) the research could not practicably be carried out without the waiver, and (4) whenever appropriate, participants will be provided with study information after participation. Minimal risk is considered to be a risk no greater than that incurred in daily life or through routine examination and testing.

Health Insurance Portability and Accountability Act

The Federal HIPAA law does not relate to biospecimens themselves, but to certain data associated with specimens. HIPAA defines 18 identifying elements as PHI.[5] Because pathology laboratory accession numbers uniquely identify patients within a health system, these numbers should be treated as PHI.[6] "Covered entities" must comply with HIPAA standards. Covered entities are defined as "health plans, health care clearinghouses, and health care providers who conduct certain financial and administrative transactions electronically."[7] Pathologists and other providers may have access to certain PHI as part of their covered entity practice role, but authorization is generally required for their access to PHI as part of a research role.

Under the current regulatory framework, three authorization methods are possible to obtain identified biospecimens and data: (1) informed patient consent and HIPAA authorization, (2) IRB-granted waiver of consent and waiver of HIPAA authorization, and (3) through a Data Use Agreement for Limited Data Sets. Research involving the use of unidentified, anonymized or coded/deidentified specimens and data may be permitted without one of these authorization methods if determined not to constitute human subjects research (except for study results to be submitted to the FDA, which defines all research using human biospecimens to be human subjects research even if the biospecimens are not identifiable).

PHI may be used in research with patient authorization allowing the covered entity to disclose the PHI for the research protocol. PHI may also be used in research if either an IRB has approved a waiver of HIPAA authorization or the covered entity and the researcher enter into a Data Use Agreement through which the covered entity may disclose a Limited Data Set. A Limited Data Set may contain only the following HIPAA identifiers: dates such as admission, discharge, service, date of birth, date of death; city, state, five-digit, or more zip code; and ages in years, months, or days or hours. IRBs may waive the requirement for patient authorization in concert with waiving the requirement for consent under the Common Rule. Under HIPAA, individuals have the right to receive an accounting of certain disclosures of PHI. If PHI is disclosed for research by the covered entity under an IRB-granted waiver of HIPAA authorization, the disclosure needs to be accounted for by, or on behalf of, the researcher. This is typically accomplished by filing an accounting of disclosure with the institution's Privacy Office.

Many research projects are undertaken using specimens and data from which the 18 HIPAA identifiers have been stripped from the specimens and data, typically by an individual working within the covered entity serving an honest broker function. An honest broker is "an individual, organization, or system acting for, or on behalf of, a covered entity to collect and provide health information to research investigators in such a manner whereby it would not be reasonably possible for the investigators or others to identify the corresponding patients-subjects directly or indirectly. The information provided to the investigators by the honest broker may incorporate linkage codes to permit information collation and/or subsequent inquiries (i.e., a 're-identification code'); however, the information linking this re-identification code to the patient's identity must be retained by the honest broker and subsequent inquiries are conducted through the honest broker."[8] To deidentify specimens and data, the honest broker would typically assign a study code to specimens and data using a coding system that is not relatable to the 18 HIPAA identifiers, release the specimens and data to the research team only by study code, and protect the link between study codes and PHI. An honest broker cannot be a member of the research team; simply providing data or specimens does not constitute involvement in the conduct of research.

These authorization mechanisms may be altered substantially in the future. Shortly before the writing of this chapter, the US Department of Health and Human Services (HHS) announced proposed revisions that would generally require consent "for secondary research with a biospecimen (for example, part of a blood sample that is left over after being drawn for clinical purposes), even if the investigator is not being given information that would enable him or her to identify whose biospecimen it is."[9] Health systems will need to monitor the potentially changing regulatory framework.

The Joint Commission, Clinical Laboratory Improvement Amendments of 1988, and the College of American Pathologists

With appropriate authorizations in place, biospecimens derived from residual portions of clinical specimens are subject to additional oversight. Per TJC all specimens obtained from patients for clinical purposes, except those specifically exempted by institutional policy, must be submitted to the pathology department for examination. Upon submission to pathology, the specimens become part of the hospital's responsibilities under the CLIA and CAP regulations. The CLIA is Federal Act pertaining to laboratory clinical testing performed on humans in the United States.[10] Rather than directly accrediting laboratories, HHS invited organizations to propose accreditation processes. A CAP process was approved such that the "accreditation process of this organization provides reasonable assurance that the laboratories accredited by it meet the conditions required by federal law and regulations."[11] Organizations additional to the CAP have been approved for laboratory accreditation, but since the CAP most widely accredits hospital laboratories, this chapter will discuss CAP requirements under CLIA (abbreviated in further discussion as CLIA/CAP).

Clinical specimens arriving in pathology are examined and representative portions of each specimen are typically fixed in formalin and processed into formalin-fixed, paraffin-embedded (FFPE) blocks (pathway labeled A in Fig. 1.1). Often for small specimens, such as biopsies, all of the tissue received in pathology is processed into FFPE blocks since it may not be evident, based solely on gross examination, what portions may be required for diagnosis versus what portions may not be needed clinically. For larger specimens, such as resection specimens composed of a grossly evident tumor and surrounding marginal grossly normal tissue, the pathologist will submit blocks for clinical purposes to document the nature of the tumor, the degree of spread of the tumor, and the status of margins. However, the remainder of the specimen may be determined not to be needed for clinical purposes. In the era before research tissue protocols were developed, this residual tissue was held for a CLIA/CAP-mandated 2-week holding period in a container/bucket, and then typically discarded/incinerated. Currently, many health systems have developed protocols for repurposing for research tissue that would otherwise be "waste" (labeled "research biospecimen pathway 2" in Fig. 1.1). A standard for determining what portion of a specimen may be procured for research has been developed by CAP which states in part that (1) the pathologist responsible for procurement determines that the sample is not necessary for diagnostic purposes, (2) formal written authorization is obtained in accordance with the requirements of HIPAA if identifiable patient information is released, and (3) the biorepository meets other relevant requirements, including but not limited to, the requirements of the institution, the directives of any applicable IRB, and laws and regulations.[12] Tissue procured for research under such protocols may be processed in various ways, such as fresh, snap frozen, and placed in stabilization media, depending on the requirements of the research protocol. Typically samples are placed in tubes/containers labeled with study codes linkable to patient identifiers only by an honest broker.

Those blocks and slides used to prepare the pathology clinical report are subject to retention requirements under CLIA/CAP. The laboratory must keep its records and histopathology slides for at least 10 years, all blocks for at least 2 years, and sufficient blocks to support the diagnosis for 10 years. Nevertheless, under CLIA/CAP such materials may be utilized for research purposes (labeled "research biospecimen pathway 3" in Fig. 1.1) if all of the following criteria are met: (1) formal written authorization is obtained in accordance with the requirements of HIPAA if identifiable patient information is released; (2) the laboratory retains sufficient blocks to support the diagnosis for the full 10-year period; (3) provision is made for retrieval by the laboratory of any blocks or material that remain after use in research, if the blocks or material are needed for diagnostic, legal, or other legitimate purposes; and (4) the laboratory meets other relevant requirements including but not limited to the requirements of the institution, the directives of any applicable IRB or similar entity, and state and local laws and regulations.[13]

These requirements place substantial responsibility on researchers and on the health system and its pathology laboratory to ensure that specimens and data used for research conform to CLIA/CAP, IRB, HIPAA, and other requirements.

OCCUPATIONAL AND ENVIRONMENTAL HEALTH REGULATIONS WHEN WORKING WITH PDX TUMORS

The evaluation and manipulation of PDX tumors for research purposes involves potential hazards that need to be minimized. There are a variety of regulations worldwide that impact the use of potentially infectious agents in the laboratory. The World Health Organization has published the Laboratory Biosafety Manual that is intended to provide a framework for countries to adhere to an international standard and this document guidance not only addresses the management of infectious organisms but also provides information on risk assessment and recombinant DNA technology.[14] Due to the fact that the guidelines in the Laboratory Safety Manual are general and not necessarily as specific as several organizations preferred, there has been a proliferation of professional organizations that have developed their own specific regulatory guidance. This has led to the creation of "embedded" biosafety guidance, assessment tools, and regulations that may vary nationally and regionally.

Oversight in the United States

In the United States, working with primary human tissues requires compliance with Occupational Safety and Health Administration's (OSHA's) Bloodborne Pathogens Standard.[15] Bloodborne pathogens are defined as infectious microorganisms present in blood that can cause disease in humans and other potentially infectious materials (OPIM) (ie, tissues or tumors). These pathogens include, but are not limited to, hepatitis B virus, hepatitis C virus, and human immunodeficiency virus. Workers exposed to bloodborne pathogens are at risk for serious or life-threatening illnesses (refer to Chapter 8 for details on the pathogens that could be associated with PDX tumors). An overview of the regulatory requirements is outlined in Fig. 1.2 and detailed in the following discussion.

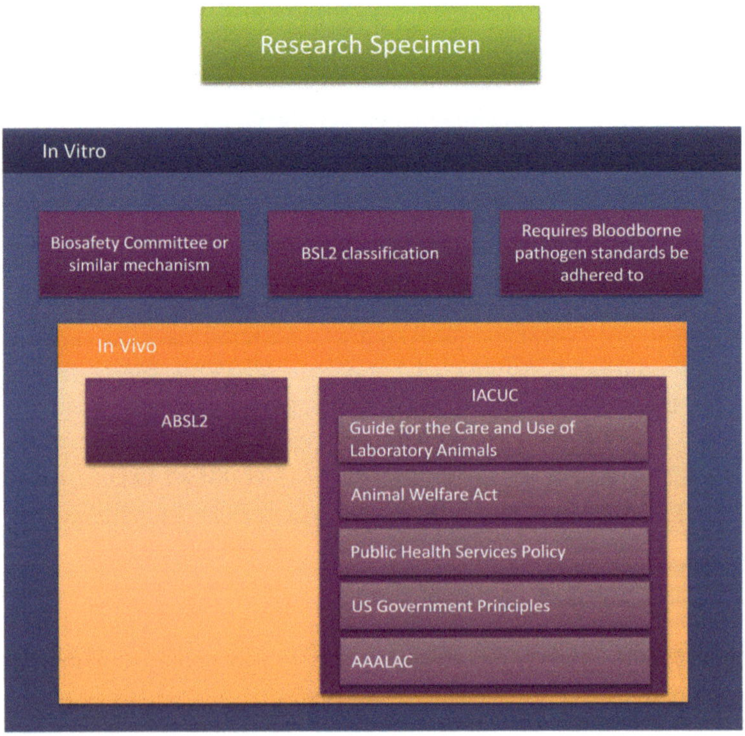

FIGURE 1.2 Regulatory oversight of research specimens in the United States. This figure outlines the major regulatory oversight involved in the use of the research specimens. In the initial in vitro evaluation stage, the oversight involves the use of biohazardous agents in the laboratory and is regulated by OSHA's Bloodborne Pathogens Standard and biosafety requirements regulated by an organizations' biosafety committee. If the specimen is then going to be used in vivo in an animal model, there is additional oversight of the biohazard as ABSL2 and the requirements that the animal procedure be evaluated by the IACUC as defined by the regulatory and oversight bodies listed.

The Bloodborne Pathogens Standard require several actions on the part of the employer. These include:

1. Establishing an exposure control plan,
2. Updating the plan annually to reflect changes in tasks, procedures, and positions that affect occupational exposure, and also technological changes that eliminate or reduce occupational exposure,
3. Implementing the use of universal precautions (treating all human blood and OPIM as if known to be infectious for bloodborne pathogens),
4. Identifying and using engineering controls,
5. Identifying and ensuring the use of work practice controls,
6. Providing personal protective equipment (PPE), such as gloves, gowns, eye protection, and masks; employers must clean, repair, and replace this equipment as needed,
7. Making available hepatitis B vaccinations to all workers with occupational exposure,
8. Making available postexposure evaluation and follow-up to any occupationally exposed worker who experiences an exposure incident,
9. Using labels and signs to communicate hazards,
10. Providing information and training to workers, and
11. Maintaining worker medical and training records.

The employer also must maintain a sharps injury log, unless it is exempt under Part 1904—Recording and Reporting Occupational Injuries and Illnesses, in Title 29 of the Code of Federal Regulations. Persons conducting research with potentially infectious materials should have a thorough understanding of these regulations and their own institution's policies.

The Biosafety in Microbiological and Biomedical Laboratories, 5th Edition, classifies human primary tissues as requiring Biosafety Level 2 precautions.[16] This means that the tissues require standard microbiological practices (including prohibiting the practice of mouth pipetting), special practices (training and awareness of hazards), safety equipment [primary barriers, such as biosafety cabinets (BSCs), and PPE—gloves, laboratory coats, safety glasses, and closed toe shores], and laboratory facilities (eyewash and handwashing sink). It is very important to clarify all of these requirements up front and ensure that all the precautions are put into place well in advance of the tissue evaluation. Ensuring compliance with these standards requires coordination between the institution's health and safety personnel, facilities personnel, and with the veterinary and animal care staff when animal studies are conducted.

Biosafety Committee

Many institutions have a biosafety committee [ie, the Institutional Biosafety Committee (IBC)[17] or similar mechanism] that reviews the use of a variety of hazards, including biological agents. IBCs were established under the National

Institutes of Health (NIH) guidelines to provide local review and oversight of nearly all forms of research utilizing recombinant or synthetic nucleic acid molecules. Over time, many institutions have chosen to assign their IBCs the responsibility of reviewing a variety of experimentation that involves biological materials (eg, infectious agents) and other potentially hazardous agents (eg, carcinogens). This additional responsibility is assigned entirely at the discretion of the institution and many institutions include all biohazards in their IBC reviews. It is essential that you contact the Environmental or Occupational Health Department that you are working with to ensure that you are following the institution's policies and procedures. If required, the biosafety committee should perform a risk assessment and establish safe practices for working with the specimens.

If the tumors are transplanted into mice, then it is common for an organization to require that they be handled via Animal Biosafety Level 2 (ABSL2) procedures while working with the animals. The ABSL2 requires that (1) access to the animal facility is restricted; (2) personnel must have specific training in animal facility procedures, the handling of infected animals, and the manipulation of pathogenic agents; (3) personnel must be supervised by individuals with adequate knowledge of potential hazards, microbiological agents, animal manipulations, and husbandry procedures; and (4) BSCs or other physical containment equipment is used when procedures involve the manipulation of infectious materials, or where aerosols or splashes may be created. Many institutions require that all injections, necropsies, and imaging be performed in a BSC where feasible. New and different regulations may come into application as the use of PDX tumors progresses to include studies in larger species or animals where this practice is not feasible.

Chemical Hazards

In addition to the biohazards associated with the primary tumor collection, evaluation, and transplantation, there are safety precautions that need to be considered when evaluating cancer therapies. Recently, the OSHA has chosen to align their Hazard Communication Standard with the Globally Harmonized System of Classification and Labeling of Chemicals so that there is a national standard for classification.[18] It is critical that all drugs and therapies that are evaluated in vitro and in vivo be explicitly evaluated to determine their potential safety hazard to the people and the environment where the study is taking place. Traditional chemotherapies have chemical hazards associated with them and ABSL2 precautions should be standard when studies involve the use of immunotherapy regimens that involve viral vectors and antibody therapies.

REGULATORY ASPECTS OF ANIMAL USE FOR THE DEVELOPMENT AND EVALUATION OF PDX TUMORS

For propagating or evaluating the PDX tumor in an animal model there are additional regulatory requirements that the project must adhere to for ensuring the humane care and treatment of the animals throughout the study and verifying that there are no alternatives to the use of animals. In most countries, the use of animals in research is regulated by local, national, and international standards. Many countries employ the use of an Oversight Body/Institutional Animal Care and Use Committee (IACUC) at the institutional level to oversee animal studies and ensure that all requirements have been considered.

Institutional Animal Care and Use Committee

The first guidance document in the United States to introduce the concept of an IACUC recommendation was the 1963 *Guide for the Care and Use of Laboratory Animals* published by the US Department of Health, Education and Welfare, Public Health Service (PHS). This document gave guidance on the composition and responsibilities of the committee for oversight of animal research and has been revised several times with the most recent version being the 8th edition.[19] The first federal US laws regulating the use of animals in research were established by US Congress through the passage of the Laboratory Animal Welfare Act in 1966 and a significant amendment in 1985 with the "Improved Standards for Laboratory Animals Act." This amendment required the Chief Executive Officer of each research facility to appoint an IACUC consisting of at least three members including a doctor of veterinary medicine and one member unaffiliated with the institution. This act also assigned the IACUC as responsible for ensuring compliance with the Animal Welfare Act (AWA).[20] (Note: Currently the AWA excludes the use of rats and mice bred for research, so it does not directly impact the PDX models that are most commonly used, but as new models in different species develop it may become more relevant.)

In parallel to the development of the AWA, the PHS Policy was being formulated in 1971 by the NIH which is a division under the PHS of the United States. This Policy currently requires that any institution that receives federal funding must provide written assurance of its compliance and describe (1) The Institutional Animal Care and Use Program, (2) The Institutional Status [Association for Assessment and Accreditation of Laboratory Animal Care International (AAALAC International) accredited or nonaccredited], and (3) the IACUC composition which must contain at least five members and be composed of a veterinarian with program responsibility, a practicing scientist, a nonscientist, and an unaffiliated member.[21]

Another set of important guidelines is the US Government Principles for the Utilization and Care of Vertebrate Animals Used in Testing, Research and Training that were developed in 1985.[22] This document stresses the importance of compliance with federal laws and has nine principles which cover the requirements regarding (1) transportation; (2) relevance to human or animal health; (3) the advancement of knowledge, or the good of society, use of alternatives, and justification of numbers; (4) minimization of pain and distress; (5) use of sedation, anesthesia, or analgesia as appropriate; (6) humane end points; (7) living conditions appropriate for the species; (8) training and qualifications of personnel performing the procedure; and that (9) any exceptions to principles (1–8) should be reviewed by an oversight body such as the IACUC for justification. These fundamental guidelines serve as a point of reference for the Guide and the PHS policy and emphasize the important role of the IACUC in the evaluation of the animal research models.

In addition to the federal laws and guidance documents listed above, a private nonprofit organization, AAALAC, was formed in the United States in 1965 with a mission to accredit animal care and use programs worldwide.[23] AAALAC site visitors do triennial site visits to facilities and provide a peer-reviewed evaluation of the animal care program at a specific institution. Although AAALAC accreditation is not a requirement, it is considered a standard of high-quality animal care across the globe.

In summary, animal research in the United States is primarily regulated, overseen, or influenced by the (1) Guide for the Care and Use of Laboratory Animals, (2) Animal Welfare Act, (3) PHS Policy, (4) Government Principles, and (5) AAALAC. In addition, there may be additional funding/regulatory agencies such as the Department of Defense, Veterans Administration, Good Laboratory Practices, private industry, or nonprofit organizations that may have specific requirements. The IACUC is the oversight body in the United States that ensures compliance with these relevant guidelines and regulations.

Oversight Bodies for Other Countries

Other countries have similar structures to the United States such as Canada with the Canadian Council on Animal Care and its requirement for an Animal Care Committee.[24] In Europe, the Council of Europe and the European Union have developed regulations and policies that oversee the use of laboratory animals and rely on the Animal Welfare Body for institutional oversight[25]; the Australian and New Zealand Council for the Care of Animals in Research and Teaching[26] require an Animal Ethics Committee to provide oversight. Most countries have some sort of oversight of animals used in research, but the specific regulations may vary slightly.[27] A common theme across countries in their evaluation of the use of animals in research is a requirement for a clear explanation of how the principles of reduction, refinement, and replacement (known as the "3R's") have been incorporated and considered in the design and evaluation of the scientific question.[28] In the context of PDX models, it is very important to demonstrate that the appropriate number of animals will be used to address the scientific question, pain and distress will be minimized, and alternatives to the use of animals have been considered and supported by a narrative.

Protocol Assessment

In the United States, in order for the IACUC to assess alignment with the regulations, guidance, and policies listed above, a protocol form is created that can capture the important information for assessment and approval of an animal study. An animal care protocol should address the following components[19]:

Protocol Component	Example for PDX Tumor
1. Rationale and purpose	Detailed description of why this particular PDX tumor is being evaluated in animals and goal of the study.
2. Step-by-step description of the procedure	Time line description of implantation of PDX tumor and evaluation of growth and potential treatment. The animal protocol must allow the IACUC/OB (oversight body) to understand all phases of the in vivo studies and impact on the animals through the entire in-life phase.
3. Alternatives, avoidance of unnecessary duplication	Description of alternatives search or assessment of why alternatives cannot be used. Verify no duplication of research.
4. Animal species and numbers justification	Specify species—justification of experimental numbers is required (statistical justification when possible).
5. Nonstandard housing requirements	Note if special housing requirements are needed (ie, special bedding, single housing, or other requirements).
6. Harm versus benefit analysis	Clear explanation of the harm to the animal and the benefit of the work to understanding and treating the type of cancer the PDX tumor represents.
7. Sedation, anesthesia, analgesia	Any sedatives, anesthesia, or analgesia required throughout the experiment must be documented—dose, frequency, and duration.
8. Surgery description	If surgery is being performed for tumor implant or catheter placement, then describe completely.
9. Postprocedural care	Describe care of the animal following tumor inoculation, surgery, or treatment with therapeutics. Explain how tumors will be monitored.
10. End points	Describe end points of the study as anticipated.
11. Intervention for unexpected outcomes	Describe interventions if there are unexpected outcomes from the tumor (size, ulceration, metastasis[a]), treatment, or surgery.
12. Euthanasia or disposition	Criteria for euthanasia and also euthanasia method to be used when animals have reached their end point.
13. Training of personnel	List all personnel on the protocol and verify training.
14. Hazardous agents/ Occupational health	List potentially hazardous agents—tumors, chemotherapies, as listed under section "Occupational and Environmental Health Regulations When Working With PDX Tumors".

[a]Most institutions have a tumor policy that specifies limits on the tumor size, metastasis, and ulceration characteristics that would be permissible. Refer to Section II, Chapter 7 Veterinary Care.

The IACUC will review and approve the Protocol based on the institutions standards and the standard approval cycle is for a duration of 3 years. There is a requirement for postapproval monitoring of the animal activities after approval, so the IACUC needs to have a mechanism in place for continuous monitoring to ensure that the study is in alignment with the protocol. If changes need to be made in between the triennial review processes, then an amendment/significant change request should be submitted to the IACUC that specifies the change that needs to be made. In addition, the IACUC has responsibility for reviewing the animal care and use program and inspecting the animal facilities semiannually.

Other Regulations

There are other regulatory agencies that may need to be considered when working with PDX models. If the investigator is required to provide analgesics to the animals, they may require a Drug Enforcement Administration registration and, depending on the state, a state-controlled substance registration.[29] Since many novel therapies may be in association with start-up or for-profit companies conflict of interest must be properly considered and addressed.

Working Across Borders

As the use of PDX tumors is expanding and international collaborations are relatively commonplace, it is important to ensure that all the proper regulations have been considered for each study. For example, a PDX animal model that receives federal funding from the United States would be subject to PHS Policy regulations even if all or a portion of the study is performed at a foreign institution. Other countries may have similar requirements, and it is important to continue to stay diligent and informed as regulations evolve. There is an effort for international harmonization of standards through organizations such as the International Council for Laboratory Animal Science[27] that will make it much more manageable in the future to work globally with our colleagues.

ACKNOWLEDGMENT

The authors thank Mr. Jonathan Henriksen for assistance with preparing figures.

REFERENCES

1. Summary of the HIPAA privacy rule. Available at: http://www.hhs.gov/hipaa/for-professionals/privacy/laws-regulations/index.html. [accessed 15.03.16].
2. Guidance for industry and FDA staff, In Vitro Diagnostic (IVD) device studies – frequently asked questions. Available at: http://www.fda.gov/downloads/MedicalDevices/.../ucm071230.pdf. [accessed 15.03.16].
3. The Belmont report. Available at: http://www.hhs.gov/ohrp/humansubjects/guidance/belmont.html. [accessed 15.03.16].
4. Informed consent for in vitro diagnostic device studies using leftover human specimens that are not individually identifiable. Available at: http://www.fda.gov/MedicalDevices/DeviceRegulationandGuidance/GuidanceDocuments/ucm078384.htm. [accessed 15.03.16].
5. How can covered entities use and disclose protected health information for research and comply with the privacy rule? Available at: https://privacyruleandresearch.nih.gov/pr_08.asp. [accessed 15.03.16].

6. Cucoranu IC, Parwani AV, West AJ, Romero-Lauro G, Nauman K, Carter AB, et al. Privacy and security of patient data in the pathology laboratory. *J Pathol Inf* 2013;**4**:4. PMID:23599904.
7. Who must comply with HIPAA privacy standards? Available at: http://www.hhs.gov/hipaa/for-professionals/faq/190/who-must-comply-with-hipaa-privacy-standards/index.html. [accessed 15.03.16].
8. National Cancer Institute Biorepositories and Biospecimen Research Branch, Glossary of terms. Available at: http://biospecimens.cancer.gov/bestpractices/got/#H. [accessed 15.03.16].
9. United States Department of Health & Human Services, Notice of Proposed rulemaking 2015-summary. Available at: http://www.hhs.gov/ohrp/humansubjects/regulations/nprm-2015summary.html. [accessed 15.03.16].
10. Public Law 100-578, 100th Congress. Available at: http://www.gpo.gov/fdsys/pkg/STATUTE-102/pdf/STATUTE-102-Pg2903.pdf. [accessed 15.03.16].
11. CLIA Program; Approval of the College of American Pathologists. Available at: http://www.gpo.gov/fdsys/pkg/FR-1995-02-09/pdf/95-3165.pdf#page=1. [accessed 15.03.16].
12. College of American Pathologists Biorepository Checklist item BAP.02400. Available for purchase from the College of American Pathologists at: http://www.cap.org/web/home/lab/accreditation/accreditation-checklists?_afrLoop=11972692687799 4#!%40%40%3F_afrLoop%3D119726926877994%26_adf.ctrl-state%3Dddh1tx5w6_55.
13. College of American Pathologists Biorepository Checklist item ANP.12500. Available for purchase from the College of American Pathologists at: http://www.cap.org/web/home/lab/accreditation/accreditation-checklists?_afrLoop=119726926877994#!%40%40%3F_afrLoop%3D119726926877994%26_adf.ctrl-state%3Dddh1tx5w6_55.
14. *Laboratory biosafety manual*. 3rd ed. Geneva: World Health Organization; 2004. Available at: http://www.who.int/csr/resources/publications/biosafety/WHO_CDS_CSR_LYO_2004_11/en/. [accessed 15.03.16].
15. OSHA's Bloodborne Pathogens Standard. Available at: https://www.osha.gov/OshDoc/data_BloodborneFacts/bbfact01.html. [accessed 12.03.16].
16. *Biosafety in Microbiological and Biomedical Laboratories (BMBL)*. 5th ed. March 13, 2015. Available at: http://www.cdc.gov/biosafety/publications/bmbl5/?ref=driverlayer.com. [accessed 12.03.16].
17. Biosafety, Institutional Biosafety Committees. Available at: http://osp.od.nih.gov/office-biotechnology-activities/biosafety/institutional-biosafety-committees. [accessed 12.03.16].
18. New OSHA Hazard Communication Standards. Available at: http://www.usfosha.com/osha-articles/new-OSHA-hazard-communication-standards.aspx. [accessed 12.03.16].
19. Guide for the care and use of laboratory animals, 8th ed. 2011; Available at: http://www.nap.edu/catalog/12910/guide-for-the-care-and-use-of-laboratory-animals-eighth. [accessed 12.03.16].
20. AWA. Animal Welfare Act of 1966 (Pub. L. 89-544) and subsequent amendments 1966. US Code vol. 7:2131-2157 et seq. http://awic.nal.usda.gov/government-and-professional-resources/federal-laws/animal-welfare-act. [accessed 12.03.16].
21. Office of Laboratory Animal Welfare, National Institutes of health, Public Health Service. *PHA policy, public health service policy on humane care and use of laboratory animals*. 2002.
22. Office of Science and Technology Policy. U.S. Government principles for the utilization and care of vertebrate animals used in testing, research and training. *Fed Regist* May 20, 1985;**50**(97). Available at: http://oacu.od.nih.gov/regs/USGovtPrncpl.htm. [accessed 12.03.16].
23. AAALAC. Available at: http://www.aaalac.org/. [accessed 12.03.16].
24. Canadian Council on Animal Care in Science. Available at: http://www.ccac.ca/en_/. [accessed 12.03.16].

25. Animal welfare body. Available at: http://www.hpra.ie/homepage/veterinary/scientific-animal-protection/animal-welfare-body. [accessed 12.03.16].
26. Australian and New Zealand Council for the Care of Animals in Research and Teaching. Available at: http://www.adelaide.edu.au/ANZCCART/. [accessed 12.03.16].
27. Guillén J. *Laboratory animals: regulations and recommendations for global collaborative research*. Amsterdam; Boston: Academic Press; 2014.
28. Russell WMS, Burch RL. *The principles of humane experimental technique*. Originally published by Methuen & Co. Ltd, London, reprinted in 1960 by Charles C. Thomas, Springfield, Illinois. 1959.
29. Title 21-food and drugs, Chapter 13-Drug abuse prevention and control. From the U.S. Government Printing Office. http://www.deadiversion.usdoj.gov/21cfr/21usc/index.html. [accessed 12.03.16].

Chapter 2

Acquisition and Storage of Clinical Samples to Establish PDX Models

M. Mattar, O. Abdel-Wahab, E. de Stanchina
Memorial Sloan Kettering Cancer Center, New York, NY, United States

COORDINATION

A number of different teams are involved in patient sample selection and acquisition; therefore, both training and coordination of the efforts of all groups involved in the program is of paramount importance to its success (Fig. 2.1).

For clinical sample acquisition, an approved institutional review board (IRB) protocol is necessary (see Section II, Chapter 1). Depending on the institution, the IRB protocol is prepared either by the hospital administration, a service core, or the principal investigator who is also in charge of the Institutional Animal Care and Use Committee (IACUC) protocol. Physicians and other professionals, such as research assistants (RAs), take care of informing prospective patients and have them consent to the correct protocol; surgeons, radiologists, pathologists, and other clinicians then need to be notified of the upcoming cases and of the modality for sample collection and retrieval. In some institutions, the whole process of collecting and delivering samples as per request may be performed by a service core (Table 2.1).

On the research side, investigators take care of IACUC protocol approvals (see Chapter 1) and determining criteria for patient selection, while skilled technical staff are in charge of sample processing, implantation, and characterization. Additional resources are then needed to make sure that clinical annotations are accurate and databases properly maintained.

Given the multiplicity of components involved in sample identification and acquisition alone, the designation of a dedicated professional, such as an RA, to spearhead coordination efforts becomes crucial.

Patient Derived Tumor Xenograft Models. http://dx.doi.org/10.1016/B978-0-12-804010-2.00008-4

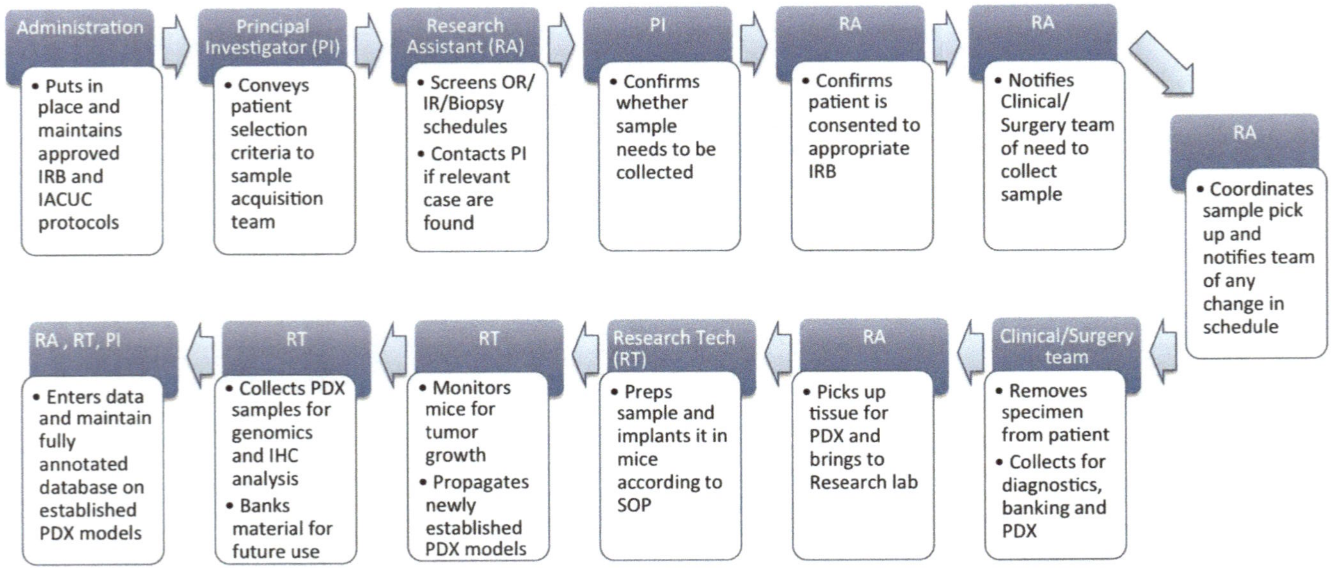

FIGURE 2.1 Flow chart detailing the necessary steps which need to be in place for the successful acquisition and processing of clinical samples in the establishment of PDX models.

TABLE 2.1 Clinical and Research Personnel Involved in Clinical Sample Acquisition and Processing

Role	Task
Administrator, PI	IRB compliance
IRB consenting professional	IRB patient consent
Dedicated research assistant or PI	Screening of cases of interest
Treating physician or physician assistant	Place request for specimen
Surgeons, radiologists, other clinicians	Sample collection procedure
Pathologists	Pathology assessment
Research assistant or research technician	Sample retrieval and transport
Research technician	Sample processing
PI or administrator	IACUC compliance
Research technician	Sample implantation and propagation
Research technician	Sample storage and distribution
PI, research technician	Data acquisition and analysis
Research assistant, research technician, IT technician	Database annotation and maintenance

IT, information technology; *PI*, principal investigator.

Equally important is the development and implementation of standard operating procedures (SOPs) to make sure personnel both on the clinical and research sides are properly trained and instructed in relevant procedures and practices so that samples are collected and processed in a documented and reproducible way.

The establishment of clear SOPs and common training programs can also help bridge knowledge gaps between basic scientists and hospital personnel and foster open communication, ultimately resulting in a more efficient and cost-effective effort.

SCREENING

Prospective selection of patients presents a challenge because it is neither feasible nor logical to attempt the establishment of patient-derived xenograft (PDX) models for every patient. Rather, patient selection is based on the interests of the investigator, and most commonly focuses on patients with disease subtypes for which treatment options do not exist or have been exhausted, or for which no current laboratory models exist.

Thus, a system for identifying samples of interest must be put into place. Investigators wishing to develop PDX models for their research will need to specify which type of patient samples they wish to obtain (tumor type, location, stage, treatment status, mutation profile). Once selection criteria have been established, samples of interest can be identified by screening the schedules for upcoming surgical resections, endoscopies, biopsies, or fluids collections (blood, ascites, and pleural effusions). Depending on the volume of samples, an individual dedicated to screening and sample pickup may be needed. Moreover, physicians, including those not directly involved with the research, assist in the prospective selection of patients by utilizing their clinical expertise to flag samples from treatment-naive patients, chemoresistant patients, and patients with unique molecular profiles. In addition, the physicians deem whether the additional tissue collection needed for PDXs is clinically safe and feasible.

In addition to satisfying patient safety concerns and investigator criteria, other factors determine whether a specimen is suitable for collection. For example, concurring conditions (such as infectious diseases that can be transmitted to the mouse, pose a risk to research personnel, or interfere with tumor take) may be the cause of concern, and may in the end lead to the exclusion of that specific patient.

Furthermore, specimens have minimum size requirements. For core needle biopsies, the lesion should be at least 1.5–2 cm, which would allow for at least two cores for PDXs in addition to the ones needed for diagnostic purposes. Although the importance of tissue quality surpasses the importance of tissue quantity, it is recommended that a minimum of two cores, approximately 10 mm in length, are obtained for implantation. Although core needle biopsies are the preferred method of noninvasive tissue acquisition since they allow for the sampling of a greater amount of tumor tissue, there have been instances of tissue being collected for PDXs from fine-needle aspirations.[1,2] Punch biopsies, which produce a 3- to 4-mm cylindrical core of tissue, are often used to obtain samples of cutaneous malignancies.[3,4] Similarly, samples of cancers of the gastrointestinal tract can be obtained via endoscopic procedures, which yield cores that are 2–3 mm.[3] Since these tissue samples are smaller than their core needle biopsy counterparts, four to six cores should be collected for PDX implantation.

For hematological malignancies, the likelihood of disease engraftment depends on the type of disease as well as the source material (peripheral blood, bone marrow, tissue biopsy) in addition to concerns regarding sample quality and quantity. Certain hematological malignancies are well known to be very challenging to achieve durable engraftment in immunocompromised mice, including NOD-SCID-gamma (NSG) mice, unrelated to initial sample considerations. In some cases, for example, with chronic lymphocytic leukemia, this is thought to be due to immunological barriers, which are incompletely understood.[5] In other cases, such as with the myelodysplastic syndromes, purification of hematopoietic stem cells[6] with potential inclusion of mesenchymal stromal cells[7] is known to be necessary to achieve engraftment. For other disorders, such as acute lymphoblastic leukemia and acute myeloid leukemias, achievement of PDX models in NSG mice has been well demonstrated and the likelihood of engraftment largely depends on the percentage of leukemic cells in the sample used for engraftment, the total cell number injected, and the method of engraftment (intrafemoral vs intraperitoneal). Generally at least 5 mL of appropriately anticoagulated peripheral blood or bone marrow aspirate blood is necessary to obtain sufficient mononuclear cell numbers from acute leukemia patients for engraftment in mice (but blast percentage is essential in determining the likelihood of engraftment).

When dealing with samples from surgical tumor resections, the lesion should be at least 2 cm, so sample acquisition for PDX will not interfere with the diagnostic analysis of the tumor.

Once a case is identified, the patient needs to sign the appropriate IRB-approved tissue acquisition consent forms. As mentioned above, coordination with both the disease management team and laboratory personnel prior to sample acquisition is integral to a successful PDX program. Ideally, a memo should be conveyed to all relevant parties days ahead of the procedure, detailing specific instructions for each team. The surgeon or interventional radiologist and their support staff, along with pathologists and their diagnostic team, need to be informed of the intricacies of the PDX collection protocols and should be made aware of specific collection conditions, tissue requirements, and the contact information for specimen pickup.

Similarly, laboratory personnel need to be notified in advance to ensure the availability of a technician with the necessary expertise to process and implant patient samples, as well as an adequate inventory of reagents and immunocompromised mice.

COLLECTION

While all specimens should be collected in aseptic conditions and processed as expeditiously as possible, specific protocols for sample collection and processing vary widely depending on the nature of the sample.

- *Surgical samples*: When surgical samples are small or diagnostic information is rapidly needed, specimens are usually sent to the pathology laboratory in sterile conditions immediately following resection. After the tissue is allocated for diagnostic and patient care uses, if enough viable tumor material exists in the remaining tissue, it can be used for PDXs. However, in cases where there are numerous related lesions or large tumors, samples can be allocated for PDX purposes intraoperatively.
- *Biopsies*: Once cores biopsies have been collected for diagnostic and therapeutic protocol purposes and deemed adequate by touch imprint cytology, additional cores can be taken for PDX.

- *Autopsies*: Wherever a "rapid autopsy program" is available, samples can also be collected from patients recently deceased. This is a very complex process that requires an additional level of coordination. Indeed, in addition to the medical staff, a number of different parties, both within the hospital (morgue, security, legal department) and outside (family members, medical examiner, funeral home) need to be involved to ensure that samples can be collected as quickly as possible.

  The initial discussion for possible patient enrollment in the study and informed consent usually takes place prior to patient death with the patient and next of kin. The final permission for autopsy remains in the hands of the patient's next of kin at the time of death. The first steps involved in carrying out a rapid autopsy procedure depend on patient location at the time of death. For patients who do not die at the hospital, timely notification of patient death is necessary to make sure that hospital personnel can start coordinating efforts to transport the body to the hospital and assemble the autopsy team within hours from the time of death. Special consideration must also be taken if the patient passed away at a facility located in another state or province, as each jurisdiction has varying guidelines on the paperwork required to transport bodies across borders. For patients who happen to die while hospitalized, this process is slightly simplified as the coordination efforts are limited to the attending physicians caring for the patient at the time of death, the morgue staff, and the research team. Tissue harvesting protocols typically consist of sampling of primary and metastatic lesions, along with some corresponding normal tissue and possibly blood samples. The collected samples are divided into aliquots that will be preserved and processed differently depending on the intended use [biobank, PDX, genomic analysis, immunohistochemistry (IHC), etc.]. A standard complete diagnostic autopsy (minus any restrictions specified in the consent form) may be performed immediately after tissue harvesting.[8]

  Rapid autopsies provide an invaluable method for tissue acquisition, especially for advanced diseases. Specifically, patients with widely disseminated disease often never undergo tumor resection; therefore, access to high-quality tumor samples from which reliable disease models can be generated is severely limited. Moreover, the ability to obtain substantially sized samples from numerous metastatic sites enhances the researchers' ability to systematically examine the cellular and molecular mechanisms that facilitate metastasis formation.[9,10]
- *Fluids*: Pleural and pericardial effusions, ascites, and bone marrow have been proved to be a valuable source of tumor cells due to their highly cellular nature. In fact, PDXs established by ascitic or pleural effusion samples often have a better take rate than the corresponding solid tumor sample.[11]
- *Blood*: For hematological malignancies, the likelihood of engraftment is related to the frequency of disease-initiating cells located in the tissue compartment being sampled and is disease dependent. For acute leukemias,

the hematological disorders in which generation of PDX models is most established, the likelihood of engraftment is most related to blast percentage and cell numbers collected. In some cases where blasts may be most enriched in bone marrow, use of bone marrow aspirate blood to collect leukemic blasts may therefore be more likely to result in successful engraftment than a similar volume of peripheral blood.

In general, surgical, biopsy, and autopsy samples should be placed in sterile media (see Table 2.2) and promptly transported to the laboratory in a cooler or on ice. Fluid samples are treated with heparin (1 mL heparin per liter of fluid) immediately following the evacuation from the patient, in order to curtail clotting and facilitate sample processing. More details on fluid sample processing can be found in Section II, Chapter 3.

In all cases, to ensure optimal engraftment rate, time is of essence. Indeed, it has been reported that prolonged "warm ischemia" (extended surgical time) and "cold ischemia" (extended time between sample resection and implantation), both adversely correlate with PDX engraftment rate.[12] Ideally, samples should be processed for implantation or storage within 30 min to 1 h of when they are collected. In case of autopsies, concerted efforts must be made so that, despite all technical and bureaucratic complexities, samples can be retrieved ideally within 8–12 h postmortem, due to the rapid decrease in cell viability following patient death.[8]

When specimens cannot be processed and implanted immediately, for example, because they are obtained from late night surgeries or shipped from outside parties, they should be placed in media that are deemed best at preserving cell viability. For instance, HypoThermosol (Biolife Solution) or similar media are purported to maximize storage stability by mitigating temperature-induced molecular cell stress response that occurs as a result of chilling and rewarming of biological material. Samples preserved in such fashion can be implanted up to 48 h from the time of explant. In our experience, this is preferable to sample cryopreservation. However, if extenuating circumstances prevent a sample from being implanted within 48 h, samples can be placed in freezing media (see Table 2.2) and stored in liquid nitrogen in an effort to preserve the vitality of the tumor cells until they can be thawed and implanted at a later time.[13] A direct comparison between take rate of the same samples when implanted immediately after resection and after cryopreservation has shown that frozen samples would only form tumors in about 50% of the cases.[12] However, tumor samples cryopreserved and stored in biobanks can still provide a very valuable source of material that can be accessed retrospectively.

DISTRIBUTION AND STORAGE

Upon collection, tumor samples may need to be distributed to different departments for research (PDX, organoids, cell lines, genomics, proteomics, histology,

TABLE 2.2 Sample Size Requirements and Recommended Collection and Storage Media for Clinical Specimens

Sample Type	Minimum Sample Size	Collection Media	Long-Term Storage Media
Surgical sample	$0.5\,cm^3$	Sterile 0.9% NaCl, or sterile media such as RPMI 1640 or DMEM, 20% FBS and antibiotics, or HypoThermosol	Up to 48 h: store at 4°C in sterile HypoThermosol; more than 48 h: store in liquid nitrogen in CryoStor or freezing media (90% FBS, 10% DMSO)
Core needle biopsy	At least two cores, 10 mm in length	Sterile 0.9% NaCl, or sterile media such as RPMI 1640 or DMEM, 20% FBS and antibiotics, or HypoThermosol	Up to 48 h: store at 4°C in sterile HypoThermosol; more than 48 h: Store in liquid nitrogen in CryoStor® or freezing media (90% FBS, 10% DMSO)
Punch biopsy	3–4 mm	Sterile 0.9% NaCl, or sterile media such as RPMI 1640 or DMEM, 20% FBS and antibiotics, or HypoThermosol	Up to 48 h: store at 4°C in sterile HypoThermosol; more than 48 h: store in liquid nitrogen in CryoStor or freezing media (90% FBS, 10% DMSO)
Whole blood (leukemia)	At least 5 mL anticoagulated peripheral blood	Tubes containing sodium heparin or EDTA	MNCs are prepared from whole blood following Ficoll density gradient separation and RBC lysis. MNCs are then saved viably in CryoStor or freezing media (90% FBS, 10% DMSO)
Whole blood (CTCs)	At least 5 mL anticoagulated peripheral blood	Tubes containing sodium heparin or EDTA	CTCs are purified from blood MNCs through a variety of methods and then may be utilized for engraftment directly or saved viably in CryoStor or freezing media (90% FBS, 10% DMSO)
Bone marrow	At least 5 mL anticoagulated bone marrow aspirate blood	Tubes containing sodium heparin or EDTA	MNCs are prepared from bone marrow aspirate blood following Ficoll density gradient separation and RBC lysis or directly following RBC lysis alone. MNCs are then saved viably in freezing media (90% FBS, 10% DMSO) or CryoStor
Effusions/ascites	At least 1000 cells	Add 1% heparin to collected fluids	Not recommended

CTC, circulating tumor cells; *DMEM*, Dulbecco's modified eagle medium; *DMSO*, dimethyl sulfoxide; *EDTA*, ethylenediaminetetraacetic acid; *FBS*, fetal bovine serum; *MNCs*, mononuclear cells; *RBCs*, red blood cells.

cytology) or banking purposes. This task is potentially problematic when specimens are small, as there may not be enough material for all purposes. It is therefore recommended that, before sample is collected, all involved agree on a prioritization list, as to avoid any delays or confusion related to tissue distribution in case of limited material.

On the other hand, in case tissue size is not a limiting factor, a portion of the specimen can also be fixed in 10% buffered formalin or equivalent for genomics or IHC analysis, flash frozen in liquid nitrogen for biochemical or genomic assays, and viably frozen as tissue or upon processing into single-cell suspension.

In case of leukemia specimens, blood separation for collection of mononuclear cells is necessary for viable storage of cells, further cell purifications, or direct engraftment.

If feasible, it is also recommended that normal tissue should be collected alongside the tumor specimen. For nonhematologic cancers, blood can serve as the source for normal tissue and germline DNA, but buccal swabs and fingernail clippings can also be considered, especially for cases involving hematological malignancies.

Although blood is a strong source of material for DNA sequencing, its use for RNA sequencing can be problematic due to the variation in messenger RNA expression among different tissue types. Ideally, a sample from a nondiseased portion of the same tissue from which the tumor sample is obtained should be collected and banked for RNA sequencing.

When blood is collected, whenever possible, it should be viably preserved, as this allows for a broader range of analyses.

Banking of normal and tumor tissue, although expensive, is generally a good investment, as models are much more valuable when PDX tumors can be compared with the corresponding patient normal and tumor tissue. For this reason, whenever possible, normal tissue samples should be banked at the time of tumor collection as subsequent access to tissue can be limited by patients lost to follow-up, transfer of care, or death.

Importantly, it is imperative that a system is in place that will allow easy retrieval of banked samples whenever needed. Records should be kept on the amount of sample and preservation method, along with clinical annotations. Ideally, this information would be stored in a comprehensive database containing thorough patient annotations and experimental data. Database creation and management will be covered in Section II, Chapter 6.

Processing of samples for implantation in mice varies greatly, depending on the tissue of origin, sample size, site, and modality of implantation. This will be discussed in detail in Section II, Chapter 3.

ACKNOWLEDGMENTS

The authors received support through grants P30 CA008748 and U54 OD020355-01 and from the Geoffrey Beene Cancer Research Center.

REFERENCES

1. Anderson WC, Boyd MB, Aguilar J, Pickell B, Laysang A, Pysz MA, et al. Initiation and characterization of small cell lung cancer patient-derived xenografts from ultrasound-guided transbronchial needle aspirates. *PLoS One* 2015;**10**:e0125255.
2. Jang SY, Bae HI, Lee IK, Park HK, Cho CM. Successful xenograft of endoscopic ultrasound-guided fine-needle aspiration specimen from human extrahepatic cholangiocarcinoma into an immunodeficient mouse. *Gut Liver* 2015;**9**:805–8.
3. Turk DJ, Kozarek RA, Botoman VA, Patterson DJ, Ball TJ. Disposable endoscopic biopsy forceps: comparison with standard forceps of sample size and adequacy of specimen. *J Clin Gastroenterol* 1991;**13**:76–8.
4. Zuber TJ. Punch biopsy of the skin. *Am Fam Physician* 2002;**65**:1155–8. 61-2, 64.
5. Bertilaccio MT, Scielzo C, Simonetti G, Ten Hacken E, Apollonio B, Ghia P, et al. Xenograft models of chronic lymphocytic leukemia: problems, pitfalls and future directions. *Leukemia* 2013;**27**:534–40.
6. Pang WW, Pluvinage JV, Price EA, Sridhar K, Arber DA, Greenberg PL, et al. Hematopoietic stem cell and progenitor cell mechanisms in myelodysplastic syndromes. *Proc Natl Acad Sci U S A* 2013;**110**:3011–6.
7. Medyouf H, Mossner M, Jann JC, Nolte F, Raffel S, Herrmann C, et al. Myelodysplastic cells in patients reprogram mesenchymal stromal cells to establish a transplantable stem cell niche disease unit. *Cell Stem Cell* 2014;**14**:824–37.
8. Embuscado EE, Laheru D, Ricci F, Yuni KJ, Witzell SD, Seigel A, et al. Immortalizing the complexity of cancer metastasis genetic features of lethal metastatic pancreatic cancer obtained from rapid autopsy. *Cancer Biol Ther* 2005;**4**:548–54.
9. Rubin MA, Putzi M, Mucci N, Smith DC, Wojno K, Korenchuk S, et al. Rapid ("warm") autopsy study for procurement of metastatic prostate cancer. *Clin Cancer Res Official J Am Assoc Cancer Res* 2000;**6**:1038–45.
10. Xie T, Musteanu M, Lopez-Casas PP, Shields DJ, Olson P, Rejto PA, et al. Whole exome sequencing of rapid autopsy tumors and xenograft models reveals possible driver mutations underlying tumor progression. *PLoS One* 2015;**10**:e0142631.
11. Verschraegen CF, Hu W, Du Y, Mendoza J, Early J, Deavers M, et al. Establishment and characterization of cancer cell cultures and xenografts derived from primary or metastatic Mullerian cancers. *Clin Cancer Res Official J Am Assoc Cancer Res* 2003;**9**:845–52.
12. Guerrera F, Tabbo F, Bessone L, Maletta F, Gaudiano M, Ercole E, et al. The influence of tissue ischemia time on RNA integrity and patient-derived xenografts (PDX) engraftment rate in a non-small cell lung cancer (NSCLC) biobank. *PLoS One* 2016;**11**:e0145100.
13. Zhang XC, Zhang JC, Li M, Huang XS, Yang XN, Zhong WZ, et al. Establishment of patient-derived non-small cell lung cancer xenograft models with genetic aberrations within EGFR, KRAS and FGFR1: useful tools for preclinical studies of targeted therapies. *J Transl Med* 2013;**11**.

Chapter 3

Methodologies for Developing and Maintaining Patient-Derived Xenograft Mouse Models

M. Mattar, O. Abdel-Wahab, J.T. Poirier, M. Scaltriti, E. de Stanchina
Memorial Sloan Kettering Cancer Center, New York, NY, United States

A supportive infrastructure including dedicated laboratory and animal facilities, regulatory approvals, skilled technical staff, and detailed standard operating procedures must already be in place at the time of sample acquisition. Details on such requirements will be discussed in Section II, Chapter 6. In this section, the methodologies involved with the processing and implantation of freshly collected tumor samples and with the maintenance and propagation of successfully established patient-derived xenograft (PDX) models will be described. In addition, the various factors that influence the likelihood of successful generation of a PDX—ranging from intrinsic properties of the patient tumor to sample handling and implantation site—will be discussed.

SAMPLE PROCESSING TECHNIQUES

Timely transportation and processing of freshly obtained specimens is crucial to maintain tumor cell viability and to allow for successful engraftment into recipient mice (see Section II, Chapter 2). Specimens should be processed and implanted in a sterile environment, such as a biosafety cabinet, to reduce the chance of bacterial and/or fungal contamination. Since these samples are derived from patients who may harbor blood-borne pathogens (see Section II, Chapter 8), it is essential that patient materials and any derived xenografts be treated in accordance with all institutional policies regarding the handling of potentially hazardous material.

Techniques for sample processing vary greatly depending on the tissue of origin and sample size (Fig. 3.1).

Tumor cells derived from fluids such as blood, pleural or pericardial effusions, and ascites are processed differently compared with samples from solid

Patient Derived Tumor Xenograft Models. http://dx.doi.org/10.1016/B978-0-12-804010-2.00009-6

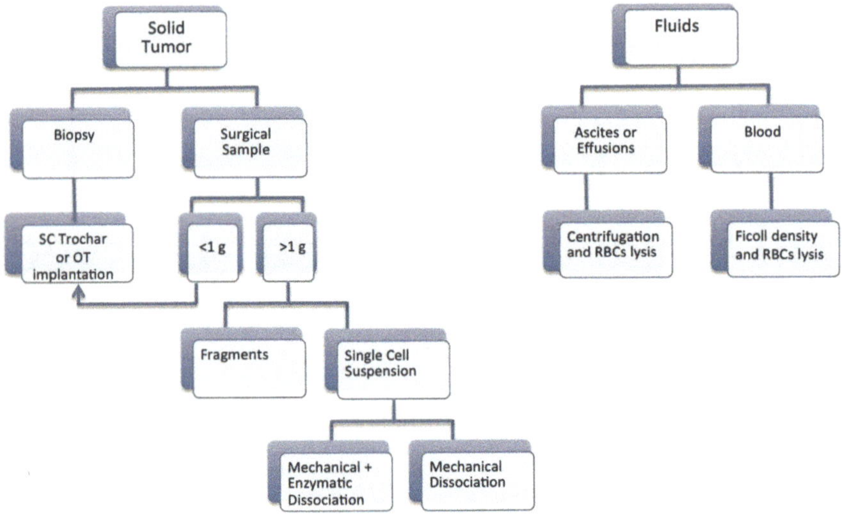

FIGURE 3.1 Processing and implantation techniques recommended based on sample origin and presentation.

tumors. Additionally, one must pay specific attention to biopsies and procedures that yield small-sized samples, due to the limitations in the amount of tumor cells that can be collected and subsequently implanted in mice. Finally, the intended implantation site and surgical techniques also dictate sample preparation. The materials and reagents needed for tissue collection, processing, and preservation are detailed in Table 3.1.

Fluids

In the case of fluids, tumor cells need to be isolated from other cell types and concentrated in a small volume, while ensuring that coagulation and cell lysis are kept to a minimum. Processing methods for samples from hematological malignancies (whole blood and bone marrow), pleural effusions, and ascites are detailed below.

Hematological Malignancies

Mononuclear cells (MNCs) are collected from peripheral blood by Ficoll density centrifugation followed by red blood cells (RBCs) lysis. MNCs can be isolated from bone marrow aspirate blood quite similarly as from peripheral blood, or may be obtained directly from RBC lysis without the preceding Ficoll separation. Depending on the planned use of the sample and disease type, unfractionated MNCs could then be used for xenografting or specific cell populations could be isolated for further purification via flow cytometric cell sorting or other means (eg, immunomagnetic cell separation).

TABLE 3.1 Media and Equipment Needed for Tissue Processing and Preservation

Technique/ Procedure	Media	Equipment
Sample collection	Tissue culture media	Cooler/ice
	Saline solution (0.9% NaCl)	Sterile containers
	PBS	Sodium heparin or ethylenediaminetetraacetic acid (EDTA)-containing tubes
	HypoThermosol	
Tissue culture	Saline solution (0.9% NaCl)	Petri dishes
	Tissue culture media with serum and antibiotics	Sterile blades, scissors, and forceps
	PBS	
Mechanical dissociation	Matrigel	Petri dishes
	Tissue culture media such as Roswell Park Memorial Institute Medium-1640 (RPMI 1640) or Dulbecco's modified Eagle medium	Sterile blades and forceps sieve with a pestle
	Saline solution (0.9% NaCl)	Conical tubes
	PBS	Centrifuge
Circulating tumor cells	Enrichment cocktail (type dependent on diagnosis)	Conical tubes
	Wash buffer (10% tissue culture media in PBS)	Centrifuge
	Ficoll–Paque Plus	
Processing ascites/pleural fluid	Heparin	Conical tubes
	Red blood cell lysis solution, ie, ammonium-chloride-potassium lysis buffer	Centrifuge
	PBS	
	Ficoll–Paque Plus	
	Matrigel	
Freezing/ preservation	Freezing media (10% DMSO + 20% FBS in media; or CryoStor)	Cryovials
		Liquid nitrogen
Enzymatic dissociation	Collagenase and hyaluronidase and trypsin/EDTA	Centrifuge
	Tumor dissociation kits (gentleMACS), which include cocktails of lysing enzymes	Conical tubes

Effusions and Ascites

Pleural and pericardial effusions and ascites (1–5 L) are collected aseptically in heparinized bottles (10 U/mL). If such bottles are not available, heparin can be added to the fluid (1 mL of heparin per liter of fluid). The bottles are centrifuged at 1500 rpm for 10 min, and washed twice with phosphate-buffered saline (PBS). If the cell pellet contains RBCs, the cells are resuspended in an RBC lysis solution (such as ammonium-chloride-potassium lysis buffer) for 5–10 min, centrifuged at 1500 rpm for 5 min, and the same steps repeated until the RBCs are no longer visible. The pellet is washed once more with PBS prior to xenografting.[1–3]

Circulating Tumor Cells

Patients with highly metastatic and aggressive tumors such as small cell lung cancer often present with high levels of circulating tumor cells (CTCs) in their blood. These levels can be in the range of hundreds to thousands of cells per milliliter, as measured by various platforms, such as Veridex's CELLSEARCH, which rely on antibody-based capture of CTCs.[4] It was reported in 2014 that these CTCs can be isolated from a blood sample and grown in immunocompromised mice.[5] These explants are referred to as CTC-derived xenografts (CDXs). This protocol describes the generation of CDXs from a clinical blood sample.[6]

1. Reserve 1 mL of whole blood and store at −20°C for germline DNA.
2. Transfer the remaining blood sample (10 mL) to a 50-mL centrifuge tube.
3. Add 500 μL CTC Enrichment Cocktail (such as RosetteSep CTC Enrichment Cocktail) containing anti-CD36 for small cell lung cancer (#15167) or anti-CD56 for breast cancer cells (#15137) to the samples, incubating for 10 min at room temperature.
4. Add an equal volume of ice-cold wash buffer (10% tissue culture media in PBS) to centrifuge tube.
5. Add 15 mL Ficoll–Paque Plus to the lower layer of a fresh 50-mL centrifuge tube.
6. Overlay the diluted blood sample on the Ficoll–Paque Plus layer.
7. Centrifuge for 20 min at 1200 relative centrifugal force (rcf).
8. Transfer the upper layer (plasma and CTC) to another centrifuge tube, add wash buffer to 50 mL.
9. Centrifuge for 10 min at 100 rcf.
10. Discard the upper layer; a pellet may not be visible.
11. Dilute the CTC with 50 μL wash buffer on ice.
12. Mix 50:50 with ice-cold Matrigel before injection.

Surgical Samples

Surgical samples are heterogeneous at the scale of gross pathology and may present with cysts, necrotic regions, and adjacent normal tissue. The viable tumor region is composed of both tumor cells and normal stromal cells that can include fibroblasts, vascular cells, and various immune infiltrates; therefore, samples need to be thoroughly examined and "cleaned" by debriding the sample of any nontumor material. Although surgeons and pathologists can assist in this, the technician responsible for sample preparation should be trained to recognize and isolate viable tumor material from adjacent normal and necrotic tissue.

Initial Sample Preparation

In general, as soon as a surgical sample arrives at the laboratory, it is placed in a Petri dish containing cold sterile saline solution (0.9% NaCl), or tissue culture media such as Roswell Park Memorial Institute Medium-1640 (RPMI-1640) or Dulbecco's modified Eagle medium, supplemented with 20% fetal bovine serum and antibiotics (see Table 3.1). Normal tissue is then excised using sterile forceps, scissors, and/or scalpels. The sample is then transferred to a new dish containing sterile media and sectioned to isolate viable tumor material. Necrotic tissue, generally characterized as dark liquefied tissue at the center of a large tumor region; cysts; and sites of hemorrhage are carefully abraded from the fully submerged sample, which is then sectioned into smaller pieces.[7]

At this point, several methods can be employed to further process the tumor specimens. Sample size and implantation method will dictate the processing protocol that should be followed. For tumor samples that are 1 g or larger, the major distinction to make is to determine whether samples should be implanted as tumor fragments, or as a single-cell suspension.

Fragments

Tumor fragments can easily be implanted both subcutaneously (SC) and orthotopically (OT) in mice. Implanting tumor fragments provide several advantages. It requires minimal manipulation of the tumor sample; therefore, loss of tumor architecture and stromal components that may be essential to tumor growth is prevented. The techniques employed to generate a single-cell suspension can be harsh resulting in the inadvertent selection of cells that are sensitized to detachment-induced apoptosis.[8] Additionally, implanting fragments is often associated with the highest take rate in multiple tumor types as it preserves the integrity and tumor heterogeneity by avoiding the stressful conditions that can occur during in vitro handling and processing.[8] Moreover, it does not require special equipment or preparation kits and it can be accomplished quickly and efficiently, limiting the risk of loss in cell viability.

In brief, tumor samples are placed in a small Petri dish with cold media and are cut into small fragments, roughly $3 \times 3 \times 3$ mm in size, and washed by gently hand agitating the dish.

If samples are intended for SC implantation, they are placed in a prechilled microcentrifuge tube along with an equal volume of Matrigel (optional). Samples are to be kept on ice and implanted in mice as soon as possible. About 10–15 fragments can be generated from a 1-g specimen. Two to three fragments are usually inserted in each implantation site (see below). Matrigel, a murine sarcoma–derived basement membrane matrix, is often utilized in tumor implantation, because it has been shown to increase engraftment efficiency.[9] This is likely due to Matrigel's structural resemblance to the complex extracellular environment and its growth factors. Tumor samples can also be implanted with human fibroblasts or mesenchymal cells to promote engraftment.[10] Of note, tumor fragments can also be preserved for long-term storage (see later), and for different applications, such as histology, nucleic acid and protein isolation, and generation of viable organoids or cell lines.[1]

Single-Cell Suspension

Tumor fragments can be further dissociated into single-cell suspensions prior to implantation. The major advantages of this technique are that single-cell suspensions can be easily injected both S.C. and OT, cell viability can be easily monitored, and specific cell subpopulations can be isolated prior to implantation. Importantly, single-cell suspensions can also be used to generate cell lines. This technique, however, tends to be more costly and time-consuming compared with implantation of simple tumor fragments, and is associated with lower tumor take rate, especially for heterogeneous tumor types.[11,12] Single-cell suspensions are usually achieved by a combination of mechanical and enzymatic dissociation procedures, as detailed below.

Mechanical Dissociation

Tissue fragments can be mechanically disrupted by either repetitive pipetting or by pressing the cells through a 600-μm sieve. In this case, the sieve is placed on top of a beaker, and tumor fragments are pressed through the sieve with a pestle. To help cells pass through the sieve, 30–50 mL of cold cell medium is poured on top of the tumor material. The content of the beaker is then poured into a 50-mL conical tube and spun at 2700 RPM for 4–5 min. The resulting cell suspension is then mixed with an equal volume of Matrigel and placed on ice until ready for implantation. The cell suspension obtained using this technique is usually composed of both single cells and cell aggregates, so it may not be suitable for intravenous injection, but can be used successfully to establish both OT and SC models.

Mechanical and Enzymatic Dissociation

Tissue fragments can be processed by mincing and enzymatic digestion with collagenase and hyaluronidase and trypsin/ethylenediaminetetraacetic acid to generate a single-cell suspension, which can then be readily implanted.[1] Tumor dissociation kits (gentleMACS), which include cocktails of lysing enzymes to be used along a mechanical dissociator, are often employed to obtain high yield of tumor cells and tumor-infiltrating lymphocytes, while preserving important cell surface epitopes.

Biopsies

Tumor material can also be obtained via core and punch biopsies and fine-needle aspirates. Due to the very limited sample size provided by these procedures, it is recommended that these specimens are implanted without additional handling. Although the risk of implanting stromal tissue is quite elevated, extensive dissociation and processing of the sample drastically reduces the number of viable tumor cells available for implantation and therefore may result in poor take rate.

IMPLANTATION TECHNIQUES

The method and site of implantation largely influences both the success rate of engraftment and the clinical relevance of a PDX model (see Tables 3.2 and 3.3).

Patient-derived samples are most commonly implanted heterotopically, usually SC in the dorsal flank of the mouse. This method of implantation is favored for logistical reasons, as it involves a simple and quick technique with low incidence of procedural complications. Additionally, it allows for easy monitoring of tumor growth and accurate measurement of tumor size. For these reasons, SC

TABLE 3.2 Heterotopic Versus Orthotopic Implantation: Advantages and Disadvantages

	Heterotopic	Orthotopic
Microenvironment	Artificial environment	Better mimics human tumor microenvironment
Heterogeneity	Dependent on tumor of origin	Dependent on tumor of origin
Metastatic potential	Seldom develop metastasis	High rate of spontaneous metastasis
Time requirements for sample implantation	Minimal	Extensive due to complex surgeries
Technical skill requirements	Minimal	Extensive due to complex surgeries
Cost	Inexpensive	Costly due to reagents, labor, and skill requirements
Assessment of tumor burden	Easily performed with calipers	Difficult, often requires specialized imaging techniques
Predictive value of patient treatment response	Good	Very good

TABLE 3.3 Factors Influencing PDX Take Rate

Potential Issues	Solutions
Hormone dependency	• Supplement mouse diet with hormones
Lack of metastasis	• Implant samples orthotopically instead of subcutaneously
Mouse illness—GVHD	• At the first sign of sickness, immediately transplant tumor into a new mouse • Implant samples into more immunodeficient mouse strain
Mouse illness, other	• At the first sign of sickness, immediately transplant tumor into a new mouse • Ensure that subpar mouse housing conditions are not causing illness • If infections frequently occur, consider prophylactic antibiotics
Sample size—limited amount of viable tumor cells available to implant	• Discuss tissue requirements with collection team to ensure tissue needs can be met
Sample quality—limited amount of viable tumor cells available to implant	• Minimize sample processing as to curtail loss of viable cells
Slow growth rate	• Implant samples into more immunodeficient mouse strain • Change method of implantation to orthotopic or subrenal capsule implantation
Time	• Ensure that all framework is in place before sample collection in an effort to minimize the unnecessary loss of time

xenografts are commonly used in studies aimed at identifying cytotoxic compounds and determining the early therapeutic efficacy of novel compounds.

On the other hand, heterotopic models may fail to most accurately represent both the primary sites and metastatic behavior of the human cancer since heterotopic xenografts are very rarely metastatic.[13,14] Additionally, heterotopic models may not be the best predictors of clinical response, as sensitivity to drugs and radiation therapy may be modulated by the tumor microenvironment.[15,16]

To circumvent these issues and generate more physiologically relevant models, tumor samples can be implanted OT into their anatomical site of origin. OT models often have high rates of spontaneous metastasis and are generally considered to more closely recapitulate the human disease and therefore be more appropriate indicators of response to therapy.[17]

Despite their advantages, OT models are substantially more expensive, labor intensive, and technically challenging to generate and may require the regular use of small animal imaging modalities, such as ultrasound, computed tomography, magnetic resonance imaging, and positron emission tomography, to keep track of tumor growth. Given that tumor progression cannot be easily monitored, it can be difficult to evaluate their response to therapy and define study end points without specialized imaging equipment.[18]

Subrenal capsule implantation is often recommended in lieu of OT implantation for "hard-to-transplant" specimens.[15,19] This relatively easy procedure is reported to yield high engraftment rates, possibly due to the fact that transplanted tissues are well contained under the renal capsule in a highly vascularized site.[20,21] Surgical techniques for implantation of tumor samples SC, in the renal capsule, and OT in the stomach wall, in the lung, and in the mammary fat pad are described in the following discussion. Additional surgery techniques are described in Section III.

In all cases, surgical procedures should be carried out by trained personnel, with the approval of the institutional regulatory body (for example, Institutional Animal Care and Use Committee, in the United States). Additionally, universal precautions for blood-borne pathogens during tissue procurement, processing, and surgical procedures should be maintained at all times. Surgeries should be conducted in an aseptic environment with sterilized instruments in an high-efficiency particulate air-filtered laminar flow hood.

Some of the commonly used implantation techniques are described in the following discussion. Please note, OT implantation procedures vary depending on the organ and tumor; however, surgical access of body cavities remain very similar, with minor variation depending on the location of the specific organ (for example, abdominal incision for stomach is more proximal compared to the incision for accessing prostate, which is more distal). Aseptic techniques should be utilized for all survival surgical procedures in animals, which includes hair removal and disinfection of the surgical site, use of sterile gloves and instruments, and use of practices that maintain a sterile surgical field. Most institutions have policies in place that require the use of accepted veterinary practices for animal anesthesia, pain relief, intraoperative monitoring, and postoperative care.

Subcutaneous Implantation

1. The animal should be anesthetized and prepared for surgery following institutional guidelines.
2. Using sterile surgical scissors, make a 5- to 10-mm vertical skin incision on the flank.
3. Insert a straight forceps gently 2 cm into the SC space to create a pocket large enough for a tumor fragment.
4. Using sterile straight forceps insert the tumor fragment previously prepared.

5. Close the skin incision using sutures, clips, or tissue glue.
6. Animals should be provided postoperative care and monitoring according to institutional guidelines.

Orthotopic Implantation in the Gastric Wall[13]

This technique can be applied to implantation in most organs accessible via laparotomy.

1. The animal should be anesthetized and prepared for surgery following institutional guidelines.
2. The skin and peritoneum is incised (midline) longitudinally for 0.5–1 cm. Use sterile dressing forceps to gently move the stomach—which lies rostral or anterior (toward the head) and dorsal to the spleen and pancreas—to the incision area using gentle traction.
3. Anchor the tumor fragment onto the suture and loosely sew it to the dorsal side of the stomach in the midsection, using two or three surgical knots. Care must be taken not to cut the lumen of the stomach with the suture needle; only the superficial layers (serosa) of the stomach should be incised using the tapered 6/0 prolene suture needle, making sure not to disrupt or damage the lumen of the stomach.
4. Apply a small amount (0.5–1.0 mL) of sterile saline to the stomach with attached tumor tissue fragment, and then use sterile tissue forceps to raise the abdominal wall and gently guide the stomach back in place within the abdominal cavity.
5. Moisten the skin and abdominal layers with saline for easier surgical closure.
6. Close the abdominal wall using 4-0 vicryl and a taper needle in an interrupted suture pattern and the skin using sterile wound clips.
7. Animals should be provided postoperative care and monitoring according to institutional guidelines.

Subrenal Capsule Implantation[19]

1. The animal should be anesthetized and prepared for surgery following institutional guidelines.
2. With the animal in right lateral recumbency, using straight forceps and scissors make a 5- to 10-mm skin incision on the left side, parallel and ventral to the spine and midway between the last rib and the iliac crest.
3. Make a similar incision in the underlying abdominal wall.
4. Externalize the left kidney and rotate it slightly so that it is held in place by the abdominal wall.
5. Make a small incision in the kidney capsule.
6. Make a shallow subcapsular pocket and place the transplant tissue into the pocket with iris forceps.
7. Keep the kidney moist with warm sterile saline and return to the abdomen.

8. Close the incision in the abdominal wall with 4-0 absorbable suture with a swaged needle and the skin using sterile wound clips.
9. Animals should be provided postoperative care and monitoring according to institutional guidelines.

Orthotopic Lung Implantation[22]

1. The animal should be anesthetized and prepared for surgery following institutional guidelines.
2. The mouse should be positioned in lateral recumbency. Using surgical scissors, carefully make a small incision (5 mm) in the area of the left lateral thorax for visualization of the left lobe of the lung.
3. Advance the needle quickly to a depth of approximately 5 mm into the left lobe of the lung between the sixth and seventh ribs and inject the cell.
4. Gently remove the needle and close the incision using sterile wound clips.
5. Animals should be provided postoperative care and monitoring according to institutional guidelines.

Mammary Fat Pad Implantation[1]

Tumor samples are implanted into the inguinal (fourth) mammary fat pad.

1. The animal should be anesthetized and prepared for surgery following institutional guidelines.
2. Make two small SC incisions in the skin to expose the fat pad: one along the midline (approximately 1.5 cm) and one a short distance down the leg (about 1 cm). Local anesthetic may be applied to the incision.
3. Expose the mammary fat pad using a sterile cotton swab, and pin the skin down using a small needle.
4. Insert the tip of a cross-action tweezer into the center of the transplantation site and make a pocket about 3 mm long. Place a tumor fragment into the pocket. Carefully remove the tweezers once the tissue has been placed.
5. Clear the mammary fat pad by using forceps and scissors paying attention not to disrupt the pocket containing the tumor fragment.
6. Close the incision with wound clips.
7. Animals should be provided postoperative care and monitoring according to institutional guidelines.

Brain Orthotopic Implantation

1. The animal should be anesthetized and prepared for surgery following institutional guidelines.
2. Place the mouse on a warm pad, and place the head in a stereotactic device.
3. Prepare the area for surgery with 10% betadine followed by 70% isopropyl alcohol.

4. Cover the animal, which has been positioned in the prone position, with sterile drape.
5. Make a 0.7-cm incision in the skin over the cranium, and dissect away the periosteum.
6. Using the stereotaxic device, drill a hole with a compact drill using a sterile bit into the skull at the entry point.
7. Inject the cell suspension using a Hamilton syringe.
8. After the injection, the syringe is left in place for approximately 3–5 min and then retracted slowly to prevent backflow of injected material, monitoring the site for leakage.
9. Animals should be provided postoperative care and monitoring according to institutional guidelines.

TUMOR TAKE RATE AND GROWTH RATE

Tumor take rates and the metastatic potential of the specimen depend on both the innate properties of the primary tumor sample and host factors including but not limited to tissue of origin, quality of sample, site of implantation, and tumor dependence on hormones,[15] as summarized in Table 3.3.

Engraftment rates can also provide prognostic insight as evident by the definitive correlation between tumor engraftment in PDXs and poorer clinical outcomes that has been observed in breast, lung, bladder, and colorectal cancer patients.[9,23–25]

Timely acquisition and implantation of the primary tumor samples is of paramount importance in maximizing the PDX take rate, as both duration of the surgery and of the interval between surgical resection and implantation in the mouse has been shown to negatively affect engraftment.[26]

Additionally, tumor engraftment is highly dependent on the mouse strain. In general, take rates are higher in more immunodeficient strains, therefore NSG (NOD/SCID/IL2Rg) mice are preferred over less immunocompromised strains such as athymic nu/nu or NOD/SCID mice.[27–29] Efforts have also been made to cotransplant human immune or stromal cells with the tumor specimen to better recapitulate tumor progression.[30–32]

Once engrafted, the growth rate of PDX models varies greatly, with some tumors forming within few weeks of implantation and others requiring up to 8 months.[33] Growth of SC tumors can be easily monitored, whereas small animal imaging techniques such as ultrasound, computed tomography, magnetic resonance imaging, and positron emission tomography need to be employed for OT and metastatic models. In the case of blood cancers, progression of disease can also be assessed by blood and bone marrow analysis.

Mice implanted with human tumor tissue need to be carefully monitored for tumor burden and other signs of distress. In general, immunocompromised mice are very susceptible to infections, so it is recommended that they be fed a diet containing antibiotics, such as sulfamethoxazole/trimethoprim or enrofloxacin, for the entire duration of the study. In some cases, SC implantation of certain tumor samples can cause general loss of health in highly immunocompromised mice. In these situations, it is at times beneficial to try to transplant the tumor into a different, less immunocompromised strain.[33]

Furthermore, animals may succumb to graft versus host disease (GVHD), as the engrafted cells start mounting an immune response against the murine host system.[10] Although not entirely preventable, the onset of GVHD can be delayed somewhat by the use of a strain of NSG mice lacking MHC-I.[34]

It is also important to keep in mind that human solid tumor xenografts in immunodeficient mice are vulnerable to spontaneous lymphomagenesis associated with Epstein-Barr virus (EBV).[35] Immunodeficient mice are also susceptible to EBV-transformed cells from the human donor.[36] This phenomenon can be recognized and avoided by routine phenotyping of primary tumors and xenografts with human lymphocytic markers.[35,36]

PROPAGATION AND PRESERVATION

Once a PDX model has been established, it can usually be retransplanted successfully.

With each transplant, stroma and necrotic tissue needs to be removed, so that only viable tumor material is implanted into the new host. Moreover, once the optimal processing strategy for a sample is determined, all samples for subsequent transplants should be processed in the same fashion.

PDX models maintained in mice and serially transplanted for several passages tend to grow faster than the early-passage samples,[12,33] likely due to the progressive substitution of human stroma to murine stroma, so it is important to keep records of each tumor model's characteristics and growth rate, including the number of times it has been passaged.

To avoid genetic or phenotypic drift, it is strongly recommended to freeze as many early-passage tumor fragments as possible, so that they can be used for future implantation. To this aim, solid tumors can be either cut into small pieces or can be processed as single-cell suspension prior to being preserved in freezing media (see Table 3.1). If the sample is processed to a single-cell suspension, ensure that the final concentration of viable cells is in the range between 10^6 and 10^7 cells per mL, as cells frozen in lower or higher cell concentration often tend to have less viability. Importantly, tissue/cell viability should be confirmed prior to freezing.

For PDX samples of hematological malignancies, serial transplantation may be achieved by collecting MNCs from bone marrow and/or splenic tissue of the primary PDX animal. Depending on the degree of human tumor involvement in these collected murine tissues, whole MNCs from the primary animal may be directly used for serial transplantation or selection for human hematopoietic cells (hCD45-positive cells) or more purified human cell populations may need to be obtained for serial transplant. The cell number required for injection in secondary transplant recipients is dependent both on the sample and the disease.

As for cell lines, samples should be placed in prechilled cryovials containing freezing media, slowly cooled, and placed in a −80°C freezer overnight prior to being moved to a liquid nitrogen tank for long-term storage as previously described.

Additional details on tumor banking and database needs for management of PDX models are discussed in Section II, Chapter 6.

ACKNOWLEDGMENTS

The authors received support through grants P30 CA008748 and U54 OD020355-01 and from the Geoffrey Beene Cancer Research Center.

REFERENCES

1. DeRose YS, Gligorich KM, Wang G, Georgelas A, Bowman P, Courdy SJ, et al. Patient-derived models of human breast cancer: protocols for in vitro and in vivo applications in tumor biology and translational medicine. *Curr Protoc Pharmacol* 2013. Editorial board, SJ Enna, Chapter 14:Unit14.23.
2. Mancini R, Giarnieri E, De Vitis C, Malanga D, Roscilli G, Noto A, et al. Spheres derived from lung adenocarcinoma pleural effusions: molecular characterization and tumor engraftment. *PloS One* 2011;**6**:e21320.
3. Verschraegen CF, Hu W, Du Y, Mendoza J, Early J, Deavers M, et al. Establishment and characterization of cancer cell cultures and xenografts derived from primary or metastatic Mullerian cancers. *Clin Cancer Res* 2003;**9**:845–52.
4. Yu M, Stott S, Toner M, Maheswaran S, Haber DA. Circulating tumor cells: approaches to isolation and characterization. *J Cell Biol* 2011;**192**:373–82.
5. Hodgkinson CL, Morrow CJ, Li Y, Metcalf RL, Rothwell DG, Trapani F, et al. Tumorigenicity and genetic profiling of circulating tumor cells in small-cell lung cancer. *Nat Med* 2014;**20**:897–903.
6. Williams ES, Rodriquez-Bravo V, Chippada-Venkata U, De Ia Iglesia-Vicente J, Gong Y, Galsky M, et al. Generation of prostate cancer patient derived xenograft models from circulating tumor cells. *J Vis Exp* 2015;**20**(105):53182.
7. Morton CL, Houghton PJ. Establishment of human tumor xenografts in immunodeficient mice. *Nat Protoc* 2007;**2**:247–50.
8. Williams SA, Anderson WC, Santaguida MT, Dylla SJ. Patient-derived xenografts, the cancer stem cell paradigm, and cancer pathobiology in the 21st century. *Lab Invest* 2013;**93**:970–82.
9. Bernardo C, Costa C, Sousa N, Amado F, Santos L. Patient-derived bladder cancer xenografts: a systematic review. *Transl Res* 2015;**166**:324–31.
10. Cassidy JW, Caldas C, Bruna A. Maintaining tumor heterogeneity in patient-derived tumor xenografts. *Cancer Res* 2015;**75**:2963–8.
11. Chen X, Liu B, Li Q, Honorio S, Liu X, Liu C, et al. Dissociated primary human prostate cancer cells coinjected with the immortalized Hs5 bone marrow stromal cells generate undifferentiated tumors in NOD/SCID-γ mice. *PloS One* 2013;**8**:e56903.
12. DeRose YS, Wang G, Lin YC, Bernard PS, Buys SS, Ebbert MT, et al. Tumor grafts derived from women with breast cancer authentically reflect tumor pathology, growth, metastasis and disease outcomes. *Nat Med* 2011;**17**:1514–20.
13. Jones-Bolin S, Ruggeri B. Orthotopic models of human gastric carcinoma in nude mice: applications for study of tumor growth and progression. *Curr Protoc Pharmacol* 2007. Editorial board, SJ Enna, Chapter 14:Unit 14.4.

14. Killion JJ, Radinsky R, Fidler IJ. Orthotopic models are necessary to predict therapy of transplantable tumors in mice. *Cancer Metastasis Rev* 1998;**17**:279–84.
15. Calles A, Rubio-Viqueira B, Hidalgo M. Primary human non-small cell lung and pancreatic tumorgraft models–utility and applications in drug discovery and tumor biology. *Curr Protoc Pharmacol* 2013. Editorial board, SJ Enna, Chapter 14:Unit 14.26.
16. Kuo TH, Kubota T, Watanabe M, Furukawa T, Kase S, Tanino H, et al. Site-specific chemosensitivity of human small-cell lung carcinoma growing orthotopically compared to subcutaneously in SCID mice: the importance of orthotopic models to obtain relevant drug evaluation data. *Anticancer Res* 1993;**13**:627–30.
17. Bibby MC. Orthotopic models of cancer for preclinical drug evaluation: advantages and disadvantages. *Eur J Cancer* 2004;**40**:852–7.
18. Sano D, Myers JN. Xenograft models of head and neck cancers. *Head Neck Oncol* 2009;**1**:32.
19. Shultz LD, Goodwin N, Ishikawa F, Hosur V, Lyons BL, Greiner DL. Subcapsular transplantation of tissue in the kidney. *Cold Spring Harb Protoc* 2014;**2014**:737–40.
20. Dong X, Guan J, English JC, Flint J, Yee J, Evans K, et al. Patient-derived first generation xenografts of non-small cell lung cancers: promising tools for predicting drug responses for personalized chemotherapy. *Clin Cancer Res* 2010;**16**:1442–51.
21. Lee CH, Xue H, Sutcliffe M, Gout PW, Huntsman DG, Miller DM, et al. Establishment of subrenal capsule xenografts of primary human ovarian tumors in SCID mice: potential models. *Gynecol Oncol* 2005;**96**:48–55.
22. Justilien V, Fields AP. Utility and applications of orthotopic models of human non-small cell lung cancer (NSCLC) for the evaluation of novel and emerging cancer therapeutics. *Curr Protoc Pharmacol* 2013;**62**. Editorial board, SJ Enna, Unit 14.27.
23. John T, Kohler D, Pintilie M, Yanagawa N, Pham NA, Li M, et al. The ability to form primary tumor xenografts is predictive of increased risk of disease recurrence in early-stage non-small cell lung cancer. *Clin Cancer Res* 2011;**17**:134–41.
24. Moon HG, Oh K, Lee J, Lee M, Kim JY, Yoo TK, et al. Prognostic and functional importance of the engraftment-associated genes in the patient-derived xenograft models of triple-negative breast cancers. *Breast Cancer Res Treat* 2015;**154**:13–22.
25. Oh BY, Lee WY, Jung S, Hong HK, Nam DH, Park YA, et al. Correlation between tumor engraftment in patient-derived xenograft models and clinical outcomes in colorectal cancer patients. *Oncotarget* 2015;**6**:16059–68.
26. Guerrera F, Tabbo F, Bessone L, Maletta F, Gaudiano M, Ercole E, et al. The influence of tissue ischemia time on RNA integrity and patient-derived xenografts (PDX) engraftment rate in a non-small cell lung cancer (NSCLC) biobank. *PloS One* 2016;**11**:e0145100.
27. McDermott SP, Eppert K, Lechman ER, Doedens M, Dick JE. Comparison of human cord blood engraftment between immunocompromised mouse strains. *Blood* 2010;**116**:193–200.
28. Quintana E, Shackleton M, Sabel MS, Fullen DR, Johnson TM, Morrison SJ. Efficient tumour formation by single human melanoma cells. *Nature* 2008;**456**:593–8.
29. Zhou Q, Facciponte J, Jin M, Shen Q, Lin Q. Humanized NOD-SCID IL2rg$^{-/-}$ mice as a preclinical model for cancer research and its potential use for individualized cancer therapies. *Cancer Lett* 2014;**344**:13–9.
30. Bankert RB, Balu-Iyer SV, Odunsi K, Shultz LD, Kelleher Jr RJ, Barnas JL, et al. Humanized mouse model of ovarian cancer recapitulates patient solid tumor progression, ascites formation, and metastasis. *PloS One* 2011;**6**:e24420.
31. Ito R, Takahashi T, Katano I, Ito M. Current advances in humanized mouse models. *Cell Mol Immunol* 2012;**9**:208–14.

32. Proia DA, Kuperwasser C. Reconstruction of human mammary tissues in a mouse model. *Nat Protoc* 2006;**1**:206–14.
33. Moro M, Bertolini G, Tortoreto M, Pastorino U, Sozzi G, Roz L. Patient-derived xenografts of non small cell lung cancer: resurgence of an old model for investigation of modern concepts of tailored therapy and cancer stem cells. *J Biomed Biotechnol* 2012;**2012**:568567.
34. Covassin L, Jangalwe S, Jouvet N, Laning J, Burzenski L, Shultz LD, et al. Human immune system development and survival of non-obese diabetic (NOD)-SCID IL2rγ^{null} (NSG) mice engrafted with human thymus and autologous haematopoietic stem cells. *Clin Exp Immunol* 2013;**174**:372–88.
35. Chen K, Ahmed S, Adeyi O, Dick JE, Ghanekar A. Human solid tumor xenografts in immunodeficient mice are vulnerable to lymphomagenesis associated with Epstein-Barr virus. *PloS One* 2012;**7**:e39294.
36. Bondarenko G, Ugolkov A, Rohan S, Kulesza P, Dubrovskyi O, Gursel D, et al. Patient-derived tumor xenografts are susceptible to formation of human lymphocytic tumors. *Neoplasia* 2015;**17**:735–41.

Chapter 4

Pathology of Patient-Derived Xenograft Tumors

J.-J. Fontaine[1], E. Marangoni[2], S. Chateau-Joubert[1], J.-L. Servely[3]
[1]Ecole Nationale Vétérinaire d'Alfort, Université Paris-Est, Maisons-Alfort, France; [2]Institut Curie, Paris, France; [3]INRA, Maisons-Alfort, France

INTRODUCTION

Since the first attempts to develop xenografts of human tumors in laboratory rodents in the middle of the 20th century, histological approaches have been used to check that the growing tissue corresponds to the expected tumor, to compare the morphological characteristics of the graft with those of the original tumor, to follow the persistence or changes in these characteristics over successive passages, and to evaluate the effects of therapeutic protocols.[1–7] New methods for investigating tumor characteristics have been developed, but pathology remains an essential tool, for both managing xenograft banks and studying their characteristics, either as an end in itself or for the preclinical evaluation of therapies.

THE VARIOUS DOMAINS OF APPLICATION OF PATHOLOGY IN PATIENT-DERIVED XENOGRAFT STUDIES

Pathology is an essential tool for studying patient-derived xenograft (PDX) tumors as models of human cancers at each step of their establishment and throughout their maintenance in successive generations of mice (Fig. 4.1A).

Characterization of Xenograft Banks

Working with PDX tumors requires the establishment and maintenance of a bank of tumors, which are implanted in mice and then serially transferred from generation to generation, unless this chain of events is interrupted by the freezing of samples. PDX are thought to reproduce the morphological characteristics of the original tumor more precisely than xenografts of established cell lines, in terms of histological and genetic profiling. They reproduce the heterogeneity of human cancers and have a better value for predicting response to treatment.[8–16]

Patient Derived Tumor Xenograft Models. http://dx.doi.org/10.1016/B978-0-12-804010-2.00010-2

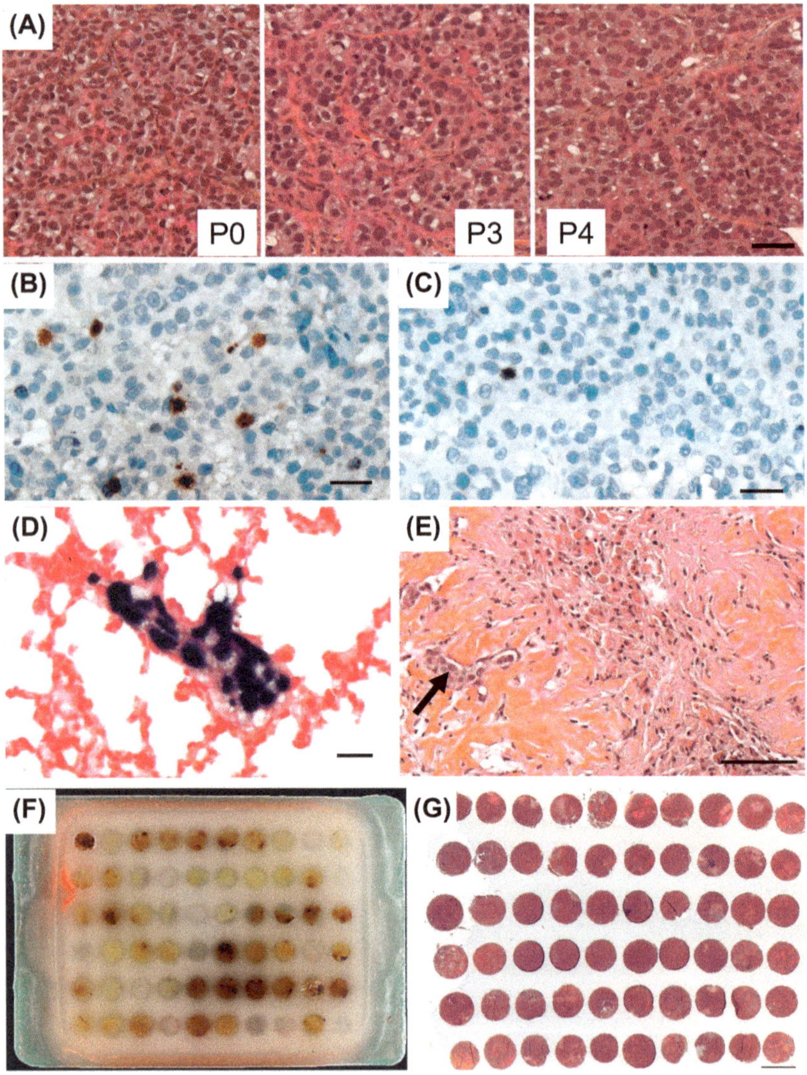

FIGURE 4.1 (A) Breast carcinoma PDX: persistence of histological characteristics from P0 to P4 (H&E staining; bar = 50 μm). (B) Immunohistochemical labeling of phosphorylated histone H3 in a breast cancer xenograft, untreated (positive nuclei are stained brown; bar = 50 μm). (C) Same tumor sampled 6 h after treatment with an anti–Aurora kinase that suppresses H3 phosphorylation (bar = 50 μm).[24] (D) Mouse lung: micrometastasis of a PDX tumor, visualized by the deep blue staining of cell nuclei after in situ hybridization with an Alu probe (bar = 20 μm). (E) Residual nodule composed of fibrous tissue and macrophages; a few tumor cells persist (*arrow*; H&E staining, bar = 100 μm). (F) TMA paraffin block, with a 10×6 matrix of 2-mm tissue cores. (G) Histological slide obtained from a TMA block (H&E staining, bar = 2 mm).

Any lesion developing at the site of implantation, either after the first engraftment (P0 in this text) or after a passage between mice (Pn) should be carefully investigated to ensure that it corresponds to the expected tumor. This is important because the lesions developing at this site may instead correspond to inflammatory lesions (eg, an abscess or a granuloma, due to a local infection or the inoculation of foreign material; Fig. 4.2A) or to unexpected tumors of murine or human origin.

Inflammatory lesions are generally easy to identify by histological methods. By contrast, for tumors, it can be more difficult to determine whether the tumor is the one expected or has a different origin. Indeed, murine tumors can develop at the site of xenografts. Most such tumors are lymphomas (Fig. 4.2B),[11] but fusiform cell sarcomas (Fig. 4.2C) are sometimes observed, and other murine tumors, such as mammary gland tumors in the subcutaneous tissue of female mice, may also be observed in rare cases. Spontaneous tumors or tumorlike lesions may also develop in distant organs and may be misinterpreted as possible metastases (eg, lung adenomas; Fig. 4.2D). Simple morphological examination of the tissue generally indicates clearly whether the tumor is of the same type as the original human tumor. This is particularly true for most carcinoma xenografts, which have a morphology very different from that of lymphomas or sarcomas. Carcinomas are generally formed by large cells, clearly arranged in cords, tubules or lobules with a prominent connective interstitium. Lymphomas (whether human or murine) consist of sheets of small round cells with scarce stroma, and sarcomas consist of streams of fusiform cells. It is therefore easy to distinguish between these different types of tumors by eye. Diagnosis may be more difficult if the original tumor is a "blue tumor," a tumor consisting of small cells with very little cytoplasm and a hyperchromatic nucleus, appearing deeply basophilic (blue in color) under a microscope at low magnification following staining with hematoxylin and eosin (H&E). Blastic tumors, such as retinoblastoma, are typically blue tumors. In such cases, tumor morphology may be difficult to interpret, particularly as the most specific characteristics of some tumors, such as the rosettes of many blastic tumors, are generally missing or poorly represented in xenografts. Anaplastic tumors, where tumor cells have little or no morphological similarity to normal cells, can also be difficult to characterize without ancillary techniques. As stated, while it is relatively easy to differentiate sarcoma from lymphoma or well-differentiated carcinoma, differentiating sarcoma xenografts from inflammatory lesions or murine sarcomas can be challenging, as these lesions can have very similar morphology.[6]

When dealing with difficult cases, or simply to confirm that a tumor really is of human origin before beginning an experiment, several different methods designed to reveal species-specific proteins or nucleotide sequences, based on immunohistochemistry or in situ hybridization, can be used to identify human or murine cells. Immunohistochemical characterization of proteins characteristic of a cell lineage is useful to specify the tissue of origin of the tumor.

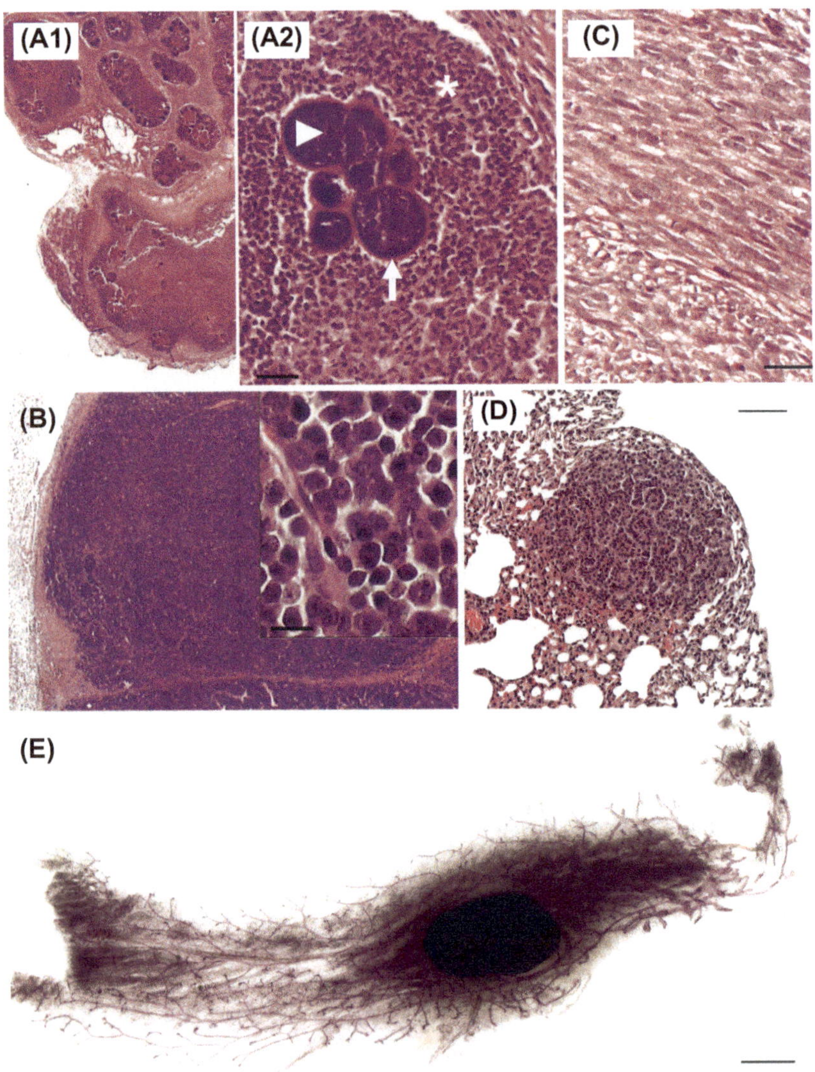

FIGURE 4.2 (A) Botryomycosis (coalescent pyogranulomas due to *Staphylococcus* infection) at the site of xenograft implantation. (A1) Low magnification, showing numerous nodular lesions embedded in fibrous connective tissue; (A2) high magnification, showing bacterial colonies (*arrowhead*), an eosinophilic rim typical of a Splendore–Hoeppli reaction (*arrow*), and degenerate neutrophils (*star*; bar = 50 μm). (B) Lymphoma developing at the site of xenograft implantation, composed of sheets of small round cells (inset: detail at high magnification; bar = 20 μm). (C) Murine sarcoma developing at the site of xenograft implantation, composed of streams of fusiform cells (bar = 50 μm). (D) Spontaneous type 2 adenoma in a mouse lung, macroscopically suspected to be a metastasis of a PDX tumor (bar = 100 μm). (E) Whole-mount technique for the visualization of a nodular lesion in a mammary fat pad (bar = 2 mm).

Particular attention should be paid to the possible development of human lymphomas at the site of engraftment of nonlymphoid tumors, mostly during initial implantation.[11] Such tumors bear the specific markers of human cells; this may lead to confusion with a true xenograft if a morphological examination of the lesion is not carried out. In PDX studies, most of the human lymphomas observed appear to develop from lymphocytes present in tissue sample used for initial engraftment. If these cells are infected with the Epstein-Barr virus (EBV), the B lymphocytes may undergo transformation to become tumor cells.[17,18] These cells are efficiently eliminated by the immune system in immunocompetent humans, whereas their engraftment in immunocompromised mice allows the malignant B cells to develop and to take the place of the initial human tumor.[11] A few cases of EBV-negative peripheral human T-cell lymphomas have also been described in the PDX context.[19] If the original human tumor was clearly different from lymphoma (eg, an adenocarcinoma), then the development of a human lymphoma is easy to manage, as a simple morphological examination is sufficient to show that the tumor growing at the engraftment site is not of the type expected and should therefore be discarded. If the original tumor was a "blue tumor," then the demonstration that the tumor found at the engraftment site is of human origin may lead to misinterpretation in the absence of further characterization, because this tumor may actually be a human lymphoma resulting from the malignant transformation of EBV-infected lymphocytes present in the initial tumor, as discussed earlier.

When a xenograft is established (PDX tumors are generally considered to be stabilized after three to five passages[20]), it should be characterized, in terms of both its histological type and its differentiation. The histological type of the tumor is generally well preserved in xenografts, so epidermoid carcinomas and tubulous adenocarcinomas, for example, have the same characteristics when they form PDX.[21] This phenotypic stability is thought to be linked to biochemical stability, because marked biochemical changes would be unlikely to result in the preservation of morphological characteristics.[6] The first question that the pathologist must address, therefore, is whether the tumor present reproduces the morphological and biochemical characteristics of the parent tissues.[17] If it does not, then it may correspond to a murine tumor, or there may have been a major change in the pattern of differentiation of the tumor, which would require further investigation.[8]

However, in some of first-generation transplants and increasingly after further passages, some tumors may tend to become less differentiated, with fewer ducts or acini in adenocarcinomas, and greater rates of mitosis, nuclear pleomorphism, and atypia.[20]

Specific morphological details may change during serial passages, with acquisition of mucin secretion or of neuroendocrine differentiation, for example, both of which are criteria for tumor progression in some carcinomas (eg, prostate cancers).[22] Similarly, the pattern of tumor differentiation may be altered by modifications to the engraftment conditions, with changes to the hormonal status of the host due to castration or hormonal supplementation, for example.[22]

Determining whether the morphology of the tumor is preserved after engraftment, serial passages or experiments are one of the difficulties faced by pathologists. Indeed, independent xenografts from the same tumor are never strictly identical, due to biological variability and intratumor heterogeneity. Even different sections of the same tumor and different regions of the same section may display morphological differences. The morphological characteristics of the cells and their nuclei, their spatial arrangement, the mitotic index and the presence of atypical mitoses, the numbers of apoptotic bodies and frequency of necrosis, the abundance of stroma, and the vasculature differ between sections and between fields. The pathologist must therefore determine whether the global pattern of the tumor is preserved and, more importantly, whether the histology of the xenografted tumor matches that of the original donor tumor. International classifications of human tumors should be used as the basis of an accurate pathological classification of xenografts, but some degree of flexibility is required, because xenografts never perfectly reproduce the morphology of the original human tumor.

When xenografts are followed over successive passages or during experiments, qualitative changes, such as a switch from a trabecular to a tubular pattern, if reproducible, can be considered significant, whereas quantitative changes, such as alterations to the mitotic index or the amount of necrosis, particularly if subtle, should be interpreted with great caution.

Another difficulty in the histological analyses of tumor xenobanks results from the partly subjective nature of the morphological analysis. If observers know the morphology of a certain type of tumor well, then their perception is finely tuned to detect small details that may become more apparent with time. The selection of a sample of stabilized PDX to be used as a reference, for comparison with new samples, is advisable, to ensure that the slides are read as objectively as possible. A digital bank of virtual slides can greatly facilitate this task. If no obvious difference between the test slide and the reference can be detected then the lesion can be considered "similar"; this does not mean that they are identical, only that no significant morphological changes can be detected.

For the first sample observed in a xenograft experiment, the reference should be a sample of the original human tumor, or at least have a morphological description as the tumor concerned in the pathology report of the patient. If no such reference is available, the pathologist can simply say that the tumor is "morphologically compatible" with a xenograft of a human tumor of a given category.

Experimentation on Tumors

Unlike extraction methods such as Western blot or PCR assays, in situ labeling methods are unique in allowing the determination of the molecular characteristics of PDX at the cellular level. It is thus possible to investigate the diversity of PDX tumors, and to identify characteristics specific to subpopulations.

Immunohistochemistry and in situ hybridization are also used in routine diagnostic procedures for characterizing lesions. The application of the same techniques to PDX tumors provides important data for model validation. Conversely, informative new in situ labeling data from experiments on PDX could be transferred to routine diagnostics in human pathology.

Stromal characteristics can be investigated in PDX tumors. In xenograft models, the stroma is produced by the host (in PDX, the human stroma disappears shortly after primary transplantation or during the first serial transplantations).[14,17] One of the advantages of PDX tumors is that they reproduce the morphological characteristics of the stroma of origin, despite their development in mice, much more accurately than xenografts of cultured cells, in which subclones not representative of the original tumor may be selected. However, the preservation of stromal characteristics is not perfect. For example, the elastosis of breast carcinomas is lost in xenografts.[20] The various components of the stroma can be identified morphologically and by immunohistochemistry, and they can be distinguished in cells (fibroblasts, inflammatory cells), vessels, and the extracellular matrix (connective fibers, such as collagen, ground substance).

The effect of anticancer treatments can be investigated by morphological studies on xenografted tumors. Morphological studies of the early phases of regression in treated xenografts can provide information about the mechanisms involved, through determinations of the extent of necrosis, changes in mitotic index or atypical mitoses, or the expression of specific markers.[23] These changes can be quantified by morphometry.[24] As xenografts grow in severely immunocompromised mice, their histological characteristics do not include pronounced inflammatory and immune reactions.

In the later phases of treatment, full clinical regression of a tumor does not necessarily mean that all the tumor cells have disappeared. Small numbers of tumor cells frequently survive and persist in the residual tissue, remaining quiescent for long periods. Their presence can be attested by histological methods, on serial or semiserial sections, to prevent a section sampling effect if residual cells are scarce (Fig. 4.1E). Extraction-based methods, such as PCR, are generally more sensitive and can be used alongside histological approaches.

Residual nodules are of particular interest as they consist of subclones of tumor cells that may enable the tumor to escape treatment. They can be labeled with markers of interest by immunohistochemistry and compared with pretreated samples, or subjected to microdissection (eg, laser capture microdissection) for molecular studies. Frozen sections or fixed and paraffin-embedded tissues may be used, after validation of the preservation of proteins and RNAs.[25–28]

Similarly, in cases in which the molecular markers of tumor cells disappear from a residual nodule, it is important to check that neoplastic cells are not detectable by histological methods and to determine the nature of the residual nodule, which may consist of fibrous tissue, macrophage infiltrate, and/or necrosis.

Orthotopic xenografts are generally considered to be better models than subcutaneous xenografts, because the microenvironment of the organ better reflects that of the original tumor.[10] Histological analyses are often required to determine whether the implantation of a xenograft is really orthotopic. Such analyses are more informative at an early stage of tumor growth, before the tumor is large enough to invade different organs and tissues. The efficiency of orthotopic engraftments should therefore be evaluated in preliminary experiments.

Histological studies are also useful for investigating the metastatic process. If large enough, metastases can be observed macroscopically on necropsy. However, as inflammatory lesions and spontaneous tumors can be confused with true metastases, each lesion should be sampled and characterized by histology (Fig. 4.2D). Smaller metastases can be detected microscopically, on serial or semiserial sections.[20] Specific labeling can facilitate the detection of human cells.

In our experience, metastases are seldom detected on the basis of gross morphology on necropsy when the tumors are grafted into the interscapular subcutaneous fat pad. Histological examination of the lung, which is small enough in mice to be fixed and embedded flat for the observation of all lung lobes on one section, frequently reveals the presence of small groups of tumor cells. It appears to be important to distinguish between tumor emboli, which obstruct small branches of the pulmonary artery without invading its wall or the surrounding parenchyma, and true metastases, which invade the parenchyma.

TECHNICAL CONSIDERATIONS

Technically, the pathology of xenograft tumors, and particularly of PDX, is no different from that of other tumors and many routine techniques can be used or easily adapted to xenografts, provided that the murine nature of the stroma is taken into account.

Histological studies of PDX tumors can be performed on formalin-fixed, paraffin-embedded tissues (FFPE), or on frozen sections. For morphological analyses and most types of in situ labeling, FFPE tissues are recommended. They best preserve the morphological features present and inactivate any infectious agents present in the human tissues (other than prion proteins). Samples can be stored for long periods in this form and can be used to constitute tissue microarrays (TMAs). Frozen sections should be retained for particular uses, such as types of immunolabeling that cannot be carried out on FFPE samples, or microdissection for molecular studies on selected subpopulations of cells. Fixatives other than formalin can be used, but the protocol must be tested and validated for the techniques to be applied thereafter.

Thus, before the first implantation and at critical steps in the experiments, portions of the tumors should be fixed for histological analysis.[21] The duration of fixation depends on the size of the sample. As samples are generally small (a few millimeters thick), we recommend 2 to 5 days of fixation at room tempera ture, followed directly by the paraffin-embedding protocol.

If it is not possible to embed the sample in paraffin rapidly enough, overfixation can be prevented by transferring the samples to 50–70% ethanol after formalin fixation.[29] However, slight changes to tumor morphology may be observed after transfer into ethanol, and immunolabeling procedures should be tested before this technique is used. In general, overfixation should be considered preferable to underfixation: morphological features are well preserved and most types of in situ labeling work on overfixed samples, after the use of antigen retrieval procedures if necessary.

It can sometimes be difficult to find and dissect small tumors within tissues (eg, for investigations of the first steps of tumor growth, or to find residual nodules after treatment). Whole-mount techniques can be used, for adipose-rich tissues, such as subcutaneous tissue or mammary glands, for the visualization of lesions and their sampling for downstream analyses (Fig. 4.2E).[30] Various fixation techniques (ethanol, paraformaldehyde) and visualization methods (staining with hematoxylin, carmine, neutral red, or fluorescent dyes) are available to improve the gross examination of the tumors; they should be evaluated according to the downstream techniques applied to the tissue samples for their histological examination.

Formalin-fixed samples are conventionally dehydrated, embedded in paraffin wax, and 4- to 5-μm sections are then cut. At least one section should be stained with H&E and observed for morphological characterization.

Specific components can be stained by histochemical methods (eg, mucins and basement membranes with periodic acid–Schiff reagent).[20] Specific fixation methods are required for some techniques (eg, specific detection of different mucins with alcian blue, at various pH values, on tissues fixed in 95% ethanol).[22] Histochemical techniques are frequently replaced by immunohistochemistry, or carried out in addition to immunohistochemistry.

The immunohistochemistry of xenografts is unusual in that the stroma is of murine origin. Consequently, in indirect techniques, mouse primary antibodies generate background staining due to the use of antimouse secondary antibodies. This background staining can be prevented by working with primary antibodies (monoclonal or polyclonal) produced in species other than mice, such as rabbit.

It is beyond the scope of this chapter to list all the possibilities for immunolabeling in the study of PDX tumors. We therefore provide just a few examples of markers or molecules:

- Cell-type markers, such as cytokeratins for epithelial cells, CD31 for blood vessels, lymphatic vessel endothelial receptor 1 for lymphatic vessels[10]
- Secretions, such as mucins[22]
- Proliferation markers, such as Ki67; apoptotic markers, such as active caspase-3, active caspase-7, or cleaved poly(ADP-ribose) polymerase; the terminal deoxynucleotidyl transferase dUTP nick end labeling technique is considered less specific on histological tissue sections[10,31–33]

- Hormone receptors, such as estrogen receptors, progesterone receptors, and human epidermal growth factor receptor 2 in breast cancers[9]
- Lymphoma markers, such as CD45 and CD19/20 for human B-cell EBV-associated lymphomas, which can also be detected by in situ hybridization for EBV[11,17,19]
- Drugs administered in vivo, such as EF5 (a nitroimidazole used in medical imaging), to detect hypoxia in the tumors[10,34]
- Markers of treatment efficacy (Figs. 4.1B and 4.1C).[24]

Special attention should be paid to checking the human origin of the tumors. Immunolabeling with monoclonal antibodies considered to be species specific (eg, detection of blood vessels of mouse origin with antimouse CD34 antibodies, or of human origin with antihuman CD31 antibodies[13,14]) can be carried out, but cross-reactions may persist, and different antibodies must be available for each type of tumor cell. We have performed in situ hybridization with probes corresponding to consensus sequences for human Alu repeats.[12,35] This approach can be applied to frozen sections or FFPE sections. As about 3–6% of the human genome consists of repetitive Alu sequences, an intense signal is obtained with all the nucleated cells. This technique is very robust to the conditions of fixation and paraffin embedding, and it can also be used to detect small metastases (Fig. 4.1D). Similarly, if necessary, murine cells could be identified by labeling with mouse-specific probes, for m-L1 genes, for example.[36] The labeling can be visualized by fluorescence methods (fluorescence in situ hybridization), immunoenzymology (chromogenic in situ hybridization), or silver-enhanced in situ hybridization.[11,21,37] Other species-specific probes, such as centromeric probes, can also be used.[11,21]

When studying PDX tumors, it is possible to generate and analyze large numbers of samples corresponding to different tumors, treatments, and/or different durations of treatment, and to study several tumors in each group. TMA approaches, which involve the sampling of small cores of FFPE tissues and their insertion into a recipient paraffin block, can be used to spare samples, to save time and money, and to improve the homogeneity of immunolabeling. Regions of interest should be selected on histological slides from the donor blocks, and several cores are then taken from each block.[11] The cores may have diameters of as little as 0.6 mm, or they may be wider (up to 5 mm). The use of narrower samples makes it possible to include larger numbers of cores in the TMA block. We generally sample 2-mm cores, as this provides sections large enough to reflect some of the heterogeneity of the tissue, in TMA blocks containing 60 cores (Fig. 4.1F and G). The sampling must be representative if morphometry is to be carried out. If only a small number of experiments are planned, then automatic TMA systems can be replaced with manual devices, which are cheap and easy to use. Some cores may be damaged during the procedure. We therefore generally take three cores from each block and then select the best two on histological slides for interpretation.

Morphometry for histological slides corresponding to PDX tumors is not significantly different from that in other contexts. It allows a more precise and more objective description of morphological characteristics and in situ labeling. The sampling of sections and of microscopic fields for analysis is critical and should be organized so as to avoid bias. Several fields from each section, and, if possible, several sections from the same tumor, from sufficiently large groups of animals, should be selected at random. The variability of the morphological characteristics of the tissue at the margins of the tumor, or close to necrotic fields or blood vessels, should be taken into account when establishing the protocol.

SUGGESTED SCHEDULES FOR HISTOLOGICAL ANALYSES

The pathological characteristics of the original human tumor are determined by the hospital pathology department. The pathological report, and/or a histological slide, should be sent to the laboratory responsible for xenograft histology studies, which can be different from the original laboratory. Alternatively, a small piece of the sample used for primary engraftment can be fixed and processed for histology.[10]

If large enough, a sample of the first growing xenograft (P0) can be sampled for histology, as inflammatory lesions and human lymphomas are more likely to develop at this step.

Histological validation of the xenograft is required when the tumor is stabilized (after three to five passages[20]), and periodically thereafter, and/or when abnormalities are detected in the doubling time of a tumor (inflammatory lesions and lymphomas generally grow faster than xenografts).

When a tumor is expanded for an experiment, an early control should be carried out to check that the expansion corresponds to the tumor desired and not to a lymphoma, and another control should be carried just before the start of the experiment. Unexpected deaths should be investigated by necropsy and histological analyses.

It is expensive to maintain xenobanks in mice in the long term. It may therefore be practical to freeze samples for storage if a tumor is not going to be used for some time. The histological features of the tumors should be checked before freezing, and after thawing and reimplantation on mice. A first control can be carried out 3 months after freezing of the tumor and before serial transfers have stopped: a few samples are grafted and subjected to histological control after their growth. If reimplantation is not successful, either because no tumor grows or because its morphological or other characteristics have changed, then the tumor should be kept alive by serial transfers and freezing should be avoided.[12]

PITFALLS

There are many pitfalls in the pathology of PDX tumors.

On necropsy, nodules may be detected at the site of xenografts or in organs distant from the xenografted tumor. All the lesions observed should be subjected to histopathological investigations. A good knowledge of histopathology is required for the correct recognition of normal structures, inflammatory lesions, and spontaneous tumors.

For instance, growing mammary buds in the subcutaneous tissue of a female mouse consist of cords of cells with no lumen. They have mitotic activity and contain many apoptotic bodies and could therefore be confused with carcinoma. A spontaneous lung adenoma could be confused with a metastasis from a carcinoma. Macrophages pigmented with melanin granules liberated by a grafted pigmented melanoma could be misinterpreted as tumor cells.

CONCLUSION

Necropsy is essential to identify the tumors, their metastases, and unexpected lesions. A histological examination should be carried out for all the lesions observed.

Histopathology is an integrative tool that is simple to use and necessary to check the retention of xenograft characteristics with transplantation and serial passages. The conventional morphological examination of routinely stained sections can be combined with immunohistochemistry and in situ hybridization, to characterize xenograft banks, to ensure that the lesions observed result from the growth of the original human tumors and to investigate changes in their characteristics due to serial passages and/or the freezing of samples, or in therapeutic trials. By focusing on the morphological and molecular characteristics of a tissue at the cellular level, histopathology provides unique insight into the organization of the tissue and the relationship between cells and their stroma, and makes it possible to detect specific characteristics of subclones of tumor cells.

As pathology requires specific techniques and equipment and a good knowledge of all the lesions that may occur in mice after xenografting, scientists carrying out xenograft studies should work with a pathology laboratory and involve pathologists early in the establishment of a xenograft bank and in the design of experimental protocols.

REFERENCES

1. Toolan HW. Successful subcutaneous growth and transplantation of human tumors in X-irradiated laboratory animals. *Proc Soc Exp Biol Med* 1951;**77**:572–8.
2. Greene HSN. The significance of the heterologous transplantability of human cancer. *Cancer* 1952;**5**:24–44.
3. Toolan HW. Transplantable human neoplasms maintained in cortisone-treated laboratory animals: H.S. #1; H.Ep. #1; H.Ep. #2; H.Ep. #3; and H.Emb.Rh. #1. *Cancer Res* 1954;**14**:660–6.
4. Chesterman FC. Heterotransplantation of human tumours and tissues. *Ann R Coll Surg Engl* 1959;**25**:39–60.
5. Detre SI, Gazet J-C. Transplantation of human tumour to immune deprived mice treated with anti-thymocyte serum. *Br J Cancer* 1973;**28**:412–6.
6. Berenbaum MC, Sheard CE, Reittie JR, Bundick RV. The growth of human tumours in immunosuppressed mice and their response to chemotherapy. *Br J Cancer* 1974;**30**:13.
7. Bailey MJ, Gazet JC, Smith IE, Steel GG. Chemotherapy of human breast-carcinoma xenografts. *Br J Cancer* 1980;**42**:530–6.

8. Bailey MJ, Gazet JC, Peckham MJ. Human breast-cancer xenografts in immune-suppressed mice. *Br J Cancer* 1980;**42**:524–9.
9. DeRose YS, Wang G, Lin Y-C, Bernard PS, Buys SS, Ebbert MTW, et al. Tumor grafts derived from women with breast cancer authentically reflect tumor pathology, growth, metastasis and disease outcomes. *Nat Med* 2011;**17**:1514–20.
10. Chaudary N, Pintilie M, Schwock J, Dhani N, Clarke B, Milosevic M, et al. Characterization of the tumor-microenvironment in patient-derived cervix xenografts (OCICx). *Cancers* 2012;**4**:821–45.
11. John T, Yanagawa N, Kohler D, Craddock KJ, Bandarchi-Chamkhaleh B, Pintilie M, et al. Characterization of lymphomas developing in immunodeficient mice implanted with primary human non–small cell lung cancer. *J Thorac Oncol* 2012;**7**:1101–8.
12. Julien S, Merino-Trigo A, Lacroix L, Pocard M, Goéré D, Mariani P, et al. Characterization of a large panel of patient-derived tumor xenografts representing the clinical heterogeneity of human colorectal cancer. *Clin Cancer Res* 2012;**18**:5314–28.
13. Hylander BL, Punt N, Tang H, Hillman J, Vaughan M, Bshara W, et al. Origin of the vasculature supporting growth of primary patient tumor xenografts. *J Transl Med* 2013;**11**:110.
14. Peng S, Creighton CJ, Zhang Y, Sen B, Mazumdar T, Myers JN, et al. Tumor grafts derived from patients with head and neck squamous carcinoma authentically maintain the molecular and histologic characteristics of human cancers. *J Transl Med* 2013;**11**:198.
15. Delitto D, Pham K, Vlada AC, Sarosi GA, Thomas RM, Behrns KE, et al. Patient-derived xenograft models for pancreatic adenocarcinoma demonstrate retention of tumor morphology through incorporation of murine stromal elements. *Am J Pathol* 2015;**185**:1297–303.
16. Depreeuw J, Hermans E, Schrauwen S, Annibali D, Coenegrachts L, Thomas D, et al. Characterization of patient-derived tumor xenograft models of endometrial cancer for preclinical evaluation of targeted therapies. *Gynecol Oncol* 2015;**139**:118–26.
17. Chen K, Ahmed S, Adeyi O, Dick JE, Ghanekar A. Human solid tumor xenografts in immunodeficient mice are vulnerable to lymphomagenesis associated with Epstein-Barr virus. *PLoS One* 2012;**7**:e39294.
18. Bondarenko G, Ugolkov A, Rohan S, Kulesza P, Dubrovskyi O, Gursel D, et al. Patient-derived tumor xenografts are susceptible to formation of human lymphocytic tumors. *Neoplasia* 2015;**17**:735–41.
19. Wetterauer C, Vlajnic T, Schüler J, Gsponer JR, Thalmann GN, Cecchini M, et al. Early development of human lymphomas in a prostate cancer xenograft program using triple knock-out immunocompromised mice. *Prostate* 2015;**75**:585–92.
20. Bailey MJ, Ormerod MG, Imrie SF, Humphreys J, Roberts JD, Gazet JC, et al. Comparative functional histopathology of human breast carcinoma xenografts. *Br J Cancer* 1981;**43**:125.
21. Cutz J-C, Guan J, Bayani J, Yoshimoto M, Xue H, Sutcliffe M, et al. Establishment in severe combined immunodeficiency mice of subrenal capsule xenografts and transplantable tumor lines from a variety of primary human lung cancers: potential models for studying tumor progression–related changes. *Clin Cancer Res* 2006;**12**:4043–54.
22. Legrier M-E, de Pinieux G, Boyé K, Arvelo F, Judde J-G, Fontaine J-J, et al. Mucinous differentiation features associated with hormonal escape in a human prostate cancer xenograft. *Br J Cancer* 2004;**90**:720–7.
23. Legrier M-E, Oudard S, Judde J-G, Guyader C, de Pinieux G, Boyé K, et al. Potentiation of antitumour activity of docetaxel by combination with trastuzumab in a human prostate cancer xenograft model and underlying mechanisms. *Br J Cancer* 2007;**96**:269–76.
24. Romanelli A, Clark A, Assayag F, Chateau-Joubert S, Poupon M-F, Servely J-L, et al. Inhibiting aurora kinases reduces tumor growth and suppresses tumor recurrence after chemotherapy in patient-derived triple-negative breast cancer xenografts. *Mol Cancer Ther* 2012;**11**:2693–703.

25. Domazet B, MacLennan GT, Lopez-Beltran A, Montironi R, Cheng L. Laser capture microdissection in the genomic and proteomic era: targeting the genetic basis of cancer. *Int J Clin Exp Pathol* 2008;**1**:475–88.
26. Matsuda Y, Fujii T, Suzuki T, Yamahatsu K, Kawahara K, Teduka K, et al. Comparison of fixation methods for preservation of morphology, RNAs, and proteins from paraffin-embedded human cancer cell-implanted mouse models. *J Histochem Cytochem* 2011;**59**:68–75.
27. Golubeva Y, Salcedo R, Mueller C, Liotta LA, Espina V. Laser capture microdissection for protein and NanoString RNA analysis. *Methods Mol Biol Clifton* 2013;**931**:213–57.
28. Priolo C, Agostini M, Vena N, Ligon AH, Fiorentino M, Shin E, et al. Establishment and genomic characterization of mouse xenografts of human primary prostate tumors. *Am J Pathol* 2010;**176**:1901–13.
29. Smith KB, Tran LM, Tam BM, Shurell EM, Li Y, Braas D, et al. Novel dedifferentiated liposarcoma xenograft models reveal PTEN down-regulation as a malignant signature and response to PI3K pathway inhibition. *Am J Pathol* 2013;**182**:1400–11.
30. Landua JD, Visbal AP, Lewis MT. Methods for preparing fluorescent and neutral red-stained whole mounts of mouse mammary glands. *J Mammary Gland Biol Neoplasia* 2009;**14**:411–5.
31. Mitiæ T, McKay JS. Immunohistochemical analysis of acetylation, proliferation, mitosis, and apoptosis in tumor xenografts following administration of a histone deacetylase inhibitor—a pilot study. *Toxicol Pathol* 2005;**33**:792–9.
32. Bressenot A, Marchal S, Bezdetnaya L, Garrier J, Guillemin F, Plénat F. Assessment of apoptosis by immunohistochemistry to active Caspase-3, active Caspase-7, or cleaved PARP in monolayer cells and spheroid and subcutaneous xenografts of human carcinoma. *J Histochem Cytochem* 2009;**57**:289–300.
33. Duan WR, Garner DS, Williams SD, Funckes-Shippy CL, Spath IS, Blomme EA. Comparison of immunohistochemistry for activated caspase-3 and cleaved cytokeratin 18 with the TUNEL method for quantification of apoptosis in histological sections of PC-3 subcutaneous xenografts. *J Pathol* 2003;**199**:221–8.
34. Evans SM, Hahn SM, Magarelli DP, Koch CJ. Hypoxic heterogeneity in human tumors: EF5 binding, vasculature, necrosis, and proliferation. *Am J Clin Oncol* 2001;**24**:467–72.
35. Just L, Timmer M, Tinius J, Stahl F, Deiwick A, Nikkhah G, et al. Identification of human cells in brain xenografts and in neural co-cultures of rat by in situ hybridisation with Alu probe. *J Neurosci Methods* 2003;**126**:69–77.
36. Hatano H, Tokunaga K, Ogose A, Hotta T, Yamagiwa H, Hayami T, et al. Origin of bone-forming cells in human osteosarcomas transplanted into nude mice—which cells produce bone, human or mouse? *J Pathol* 1998;**185**:204–11.
37. Li H, Wozniak A, Sciot R, Cornillie J, Wellens J, Van Looy T, et al. Pazopanib, a receptor tyrosine kinase inhibitor, suppresses tumor growth through angiogenesis in dedifferentiated liposarcoma xenograft models. *Transl Oncol* 2014;**7**:665–71.

Chapter 5

Genetic Profiling of Tumors in PDX Models

J.T. Poirier[1,2]

[1]*Memorial Sloan Kettering Cancer Center, New York, NY, United States;* [2]*Weill Cornell Medical College, New York, NY, United States*

INTRODUCTION

Genomic profiling of patient-derived xenografts (PDXs) is in many ways similar to genomic profiling of human tumors. All standard best practices for sequencing of human tumors should be followed for optimal results, with the addition of the recommendations outlined in this chapter. Additionally, genomic sequencing of PDXs should be done in a way that is consistent with all local laws and institutional policies governing patient privacy. In most cases, informed consent and institutional review will be required not only for collection of tissues for research purposes but also for downstream genetic analysis as inappropriate use of this data can present a privacy concern.

A critical aspect of any PDX program is the necessity to obtain normal tissue from the donor patient. This allows germline variants to be distinguished from somatic variants at the analysis step. Normal tissue can come from a variety of sources and tissue types. The simplest approach to obtain normal DNA for solid tumors is to request collection of an additional 3 mL of blood in an ethylenediaminetetraacetic acid tube. Whole blood can be collected during surgery, or at any time during follow-up if the patient is having blood drawn for reasons related to medical treatment. This whole blood can be aliquoted and stored at −20°C, to be used in the future if the PDX successfully engrafts. It is encouraged to collect blood contemporaneous to tumor tissue acquisition, as it may be difficult or impossible to obtain this research material at a future date.

Normal tissue may also be obtained from an institutional pathology service. Many institutions have a dedicated frozen tissue banking service that collects and banks tumor and adjacent normal tissue from surgical resections which can be a useful source of normal tissue. Fresh frozen tissue is preferred, but if such tissue is not available, permanent formalin-fixed, paraffin embedded tissue may be sufficient. Unlike collection of small amounts of blood,

Patient Derived Tumor Xenograft Models. http://dx.doi.org/10.1016/B978-0-12-804010-2.00011-4

which may be exempt from regulatory approval, use of banked tissues may be subject to a separate institutional review, further complicating tissue acquisition. Given these realities, whole blood is usually the ideal source of normal DNA for solid tumors.

The primary barrier to successful genomic characterization of established PDXs is the presence of contaminating mouse DNA. This DNA can arise from small amounts of mouse tissue such as skin, hair, or viscera carried over during tumor excision or from stromal cells comprising immune infiltrates and vasculature resident within the tumor itself. These cells can contribute greater than 50% of the total DNA in the tumor by mass; however, this number is highly variable and depends greatly on the histological type from which the tumor was established. In general, the stromal content for each PDX is stable between passages—even if tumor cells are purified between passages—as new stroma is recruited from the recipient mouse. The presence of contaminating mouse DNA presents two distinct challenges for next-generation sequencing: spurious mapping of mouse reads to the human reference genome and sequencing of mouse reads that are not mapped to the human reference. The former may result in false-positive mutation calls, if sequence identity is low, or, under some circumstances, blind spots if identity is high, while the latter results in wasted sequencing resources and loss of depth of coverage. It is important to note that use of a human-specific enrichment technique such as whole exome capture or PCR amplicon sequencing is not sufficient to eliminate contaminating mouse DNA sequences, especially in the case of high sequence identity.

The challenge of contaminating mouse DNA can be addressed using a combination of two techniques: purification at the cellular level and bioinformatic depletion of reads mapping to the mouse genome. In this chapter, we discuss these approaches, their advantages and disadvantages, as well as quality control techniques that should be a part of any characterization efforts. For many PDX users, a combination of techniques may be most appropriate for their needs.

LABORATORY TECHNIQUES

When excising solid tumors, great care should be taken to avoid carryover of mouse skin, hair, fluids, or viscera. The field used for tumor removal should be kept clean and surgical tools should be cleaned and maintained between necropsies to prevent carryover. During necropsy, it is often helpful to apply 70% ethanol on the area of the initial incision to reduce carryover of fur and blood. It may also be useful to employ a separate set of surgical tools for tumor exposure and removal.

In the case of solid tumors, cells must be dissociated and disaggregated into a single-cell suspension prior to further attempts at purification. Mechanical mincing followed by gentle enzymatic dissociation as described in the following discussion are recommended.

Purification

Purification of human tumor cells can usually only be performed on fresh tumor or cell suspensions that have been viably cryopreserved in freezing media. Flash frozen tissue cannot be used for these separation techniques.

Fluorescence-Activated Cell Sorting

Fluorescence-activated cell sorting (FACS) can be used to obtain very pure populations of cells from leukemia and solid tumor PDXs, but first requires either red cell lysis or in the case of solid tumors, processing into a single-cell suspension followed by red cell lysis. FACS has the advantages of being capable of giving high purity as well as having the capacity to sort cell populations based on several parameters at once; however, FACS is limited by the requirement for expensive equipment, specialized operators, and high cost relative to other approaches.[1] Reasonable purity can be obtained simply by setting conservative gates that exclude clumping or dead cells (as assessed by uptake of a vital dye such as propidium iodide, 4′,6-diamidino-2-phenylindole, or 7-aminoactinomycin D) and negatively select for a mouse-specific cell surface marker such as $H2K^d$ (MHC class I alloantigen).[2] Additional purity can be obtained by positively gating for a human-specific marker such as epithelial cell adhesion molecule (EpCAM) for epithelial tumors or CD19 for B-cell malignancies.[3,4] Other markers or combination of markers may be used as appropriate for the model in question. A postsort purity check can be used to confirm the purity of the resulting sorted populations. FACS users should be aware that it is critical to thoroughly flush and wash any FACS instrument, particularly if it is a shared resource used by multiple groups.

Immunomagnetic

Immunomagnetic depletion of mouse cells can also be effective at reducing subsequent stromal DNA contamination. Immunomagnetic purification is based on the principle of magnetic separation. Superparamagnetic iron oxide beads are functionalized with an antibody or antibody cocktail and allowed to bind to cells in suspension. This allows cells of interest to be separated using a gentle magnetic field. Various kits exist from commercial vendors that rely on either positive selection or negative selection. We have tested both approaches and find that negative selection (depletion of murine cells) results in the highest final purity under the broadest range of contamination levels. Negative selection is further preferred in that a single approach can be effective at increasing purity regardless of the expression of a specific target antigen, such as EpCAM, which may not be universally expressed. In our experience, negative selection results in comparable purity to FACS with added flexibility and reduced overall cost.

Quality Control

Although the cost of next-generation sequencing has plummeted over the past decade, these experiments still remain resource intensive. Therefore, it is essential to pay close attention to quality control prior to investing in a next-generation sequencing project. Standard DNA quality control measures should be taken in confirming sufficient DNA quantity and quality for a successful sequencing experiment. Bioanalyzer or agarose gel quality control (QC)

Xenograft Fluorescence-Activated Cell Sorting (FACS) Standard Operating Procedure

Human xenografts grown in immunocomprimised hosts are comprised of both tumor cells and mouse stroma which can include multiple different cell types that make up the vascular support, immune infiltrate and fibroblast component of the tumor. When performing analytical FACS on xenograft cells, it is important to differentiate the species of origin of these cells, which can be done with species-specific antibodies. This approach can also be useful when it is desired to sort a pure population of cells for downstream analysis or to exclude a population of cells, such as mouse macrophages, that carry murine viruses such as lactate dehydrogenase elevating virus (LDHV).

Materials

Reagents

FACS buffer (phosphate buffered saine [PBS] containing 1% FBS and 1 mM EDTA)
75 mm Petri dish
Fresh sterile razor blade
Accutase solution (BD #561527)
DNase 1 (Sigma #D4263)
Ammonium-chloride-potassium (ACK) lysis buffer
TruStain FcX blocking solution (BioLegend # 422302)
$H2K^d$-PE (e.g. BD Pharmingen SF1-1.1)
Secondary human-specific marker (e.g. CD56-APC)
DAPI
Ice

Equipment

Biosafety Level-2 (BSL-2) safety cabinet
Clinical centrifuge
Vacuum source and glass Pasteur pipettes
50 mL conical tube

Micropipettes and pipette tips
Serological pipettes and pipette aids
70 μm mesh cell strainer
FACS tubes

Samples

Dissociated PDX tumor cells or fresh PDX tumor tissue in PBS on ice

Procedure

Sample Preparation

Note: All steps should be performed in a Biosafety level-2 (BSL-2) biosafety cabinet

1. If you already have dissociated PDX tumor cells, skip to step 6, otherwise proceed with steps 2–5.
2. Aspirate PBS from PDX tumor tissue using a Pasteur pipette and add 10 mL of Accutase solution (BD #561527) containing 100 Kunitz Units DNase I (Sigma #D4263) at room temperature
3. Decant the contents into a sterile 75 mm dish and finely mince the tumor tissue with a sterile razor blade, taking care to break all visible clumps
4. Collect the digesting mixture in a 50 mL conical tube and allow digestion to proceed for an additional 5 minutes at room temperature
5. Pass the mixture through a 70 μm mesh cell strainer, washing the dish and cell strainer with 20 mL of cold FACS Buffer, bringing the volume to 30 mL
6. Spin down the dissociated tumor cells at 200 rcf for 5 minutes and wash once with ice cold FACS Buffer
7. Optional step: Re-suspend the tumor cell pellet in 5 mL of ACK lysis buffer, gently creating a homogenous suspension and allow red cells to swell and lyse for 3–5 minutes at room temperature
8. Quench the lysis with 20 mL of FACS Buffer and spin down at 200 rcf
9. Re-suspend the pellet in 10 mL of FACS Buffer
10. Using trypan blue as a viability dye, determine a rough estimate of yield
11. Prepare the following FACS tubes for sorting in 1 mL FACS Buffer:
    a. unstained sample for FSC/SSC control
    b. sample stained with DAPI alone for single channel compensation
    c. DAPI will be added last for a final concentration of 1 nM
12. For samples that will be stained with conjugated antibodies, proceed to blocking non-specific sites with Human TruStain FcX blocking solution (BioLegend # 422302)
13. It is recommended that this be used at 5 μL per 100 μL of cell suspension without a clear indication of saturation potential. Therefore, samples will be concentrated to 500 μL in FACS buffer and 20 μL of blocking solution will be added to each tube being stained
14. Incubate at room temperature for 5 minutes and then proceed directly to staining
15. Incubate samples on ice, protected from light, for one hour
16. Wash cells with 10 mL of FACS buffer
17. Repeat wash steps two additional times, and re-suspend the final sample to be sorted to roughly 10-20 million cells/mL in FACS buffer. The target isolated population will be greater than 99% pure against $H2K^d$-phycoerythrin

should demonstrate that the DNA is not degraded and is in the size range of 10–20 kb. The DNA should be in a buffer that is free of contaminants such as PCR inhibitors. It is highly recommended to check for contaminating mouse DNA sequences prior to next-generation sequencing, which can also detect spontaneous murine lymphomas that appear to be human PDXs. We describe species-specific PCR amplicon length (ssPAL), a technique developed by the laboratories of Jim Eshleman and Sarah Wheelan.[5] This PCR-based assay is also useful for confirming overall DNA quality, as amplification will fail in the presence of poor-quality DNA.

Species-Specific PCR Amplicon Length

ssPAL is an approach to quantitation of human and mouse DNA content that relies on the amplification of nearly identical amplicons within the two reference genomes that differ only by the presence of a short indel (insertion and deletion). The result of this amplification reaction in an admixed sample is two PCR products of slightly differing lengths. These peaks can be resolved and quantitated by capillary electrophoresis, allowing for relative quantitation of the

Species-Specific PCR Amplicon Length (ssPAL) Standard Operating Procedure Analysis

The purpose of this technique is to evaluate the percentage of murine cells versus human cells in a given tissue. This procedure consumes the tissue since DNA extraction is required. By averaging the results of the two primer pairs used to perform ssPAL, an accurate calculation of the percentage of mouse versus human DNA is achieved.

Materials

Reagents

Primer pair 5: PCR products are 272 (human) and 278 (mouse) bp long
- F: 5′-TCATTGGCTTAAAATGTGT-3′
- R: 5′-**FAM**-TTTATTTTAAGGGGTTGTAATG-3′

Primer pair 43: PCR products are 211 (human) and 206 (mouse) bp long
- F: 5′-CTATTCCTATAGCACAAAGG-3′
- R: 5′-**FAM**-GATGGTGTACACCCATCATG-3′

Phusion high fidelity PCR master mix (New England Biolabs cat. no. M0531S)
Molecular Biology Grade Water (Hyclone cat. no. SH40003-12)

Equipment

PCR machine

Samples

100 ng xenograft DNA per PCR reaction

Reagent Setup

Dilute samples with nuclease free H_2O to get a 100 ng/μL DNA concentration

Procedure

PCR reaction

1. Prepare one master mix for each primer pair by adjusting the quantities below based on the number of samples

25 μL Phusion master mix
1.5 μL Dimethyl sulfoxide (DMSO)
2.5 μL Forward PCR primer at a 10 μM concentration
2.5 μL Reverse PCR primer at a 10 μM concentration
17.5 μL H_2O

2. Add 49 μL of master mix to each PCR tube then add 1 μL DNA to corresponding tube
3. Run PCR using the following conditions:

98 °C for 5′
35 cycles – 98 °C for 30″, 52 °C for 30″, 72 °C for 30″
72 °C for 10′
Hold 4 °C

4. Check the PCR product on an agarose gel. It will not be possible to resolve the two bands for mouse and human, but you should be able to see a single clear band.
5. Once PCR is complete dilute each sample by adding 1 μL PCR product to 32 μL H_2O. Mix well.

Sample preparation for sizing by capillary electrophoresis

1. Add 18 μL H_2O to the number of PCR tubes needed for your samples
2. Add 1 μL of diluted PCR product from primer pair 43 and 1 μL of diluted PCR product from primer pair 5 to the same tube

Peak Scanner analysis

1. Open peak scanner and start new project
2. Use "add files" button to upload the trace files
3. Set the size standard to "GS500(-250)Liz" for each file
4. Click analyze
5. Peak heights are proportional to DNA content
6. Once you've obtained the DNA percentages for primer pair 5 and 43, average them together to obtain the final DNA percentage.

Notes

- The peak height should not exceed the cutoff line of 32,000. If it does, you may need to dilute your PCR product further due to saturation.
- The calculated DNA percentages for primer pair 43 and 5 will usually differ from each other by about 10%, which is why we average both values at the final step
- The mouse peak height is multiplied by 0.85 to correct for genome size.

abundance of mouse and human DNA in a given sample. The assay is simple, cost-effective, and easy to interpret.

BIOINFORMATIC TECHNIQUES

The techniques described below are compatible with both purified cells and mixed populations of human and mouse cells. However, it must be stated that it will be impossible to deconvolute the origin of reads that map to regions of high sequence identity between the human and mouse genomes. This may result in regions of low coverage in conserved regions that impair mutation calling and copy number assignment at the basic level as well as more advanced analysis, such as allele-specific copy number calls or clonal reconstructions.

Computational Requirements

Ideally, the user will have access to high-performance computing resources that include high-performance storage, Ethernet-connected cluster nodes, and a job scheduling environment. For reasons described in detail below, the techniques described in this section require a Linux system running a 64-bit kernel as well as a 64-bit aligner such as BWA.[6,7] As a major bottleneck for alignment is storage, high-performance data storage is preferred.

Alignment

Hybrid Genome Preparation

Several approaches have been described for sequencing human xenografts. Early approaches focused on the concept of sequentially aligning sequenced reads to both the human and mouse genome, and then filtering the final reads based on a percent identity cutoff or by classification of reads to either human or mouse genome based on *k*-mer decomposition prior to alignment.[8–10] An alternative approach that requires no assignment of threshold limits is to align sequenced reads to a hybrid human/mouse reference genome in which the mouse portion serves as bait sequence.[11] Reads mapping to mouse contiguous consensus sequences (contigs) are subsequently discarded after alignment. However, unlike sequential alignment approaches, the hybrid genome approach requires more available RAM in order to maintain the larger hybrid genome in memory. Moreover, a hybrid human/mouse genome exceeds the at most 4 GB of addressable memory on 32-bit chipsets, necessitating the use of a 64-bit chipset, binary and operating system for alignment. A distinct advantage of the hybrid genome approach is in performance: it takes less than half of the compute time required for sequential alignment.

To generate a hybrid genome, the reference genomes for both human and mouse must be downloaded in FASTA format. Reference genomes for various assemblies are available from both the GENCODE project and Illumina, among other sources. The human and mouse reference genomes share some overlapping contig names (eg, chr1, chr2, chr3,...). Therefore, the mouse contigs must all be tagged with a unique identifier prior to merging the hybrid genome (eg, mm_chr1, mm_chr2, mm_chr3) in order to later distinguish mouse and human reads mapped to contigs of the same name. In the Linux example shown below, hg.fa, which represents a human genome reference FASTA sequence, is first copied to a new FASTA file, hybrid.fa, using the cp command. The sed command is then used to concatenate a mouse reference genome, mm.fa, to the end of hybrid.fa while simultaneously tagging each chromosome with "mm_," to indicate that these contigs are of murine origin.

```
cp hg.fa hybrid.fa
sed 's/chr/mm_chr/' mm.fa >> hybrid.fa
```

The resulting FASTA file can be used to generate a hybrid genome reference index file for use with your aligner of choice. Critically, if this approach is taken, it is necessary to align both the PDX sample and matched normal sample to the same hybrid genome. Regions of high sequence identity between human and mouse genomes will result in reads for a specific region that cannot be uniquely mapped. If the normal sample does not have similar mapping irregularities, it can result in a distorted impression of apparent copy number loss in the tumor sample, manifesting as focal deletions.

Eliminating Mouse Reads From Analysis

Mouse reads can be eliminated from analysis in several ways. Perhaps the most convenient way is to provide a list of genomic regions to be focused on by downstream analysis tools in BED (Browser Extensible Data) format. For example, for whole genome shotgun sequencing, it may be sufficient to provide a list of each of the human chromosomes, disregarding mouse contigs tagged with "mm_" eg,:

```
chr1
chr2
chr3
...
```

Your analysis may already be focused on specific genomic regions, such as in whole exome capture sequencing, or targeted capture sequencing. BED files for commercial kits are provided by the manufacturer. If this is the case, the appropriate capture regions specified already exclude the "mm_" tagged contigs and reads mapping to these regions will be disregarded from analysis.

Quality Control

After alignment is complete, perhaps the most important and difficult to predict quality control measure is average depth of coverage of the region of interest. A specific target depth of coverage can be estimated based on the size in base pairs of the region to be sequenced and the number of reads to be sequenced. PDX users should additionally use estimates of human DNA content from ssPAL to inform their target estimates. For example, if a DNA sample consists of 50% murine DNA, you may need to sequence twice as many reads to achieve the target depth of coverage as would be necessary in a pure sample. The need for this extra sequencing is obviated by sample purification.

After sequencing, actual depth of coverage of the target regions should be calculated and compared to the expected depth of coverage. If depth of coverage is lower than expected, additional data may need to be collected. It may also be useful to perform a low-depth sequencing experiment to estimate the level of murine DNA contamination in the final library. This is particularly useful when multiple PDXs are to be sequenced in a batch and multiplexing is available.

ACKNOWLEDGMENTS

The authors received support through grants P30 CA008748 and U54 OD020355-01 and from the Geoffrey Beene Cancer Research Center.

REFERENCES

1. Mattanovich D, Borth N. Applications of cell sorting in biotechnology. *Microb Cell Fact* 2006;**5**:12.
2. Liu H, Bockhorn J, Dalton R, Chang YF, Qian D, Zitzow LA, et al. Removal of lactate dehydrogenase-elevating virus from human-in-mouse breast tumor xenografts by cell-sorting. *J Virol Methods* 2011;**173**(2):266–70.
3. Caligaris-Cappio F, Bergui L, Tesio L, Pizzolo G, Malavasi F, Chilosi M, et al. Identification of malignant plasma cell precursors in the bone marrow of multiple myeloma. *J Clin Invest* 1985;**76**(3):1243–51.
4. De Leij L, Helrich W, Stein R, Mattes MJ. SCLC-cluster-2 antibodies detect the pancarcinoma/epithelial glycoprotein EGP-2. *Int J Cancer Suppl* 1994;**8**:60–3.
5. Lin MT, Tseng LH, Kamiyama H, Kamiyama M, Lim P, Hidalgo M, et al. Quantifying the relative amount of mouse and human DNA in cancer xenografts using species-specific variation in gene length. *BioTechniques* 2010;**48**(3):211–8.
6. Li H, Durbin R. Fast and accurate long-read alignment with Burrows-Wheeler transform. *Bioinformatics* 2010;**26**(5):589–95.
7. Li H, Durbin R. Fast and accurate short read alignment with Burrows-Wheeler transform. *Bioinformatics* 2009;**25**(14):1754–60.
8. Schmieder R, Edwards R. Fast identification and removal of sequence contamination from genomic and metagenomic datasets. *PLoS One* 2011;**6**(3):e17288.
9. Rossello FJ, Tothill RW, Britt K, Marini KD, Falzon J, Thomas DM, et al. Next-generation sequence analysis of cancer xenograft models. *PLoS One* 2013;**8**(9):e74432.

10. Conway T, Wazny J, Bromage A, Tymms M, Sooraj D, Williams ED, et al. Xenome–a tool for classifying reads from xenograft samples. *Bioinformatics* 2012;**28**(12):i172–8.
11. Tso KY, Lee SD, Lo KW, Yip KY. Are special read alignment strategies necessary and cost-effective when handling sequencing reads from patient-derived tumor xenografts? *BMC Genomics* 2014;**15**:1172.

Chapter 6

Running a PDX Core Laboratory or a PDX Support Program

A. Krivtsov[1], M. Mattar[1], R.K. Uthamanthil[2], E. de Stanchina[1]
[1]Memorial Sloan Kettering Cancer Center, New York, NY, United States; [2]Fred Hutchinson Cancer Research Center, Seattle, WA, United States

Patient-derived xenografts (PDXs) and organoid models are contributing to substantial advances in our understanding of the physiological impact of genetic variation in a variety of human diseases and have been successfully used to discover novel biomarkers and as tools for the development of new therapies for advanced and drug-resistant tumors. However, the process of establishing and propagating such models so that they can be used in preclinical studies is expensive and fraught with procedural and technical challenges. Thus it may be beneficial for large academic institutions to set up a centralized PDX Core to promote seamless coordination between clinical and research teams and integration of components of basic science research, genomic information, clinical data, and mouse model technology.

INFRASTRUCTURE

For a PDX Core to function effectively and cost-efficiently, in addition to dedicated and skilled personnel on both the clinical and research side (see also Section II, Chapter 2), critical infrastructural components must already be in place. In particular, both laboratory and animal research space has to be carefully planned.

Regulatory and Administrative Infrastructure

As described in other chapters in this section, meeting regulatory requirements (Section II, Chapter 1) as well as occupational health and safety considerations (Section II, Chapter 8) are critical in working with human tissues and animals. Most medium to large research institutions have their own well-structured programs supporting these aspects, whereas some smaller institutions or hospitals rely instead on the regulatory infrastructure of

Patient Derived Tumor Xenograft Models. http://dx.doi.org/10.1016/B978-0-12-804010-2.00012-6

larger programs with which they establish close working relations. Considering the high cost of PDX programs (see below and Section IV, Chapter 1), it is important that proper finance and grant management infrastructure is also put in place.

Vivarium

The physical space within which mice are housed and the housing environment are key areas to consider. The quality and efficiency of the vivarium directly and indirectly influence the quality and efficiency of the PDX program. The process of establishing and maintaining a pathogen-free and clean environment for mice in research is complex and labor intensive. Running an efficient vivarium involves managing a complex system of people, processes, and technology in an environment of constantly changing regulations, scientific needs, and financial constraints. A centralized vivarium design typically increases the efficiency of the program and reduces the potential for pathogen outbreaks in the barrier. Procedures and standards need to be established and implemented to guarantee that the mice are housed in a pathogen-free environment, with standard room temperature, humidity, and air pressure differential. Additionally, animal rooms housing PDX models, and procedural suites where patient specimens are handled, will need to be equipped as biosafety level 2 areas, because of the risk of exposure to potentially infectious material. Ideally, the vivarium should also be equipped with small animal imaging [computed tomography (CT), positron emission tomography (PET), magnetic resonance imaging (MRI), bioluminescence, ultrasound, X-ray] capabilities, essential for monitoring the growth of orthotopic models.

The per diem cost, which is the typical way the vivarium maintenance costs are charged back to investigators, vary widely among institutions depending on their location (http://www.aclam.org/Content/files/files/Forum2012/ACLAM_Forum_2012_Macy.pdf), size of the vivarium, institutional subsidies, and other factors including labor costs. Proper veterinary care of mice (see Section II, Chapter 7) includes support for strain-specific concerns, disease prevention, as well as management of research-related health issues. Stringent monitoring against pathogens that compromise rodent health and/or act as confounding factors in research are critical for the success of the program.

Laboratory Space

Particular attention will need to be paid to ensure the availability of a fully equipped tissue culture room for processing freshly collected samples for implantation and banking, and establishing cell lines and organoids. Ideally, space for histology equipment (tissue processor, embedding station, slide preparation, and staining) will also be allocated nearby, for easy and seamless processing of PDX samples for immunohistochemistry (IHC) analysis.

Biobank and Data Center

Ample space will need to be designated for storage of viable specimens (in liquid nitrogen tanks) and of samples set aside for genomic and histologic analysis. Ideally, a barcoding system for sample inventory and tracking will be set in place for easy cataloging and retrieval of archived samples. This function becomes crucial as the collection of established PDX models grows larger, and samples may need to be stored in separate locations. For each model, at any time it should be possible to easily query the number of samples available for future propagation, along with their location in the biobank, and whether there is any corresponding material set aside for molecular or histologic analysis. Therefore, a data center for annotation and storage of data on all PDX-related activities will also need to be set up. Database requirements will be covered in greater detail later on in this chapter.

Mouse Hospital

Experiments involving PDXs are usually very laborious and costly (see later). Thus, thorough upfront planning and skillful execution of every aspect of a study are of utmost importance to its success and reproducibility. For these reasons, whenever possible, expansion of PDXs for efficacy studies should be overseen by specialized personnel, familiar with the characteristics of each disease model and well versed in all technical aspects of tumor transplantation, drug administration, and clinical and efficacy assessments. In fact, in many academic institutions, PDX programs are managed within a larger infrastructure, commonly referred to as the "mouse hospital."[1]

Mouse hospitals are usually designed to closely resemble a patient hospital, where patient care is administered through integrated services including access to a research Pharmacy (drug purchasing, stability analysis, formulation, vialing), Analytical Chemistry laboratory (for pharmacokinetics studies), Anatomical Imaging services (MRI, PET/CT, bioluminescence/fluorescence, Ultrasound, X-ray), Interventional Radiology, Pathology (hematology and clinical chemistry assays, biopsy, necropsy, histopathology), Genomics laboratory, and Data storage and analysis. It is important to note that mouse hospital personnel are usually trained in and required to follow detailed standard operating procedures (SOPs) in all aspects of their work. This is crucial to ensure that studies are carried out in a consistently uniform and reproducible manner.[1]

In particular, SOPs should be in place for all aspects of patient sample acquisition, processing, implantation, propagation, storage, and distribution. Staff should also be trained on technical SOPs related to animal care (husbandry, drug administration, blood sampling, imaging, surgery and postsurgical care, etc.). Moreover, additional SOPs may be established to detail formulation; storage, stability, and administration schedule for each compound used in a PDX study; and processing of collected samples for hematology, clinical chemistry, pharmacokinetic, biochemistry, histology, and genomic analyses.

Finally, for each PDX study carried out within the mouse hospital, a detailed study protocol, with clear indication of all data that should be collected during the study should be agreed upon with the investigators and distributed to all the staff involved in the study.

PERSONNEL

As discussed in Section II, Chapter 2, a large number of dedicated staff are usually involved at different levels to assure the smooth functioning of a PDX operation. On the administrative side, staff need to ensure regulatory requirements (Institutional Review Board, patient consent forms, Institutional Animal Care and Use Committee, Institutional Biosafety Committee) are met, legal documents (Material Transfer Agreements, sponsored research agreements, software licenses, other contracts) are in place, and the budget (grant support, fee-for-service agreements) is well managed. Research support on the clinical side takes care of sample accrual (patient selection, coordination with surgery schedules, specimen collection), PDX database annotation, and interface with clinical applications. The PDX laboratory branch meanwhile devises and implements SOPs for sample processing, storage and implantation, model maintenance, PDX characterization and distribution, and execution of preclinical research studies (see also Section II, Chapter 2, Table 2.1).

Education and Training

The key to successful implementation of a PDX Core is the development and implementation of training programs for personnel involved in each aspect of this complex operation. Indeed, it is essential that all staff be properly qualified and instructed in relevant procedures and practices pertinent to their specific assignments. Hands-on classes on sample acquisition and processing, animal handling, specialized techniques, and surgical procedures should be offered, along with lectures on data acquisition and analysis. As mentioned above, the establishment of well-designed SOPs can greatly help in training and education of dedicated personnel, and it is integral to achieving uniformity and reproducibility. This is of particular relevance when PDX models are distributed to collaborators, as even small changes in procedures may lead to discrepancies and thus, difficulties in data comparison across multiple laboratories and institutions.[1]

DATA STORAGE AND MANAGEMENT

Effective storage and management of data related to the phenotypic and genomic characterization of PDX models involves the seamless integration of numerous aspects of both clinical and laboratory processes and is inextricably linked to the success of a PDX Core Program, as it maximizes the utility and potential applications of the models.

Thus, a comprehensive yet dynamic database, that can be tailored to the needs of multiple investigators must be developed and implemented. This dedicated database (which, in the United States, must be Health Insurance Portability and Accountability Act compliant) will serve as an interface for collecting, storing, and tracking raw experimental data obtained from several sources including tissue collection, biobanking, molecular and genomic analysis, and in vivo and in vitro experiments. Importantly, the database should be kept on a secure server that is routinely backed up.

The database will function by integrating various modules to allow researchers to accomplish several goals including management of raw data, tracking of experimental data, and clinical annotation of samples and models. Ideally, this database would be hosted on a dedicated internal server, where data are securely stored and regularly backed up. In addition, the database should be searchable and accessible to multiple users. However, a different level of access should be set in place, to make sure that privileged information, along with data entry/modification rights, are accessible only to authorized users.

Although the database obviously needs to be developed based on the investigators' current needs, it is ideal if it is built in such a way that it can be modified and expanded modularly to accommodate novel requirements as they arise. Most of the data input fields should be predetermined, while the number of free text fields should be minimized. These guidelines enforce standardized data recording and allow for all records to be searchable.

Annotation of Patient Samples

Patient samples should be thoroughly clinically annotated. Data capture can start as soon as a patient is enrolled for sample collection. Once patient consent is confirmed, basic demographic and diagnostic information along with relevant medical history can be entered into the database.

- *The diagnostic information* should include the date of diagnosis, disease status (ie, de novo, refractory, recurrent), evidence (if any) of metastatic sites, and any additional information that may be available on tumor subtype, grade and stage, and mutational status.
- *The relevant medical history* should include personal and family history of malignancies, preoperative scans and relevant laboratory results, previous treatments and treatment responses, disease-specific risk factors (ie, smoking history, *Helicobacter pylori* infection, reproductive history), and any other notable risk factors. Some parameters will depend on the tumor type. For example, the disease-specific risk factors or histological classification should be presented as drop-down lists whose values are shown according to the selected tumor type.

  Ideally, most of the clinical data would be directly migrated from the institutional electronic medical records in order to ensure the standardization of data recording and reduce errors due to manual entry. Moreover, given that manual data entry can be exceedingly laborious and time-consuming, the automatic migration of data will simultaneously assure timely data entry and easier management of large set databases.

- *Additional clinical information* will be collected from patients whose samples successfully engraft. This will include patient vital status, date of follow-up, and date of death (if applicable), along with a history of subsequent treatments and treatment responses, relevant laboratory reports, imaging results, and any other significant events. Any additional sample collection from the same patient would also be recorded. These follow-up annotations can prove very valuable, particularly when analyzing data from coclinical trials.[1,2]

Annotation of PDX Samples

PDX samples should be as thoroughly annotated as the corresponding patient samples, starting at the time of sample collection.

- *Collected sample information*: During sample collection, information should be recorded about both the collection process and the quality of the collected sample. This should include the date of sample collection, type of procedure performed to obtain the sample, duration of the entire procedure, preferably name of the doctor/team that performed the said procedure, and time elapsed from sample resection/collection, to delivery to the laboratory for processing, to final implantation in mice, appropriately accounting for any lags. Additionally, details on sample quality should include details on anatomical site from which the sample was collected, amount of sample, primary or metastatic classification, visual appearance (ie, areas of necrosis, stromal component, small sample size), and any other pertinent notes about the primary tissue. These records can be analyzed when examining tumor take rates and can help identify factors that may contribute to poor engraftment.
- *In-life PDX information*: Once a patient sample is implanted in animals, a record needs to be entered for each xenografted animal and updated through its life cycle. Basic information such as animal strain, age, sex, and source (including vendor purchase requisition ID, when available), and any nonstandard husbandry conditions (ie, special diet) should be entered in predetermined fields, along with animal and cage identification and housing location. At all times, animals enrolled in studies should be associated with a "status," which describes their current condition (ie, implanted, on experimental protocol, ready for transplantation, sacrificed, found dead). Essential information regarding sample implantation should be recorded as well. This will include sample origin and processing method, site of sample implantation, name of the technician performing the procedure and in charge of animal care, and any special husbandry conditions (ie, antibiotics, hormones). Clinical signs (ie, weight loss, tumor ulceration, graft versus host disease) along with tumor volume measurements should be recorded. Ideally, a tumor growth chart should be automatically generated and associated with the animal records, for easy visualization of PDX model growth. Any additional notes relating to tumor appearance and growth rate should be recorded in a free text field. Depending on the model, information such as in-life clinical pathology data

(for leukemia models) or imaging (for orthotopically implanted tumors) would also need to be included. Finally, the date and reason of animal death should also be recorded. This ideally should prompt the system to generate a few yes or no questions that will lead to the generation of a summary table for each animal/model (ie, Did the tumor grow? Was the model transplanted? Was this the first transplant? Was this model used in a preclinical study?).

- *PDX-generated samples*: Once animals are sacrificed and tumors collected, very accurate records should be kept of all that is done with the tumor material. It is recommended that, whenever possible, tumor material should be viably preserved for future transplantation; additionally, samples may be preserved in formalin or flash frozen for further analyses, or used to establish cell lines. Ideally, each collected sample will have a barcode, so that information on the number of aliquots and their exact location will also be stored in the database within its biobank section. This way, it is easy to keep track of how many samples are available for each model at any given time. Taking into consideration that PDX models may constitute a limited resource, and that serial PDX transplantation can result in genetic drift, PDX distribution should be circumspectly planned. Whenever samples are distributed to collaborators, records of which aliquots were shared and of the subsequent analyses performed on the shared samples should also be noted.

Annotation of Histology and Genomic Data

PDXs can effectively recapitulate the human disease by retaining the morphological and genomic characteristics of the human tumor. Therefore, the database should contain an IHC section with pathology reports and pictures of associated slides for both the patient samples and the corresponding PDX. Side-by-side comparisons will allow investigators to easily confirm the morphological continuities between the patient tumor and the PDX.

Similarly, the database should facilitate visualization and analysis of cancer genomics data by integrating data that may have been captured for both patient (tumor and normal) and corresponding PDX samples through multiple platforms (whole-genome, exome, and transcriptome sequencing; epigenomics and metagenomics; and capture-based targeted sequencing assays such as MSK-IMPACT[3]). The database could then be used to facilitate comparative cross-species and longitudinal analyses of samples from the same patient or patient-derived model, and will allow investigators to quickly identify PDX models with specific genomic signatures and select the ones that may be most appropriate for their in vivo studies.

Annotation of In Vitro, Ex Vivo, and Preclinical Data

The tumor material from a PDX model can also be used to establish cell lines and organoids and for ex vivo analyses.[4] As mentioned above, this information should also be collected in the database, along with details on the growth and preservation conditions, and any additional available data (genomic analysis, results of drug screening assays, etc.). Similarly, results of preclinical and coclinical trials[1] conducted in established PDX models should be uploaded in the database.

Query Capabilities and Data Access

Making every annotated field in the database searchable will allow investigators to perform different types of queries, both broad (ie, how many PDXs are available of a specific cancer subtype, or with a certain genomic alteration) and narrow (ie, how many vials of a certain PDX are in the freezer, how many PDX models are currently growing in mice). Importantly, access to data will need to be regulated; the PDX Core team and database managers will have the ability to view, create, and delete the data in each of the fields, whereas external collaborators may be able to search and view only a limited number of categories that are of general interest, such as the number of PDX models of any tumor subtype, models resistant to a specific targeted therapy, or models with a defined genetic alteration.

This makes the database an ideal avenue for collaborative projects and can maximize the utility of each PDX model.

COST ANALYSIS CONSIDERATIONS

Establishing and maintaining libraries of PDX models is an expensive endeavor. Costs will vary significantly in different institutions, depending on the available infrastructure, local cost of labor and reagents, and level of institutional support. Main costs to consider are summarized in Table 6.1 and discussed in the following sections.

Cost of Mice

Mouse charges, which include purchasing, breeding, and per diem costs, are often one of the most expensive components of a PDX program budget, as mice are used for both PDX model development and propagation and for preclinical studies. PDX programs typically use a large number of immunocompromised mice, such as NSGs. Depending on the source and usage, immunocompromised strains can be very expensive to obtain and difficult to maintain. When purchased from an accredited vendor, such as Jackson Laboratories, prices vary between $100 and $200 or more depending on the chosen strain (www.jax.org).

Large PDX programs in nonprofit or academic institutions may be able to offset some of these costs by breeding the mice in-house, upon approval of specific contracts with the breeder. However, feasibility and the cost savings may vary widely based on multiple factors including availability of a high-quality barrier mouse facility with dedicated breeding rooms, cost of husbandry (mouse per diem charges), genetic monitoring, and labor (salary of the technician in charge of maintaining the colony), as well as the size of the program. It is important to note that breeding programs should always be managed by experienced personnel, to avoid potential issues with the colonies, such as genetic drift.[5]

TABLE 6.1 List of Services Associated With the Establishment and Propagation of PDX Models, and Estimate of Corresponding Cost/Model

Item or Service	Average Cost
Mice purchase	$100–200/mouse
Veterinary and husbandry charges	>$l/cage/day
Mice imaging	$0–200/mouse
Surgery/procedure suites	$0–10/mouse
Reagents/consumables	$10–50/model
Biobanking of patient and PDX samples	$50–100/model
Labor—research technician	$100–1000/model
Labor—database manager	$100–500/model
Histopathology	$50–500/model
Sequencing	$500–1000/model
Administrative costs (IRB, IACUC, IBC, MTAs)	$0–50/model
Data analysis	$0–500/model
Other infrastructural costs (software licenses, data server charges, laboratory space charges)	$0–50/model

It is important to note that cost of establishing a new model will vary significantly even within the same laboratory depending on a number of variables: How many mice are initially implanted with the patient specimen? How is the sample implanted (subcutaneously or orthotopically)? How is tumor growth monitored (tumor volume measurement by caliper, imaging, blood/bone marrow analysis)? How long it takes for the tumor to grow? What type of molecular characterization is performed? In our experience, the average cost is ~$1000–1500/model, not including the cost of IHC or genomic analysis.
IRB, Institutional Review Board; *IACUC*, Institutional Animal Care and Use Committee; *IBC*, Institutional Biosafety Committee; *MTA*, Material Transfer Agreement.

Additionally, breeding costs can also be affected by the fact that investigators often choose to use only mice of one sex for PDX propagation and preclinical experiments. This may be due to both practical and scientific reasons. In general, because of aggressive behavior and fighting, male mice often need to be housed in single cages, with increase in per diem charges. Fights originating from aggressiveness can also lead to ulceration of subcutaneous tumors and possible loss of precious samples. Therefore, female mice are quite often preferred. Scientific reasons also can drive sex selection. While gender-related cancer models might need mice of specific gender (eg, male mice for prostate cancer and females for ovarian cancer), it is becoming increasingly apparent that take rates of various tumors may also depend on the mice gender. For example, hematopoietic stem cell engraftment is significantly more efficient in female mice than in male mice.[6] On the other hand, hepatocellular carcinomas engraft faster and produce larger tumors in male mice.[7]

A number of resources, such as the Jackson Laboratory Resource Manual *Breeding Strategies for Maintaining Colonies of Laboratory Mice* (www.jax.org) are available to help determine whether it is worth to consider establishing an in-house breeding program, depending on the number of mice/sex/week that would be needed for PDX studies.

Cost of Infrastructures

A well-run animal facility with excellent husbandry standards is critical for breeding and maintenance of immunocompromised mice. Minimum requirements include sterilized caging, bedding, feed, and water; individually ventilated caging or other closed systems supplying (high-efficiency particulate air or other high-efficiency filters) filtered air; well-designed procedure suites/spaces; proper personal protective equipment; and husbandry and veterinary care SOPs. PDX programs within such facilities are usually charged a per diem cage cost. In addition, use of specialized procedure rooms or imaging equipment within the animal facility may be charged separately.

Substantial costs are also associated with maintenance of biobank programs that will take care of storing patient and PDX-related specimens in dedicated repositories. Costs will vary significantly depending on the size of the operation and the amount of support (space, purchase, and maintenance of freezers and liquid nitrogen tanks) provided by each institution.

Cost of Labor

As already mentioned earlier and in Chapter 2 of this section, skilled personnel are needed in all aspects of PDX establishment. Salaries of clinical and administrative staff may be covered by other institutional sources, and cost of veterinary staff may be included in animal per diem charges. However, salaries of skilled research technicians involved in establishing, maintaining, and propagating PDX models, and of staff in charge of data entry and database maintenance, are usually the responsibility of the PDX lab and therefore need to be taken into account.

Cost of PDX Model Characterization

To be most useful, PDX models need to be well characterized both histologically and molecularly. Thus, PDX samples are often processed for histopathology, biochemistry, proteomics, and genomic analysis. The depth as well as breadth of analysis depends on the specific research focus, but in all cases access to specialized infrastructures and qualified personnel is required. Histopathology characterization may be limited to H&E staining to assess tissue morphology, but it would also normally include a panel of IHC markers to match the patient data. Similarly, genomic analysis techniques and associated costs vary widely, from target-specific PCR to whole-genome next-generation sequencing (NGS). In most cases it is also necessary to take into consideration the cost of genomic characterization of the corresponding patient sample (ideally both tumor and normal tissue), since health insurance coverage of tumor genomic analysis varies significantly. For example, many comprehensive cancer centers analyze patient tumors for mutations in a list of specific genes[3]; however, the numbers of genes and type of analysis in the list varies based on institution policies and patient health care insurance coverage. Although NGS is considered ideal for global genetic screening of tumors as well as a standard platform across PDX programs, until recently NGS was not covered by health insurance programs. However, some recent changes in the United States are exciting. For example, In January 2016, Independence Blue Cross and NantHealth announced the nation's first insurance coverage for a comprehensive whole-genome and proteome molecular diagnostic platform (GPS Cancer) to diagnose molecular alterations in an individual's cancer, and to identify personalized therapeutic regimens (http://www.businesswire.com/news/home/20160111006104/en/Nation%E2%80%99s-Insurance-Coverage-Next-Generation-Genome-Sequencing-Proteomic).

Finally, costs associated with data analysis cannot be overlooked, as highly qualified personnel, such as board-certified pathologists and bioinformatics analysts, need to be consulted, and sophisticated software and instrumentations need to be employed.

Cost of Data Management

Recording, storing, managing, and securing data is an important part of any PDX program. Although many small PDX research programs can initially manage most of the data by using standard spreadsheets and other basic software (such as FileMakerPro), as programs grow larger or extend in time, a well-designed database with very good interactive and search capabilities becomes necessary. Unfortunately, most commercially available laboratory and biospecimen management software applications do not meet all the needs for supporting a PDX program. Many large programs have resorted to using multiple software products to meet the needs, whereas some institutions have invested considerable resources in developing powerful software solutions that will meet most of the needs of a complex PDX research program.[2]

In conclusion, establishing a PDX program can be a challenging task financially, technically, and organizationally. For large institutions, a centralized PDX Core capable of combining existing resources with new infrastructure to create an integrated organization can be a solution that is both cost-effective and efficient. This in turn can lead to better use of the established PDX models and increased collaborative efforts and, ultimately, scientific advances.

ACKNOWLEDGMENTS

The authors received support through grants P30 CA008748 and U54 OD020355-01 and from the Geoffrey Beene Cancer Research Center. Additionally, the authors would like to thank Andrea Bertotti and his colleagues for very valuable discussions on implementation of comprehensive PDX databases.

REFERENCES

1. Clohessy JG, de Stanchina E. Infrastructure needs for translational integration of mouse and human trials. *Cold Spring Harb Protoc* 2013;**2013**:1109–14.
2. Bertotti A, Papp E, Jones S, Adleff V, Anagnostou V, Lupo B, et al. The genomic landscape of response to EGFR blockade in colorectal cancer. *Nature* 2015;**526**:263–7.
3. Hyman DM, Solit DB, Arcila ME, Cheng DT, Sabbatini P, Baselga J, et al. Precision medicine at Memorial Sloan Kettering Cancer Center: clinical next-generation sequencing enabling next-generation targeted therapy trials. *Drug Discov Today* 2015;**20**:1422–8.
4. Corben AD, Uddin MM, Crawford B, Farooq M, Modi S, Gerecitano J, et al. Ex vivo treatment response of primary tumors and/or associated metastases for preclinical and clinical development of therapeutics. *J Vis Exp* 2014:e52157.
5. Casellas J. Inbred mouse strains and genetic stability: a review. *Animal* 2011;**5**:1–7.
6. Notta F, Doulatov S, Dick JE. Engraftment of human hematopoietic stem cells is more efficient in female NOD/SCID/IL-2Rgc-null recipients. *Blood* 2010;**115**:3704–7.
7. Martin-Padura I, Agliano A, Marighetti P, Porretti L, Bertolini F. Sex-related efficiency in NSG mouse engraftment. *Blood* 2010;**116**:2616–7.

Chapter 7

Veterinary Care

T. Brabb[1], P.T. Tinkey[2]
[1]*University of Washington, Seattle, WA, United States;* [2]*The University of Texas MD Anderson Cancer Center, Houston, TX, United States*

INTRODUCTION

Many strains and lines of immunodeficient mice are available for cancer research and include mice with single mutations [eg, nude, severe combined immunodeficiency (SCID), beige, X-linked immunodeficient, recombination activating gene 1 (*Rag1*), and 2 (*Rag2*) null] and those with combined mutations [eg, nonobese diabetic (NOD)-SCID-*IL2g* null (NSG), NOD-*Rag-IL2g* null, and NOD-SCID-*IL2g* null + human cytokine expression]. These models have different degrees of impaired immune function resulting in moderate to profound immunodeficiency, which makes them susceptible to numerous pathogens, opportunistic infections, and unique health conditions. Specialized systems of husbandry and health care are required for successful maintenance and research use of these models.

This chapter will review best practices and procedures involved in caring for highly immunodeficient and humanized mice used in cancer research. We will discuss murine pathogens and opportunists, facility infrastructure, and the unique health conditions encountered in humanized and patient-derived tumor xenograft (PDX) models, including mouse strain–specific diseases, graft-versus-host disease (GVHD), radiation toxicity, chemotherapy toxicity, and tumor development.

PATHOGENS AND OPPORTUNISTS

Most facilities exclude known murine pathogens but maintain mice that do not have defined microbiomes.[1] Rodents housed in uncovered cages in barrier rooms develop a complex microflora that include microbes from the environment, other mice, and people. These agents, including *Pseudomonas aeruginosa*, β-hemolytic streptococci, *Staphylococcus aureus*, and *Pneumocystis murina*, can be opportunistic pathogens in highly immunodeficient mice.[2] Surveys of colony surveillance samples submitted to diagnostic laboratories show that several murine pathogens and opportunistic agents are still

Patient Derived Tumor Xenograft Models. http://dx.doi.org/10.1016/B978-0-12-804010-2.00013-8

relatively prevalent in research facilities.[3] The most commonly identified agents included viruses, bacteria, fungi, and various parasitic organisms.[3,4]

Murine viruses that remain problematic in research facilities include, in order of prevalence, mouse norovirus, mouse parvoviruses (minute virus of mice and mouse parvovirus), and mouse hepatitis virus[3]; lactate dehydrogenase–elevating virus and lymphocytic choriomeningitis virus are less prevalent but remain problematic when they occur.[5] These viruses are difficult to eradicate from mouse colonies because the viruses may be environmentally resistant or may persist in the host with long-term shedding. In some viruses with multiple strains (eg, parvoviruses), infection with one strain may not provide cross-protection against other strains.[2,5] In most cases, these viruses do not cause disease in immunocompetent mice, but significant clinical illness has been reported sporadically in mice with immune system defects as well as interference with tumor xenograft models. These illnesses include pneumonia and meningoencephalitis caused by mouse norovirus in *Stat1* and *IFN alpha/beta* receptor-deficient mice,[1] decreased neoplastic cell growth and altered immune system function resulting from mouse parvovirus infection,[1,5] and wasting disease caused by mouse hepatitis virus.[1] Lactate dehydrogenase–elevating virus is notorious as the most common contaminant of murine cell lines and biological materials in mice and causes significant alteration of macrophage and immune function in immunocompetent mice.[5] While most viruses are of concern owing to their ability to cause disease or alter research results in mice, the primary relevance of lymphocytic choriomeningitis virus is for its zoonotic potential to cause meningitis in humans.[5]

Opportunistic infections with bacteria that are not routinely excluded from barrier facilities are a common cause of morbidity and mortality among immunodeficient mice. Reviews of the literature show that *Helicobacter*, *Pasteurella pneumotropica*, and *S. aureus* are still prevalent in laboratory mouse populations, and reports of disease caused by *Staphylococcus xylosus, Enterococci*, and opportunists like *Staphylococcus paucimobilis* are increasing.[6,7] In immunocompromised mice, many of these bacteria have been reported to cause systemic infections including dermatitis (caused by *Corynebacterium bovis*[8] or *S. xylosus*[9,10]), genital tract infections (caused by *P. pneumotropica*,[1,5] *Klebsiella oxytoca*,[11] or *Enterococci*[11]), and multiorgan abscesses (caused by *S. aureus* or *P. pneumotropica*). Several species of *Helicobacter* naturally infect mice, including *Helicobacter hepaticus*, *Helicobacter bilis*, *Helicobacter muridarum*, and *Helicobacter rodentium*. *Helicobacter hepaticus* is most prevalent in mouse colonies and produces various clinical signs ranging from none to enterocolitis to hepatic neoplasia.[12,13] Long-term antibiotic treatment is used to reduce mortality in colonies of highly immunodeficient rodents but may inadvertently increase susceptibility to opportunistic bacterial colonization and morbidity.[14]

The bacteria present in biofilm in watering systems include *P. aeruginosa*, *Ralstonia* spp., and other gram-negative, nonfermenting bacteria that may cause sporadic disease in highly immunodeficient mice.[15,16] *Pseudomonas aeruginosa* has been identified as the cause of bacteremia with multiorgan infection and mortality in MyD88-deficient mice.[17,18] *Ralstonia pickettii* has been identified as the cause of otitis media with ataxia and mortality in immunocompromised mice.[19,20]

The genus *Pneumocystis* contains a diverse group of fungi that inhabit several species of animals.[12] *Pneumocystis murina* is a major opportunistic infection in immunodeficient mice, and outbreaks of *Pneumocystis* pneumonia have been reported in barrier facilities in which immunocompetent and immunodeficient mice were cohoused in the same facility.[21,22] Treatment of infected animals with trimethoprim/sulfamethoxazole reduces mortality but does not eliminate the fungus. Effective elimination of the fungus requires rederivation of infected lines, depopulation, and stringent barrier practices to prevent reentry of the organism.[23]

Pathogenic intestinal protozoa, such as *Giardia*, *Eimeria*, and *Cryptosporidium*, are rarely reported in modern barrier facilities. Immunodeficient mice occasionally display large growths of intestinal flagellates throughout the gastrointestinal tract; these are generally seen as incidental findings in histopathology and have not been reliably associated with clinical disease.[1] *Spironucleus muris* is a flagellated protozoan that colonizes the gastrointestinal tract of rodents and is considered an opportunistic pathogen of mice.[12] Severe *S. muris* infections have been reported to cause diarrhea, weight loss, and unthriftiness, with mortality rates that vary from 20% to 50%.[5] However, the ability of *S. muris* to cause disease in mice is unclear; although some studies have reported clinical disease, others have reported no disease or research effects in infected mouse colonies, including colonies with breeding populations of immunodeficient mice.[24]

Facilities for housing immunodeficient mice must have infrastructure, caging, and management practices designed to exclude murine pathogens and opportunistic agents. Sources of infection include other mice, fomites, human handlers, food, water, and biological materials. Frequent movement of animals between institutions increases the potential for entry of pathogens and opportunists into barrier facilities.[1,4,25]

Barrier facilities employ many standard practices that are adequate to protect nude and SCID mice but may not be adequate for NSG or other highly immunodeficient mice.[26] High-level barrier practices recommended for severely immunodeficient lines/strains include a separate or isolated facility; separate entry portals for personnel, animals, and supplies; high-volume cage sanitation/sterilization facilities; and interior procedural space for animal activities. In some cases, the use of flexible film isolators may be needed for facilities in which populations of immunodeficient mice cannot be effectively separated from those of immunocompetent mice.

Recommended facility management practices include restricted entry of animals on the basis of health assessment; restricted personnel access with showering and/or protective clothing requirements for entry; use of positive-pressure individually ventilated caging systems; sterilization of all caging, food, bedding, water, and supplies in direct contact with animals; sanitation or sterilization of all materials entering the barrier; acidification of drinking water; frequent cage changes (>1 time/week); and the use of strict microisolator techniques when handling mice.[26,27] Watering systems can develop biofilm composed of various bacterial organisms.[15,19] The advantages of these systems[28,29] compared with water bottles must be weighed against the risk of increased microbial exposure to highly sensitive mouse populations.

Health surveillance programs are used to identify the presence of pathogens and opportunists. The surveillance strategy used in most facilities consists of quarterly testing of colonies using dirty bedding exposure of immunocompetent sentinel mice from commercial vendors.[4] Although adequate to identify most common murine pathogens, these systems may not effectively identify opportunistic or emerging murine pathogens. Paradoxically, the same isolation caging systems that are highly effective in maintaining biosecurity at a cage level also interfere with the ability to detect agents that are present but at low prevalence or those that are not easily transmitted using the dirty bedding sentinel system.[25] Enhanced biosecurity measures should employ sentinel protocols designed to find agents that do not transfer well to sentinels by the dirty bedding method, such as direct testing of colony mice and environmental monitoring using molecular biological screening methods such as polymerase chain reaction. All potential sources of entry of pathogens and opportunists should be included in the surveillance program. In 2008, 15% of surveyed institutions (primarily in academic research centers) reported contaminated biological materials as the source of disease outbreaks in their facilities and listed mouse parvovirus, lactate dehydrogenase–elevating virus, and mouse hepatitis virus as the most common contaminants.[4] Thus, additional surveillance measures should include routine screening of cell lines and rodent biological products.[4,24]

MOUSE STRAIN–SPECIFIC DISEASES

In addition to immunodeficiency, the strain of the recipient mouse can present clinical challenges because each strain has its own unique spontaneous diseases. Some of the immunodeficiency-inducing genetic mutations cause additional clinical issues, and secondary model refinements, such as engraftment of human immune systems, contribute further to disease.

NOD mice are a robust inbred strain with good breeding performance but are prone to developing type 1 diabetes depending on the environment and the mouse's age, sex, and related genetic defects.[30] Because NOD mice have defective natural killer cell function, the *SCID* and *Rag* mutations are often crossed to this strain, which eliminates the development of diabetes. NOD/ShiLtJ- and NOD-derived mice are prone to spontaneous development of osteosarcomas, occurring at a rate of 11.5% and 7%, respectively, according to one study.[31]

Nude mice are commonly available on an outbred background, a BALB/c background, and a C57BL/6 background. BALB/c mice are often aggressive and are likely to fight, whereas C57BL/6 mice are generally less likely to fight but are susceptible to hydrocephalus, microphthalmia, and other clinical diseases.[30] The background strain should be considered when spontaneous clinical disease is being predicted in an Institutional Animal Care and Use Committee (IACUC) protocol or is being diagnosed.

The most prominent example of a genetic mutation contributing to disease unrelated to immunodeficiency is thymic lymphoma in SCID mice. Clinical signs include loss of body condition, weakness, and dyspnea.[32,33] The incidence of lymphoma varies with the genetics of the mouse and the background strain. In NOD-SCID mice, the incidence can be as high as 67% (24/36),[34] which lowers the mean life span of these mice to 8.5 months and makes long-term engraftment studies inappropriate in this model.[35] Adding *IL2R* gamma chain deficiency to the NOD-SCID background (NOG mice) nearly eliminates thymic lymphoma (16 out of 2406)[32] and extends the mean life span to approximately 22 months (89 weeks).

The spontaneous development of lymphoma in NOD-SCID mice should not be confused with lymphoma of human origin that develops from reactivation of latent Epstein-Barr virus (EBV) in intratumoral passenger B lymphocytes following their xenotransplantation as part of patient-derived solid tumors. EBV-related lymphomas, which replace the intended tumor, have been reported in immunodeficient mice receiving PDX prostate tumors[36,37]; hepatocellular carcinoma[38]; non–small cell lung cancer[39]; breast, colon, or renal cancer[40]; or gastric cancer.[41] The incidence of EBV-related lymphoma may vary with both the type of tumor and the immunodeficiency of the recipient mouse, with an incidence of lymphoma ranging from 80% during the first 3 months after initial implantation of human prostate tumors in one model[36] to 11% in a different study.[37] In many cases, EBV-driven lymphomas are metastatic and spread to the spleen, lymph nodes, liver, or lungs following subcutaneous transplantation.[33,40] Since there is a high latent EBV infection rate (up to 90%) in humans and since B lymphocytes are commonly present in solid tumors,[38,42] lymphoma of mouse origin (generally thymic) must be differentiated from EBV-driven B-cell lymphoma of human origin.

Nude mice also have unique spontaneous disease related to the primary mutation. The defect in the *Foxn1* gene leads to abnormal development of the thymic epithelium, immunodeficiency, and abnormal development of other epithelial structures, including hair, nails, and eyelashes.[43,44] These defects may result in various clinical effects, including poor thermoregulation and increased susceptibility to skin and eye infections.[9,45,46] To minimize these issues, nude mice should be provided with nesting material that does not affect the eyes and a warm cage environment. Conjunctivitis can be treated by flushing the eyes with saline and, when necessary, treating secondary bacterial infections with topical drops. Anasarca secondary to glomerulonephritis also can occur in nude mice.[47,48]

HUMANIZED MICE AND GRAFT-VERSUS-HOST DISEASE

The addition of a human immune system to immunodeficient strains results in GVHD in nearly all the currently used models, although the rate of GVHD development varies with the model.[49,50] GVHD develops first in the skin on the head in most mice. Conjunctivitis and blepharitis are the first clinical signs in mice with engrafted human fetal bone marrow, liver, and thymus (BLT mice), followed by alopecia of the head, which progresses to full body alopecia and dermatitis.[49] In addition to invading the epidermis, dermis, and subcutaneous areas, lymphocytes from the graft invade the lungs in most animals (although clinical signs of lung disease are not typically noted), the gastrointestinal tract (primarily the colon), and the parotid gland. Establishment of clinical end points, such as ulcerative dermatitis and weight loss criteria, is key for managing these animals, as the clinical symptoms rarely respond to symptomatic treatment. Newer humanized models, such as MI(S)TRG mice (Rongvaux et al., Nature Bitechnology, 2014) demonstrate more powerful humanized system; however, these mice are susceptible to GVHD-related anemia, leading to death in a few weeks after establishment of a functional human immune system.

RADIATION

Irradiation of recipient xenograft mice may be part of the conditioning step in creating the model or may be part of the study's treatment protocol. The background strain of the mouse and dose must be carefully considered in all systems.[51] Sublethal irradiation of humanized mice to increase the acceptance of grafts can lead to cataracts in the recipients[52] and can increase the incidence of spontaneous lymphoma in certain strains of mice.[52,53] Sublethal radiation as low as 3 Gy in NOD-SCID mice has been associated with tooth defects, where the lower incisors erupt normally but are weak, deformed, and prone to fracture.[54] Affected mice have difficulty eating, lose weight, and can die prematurely from this complication. Successful treatment involves either lowering the dose of radiation or trimming the teeth. Providing nutrient hydrogels or moist food on the floor and close monitoring including weighing the animals daily provides effective supportive care for animals that received high doses of radiation or strains that have increased sensitivity to irradiation.

Local radiation side effects include necrosis of normal tissues and tumor tissues and off-target effects.[55] Generalized disease parameters associated with systemic responses, generalized cytokine responses, and localized skin and tissue injury all should be monitored in these models.

CYTOTOXIC CHEMOTHERAPEUTIC DRUGS AND TREATMENTS

One of the many uses of xenografts is to determine optimal treatment regimens. Chemotherapeutic agents can be associated with numerous side effects, including local tissue irritation at the injection site, gastrointestinal disease, renal disease, infection, and anemia.[56–58] During the treatment protocols, careful monitoring of hydration, body condition scoring and body weight (or food intake), diarrhea, and anemia is essential to maintain these models.[58] Anemia is often best assessed in mice by close examination for a pale color in the distal plantar surface of the toes. Microhematocrit tubes (25 μL) can be used to monitor hematocrit levels; however, the blood loss during blood draws for monitoring must be balanced with the information gained.[58]

As with all drug administration protocols, care must be taken to choose the appropriate route, dose, volume, and vehicle when administering chemotherapeutic drugs.[59] Some drugs, depending on the formulation, can be locally irritating and thus should be given intravenously rather than by another parenteral route. For example, doxorubicin, which is known to cause significant extravasation reactions in humans and dogs, causes sterile peritonitis when given intraperitoneally to mice; however, the liposomal formulation does not induce peritonitis and eliminates this complication.[60,61] Preprotocol screening of agents is essential to ensure that dosing has been adjusted for species differences. For new agents, dose optimization studies should be undertaken with care and should involve frequent monitoring and small group sizes.[58] Volumes used depend on the route of administration and must be within standard best practices guidelines.[59] The choice of vehicle for hard-to-solubilize compounds is critical in mice because their small size can make the use of common agents problematic when administered in certain concentrations and by certain routes.[62,63]

New nanoparticle therapies, involving various drugs attached to nanoparticles or the use of nanoparticles to target radiation or heat to the tumor, have been associated with toxicity depending on the nanoparticles' size, shape, charge, surface ligands, composition, and immunogenicity.[64,65] While certain parameters related to size, shape, and charge have been established for in vivo toxicity of nanoparticles, surface ligands individualize each newly designed particle, and evaluation for toxicity is critical.[66] As the nanoparticle interacts with physiologic substances (eg, blood) in vivo, the surface characteristics of the particle can change, with unexpected results.[64] Thus, new formulations should be evaluated in vitro and then carefully tested in small groups with adequate pathology support before being used in trials to evaluate efficacy.[66] Toxicity can develop as early as hours after injection, so careful monitoring is important in trials. Batch-to-batch variation can occur when producing nanoparticles as well as dissociation during transportation; thus, careful quality control is essential to avoid unexpected toxicity.[67]

ENGRAFTED TUMORS

Clinical signs associated with the growth and metastasis of the tumor can vary with the character of the engrafted tumor cells, the treatment, the host, and the implantation site.[58] The character of the tumor cells themselves can result in numerous clinically important outcomes. Most IACUCs have developed size and surface ulceration limitations for tumors; however, unpredictable tumor growth, which is common in PDX tumors, can make complying with these standards challenging.[58] Rapidly growing tumors develop necrotic centers and ulcerated surfaces. Frequent monitoring after each new cell line is implanted and clear end points can minimize the effect of these complications. Treatment protocols may need to be adjusted to conform to various conditions, making flexibility in timing critical as IACUC protocols are developed.

In addition to growth characteristics, some tumors can result in systemic disease owing to metastasis or generalized electrolyte and cytokine abnormalities.[58] While metastasis is often desired in neoplasia models to better mimic the human condition, metastasis rarely occurs in mouse models.[68] Recognizing metastasis and subsequent disease is essential to limit clinical consequences.

Clinical assessment of pain, and even disease, in mice can be challenging.[69] Typically, tumor size, body condition scoring,[70] and mobility parameters have been used to monitor clinical outcomes of tumor transplantation[58]; however, for some tumor models, monitoring body temperature and food and water intake (at the cage level for group-housed animals) may provide reliable clinical indicators of disease.[71] Generalized symptoms of disease such as tumor-related cachexia can occur in some models.[72,73]

Treatment protocols can result in changes in the tumors themselves. For instance, ulceration and focal necrosis of tumors can occur owing to specific therapies such as intratumoral injection of monoclonal antibodies or immunotherapies.[74–76] These outcomes should be considered during end point development. Supportive care and systemic antibiotics may be needed to minimize secondary bacterial infections of ulcerated or necrotic tumors in an immunodeficient host.

Although subcutaneously implanted tumors are relatively easy to monitor, care should be taken to place subcutaneous tumors in a location that will not impair normal mobility. Careful training of individuals who inject the tumor cells and, in some cases, using short-acting anesthesia to facilitate consistent placement will minimize placement complications for subcutaneous tumors. Imaging modalities can be utilized to monitor tumors in nonsuperficial sites.

For tumors not planted subcutaneously, complications associated with the tumor site need to be considered. Intramuscular injections should be used only when specific scientific justification of this site is made and the volume of tumor cells injected is modified appropriately owing to the likely negative effect on movement and associated pain.[58] Footpad injections have similar concerns. Orthotopic tumor transplantation is popular, as these models may better mimic human disease processes.[58,77] However, implanting tumors within some organs can result in secondary disease processes and painful outcomes. For instance, implanting glioblastoma cells into the brain can result in morbidity as the tumor expands; behavior tests may facilitate early detection.[78] Implanting tumors within the bone marrow to model osteosarcomas or metastasis of solid tumors can result in pathological fractures, as tumors result in osteolysis.[79] For orthotopic and metastatic models, the solution to avoiding clinical disease often lies in careful monitoring that is tailored to each site and using imaging modalities.

Monitoring growth of tumors in PDX mouse models is critical for both the welfare of the animal and the collection of research data. Several imaging modalities are available to monitor tumor growth and development in rodent models. These modalities include microcomputed tomography, magnetic resonance imaging, positron emission tomography, optical imaging, and high-resolution ultrasonography. Each system has different advantages and disadvantages in quality of tissue differentiation, ability to image physiologic processes, cost, availability, and expertise required to operate the system.[80–82]

CONCLUSION

This chapter summarizes the recommended facility and health management practices in the use of highly immunodeficient mice in cancer research. These specialized humanized and PDX models are susceptible to diseases and unique research-related conditions, including pathogens, mouse strain–specific diseases, GVHD, radiation toxicity, chemotherapy toxicity, and tumor development. Researchers must be familiar with these conditions and develop programs that provide high-level biosecurity, health surveillance, and systems to monitor tumor progression to utilize these models effectively. The use of primary patient tissues implanted directly into immunodeficient mice, which may permit the passage of human pathogens, represents additional unique challenges in the use of these models. The next chapter will review special considerations for the use of PDX models in occupational health and safety programs.

REFERENCES

1. Treuting PM, Clifford CB, Sellers RS, Brayton CF. Of mice and microflora: considerations for genetically engineered mice. *Vet Pathol* 2012;**49**:44–63.
2. Shek WR. Role of housing modalities on management and surveillance strategies for adventitious agents of rodents. *ILAR J* 2008;**49**:316–25.
3. Pritchett-Corning KR, Cosentino J, Clifford CB. Contemporary prevalence of infectious agents in laboratory mice and rats. *Lab Anim* 2009;**43**:165–73.
4. Carty AJ. Opportunistic infections of mice and rats: Jacoby and Lindsey revisited. *ILAR J* 2008;**49**:272–6.
5. Percy DH, Barthold SW. Mouse. In: *Pathology of laboratory rodents and rabbits*. Blackwell Publishing Professional; 2008. p. 3–124.
6. Brayton CF, Treuting PM, Ward JM. Pathobiology of aging mice and GEM: background strains and experimental design. *Veterinary Pathol Online* 2012;**49**:85–105.
7. Benga L, Benten WPM, Engelhardt E, Gougoula C, Sager M. Spontaneous bacterial and fungal infections in genetically engineered mice: is *Escherichia coli* an emerging pathogen in laboratory mouse? *Berl Munchener tierarztliche Wochenschr* 2015;**128**:278–84.

8. Burr HN, Lipman NS, White JR, Zheng J, Wolf FR. Strategies to prevent, treat, and provoke *Corynebacterium*-associated hyperkeratosis in athymic nude mice. *J Am Assoc Lab Anim Sci* 2011;**50**:378–88.
9. Russo M, Invernizzi A, Gobbi A, Radaelli E. Diffuse scaling dermatitis in an athymic nude mouse. *Veterinary Pathol Online* 2013;**50**:722–6.
10. Won YS, Kwon HJ, Oh GT, et al. Identification of *Staphylococcus xylosus* isolated from C57BL/6J-Nos2 (tm1Lau) mice with dermatitis. *Microbiol Immunol* 2002;**46**:629–32.
11. Foreman O, Kavirayani A, Griffey S, Reader R, Shultz L. Opportunistic bacterial infections in breeding colonies of the NSG mouse strain. *Veterinary Pathol Online* 2011;**48**:495–9.
12. Baker DG. Natural pathogens of laboratory mice, rats, and rabbits and their effects on research. *Clin Microbiol Rev* 1998;**11**:231–66.
13. Chichlowski M, Hale LP. Effects of *Helicobacter* infection on research: the case for eradication of *Helicobacter* from rodent research colonies. *Comp Med* 2009;**59**:10–7.
14. Bleich A, Kirsch P, Sahly H, et al. *Klebsiella oxytoca*: opportunistic infections in laboratory rodents. *Lab Anim* 2008;**42**:369–75.
15. Molk DM, Karr-May CL, Trang ED, Sanders GE. Sanitization of an automatic reverse-osmosis watering system: removal of a clinically significant biofilm. *J Am Assoc Lab Anim Sci* 2013;**52**:197.
16. Lee J, Lee C, Hugunin K, Maute C, Dysko R. Bacteria from drinking water supply and their fate in gastrointestinal tracts of germ-free mice: a phylogenetic comparison study. *Water Res* 2010;**44**:5050–8.
17. Moritz MM, Flemming HC, Wingender J. Integration of *Pseudomonas aeruginosa* and *Legionella pneumophila* in drinking water biofilms grown on domestic plumbing materials. *Int J Hyg Environ Health* 2010;**213**:190–7.
18. Villano JS, Rong F, Cooper TK. Bacterial infections in Myd88-deficient mice. *Comp Med* 2014;**64**:110.
19. Berard M, Medaille C, Simon M, Serre S, Pritchett-Corning K, Dangles-Marie V. *Ralstonia pickettii*-induced ataxia in immunodeficient mice. *Comp Med* 2009;**59**:187.
20. Ryan M, Adley C. *Ralstonia* spp.: emerging global opportunistic pathogens. *Eur J Clin Microbiol Infect Dis* 2014;**33**:291–304.
21. Percy D, Barta J. Spontaneous and experimental infections in scid and scid/beige mice. *Lab Anim Sci* 1993;**43**:127–32.
22. Dagnæs-Hansen F, Poulsen K. *Pneumocystis murina* infection in immunodeficient mice in a closed barrier unit: a case report. *Scand J Lab Anim Sci* 2011;**38**:91–6.
23. Charles River Research Models and Services. *Pneumocystis technical sheet.* Charles River Laboratories; 2011.
24. Perdue KA, Copeland MK, Karjala Z, Cheng LI, Ward JM, Elkins WR. Suboptimal ability of dirty-bedding sentinels to detect *Spironucleus muris* in a colony of mice with genetic manipulations of the adaptive immune system. *J Am Assoc Lab Anim Sci* 2008;**47**:10–7.
25. Clifford CB, Watson J. Old enemies, still with us after all these years. *ILAR J* 2008;**49**:291–302.
26. The Jackson Laboratory. *Nsg mouse portfolio: housing and breeding consideration for NSG mice*. The Jackson Laboratory; 2015.
27. Yeadon J. *What type of housing conditions do immunodeficient mice need?*. Jax Blog. Jax Home: The Jackson Laboratory; 2013.
28. Hessler J, Lehner N. *Planning and designing research animal facilities*. Academic Press; 2011.
29. Kiermayer C, Hoehne-Hückstädt UM, Brielmeier M, Brütting M, Ellegast R, Schmidt J. Musculoskeletal load in and highly repetitive actions of animal facility washroom employees. *J Am Assoc Lab Anim Sci* 2011;**50**:665–74.

30. Brayton C. *Spontaneous diseases in commonly used mouse strains and stocks*. 2015. MPD: Brayton1 Mouse Phenome Database Website.
31. Kavirayani AM, Foreman O. Retrospective study of spontaneous osteosarcomas in the nonobese diabetic strain and nonobese diabetic-derived substrains of mice. *Vet Pathol* 2010;**47**:482–7.
32. Kato C, Fujii E, Chen YJ, et al. Spontaneous thymic lymphomas in the non-obese diabetic/Shi-scid, IL-2R gamma (null) mouse. *Lab Anim* 2009;**43**:402–4.
33. Custer RP, Bosma GC, Bosma MJ. Severe combined immunodeficiency (SCID) in the mouse. Pathology, reconstitution, neoplasms. *Am J Pathology* 1985;**120**:464–77.
34. Prochazka M, Gaskins HR, Shultz LD, Leiter EH. The nonobese diabetic scid mouse: model for spontaneous thymomagenesis associated with immunodeficiency. *Proc Natl Acad Sci USA* 1992;**89**:3290–4.
35. Shultz LD, Schweitzer PA, Christianson SW, et al. Multiple defects in innate and adaptive immunologic function in NOD/LtSz-scid mice. *J Immunol* 1995;**154**:180–91.
36. Wetterauer C, Vlajnic T, Schuler J, et al. Early development of human lymphomas in a prostate cancer xenograft program using triple knock-out immunocompromised mice. *Prostate* 2015;**75**:585–92.
37. Lin D, Wyatt AW, Xue H, et al. High fidelity patient-derived xenografts for accelerating prostate cancer discovery and drug development. *Cancer Res* 2014;**74**:1272–83.
38. Chen K, Ahmed S, Adeyi O, Dick JE, Ghanekar A. Human solid tumor xenografts in immunodeficient mice are vulnerable to lymphomagenesis associated with Epstein-Barr virus. *PLoS One* 2012;**7**:e39294.
39. John T, Yanagawa N, Kohler D, et al. Characterization of lymphomas developing in immunodeficient mice implanted with primary human non-small cell lung cancer. *J Thorac Oncol Off Publ Int Assoc Study Lung Cancer* 2012;**7**:1101–8.
40. Bondarenko G, Ugolkov A, Rohan S, et al. Patient-derived tumor xenografts are susceptible to formation of human lymphocytic tumors. *Neoplasia* 2015;**17**:735–41.
41. Fujii E, Kato A, Chen YJ, Matsubara K, Ohnishi Y, Suzuki M. Characterization of EBV-related lymphoproliferative lesions arising in donor lymphocytes of transplanted human tumor tissues in the NOG mouse. *Exp Anim* 2014;**63**:289–96.
42. Thorley-Lawson DA, Allday MJ. The curious case of the tumour virus: 50 years of Burkitt's lymphoma. *Nat Rev Microbiol* 2008;**6**:913–24.
43. Mecklenburg L, Tychsen B, Paus R. Learning from nudity: lessons from the nude phenotype. *Exp Dermatol* 2005;**14**:797–810.
44. Mecklenburg L, Paus R, Halata Z, Bechtold LS, Fleckman P, Sundberg JP. FOXN1 is critical for onycholemmal terminal differentiation in nude (Foxn1) mice. *J Invest Dermatol* 2004;**123**:1001–11.
45. McGarry MP, Bahny L, Jividen J, Williams P, Mirand EA, Murphy GP. Particulate matter induced periorbital abscess in gnotobiotic athymic nu/nu (nude) mice. *Lab Anim Sci* 1976;**26**:956–8.
46. Gaskill BN, Winnicker C, Garner JP, Pritchett-Corning KR. The naked truth: breeding performance in nude mice with and without nesting material. *Appl Anim Behav Sci* 2013;**143**:110–6.
47. Viguera C, Ward JM, Nims RM, Wenk ML, Strandberg JD. Clinical and pathologic conditions of female nude (athymic) mice in two conventional maintained colonies. *J Am Vet Med Assoc* 1978;**173**:1198–201.
48. Pritchett-Corning KR, Girod A, Avellaneda G, Fritz PE, Chou S, Brown MJ. *Handbook of clinical signs in rodents and rabbits*. Wilmington: Charles River Laboratories; 2011.

49. Greenblatt MB, Vrbanac V, Tivey T, Tsang K, Tager AM, Aliprantis AO. Graft versus host disease in the bone marrow, liver and thymus humanized mouse model. *PLoS One* 2012;**7**:e44664.
50. Brehm MA, Wiles MV, Greiner DL, Shultz LD. Generation of improved humanized mouse models for human infectious diseases. *J Immunol Methods* 2014;**410**:3–17.
51. Duran-Struuck R, Dysko RC. Principles of bone marrow transplantation (BMT): providing optimal veterinary and husbandry care to irradiated mice in BMT studies. *J Am Assoc Lab Anim Sci* 2009;**48**:11–22.
52. Ainsbury EA, Bouffler SD, Dorr W, et al. Radiation cataractogenesis: a review of recent studies. *Radiat Res* 2009;**172**:1–9.
53. Bannik K, Rossler U, Faus-Kessler T, et al. Are mouse lens epithelial cells more sensitive to gamma-irradiation than lymphocytes? *Radiat Environ Biophys* 2013;**52**:279–86.
54. Larsen SR, Kingham JA, Hayward MD, Rasko JE. Damage to incisors after nonmyeloablative total body irradiation may complicate NOD/SCID models of hemopoietic stem cell transplantation. *Comp Med* 2006;**56**:209–14.
55. Perez-Torres CJ, Engelbach JA, Cates J, et al. Toward distinguishing recurrent tumor from radiation necrosis: DWI and MTC in a gamma knife–irradiated mouse glioma model. *Int J Radiat Oncol Biol Phys* 2014;**90**:446–53.
56. Kayl AE, Meyers CA. Side-effects of chemotherapy and quality of life in ovarian and breast cancer patients. *Curr Opin Obstet Gynecol* 2006;**18**:24–8.
57. MacDonald V. Chemotherapy: managing side effects and safe handling. *Can Veterinary J* 2009;**50**:665–8.
58. Workman P, Aboagye EO, Balkwill F, et al. Guidelines for the welfare and use of animals in cancer research. *Br J Cancer* 2010;**102**:1555–77.
59. Turner PV, Brabb T, Pekow C, Vasbinder MA. Administration of substances to laboratory animals: routes of administration and factors to consider. *J Am Assoc Lab Anim Sci* 2011;**50**:600–13.
60. Gabizon AA. Pegylated liposomal doxorubicin: metamorphosis of an old drug into a new form of chemotherapy. *Cancer Invest* 2001;**19**:424–36.
61. Krysko DV, Kaczmarek A, Krysko O, et al. TLR-2 and TLR-9 are sensors of apoptosis in a mouse model of doxorubicin-induced acute inflammation. *Cell Death Differ* 2011;**18**:1316–25.
62. Neervannan S. Preclinical formulations for discovery and toxicology: physicochemical challenges. *Expert Opin Drug Metab Toxicol* 2006;**2**:715–31.
63. Gad SC, Cassidy CD, Aubert N, Spainhour B, Robbe H. Nonclinical vehicle use in studies by multiple routes in multiple species. *Int J Toxicol* 2006;**25**:499–521.
64. Singh S, Sharma A, Robertson GP. Realizing the clinical potential of cancer nanotechnology by minimizing toxicologic and targeted delivery concerns. *Cancer Res* 2012;**72**:5663–8.
65. Khlebtsov N, Dykman L. Biodistribution and toxicity of engineered gold nanoparticles: a review of in vitro and in vivo studies. *Chem Soc Rev* 2011;**40**:1647–71.
66. Dam DH, Culver KS, Kandela I, et al. Biodistribution and in vivo toxicity of aptamer-loaded gold nanostars. *Nanomedicine* 2015;**11**:671–9.
67. Wu L, Zhang J, Watanabe W. Physical and chemical stability of drug nanoparticles. *Adv Drug Deliv Rev* 2011;**63**:456–69.
68. van Marion DM, Domanska UM, Timmer-Bosscha H, Walenkamp AM. Studying cancer metastasis: existing models, challenges and future perspectives. *Crit Rev Oncol/Hematol* 2015. http://dx.doi.org/10.1016/j.critrevonc.2015.08.009. Available online: 10 August, 2015, ISSN: 1040-8428.
69. Miller AL, Leach MC. The mouse grimace scale: a clinically useful tool? *PLoS One* 2015;**10**:e0136000.

70. Ullman-Cullere MH, Foltz CJ. Body condition scoring: a rapid and accurate method for assessing health status in mice. *Lab Anim Sci* 1999;**49**:319–23.
71. Hunter JE, Butterworth J, Perkins ND, Bateson M, Richardson CA. Using body temperature, food and water consumption as biomarkers of disease progression in mice with Eμ-myc lymphoma. *Br J Cancer* 2014;**110**:928–34.
72. Kamoshida S, Watanabe K, Suzuki M, et al. Expression of cancer cachexia-related factors in human cancer xenografts: an immunohistochemical analysis. *Biomed Res* 2006;**27**:275–81.
73. Baumgarten AJ, Fiebig HH, Burger AM. Molecular analysis of xenograft models of human cancer cachexia–possibilities for therapeutic intervention. *Cancer Genomics Proteomics* 2007;**4**:223–31.
74. Zhang B, Zhang Y, Bowerman NA, et al. Equilibrium between host and cancer caused by effector T cells killing tumor stroma. *Cancer Res* 2008;**68**:1563–71.
75. Zhang B, Karrison T, Rowley DA, Schreiber H. IFN-gamma- and TNF-dependent bystander eradication of antigen-loss variants in established mouse cancers. *J Clin Invest* 2008;**118**:1398–404.
76. Johanson V, Ahlman H, Bernhardt P, et al. A transplantable human medullary thyroid carcinoma as a model for RET tyrosine kinase-driven tumorigenesis. *Endocrine-Related Cancer* 2007;**14**:433–44.
77. Hoffman RM. Patient-derived orthotopic xenografts: better mimic of metastasis than subcutaneous xenografts. *Nat Rev* 2015;**15**:451–2.
78. Wasilewska-Sampaio AP, Santos TG, Lopes MH, Cammarota M, Martins VR. The growth of glioblastoma orthotopic xenografts in nude mice is directly correlated with impaired object recognition memory. *Physiol Behav* 2014;**123**:55–61.
79. Raheem O, Kulidjian AA, Wu C, et al. A novel patient-derived intra-femoral xenograft model of bone metastatic prostate cancer that recapitulates mixed osteolytic and osteoblastic lesions. *J Transl Med* 2011;**9**:185.
80. James ML, Gambhir SS. A molecular imaging primer: modalities, imaging agents, and applications. *Physiol Rev* 2012;**92**:897–965.
81. Lyons SK. Imaging mouse models of Cancer. *Cancer J* 2015;**21**:152–64.
82. Wang Y, Tseng J-C, Sun Y, Beck AH, Kung AL. Noninvasive imaging of tumor burden and molecular pathways in mouse models of cancer. *Cold Spring Harb Protoc* 2015;**2015**. http://dx.doi.org/10.1101/pdb.top.069930.

Chapter 8

Occupational Health and Safety

L.A. Colby[1], E. Corwin[2]
[1]*University of Washington, Seattle, WA, United States;* [2]*Seattle Genetics, Bothell, WA, United States*

INTRODUCTION[1–4]

Patient-derived tumor xenograft (PDX) mouse models are uniquely suited for many areas of research due to their ability to accept and allow the proliferation of human-origin tissues. Although a permissive host immune system is an absolute model requirement, it is also the model feature from which most occupational health concerns arise. These concerns are intensified with humanized PDX mouse models in which the murine immune system has been modified to permit human immune system function.

Numerous institutional entities share the responsibility of ensuring personnel safety during the conduct of biomedical research. These entities and the applicable regulations are described in depth in Section II, Chapter 1.

Multiple occupational health issues must be considered for personnel working with mice in all research settings including physical injuries (eg, animal bites and scratches, pinch and crush injuries), ergonomic injuries, laboratory animal allergen exposure, noise exposure, use or administration of hazardous chemicals or biologic organisms, and exposure to zoonotic pathogens from animals. Although these issues certainly apply to the use of PDX mouse models, they are not specifically addressed in this chapter as they are described elsewhere. Rather, this chapter emphasizes occupational health concerns specific to PDX mouse models.

PDX MOUSE MODELS: UNIQUE OCCUPATIONAL HEALTH CONCERNS[5–10]

A wide range of personnel may have direct or indirect contact with PDX mice and/or their immediate environment (eg, caging). These include laboratory personnel directly handling the mice, their fluids, or their tissues; animal husbandry personnel including those responsible for cage washing and carcass disposal; and veterinary care personnel.

Both wild and laboratory mice can maintain persistent infections of select zoonotic agents (eg, lymphocytic choriomeningitis virus, hantavirus, and *Leptospira*

Patient Derived Tumor Xenograft Models. http://dx.doi.org/10.1016/B978-0-12-804010-2.00014-X

spp). Fortunately, PDX mouse model studies are almost exclusively conducted utilizing mice of a well-defined health and pathogen status and maintained in modern animal facilities with active animal health surveillance programs as well as robust employee health programs.

Zoonotic agents have been largely eliminated from barrier-maintained mouse colonies through routine colony health monitoring programs, mandatory screening of imported animals and biologic materials (eg, serum, cell and tissue cultures), and physical exclusion of disease vectors (eg, insects). However, severely immunocompromised mice, such as those used in PDX research, present additional challenges as select infectious agents may not be readily detected with use of common diagnostic tests. Infectious agents may also be capable of proliferating unchecked within the animal host, resulting in abnormally high concentrations of the organism within the body or excretions. Furthermore, once a disease agent becomes established in a colony of immunocompromised mice, eradication of the agent from the colony can be extremely difficult or impossible.

PDX mouse models are associated with additional occupational health concerns, including the following:

- Established human tumor tissue cultures are often not screened for infectious agents prior to their use or distribution. When used, screening panels are often limited in scope.
- Many infectious diseases are endemic in the human population. This is especially significant in cancer patients, who may themselves be immunocompromised and therefore more susceptible to infections, and are not commonly screened for infectious agents prior to their tissue harvest.
- Many research protocols do not allow sufficient time to test xenografts samples for pathogens prior to their implantation in recipient mice.
- Humanized mouse models may be able to support a productive infection and/or persistent viremia not otherwise possible in a murine host.

INFECTIOUS AGENTS OF CONCERN[5,11–13]

It is difficult to clearly define the infectious agents of greatest occupational health concern with PDX mouse models; this determination must consider both an agent's estimated prevalence within the human population and the consequence of infection.

If the true prevalence of common, significant infectious agents within the population were known, then one could roughly estimate the prevalence of infectious agents in human-derived tissues. Unfortunately, reliable prevalence rates are unknown. While national infectious disease reporting programs exist in the United States and other countries, they apply only to a limited number of diseases and likely underestimate the true prevalence of those diseases. Similarly, it is not possible to anticipate every infectious agent present in human tissues. Therefore, the conduct of a risk assessment is necessary to evaluate potential health risks associated with PDX model systems. The risk assessment should consider the wide range of infectious agents that may be present, potential routes of exposure and transmission with common procedures, and strategies for personnel risk reduction.

A brief review of select infectious agents (ie, human oncogenic viruses, those associated with Occupational Safety and Health Administration's (OSHA) Bloodborne Pathogens Standard, and those purposefully excluded from the US donor blood supply) (Table 8.1) is included in the last section. These were selected as they are representatives of the infectious agents that may contaminate human xenografts within the United States. It should be recognized that the infectious agents most likely to contaminate human xenografts will vary between xenograft donor populations in different countries and regions around the world to at least partially reflect the prevalence of disease within a population.

Ensuring Human Safety

Many occupational health issues (eg, physical and ergonomic injuries, laboratory animal allergen exposure, hazardous chemical exposure) must be considered for personnel working with mice. Immunocompromised mice and humanized mice present additional concerns due to risks associated with infectious disease agents. Currently, the true risk associated with PDX-recipient mice is unknown. Therefore, precautions should be employed to minimize potential exposure events of research and animal husbandry personnel. Additionally, a well-defined occupational health plan must be in place to address postexposure treatment, postexposure prophylaxis, monitoring, and potential transmission to other human contacts. At a minimum, an occupational health plan should include standard OSHA protocols related to potential bloodborne pathogens (BBPs) exposure in the health care workplace. Further consideration should be given to the type of human tissue/tumor regarding the presence of specific infectious agents.

Considerations with Sample Handling and Collection[1]

It is the authors' opinion that in a PDX mouse model system, the direct handling of primary human tissue (ie, tissues obtained directly from a human patient without subsequent testing and/or culturing and expansion) poses the greatest occupational health risk due to the potential presence of undetected infectious agents. All human tissues should be considered infectious and thus, standard precautions and use of personal protective equipment are imperative. Likewise, tissues and fluids (both of human and mouse origin) obtained from mice, pre- and postmortem following xenotransplantation, should be regarded as potentially infectious. A minimum of biosafety level 2 (BSL-2) and animal biosafety level 2 (ABSL-2) containment practices are recommended.

TABLE 8.1 Select Infectious Agents of Concern in PDX Mouse Models Implanted With Human-Derived Xenografts

	Origin of Concern		
Infectious Agent	**Preamble to Bloodborne Pathogens Standard**	**Excluded From US Donated Blood Supply**	**Virus-Associated Neoplasia (*Resultant Neoplasia*)**
Arboviral infections (eg, Colorado tick fever virus, West Nile virus)	✔	✔ (West Nile virus)	
Babesiosis (*Babesia microti*)	✔		
Brucellosis (*Brucella spp*)	✔		
Chagas disease (*Trypanosoma cruzi*)		✔	
Creutzfeldt-Jakob disease	✔		
CMV	✔		✔ *(Neuroblastoma)*
EBV	✔		✔ *(Burkitt lymphoma, nasopharyngeal carcinoma, posttransplant lymphomas, Hodgkin disease)*
HBV	✔	✔	✔ *(Hepatocellular carcinoma)*
HCV	✔	✔	✔ *(Hepatocellular carcinoma)*
HHV-8			✔ *(KS; primary effusion lymphoma, with HIV; Castleman disease)*
HIV	✔	✔ (HIV-1 and -2)	✔ *(Lymphoma, primary effusion lymphoma, in particular)*

TABLE 8.1 Select Infectious Agents of Concern in PDX Mouse Models Implanted With Human-Derived Xenografts—cont'd

	Origin of Concern		
Infectious Agent	**Preamble to Bloodborne Pathogens Standard**	**Excluded From US Donated Blood Supply**	**Virus-Associated Neoplasia (*Resultant Neoplasia*)**
HPV	✔		✔ *(Cervical cancer, head and neck cancers, anogenital cancers, skin cancers in patients with epidermodysplasia verruciformis)*
HTLV-1	✔	✔	✔ *(Adult T-cell leukemia)*
HTLV-2		✔	
Leptospirosis (*Leptospira*)	✔		
Malaria (*Plasmodium* spp.,)	✔		
Tick-borne relapsing fever (*Borrelia*)	✔		
Syphilis (*Treponema pallidum*)	✔	✔	
Viral hemorrhagic fevers	✔		
West Nile virus (an arbovirus)		✔	

Considerations with Animal Handling and Husbandry Procedures

Multiple factors must be considered in managing occupational health risks associated with animal handling and husbandry practices with PDX mouse models. The immune status of the mouse xenograft recipient directly influences its ability to maintain (and possibly amplify) a xenograft-acquired pathogen. In addition, all potential routes of pathogen shedding (eg, urine, feces, saliva) should be recognized. This is especially important in the management of animal-related injuries (eg, animal bites and scratches, equipment-related injuries) as well as the handling and disinfection of equipment (eg, research and veterinary instruments) and animal environments (eg, caging) utilized by research, veterinary, and animal husbandry and cagewash personnel. BSL-2 and ABSL-2 practices should be strongly considered.

Conclusion

Numerous occupational health risks exist when working with PDX-transplanted mice, as tissue donors are often asymptomatic and are screened for very few, if any, disease agents prior to xenografts collection. Furthermore, xenografts are infrequently tested as part of the implantation and passage process. Thus, it is reasonable to assume that human-derived xenografts may be contaminated with an infectious organism. A risk exists for these infectious organisms to be transmitted to PDX-recipient mice that, by purposeful design, are immunocompromised or humanized. Moreover, given their unique immune system characteristics, it may be possible for infectious organisms to be amplified and/or shed in ways not expected in immunocompetent mice. Given current practices and understanding of associated risks, a minimum of BSL-2 and ABSL-2 containment should be employed during the conduct of research directly utilizing human-derived xenografts and PDX mouse models, including the collection and handling of biological samples obtained from the mice and all husbandry and veterinary care activities.

Mouse strains will continue to be developed and refined to more closely emulate the human immune system and therefore serve as better model systems. As a consequence, assessment of the occupational health risks inherent to their use in PDX model systems must likewise evolve.

POTENTIAL INFECTIONS AGENTS

Tumor-Associated Viruses[14]

By definition, a virus is considered oncogenic if it is found in the presence of the tumor tissue, the virus was present before disease onset, the virus persists in the host organism at appropriate sites, and the disease can be averted by prevention of viral infection. By these criteria, several human oncogenic viruses have been identified. Recently, a commercial laboratory evaluating human tumors submitted for pathogen screening found human` papilloma virus (HPV) 16 to be the most prevalent viral contaminant followed by Epstein-Barr virus (EBV).[11] While the prevalence of HPV likely depends on the relative percentage of certain types of cancers in the tested samples, this finding underlies the high risk of handling xenograft donations given that HPV is a high-risk oncovirus that can be transferred by fomites or skin contact.

For ease of identification in the case of an accidental exposure, the following section is organized by tumor type.

Hepatocellular Carcinoma[15–19]

The hepatitis B virus (HBV) and hepatitis C virus (HCV) are both closely associated with hepatocellular carcinoma (HCC). Among patients in the United States diagnosed with HCC, 50–60% are infected with HCV, 10–15% with HBV, less than 5% with both viruses, and 30–35% with neither.

Neither HBV nor HCV is capable of infecting wild-type mice. However, at least one study has shown that although the sera of mice implanted with HBV- and HCV-positive HCC tumors consistently tested negative for DNA (HBV) or RNA (HCV), HBV DNA was detected in all surviving xenografts of HBV-positive tumors. HCV RNA was not maintained in the tumor xenografts in this study.

HBV can be transmitted via sexual intercourse, shared needles and syringes, contact with infected blood or wounds, needlestick and sharps injuries, sharing personal care items, during birth and breastfeeding, as well as through blood transfusion and solid organ transplantation.

The highest risk of transmission in the workplace is through direct or indirect exposure to blood. All exposed workers should be monitored clinically and with serologic testing.

Postexposure prophylactic treatment of nonimmunized individuals with HBV and hepatitis B immunoglobulin should be offered following a workplace injury, preferably within 24h.

Like HBV, the highest risk of HCV transmission in the workplace is through exposure to blood. The transmission of HCV via blood exposure, however, is much less efficient than with HBV, with a seroconversion rate of just 1.8% for a percutaneous exposure.

There is currently no vaccine available to prevent infection with HCV. Postexposure management consists of early identification of infection by clinical monitoring and serologic testing for anti-HCV antibodies.

Urogenital, Anogenital, and Oropharyngeal Cancers[20,21]

The HPV is associated with 90% of anal and cervical cancers, 70% of vaginal and vulvar cancers, 60% of penile cancers, and 70% of cancers of the oropharynx. Transmission occurs via sexual intercourse, but the virus can be transferred via fomites or skin contact as well.

The virus is capable of propagation in immunocompromised mice. Although there are no data regarding the use of either vaccine for postexposure prophylaxis following workplace exposure, the Gardasil and Cervarix vaccines both protect against all oncogenic strains of the virus.

Lymphoma[14,16,18,21–24]

At least three distinct viruses have been associated with the development of lymphoma in humans: EBV, human T-cell lymphoma virus types 1 and 2 (HTLV-1 and HTLV-2), and human herpes virus 8 (HHV-8).

EBV is associated with B-cell lymphomas as well as Hodgkin lymphoma and T-cell lymphomas. EBV is also associated with 90–100% of cases of

Burkitt lymphoma arising in patients immunocompromised due to AIDS or due to immunosuppression following solid organ transplantation. The prevalence of EBV is as high as 80–90% of most adult populations, and the virus can be transmitted in multiple ways including via blood exposure in the workplace.

The EBV genome has been found within Reed–Sternberg cells, which are diagnostic for Hodgkin lymphoma and in a small subset of T-cell lymphomas.

Although the EBV genome is detected in these malignancies, only a small percentage of cells shed virus. However, high EBV viral loads have been detected in peripheral blood mononuclear cells from patients with EBV-related lymphomas.

Infection with EBV causes the acute illness known as mononucleosis which is diagnosed by serology. Other acute illnesses associated with EBV include Guillain-Barré syndrome, viral meningitis, encephalitis, optic neuritis, transverse myelitis, and acute cerebellar ataxia. Diagnosis of acute infection is made by serology and treatment is supportive.

HTLV-1 is considered the etiologic agent in most cases of acute T-cell lymphoma/leukemia. HTLV-2 has been associated with T-cell hairy cell leukemia and cutaneous T-cell lymphoma, although a causal link has not been clearly established. The prevalence of both viruses varies around the globe.

Transmission is primarily bloodborne, and while blood donors are screened for HTLV-1 and 2; there is no vaccine or postexposure prophylaxis. The latency period for the development of HTLV-1 malignancies is long, typically 20–30 years after the initial infection. To date, there is no antiviral therapy considered standard of care for asymptomatic carriers of HTLV or patients diagnosed with HTLV-1–related malignancies or nonmalignant diseases.

HHV-8, also known as Kaposi sarcoma–associated herpesvirus, is a member of the HHV family. It is an oncogenic virus associated with the human immunodeficiency virus (HIV)–associated lymphoproliferative diseases known as primary effusion lymphoma (PEL) and multicentric Castleman disease (MCD). MCD and PEL are found almost exclusively in HIV-positive patients. HHV-8 DNA is found in 67% of lymph nodes affected by MCD and patients with active disease are almost universally viremic.

The HHV-8 virus has varying rates of prevalence across the world and across different subpopulations. Transmission routes include blood borne, vertical and horizontal, organ transplantation, and sexual. Neither does a vaccine exist for prevention nor is any postexposure prophylaxis recommended.

Diagnosis of HHV-8 acute infection is by serologic testing. Treatment in immunocompetent patients is supportive. Antiviral agents active against HHV-8 in combination with immune system reconstitution with highly active antiretroviral therapy is typically used in HIV-positive patients.

Nasopharyngeal Carcinoma[14,18]

Nasopharyngeal carcinoma is highly associated with the EBV virus, detailed in the preceding section.

Kaposi Sarcoma[23,25]

Kaposi sarcoma (KS) is a highly vascular tumor with a very low incidence, predominantly in men of Middle Eastern and Mediterranean origin, until the rise of the AIDS epidemic when its incidence increased greatly. The HHV-8 virus is found uniformly in classical and endemic KS, HIV-associated KS, and iatrogenic KS (immunosuppressed patients, such as transplant recipients).

Glioblastoma, Medulloblastoma, and Neuroblastoma[26–28]

Recent reports have identified an association between the human cytomegalovirus (CMV) and tumors of the central and peripheral nervous systems including glioblastomas, medulloblastomas, and neuroblastomas. These studies have not conclusively demonstrated that the viral particles found in the tumors are infectious.

CMV is highly prevalent around the world. Transmission occurs through contact with body fluids, sexual contact, blood transfusions, and organ transplants.

Acute infection with CMV causes a mononucleosis-like syndrome with fever as well as a mild hepatitis and is diagnosed by serology. Treatment is supportive in immunocompetent hosts. Acute infection in immunocompromised individuals can be severe. Infection in pregnant woman can cause congenital malformations in the fetus.

HIV/AIDS Related and Nonrelated Malignancies[29,30]

KS, non–Hodgkin lymphoma [Burkitt and central nervous system (CNS) lymphoma], and invasive cervical cancer all constitute AIDS-defining illnesses in HIV-positive patients. As described above, each of these malignancies are highly associated with distinct viruses that are considered oncogenic. Coincident infection with HPV, HBV, and HPC is also common in HIV-positive patients due to shared routes of transmission and risk factors, leading to an increased incidence of cancers related to these viruses.

In 2015, 35 million people worldwide were infected with HIV, with an incidence of over 1.2 million people in the United States. The virus can be transmitted via sexual intercourse, contact with blood or body fluids, transfusion, shared needles, from mother to fetus, and through needlestick and sharps injuries in the workplace. Blood donors are universally screened and tested for HIV, and the incidence of HIV transmission through blood transfusion is now approximately 1 in 1.5 million.

The occupational transmission risk is quite low, estimated at 0.23%. Although no vaccine exists to prevent AIDS, postexposure prophylaxis (PEP) is quite effective in preventing infection with different regimens of PEP recommended based upon the exposure type.

Other Infectious Agents of Concern

Arboviral Infections[31–34]

Arboviruses replicate in and are transmitted to vertebrate hosts by blood-sucking arthropods (eg, mosquito and ticks). Transmission of arboviruses present in the

United States (West Nile Virus, Colorado tick fever, dengue) has been documented by blood transfusions and organ donations. The tick-borne Colorado tick fever virus is specifically mentioned in the Bloodborne Pathogens Standards as it infects and remains infectious within red blood cells for prolonged periods. Due to the continuing spread of the West Nile virus infections across the United States, a national blood donor testing program has been instituted.

Human disease characteristics vary by the infecting agent. Asymptomatic infections or infections with mild flulike symptoms are common. However, severe neurologic disease and death may occur. Treatment is largely supportive.

Babesiosis (Babesia microti)[35–38]

Babesiosis is a potentially fatal, tick-borne parasitic disease defined by *Babesia microti* infection of red blood cells. Numerous species, including humans and mice, are naturally susceptible to infection. The frequency of human disease transmission through transfusion has increased since it was first recognized in the 1980s. Both vertical and horizontal disease transmission are suspected in the mouse.

Human infections may be asymptomatic, characterized by a mild-to-moderate flulike illness, or severe relapsing disease or death. Severe disease most commonly occurs in immunocompromised or splenectomized individuals. Diagnosis is by microscopic identification of the organism on blood smears and through serology and polymerase chain reaction testing. Treatment includes antimicrobial therapy with or without the antimalarial drug, quinine.

Brucellosis (Brucella *spp.*)[39]

Brucellosis is the world's most widespread zoonosis and is caused by infection with bacterium of the genus *Brucella. Brucella* species are highly adapted to select animal host species, although infections do regularly occur in nontarget host species (eg, humans). Inadvertent murine brucellosis infection is not a concern in modern animal care programs. However, the US population is at risk of brucellosis from livestock and wildlife reservoirs.

Although asymptomatic infections do occur, clinical signs of human infection frequently include undulating fevers, sweating, headaches, myalgia, and generalized lymphadenopathy. Disease may progress to become debilitating or fatal. Transmission occurs by direct contact through broken skin, mucous membrane exposure, ingestion, and by aerosol. Human transmission has occurred through blood transfusion. Diagnosis is most frequently through serology in conjunction with secondary testing methods. Treatment predominantly consists of antibiotic therapy.

Chagas Disease (Trypanosoma cruzi)[40,41]

Chagas disease is endemic to some regions of the Americas, predominantly Latin America, and is caused by the flagellate protozoan parasite, *Trypanosoma cruzi.*

Undiagnosed human infections are common due to extended latent infections. Acute disease is often asymptomatic but may present as fever, lymphadenopathy, hepatosplenomegaly, and/or skin rash and may progress to myocarditis, encephalitis, or even death.

Natural disease transmission occurs predominantly by direct contact with contaminated feces of the insect vectors (Reduviidae family) or by their bite. Humans and domestic and wild animals serve as disease reservoirs. *T. cruzi* has been transmitted by transfusion and organ transplantation in the United States where all blood donors are screened for the disease. Diagnosis is most commonly by serology. Optimal disease treatment varies by the stage of the disease and patient characteristics.

Creutzfeldt-Jakob Disease[42–45]

Creutzfeldt-Jakob disease is a transmissible spongiform encephalopathy with approximately 300 cases diagnosed annually in the United States. The causative agent is a misfolded, self-replicating, cellular protein (prion). This progressive, uniformly fatal, neurodegenerative disease may have a prolonged incubation period (months to years) with death occurring within a year of clinical sign development. Prions are transmissible across some mammalian species including transgenic mice. Disease transmission has resulted from blood transfusion from asymptomatic human carriers and are suspected to have occurred in the United States. Human disease is causally associated with a prion disease of cattle, Bovine Spongiform Encephalopathy (BSE). As a result, individuals who have lived for more than 3 months in a country where BSE is common are deferred as blood donors in the United States. Definitive diagnosis requires immunohistochemical evaluation of brain tissue collected by biopsy or at autopsy. Effective treatments do not exist.

*Leptospirosis (*Leptospira*)*[2,10,46,47]

Leptospirosis is a zoonotic disease common to domestic animals and wildlife. Disease results from infection with spirochete bacteria of the genus *Leptospira.* Numerous serovars of *Leptospira* exist, each adapted to one or more host species.

Leptospirosis in humans is highly variable ranging from asymptomatic to severe infection and death. Human infections do occur in the United States, with higher incidences observed in areas where humans live in close association with wild rodents. *Leptospira* is a recognized BBP and serologic evidence of infection is documented in the US blood donor population. Endemic infections have been sustained in laboratory mouse colonies with presumed transmission to animal handlers.

Diagnosis is primarily by serologic testing and treatment is largely supportive.

*Malaria (*Plasmodium *spp.)*[37,48–54]

Human malaria is caused by infection with one of five species of the genus *Plasmodium*, namely, *Plasmodium falciparum, Plasmodium vivax, Plasmodium ovale, Plasmodium malariae,* or *Plasmodium knowlesi*. Common clinical manifestations include cyclic fever and chills, headaches, fatigue, malaise, myalgia, and nausea. Severe anemia, acute renal failure, acute respiratory distress syndrome, coagulopathies, hypotension, and neurologic abnormalities may develop.

Natural human infection can only be acquired from female mosquitoes of the genus, *Anopheles*. The vast majority of US human cases are diagnosed in individuals who have traveled to endemic areas (eg, tropics and subtropics), although congenital infections and infections from exposure to blood or blood products do occur. Seven cases of transfusion-related malaria transmission have been documented in the United States. As a result, potential US blood donors with travel history to endemic areas are deferred from donation for a minimum of 3 years. Organ transplantation–associated malaria transmission has occurred. Experimentally, long-lasting parasitemia has been demonstrated in humanized mouse models.

Diagnostic methods include microscopic identification of the parasite and molecular assays. Antimalarial drugs are key to treatment.

*Tick-Borne Relapsing Fever (*Borrelia*)*[55–58]

Tick-borne relapsing fever is endemic in multiple countries including the western United States. Disease results from infection with a bacterial spirochete of the *Borrelia* species. Infected individuals frequently have a history of contact with or close proximity to animal reservoirs of the spirochete agent and their associated soft tick vectors (genus *Ornithodoros*). Persistent infection of some *Borrelia* sp can be maintained in experimentally infected mice. Natural transmission occurs when an infected tick feeds on a susceptible host. Human disease transmission has also occurred through transfusion and contact with contaminated blood.

Disease is characterized by recurring episodes of fever and nonspecific symptoms which may progress to severe respiratory, renal, hematologic, and CNS involvement. The disease tends to be more severe and prolonged in young children and in pregnant women, frequently resulting in abortion or stillbirths. In the United States, mortality is rare, most commonly occurring in the fetus or neonate.

Diagnosis is most commonly by serologic (eg, enzyme-linked immunosorbent assay) and molecular assays. Treatment includes extended antibiotic administration.

*Syphilis (*Treponema pallidum*)*[59–63]

Human syphilis is caused by the bacteria, *Treponema pallidum*. Acute and latent (asymptomatic) infections occur. Signs and symptoms of disease include ulcers, skin rashes, mucocutaneous lesions, lymphadenopathy, CNS impairment, cardiovascular disorders, auditory or ophthalmic abnormalities, and paresis.

Transmission is by sexual transmission, congenitally, and through exposure to unhygienic conditions. Disease transmission has occurred through blood transfusion resulting in US federal regulations that require routine screening of blood donations. Syphilis has been transmitted through organ transplantation, and the current US policy requires the screening of all deceased organ donors for infection.

Diagnosis is by serology or molecular assays. Penicillin G is the preferred treatment.

Viral Hemorrhagic Fevers[2,33,64,65]

Hemorrhagic fever viruses are RNA viruses that produce a clinical syndrome in humans characterized by high fever, epistaxis, ecchymosis, diffuse hemorrhage, hypotension, and shock. Natural disease transmission has been increasing around the globe and involves arthropod vectors, direct contact with the excreta of infected rodents, or contaminated blood or bodily fluid. Infection with many of these viruses (eg, yellow fever, dengue, hantaviruses) occurs in the United States and/or in US tourists with prior travel to endemic areas. Other viruses (Marburg and Ebola viruses) could be diagnosed in the US population (eg, following travel-associated exposure), but are highly unlikely. Transmission of select hemorrhagic fever viruses have been documented through transfusions and tissue transplants from contaminated donors.

REFERENCES

1. U.S. Dept. of Health and Human Services. *Biosafety in microbiological and biomedical laboratories*. 5th ed. 2010. Washington.
2. Fox JG, Otto G, Colby LA. Selected zoonoses. In: Fox JG, Anderson LC, Otto G, Pritchett-Corning K, Whary M, editors. *Laboratory animal medicine*. 3rd ed. Academic Press; 2015. p. 1313–70.
3. Rabinowitz PM, Lefkowitz RY, Conti LA, Redlich CA, Weigler BJ. Occupational health of laboratory animal workers. In: Fox JG, Anderson LC, Otto G, Pritchett-Corning K, Whary M, editors. *Laboratory animal medicine*. 3rd ed. Academic Press; 2015. p. 1382–402.
4. Swearengen JR, Carpenter CB. Working safely with experimental animals exposed to biohazards. In: Fox JG, Anderson LC, Otto G, Pritchett-Corning K, Whary M, editors. *Laboratory animal medicine*. 3rd ed. Academic Press; 2015. p. 1297–312.
5. Adams D, Fullerton K, Jajosky R, Sharp P, Onweh D, Schley A, et al. Summary of notifiable infectious diseases and conditions – United States, 2013. *MMWR Morb Mortal Wkly Rep* 2015;**62**(53):1–122.
6. Akkina R. New generation humanized mice for virus research: comparative aspects and future prospects. *Virology* 2013;**435**(1):14–28.
7. Centers for Disease Control and Prevention (CDC). Notes from the field: lymphocytic choriomeningitis virus infections in employees of a rodent breeding facility–Indiana, May–June 2012. *MMWR Morb Mortal Wkly Rep* 2012;**61**(32):622–3.
8. Brehm MA, Shultz LD, Greiner DL. Humanized mouse models to study human diseases. *Curr Opin Endocrinol Diabetes Obes* 2010;**17**(2):120–5.

9. Araki K, Yoshimatsu K, Lee B-H, Kariwa H, Takashima I, Arikawa J. Hantavirus-specific CD8(+)-T-cell responses in newborn mice persistently infected with Hantaan virus. *J Virol* 2003;**77**(15):8408–17.
10. Stoenner HG, Maclean D. Leptospirosis (ballum) contracted from Swiss albino mice. *AMA Arch Intern Med* 1958;**101**(3):606–10.
11. Riley LK, Livingston RS. Pathogen contamination of human tumors and patient-derived xenografts. In: *Poster, 66th national meeting of the american association of laboratory animal science, Phoenix, AZ.* 2015.
12. *OSHA bloodborne pathogens standard.* 2015. https://www.osha.gov/pls/oshaweb/owadisp.show_document?p_table=STANDARDS&p_id=10051.
13. Zou S, Stramer SL, Dodd RY. Donor testing and risk: current prevalence, incidence, and residual risk of transfusion-transmissible agents in US allogeneic donations. *Transfus Med Rev* 2012;**26**(2):119–28.
14. Macnab JCM, Onions D. Tumor viruses. [Internet]. In: Baron S, editor. *Medical microbiology*. 4th ed. Galveston (TX): University of Texas Medical Branch at Galveston; 1996www.ncbi.nlm.nih.gov/books/NBK7998/.
15. Centers for Disease Control and Prevention. *Hbv FAQs for health professionals*. 2015. http://www.cdc.gov/hepatitis/hbv/hbvfaq.htm#overview.
16. Centers for Disease Control and Prevention. *Hcv FAQs for health professionals*. 2015. http://www.cdc.gov/hepatitis/hcv/hcvfaq.htm#section1.
17. El-Serag HB. Epidemiology of viral hepatitis and hepatocellular carcinoma. *Gastroenterology* 2012;**142**(6):1264–73.
18. Hjalgrim H, Friborg J, Melbye M. The epidemiology of EBV and its association with malignant disease. In: Arvin A, Campadelli-Fiume G, Mocarski E, Moore PS, Roizman B, Whitley R, et al., editors. *Human herpesviruses: biology, therapy, and immunoprophylaxis*. Cambridge: Cambridge University Press; 2007. [Chapter 53].
19. Armengol C, Tarafa G, Boix L, Solé M, Queralt R, Costa D, et al. Orthotopic implantation of human hepatocellular carcinoma in mice: analysis of tumor progression and establishment of the BCLC-9 cell line. *Clin Cancer Res* 2004;**10**(6):2150–7.
20. Centers for Disease Control and Prevention. *HPV-associated cancers statistics*. 2015. http://www.cdc.gov/cancer/hpv/statistics/.
21. Sunil M, Reid E, Lechowicz MJ. Update on HHV-8-associated malignancies. *Curr Infect Dis Rep* 2010;**12**(2):147–54.
22. Oksenhendler E, Carcelain G, Aoki Y, Boulanger E, Maillard A, Clauvel JP, et al. High levels of human herpesvirus 8 viral load, human interleukin-6, interleukin-10, and C reactive protein correlate with exacerbation of multicentric Castleman disease in HIV-infected patients. *Blood* 2000;**96**(6):2069–73.
23. Ablashi DV, Chatlynne LG, Whitman JE, Cesarman E. Spectrum of Kaposi's sarcoma-associated herpesvirus, or human herpesvirus 8, diseases. *Clin Microbiol Rev* 2002;**15**(3):439–64.
24. Roucoux DF, Murphy EL. The epidemiology and disease outcomes of human T-lymphotropic virus type II. *AIDS Rev* 2004;**6**(3):144–54.
25. Chang Y, Cesarman E, Pessin MS, Lee F, Culpepper J, Knowles DM, et al. Identification of herpesvirus-like DNA sequences in AIDS-associated Kaposi's sarcoma. *Science* 1994;**266**(5192):1865–9.
26. Wolmer-Solberg N, Baryawno N, Rahbar A, Fuchs D, Odeberg J, Taher C, et al. Frequent detection of human cytomegalovirus in neuroblastoma: a novel therapeutic target? *Int J Cancer J Int Cancer* 2013;**133**(10):2351–61.
27. Söderberg-Nauclér C, Johnsen JI. Cytomegalovirus in human brain tumors: Role in pathogenesis and potential treatment options. *World J Exp Med* 2015;**5**(1):1–10.

28. Centers for Disease Control and Prevention. *Cytomegalovirus (CMV) and congenital CMV infection*. 2015. http://www.cdc.gov/cmv/clinical/features.html.
29. Kuhar DT, Henderson DK, Struble KA, Heneine W, Thomas V, Cheever LW, et al. Updated US Public Health Service guidelines for the management of occupational exposures to human immunodeficiency virus and recommendations for postexposure prophylaxis. *Infect Control Hosp Epidemiol* 2013;**34**(9):875–92.
30. Centers for Disease Control and Prevention. *HIV in the United States*. 2015. http://www.cdc.gov/hiv/statistics/basics/ataglance.html.
31. Kumar D, Prasad GVR, Zaltzman J, Levy GA, Humar A. Community-acquired West Nile virus infection in solid-organ transplant recipients. *Transplantation* 2004;**77**(3):399–402.
32. Leiby DA, Gill JE. Transfusion-transmitted tick-borne infections: a cornucopia of threats. *Transfus Med Rev* 2004;**18**(4):293–306.
33. Pozzetto B, Memmi M, Garraud O. Is transfusion-transmitted dengue fever a potential public health threat? *World J Virol* 2015;**4**(2):113–23.
34. Dodd RY, Foster GA, Stramer SL. Keeping blood transfusion safe from West Nile virus: American red cross experience, 2003 to 2012. *Transfus Med Rev* 2015;**29**(3):153–61.
35. Konopka E, Siński E. Experimental infection of mice with *Babesia microti*: characterization of parasitemia. *Wiad Parazytol* 1996;**42**(4):395–406.
36. Tonnetti L, Eder AF, Dy B, Kennedy J, Pisciotto P, Benjamin RJ, et al. Transfusion-transmitted *Babesia microti* identified through hemovigilance. *Transfusion* 2009;**49**(12):2557–63.
37. Cox FE. Babesiosis and malaria. In: Palmer SR, Soulsby L, Torgerson P, Brown WG, editors. *Oxford textbook of zoonoses: biology, clinical practice, and public health control*. 2nd ed. New York: Oxford University Press; 2011. p. 589–95.
38. Bednarska M, Bajer A, Drozdowska A, Mierzejewska EJ, Tolkacz K, Welc-Falęciak R. Vertical transmission of *Babesia microti* in BALB/c mice: preliminary report. *PLoS One* 2015;**10**(9):e0137731.
39. Doganay M, Aygen B, Eşel D. Brucellosis due to blood transfusion. *J Hosp Infect* 2001;**49**(2):151–2.
40. Moraes-Souza H, Bordin JO. Strategies for prevention of transfusion-associated Chagas' disease. *Transfus Med Rev* 1996;**10**(3):161–70.
41. Castro E. Chagas' disease: lessons from routine donation testing. *Transfus Med Oxf Engl* 2009;**19**(1):16–23.
42. Prusiner SB. Prions. *Proc Natl Acad Sci USA* 1998;**95**(23):13363–83.
43. Wroe SJ, Pal S, Siddique D, Hyare H, Macfarlane R, Joiner S, et al. Clinical presentation and pre-mortem diagnosis of variant Creutzfeldt-Jakob disease associated with blood transfusion: a case report. *Lancet* 2006;**368**(9552):2061–7.
44. National Institute of Neurological Disorders and Stroke (NINDS). *Creutzfeldt-Jakob disease fact sheet*. 2015. http://www.ninds.nih.gov/disorders/cjd/detail_cjd.htm.
45. Lee J, Hyeon JW, Kim SY, Hwang K-J, Ju YR, Ryou C. Review: laboratory diagnosis and surveillance of Creutzfeldt-Jakob disease. *J Med Virol* 2015;**87**(1):175–86.
46. Lettieri C, Moon J, Hickey P, Gray M, Berg B, Hospenthal D. Prevalence of leptospira antibodies in U.S. Army blood bank donors in Hawaii. *Mil Med* 2004;**169**(9):687–90.
47. Haake DA, Levett PN. Leptospirosis in humans. *Curr Top Microbiol Immunol* 2015;**387**:65–97.
48. Arnold L, Tyagi RK, Meija P, Swetman C, Gleeson J, Pérignon J-L, et al. Further improvements of the P. falciparum humanized mouse model. *PLoS One* 2011;**6**(3):e18045.
49. Kotton CN. Transplant tourism and donor-derived parasitic infections. *Transpl Proc* 2011;**43**(6):2448–9.

50. Cullen KA, Arguin PM. Malaria surveillance–United States, 2012. *Morb Mortal Wkly Rep Surveill Summ* 2014;**63**(12):1–22.
51. Centers for Disease Control and Prevention. *Malaria: disease*. 2015. http://www.cdc.gov/malaria/about/disease.html#uncomplicated.
52. O'Brien SF, Delage G, Seed CR, Pillonel J, Fabra CC, Davison K, et al. The epidemiology of imported malaria and transfusion policy in 5 nonendemic countries. *Transfus Med Rev* 2015;**29**(3):162–71.
53. Roth JM, Korevaar DA, Leeflang MMG, Mens PF. Molecular malaria diagnostics: a systematic review and meta-analysis. *Crit Rev Clin Lab Sci* 2015:1–19.
54. World Health Organization. *Guidelines for the treatment of malaria*. 3rd ed. 2015. http://www.ncbi.nlm.nih.gov/books/NBK294440.
55. Cutler SJ. Possibilities for relapsing fever reemergence. *Emerg Infect Dis* 2006;**12**(3):369–74.
56. Dworkin MS, Schwan TG, Anderson DE, Borchardt SM. Tick-borne relapsing fever. *Infect Dis Clin North Am* 2008;**22**(3):449–68. viii.
57. Larsson C, Andersson M, Bergström S. Current issues in relapsing fever. *Curr Opin Infect Dis* 2009;**22**(5):443–9.
58. El-Bahnsawy MM, Labib NA, Abdel-Fattah MA-H, Ibrahim AMA, Morsy TA. Louse and tick borne relapsing fevers. *J Egypt Soc Parasitol* 2012;**42**(3):625–38.
59. Orton S. Syphilis and blood donors: what we know, what we do not know, and what we need to know. *Transfus Med Rev* 2001;**15**(4):282–91.
60. Shockman S, Buescher LS, Stone SP. Syphilis in the United States. *Clin Dermatol* 2014;**32**(2):213–8.
61. Kaur G, Kaur P. Syphilis testing in blood donors: an update. *Blood Transfus* 2015;**13**(2):197–204.
62. Theodoropoulos N, Jaramillo A, Penugonda S, Wasik C, Brooks K, Ladner DP, et al. Improving syphilis screening in deceased organ donors. *Transplantation* 2015;**99**(2):438–43.
63. Workowski KA, Bolan GA. Sexually transmitted diseases treatment guidelines. *MMWR Recomm Rep 2015* 2015;**64**(RR-03):1–137.
64. Wiwanitkit V. Unusual mode of transmission of dengue. *J Infect Dev Ctries* 2010;**4**(1):51–4.
65. Schmidt M, Geilenkeuser W-J, Sireis W, Seifried E, Hourfar K. Emerging pathogens – how safe is blood? *Transfus Med Hemotherapy* 2014;**41**(1):10–7.

Section III

PDX Models for Tumors of Various Organ Systems

Chapter 1

Pediatric and Adult Brain Tumor PDX Models

A.D. Strand[1], E. Girard[1], J.M. Olson[1,2,3]
[1]*Fred Hutchinson Cancer Research Center, Seattle, WA, United States;* [2]*Seattle Children's Research Institute, Seattle, WA, United States;* [3]*University of Washington, Seattle, WA, United States*

BACKGROUND

Brain cancer is a uniquely frightening and personal disease, as it strikes at the tissue that controls both our body and personal identity. Treatment remains a challenge for a variety of reasons. Attempts to spare normal brain, particularly in pediatric cancer, often limit surgical and radiologic options. The blood–brain barrier (BBB) prevents most chemicals, including drugs that are intended to be therapeutic, from entering the brain. Even if therapies can get past the BBB, many types of brain cancer are intrinsically chemo- and radioresistant.

Currently, 90% of therapeutic drug candidates that look promising in the laboratory fail in human clinical trials, which suggest that our brain cancer models need improvement. Tissue culture cell lines have long served as the primary model system. The limitations of tissue culture lines have long been recognized, so in vivo alternatives, mainly laboratory mice, have come to the fore. Genetically engineered mouse models allow clinical researchers to study several types of brain cancer. However, the creation of relevant genetically engineered mouse models is time-consuming and requires a great deal of understanding of the biology of cancer. Cell line xenografts are commonly used, but carry the limitations of cells that have been grown under nonphysiologic tissue culture conditions for prolonged periods. Patient-derived xenograft (PDX) models offer a way to create models representing types of cancer that are less well understood, with the added feature (or flaw) that the model represents an individual's unique tumor. The generation of genomically curated PDX mouse models and careful translational experiments may modernize nonclinical pharmacology studies in a manner that reduces the failure rate of human clinical trials that include children or adults with brain tumors.

In the case of brain cancers, pediatric and adult cancers have distinct biological differences and require different models. Anatomically the brain is

Patient Derived Tumor Xenograft Models. http://dx.doi.org/10.1016/B978-0-12-804010-2.00015-1

separated into a top (supratentorial) and bottom (infratentorial) compartment. In adults, most tumors are supratentorial. In contrast to adult tumors, most pediatric tumors occur in the posterior fossa (cerebellum or brainstem), which are located in the infratentorial compartment. Adult brain cancers occur after the brain is fully developed. In this setting, cancer is largely a disease of aging and most cancers are glial in origin. Pediatric brain cancer is a developmental disease and tumors of neural origin are more common in children.

Because the brain lacks pain receptors and because glioma cells are highly migratory, adult brain tumors are often quite advanced at the time of diagnosis. The extent of surgical resection makes a significant difference in patient outcome, with patients undergoing >90% resection experiencing a significant survival advantage.[1,2] It is assumed that radiation and chemotherapy are more effective for microscopic disease than bulky disease, hence outcomes are improved when most of the bulky tumor is removed, even when microscopic disease remains.

Although brain tumors are relatively uncommon, representing only 1.4% of all cancers, brain tumors further challenge drug hunters because of their diversity; there are over 20 types of adult brain cancer and over 20 types of pediatric brain cancer—with essentially no biological overlap between the two age groups even in cancers of the same type.

Diagnosis and classification of pediatric brain tumors represent a particular quandary for neuro-oncologists at this point in time because molecular studies imply that pathology-based classification may have conflated multiple distinct types of brain tumors. As tumor categories that were already rare become further split into molecular subtypes, it will be more difficult to conduct statistically meaningful human clinical trials. For that reason, PDX mice will be critical for prioritizing and advancing effective therapeutics.

METHODOLOGIES AND MODELS

Technical Considerations

Xiao-nan Li at Texas Children's Hospital modernized techniques to create orthotopic PDX models of pediatric brain tumors.[3,30] He recognized that it was essential to implant the tumors rapidly after the cells were separated from their blood supply in human patients. Engraftment rates in his hands approached 80% when cells were implanted within 2h of resection versus approximately 20–30% for cells that were separated from the blood supply for longer periods.[3] Brain tumor cells generally survive poorly once disconnected from endogenous blood supply, so time is of essence when creating these models.

Although each laboratory has preferences as to whether tumor tissue fragments or disperse single-cell suspensions should be implanted, there are no data that clearly indicates that one approach is superior to the other. Generally, the use of proteolytic or glycolytic enzyme concoctions to disperse the cells is frowned upon because the process cleaves growth factor receptors and other important cell surface proteins. It is also important to consider the media and additives used for transport of the cells/tissues and to avoid exposure to differentiating agents (eg, retinoids) that are common in serum and some commercial media preparations. In cases where implantation occurs after shipping or delay, some have found that cryopreserving cells is helpful.[4]

Protocols for tumor preparation, implantation (subcutaneous as well as orthotopic/intracranial) are described in various publications.[3–35] Flank models are easier to generate and monitor than orthotopic models but at the expense of implanting the tumors in a subcutaneous microenvironment rather than a brain (albeit mouse) microenvironment.

Most of the techniques for orthotopic transplantation vary slightly. Many laboratories use stereotactic equipment to precisely implant human tumor cells into the designated location in mouse brain.[36] The advantage to this approach is that the implantation site can be controlled in all three planes. The disadvantage is that it is time-consuming and thus expensive. Our laboratory is able to consistently establish orthotopic PDX models at a rate of approximately 30 mice per hour by using the technique of inserting a 20-μL pipette tip containing cancer cells through a 0.9-mm-diameter burr hole created with a handheld drill. An important element is a careful placement of the burr hole, which is a placed approximately 2 mm lateral (right) of the sagittal suture and 2 mm posterior to the lambdoid suture for cerebellar implantation. Implantation in the right cerebral hemisphere should be done approximately 1 mm lateral of the sagittal suture and 1.5 mm anterior to the lambdoid suture.

Approximately 20% of the human pediatric brain tumor lines that we passage in mice have eventually given rise to mouse brain tumors rather than human brain tumors. This phenomenon has been previously reported by others.[37] The mechanism of transformation is unknown and represents an interesting avenue for future research. In the meantime, it is critical to monitor for this possibility and to preserve early passages in case the transformation occurs later and the line needs to be restarted. Importantly, we observe that the mouse tumors grow much faster than human tumors, so we typically keep mice that are asymptomatic alive beyond the time that mice are sacrificed for early signs of tumors, in case the early symptomatic mice are carrying mouse tumors and the later symptomatic mice continue to grow human tumors.

TUMOR BIOLOGY

Adult Brain Tumors: Pathology and Molecular Drivers

Traditionally, adult gliomas were classified by the World Health Organization (WHO) by pathologic grade[38]; however, this is being supplanted by molecular-based characterization,[39–41] which will be summarized here.

Isocitrate dehydrogenase (IDH1 or IDH2) mutation and chromosome 1p/19q codeletion: These tumors are typically WHO grade II oligodendrogliomas that also contain a mutation of the TERT gene promoter. Concurrent genetic mutations include mutations in the CIC, FUBP1, NOTCH1 and PIK3CA, or PIK3R1 genes. The CDKN2A/B gene or a portion of chromosome 4 is deleted in a subset of tumors. The mean age at diagnosis is 44–45 years and the median survival is >8 years.

IDH mutation without 1p/19q codeletion: These tumors are astrocytic or oligoastrocytic and more often grade II than grade III. The TERT promoter is mutated in a subset and is often associated with mutations of the TP53 and ATRX genes. Chromosomal gains include 7q and 8q24 (MYC) and losses include CDKN2A/B. Median age at diagnosis is the late thirties to midforties, and survival tends to be >6 years.

IDH wild type: These tumors tend to be high grade (III or IV), and the prognosis is poor (typically <2 years median). These tumors are pathologically called anaplastic astrocytomas (Gr III) or glioblastomas (grade IV). EGFR, NF1, and PTEN gene mutations are frequently associated with these tumor phenotypes and those with a TERT promoter mutation also tend to have mutations in RB1, PIK3CA, or PIK3R1. Copy number alterations include chromosomes 7 or 19, EGFR amplification, and homozygous deletion of CDKN2A/B.

Pediatric Brain Tumors: Pathology and Molecular Drivers

Over 20 types of brain tumors occur in children, and the molecular underpinnings have been established for most of these.[42]

Pediatric high-grade gliomas (HGGs) differ from adult counterparts at both the genetic and epigenetic level.[42–44] The H3.3K27M histone tail mutation occurs in young children with midline HGGs[45–47] and is associated with mutations in TP53, ATRX, ACVR1 (diffuse intrinsic pontine gliomas), or FGFR1 (thalamic location), as well as PDGFRA amplifications.[48] The H3.3G34V/R histone tail mutation occurs in adolescents with cerebral hemisphere HGGs and is associated with TP53 and ATRX mutations.[48] Proneural and mesenchymal HGGs driven by PDGFRA amplification and NF1 mutation, respectively, occur in cerebral hemispheres and both types are associated with TP53 mutations, CDKN2A/B deletions, and EGFR amplification.[48] Unfortunately, all these pediatric HGGs have a short median survival time of 6–12 months.

Located in the cerebellum and of neural origin, medulloblastomas are classified into four distinct molecular subtypes: Wnt, sonic hedgehog (shh), group 3, and group 4. Wnt tumors arise from the rhombic lip and are typically driven by mutations in CTNNB1, often accompanied by monosomy 6. The median age is 10 years and the median 5-year event-free survival is 90%, whereas the median 5-year survival for other subgroups of medulloblastoma range from 40 to 70%.[48]

Shh medulloblastomas arise from cerebellar granule cells and are sharply divided by age. Infant shh (0–4 years) typically express SUFU or PTCH1 mutations.[49] Childhood (4–17 years) shh tumors occur in individuals with Li–Fraumeni syndrome (TP53 germline mutations).[49] Outcome for these childhood patients is poor if GLI2 or MYCN is amplified. Adult (>17 years) shh tumors typically harbor SMO (smoothened gene) mutations and activation of PI3K/AKT/mTOR networks, and these patients have an intermediate outcome.[49]

Groups 3 and 4 medulloblastomas are molecularly heterogeneous subclasses of tumors with subsets of tumors expressing various combinations of isochromosome 17q, loss of chromosome 11, MYCN amplification, activation of GFI1/1B, mutations of SMARCA4, and mutations in genes that encode chromosome-modifying proteins.[48] Ependymomas derive from ependymal cells in the supratentorium, posterior fossa, or spinal cord. Supratentorial tumors are thought to be driven by RELA gene fusions or Yap1 fusions. Posterior fossa ependymomas fall into two molecular subgroups named Group A (most common, notable for epigenetic changes) and Group B (less common, no reoccurring mutations or amplifications).[48]

Atypical teratoid rhabdoid tumors primarily affect infants and toddlers and carry a poor prognosis. The absence of the SMARCB1 protein in these tumors is pathognomonic for this disease.[50]

The need for improved therapies has driven the quest to develop more predictive preclinical models. Many clinical and translational medicine programs now engage in PDX mouse–generating activities. Many of the models have not yet been published. Table 1.1 provides references to articles that have been published on brain tumor PDX models and websites at which others can be obtained. This list focuses on contemporary efforts and is not comprehensive. We are grateful to the pioneers who developed brain tumor xenograft models in the 20th century and apologize to those whose work is not cited below.

GENOMIC CHARACTERIZATION

Whenever possible, it is important to retain tumor tissue from the patient for genomic analyses to assess the fidelity of the mouse models to the original patient tumor. Obtaining nonneoplastic tissue (eg, blood samples) from the patient enables determination of cancer-specific mutations.

Two levels of genomic analyses are important in a robust PDX model program. The first ensures that inadvertent tube swaps or mouse swaps are detected and addressed. Undetected, such swaps can create significant risk to downstream users. One approach is to use a commercial "paternity" test kit to rapidly ensure that each batch of mice or frozen material from mice carries the same genetic "barcode" as the original patient sample (Promega PowerPlex Fusion and similar kits). The second level of genomic analysis involves genome sequencing, 450K methylation studies, or other genomic characterization to assess the molecular subclass of tumor. As translational research laboratories

TABLE 1.1 Brain Tumor Mouse Models

Tumor Type	Adult GBM	Pediatric Glioma	Ependymoma	ATRT	PNET	Medulloblastoma	Medulloblastoma
Model name	U87 (hu)	F98	Epd210FH	ATRT310FH	PNET109FH	Med311FH	DMB012
	U251 (hu)	9L	Epd710FH	ATRT312FH	PNET113FH	Med314FH	RCMB018
	G126 (mu)	C6			PNET212FH	Med2112FH	RCMB024
	Published PDX	Gli113FH				Med210FH	RCMB025
	aGBM110FH					Med313FH	RCMB32
						Med913FH	RCMB020
						Med610FH	RCBM028
						Med1512FH	RCMB40
						Med411FH	DMB006
						Med2312FH	RCMB38
						Med1712FH	RCMB41
						Med813FH	RCMB37
						Med512FH	RCMB35
						Med113FH	RCMB31
						Med114FH	
						Med211FH	

Cell source	Varies, frequently tissue culture immortalized cells or neurospheres of PDX cells	Orthotopic implant directly from patient or mouse to mouse without culturing. Other laboratories implant cultured samples	Orthotopic implant directly from patient or mouse to mouse without culturing	Orthotopic implant directly from patient or mouse to mouse without culturing	Orthotopic implant directly from patient or mouse to mouse without culturing	Orthotopic implant directly from patient or mouse to mouse without culturing	Orthotopic implant directly from patient or mouse to mouse without culturing
Cells for implant	$1–1.5 \times 10^6$ (hu)	1×10^5	1×10^5	1×10^5	1×10^5	1×10^5	2×10^6
	2×10^4 (mu)						
	$1–3 \times 10^5$ (PDX)						
Implantation method	Stereotactic guided surgery	Stereotactic guided surgery	Stereotactic guided surgery	Stereotactic guided surgery	Stereotactic guided surgery	Stereotactic guided surgery	Stereotactic guided surgery
Mouse strain	Athymic nude	NSG	NSG	NSG	NSG	NSG	Nu/Nu
Tumor latency	Cell lines: 17–30 days PDX models: 2–6 months	3–6 months	2–5 months	2–4 months	2–6 months	2–8 months	2–8 months
Internet resources	jax.org crownbio.org	btrl.org	btrl.org	btrl.org	btrl.org	btrl.org	
Additional references	5–8,11,13,14,20, 21,23,25,26,28	3,4,19,29,31	16,17,30	9,10,27	9	3,9,12,15,18,43, 44,30	32–35

ATRT, Atypical teratoid rhabdoid tumors.

focus on certain molecular subgroups of patients, knowing the genomic details of each mouse line is invaluable.

Preclinical Applications

As with all PDX models, brain tumor PDX models are used for drug discovery and development, particularly in vivo pharmacological assessment of drug efficacy at maximally tolerated doses (MTDs). In this section, we focus on the unique challenges of brain tumors that distinguish them from all other cancers and how this impacts decisions in PDX-based translational oncology programs.

The BBB represents a unique challenge in developing effective chemotherapies for brain cancer. The capillary endothelial cells of nearly all organs (except brain and testes) contain fenestrations and pores that allow free passage of most drugs and small proteins into the tissue. In contrast, brain capillaries lack fenestrations and pores. Furthermore, the endothelial cells lining the blood vessels in the brain are linked together by tight junctions. This physical barrier physically prevents most drugs from entering the brain parenchyma. In addition, the BBB endothelium contains transporters such as P-glycoprotein, which actively transports substrates out of the endothelial cells. Drugs that cross the BBB to achieve levels in the brain that are >10% of the levels achieved in peripheral tissues are considered to have "good" CNS penetration. For a typical chemotherapeutic agent, this would mean that if a drug is administered at its MTD, brain tumor cells would need to be 10 times more sensitive to the drug than a peripheral cancer in order for the drug to be equally effective in brain tumors as in peripheral cancers. This is a very high bar and is part of the reason that certain brain tumors are frequently fatal.

In some patient brain tumors, the BBB is disrupted, as evidenced by the fact that gadolinium contrast enters the tumor tissue and illuminates the tumor on magnetic resonance imaging (MRI). In these tumors, the intratumoral concentration of chemotherapy is more likely to be near the levels achieved in peripheral tissues. Unfortunately, even in brain tumors with disrupted BBB, cancer cells in the leading edge may be protected by intact BBB and these cells will repopulate the tumor after surgical resection and chemotherapy.

One theoretical advantage of genetically engineered brain tumor mouse models is that the BBB generally remains intact until the tumor reaches a certain stage of growth at which time heterogeneous or homogeneous disruption may occur. Some argue that because the BBB must be disrupted at the time of tumor cell implant in PDX mice, the BBB cannot be considered intact in PDX models. Surprisingly, many PDX models do appear to have an intact BBB, which reduces drug penetration. In many cases, these endothelial cells express P-glycoprotein pumps that sharply limit drug access to the tumors.[51] In these situations, it is common for a drug to cause significant cytoreduction of tumors that are implanted in the flank yet fail to affect tumors that are implanted orthotopically in the brain.[52–54] In some cases, the resistance of the orthotopic brain tumors can be overcome by genetically or pharmacologically inhibiting the P-glycoprotein pumps.[52–54] This is not a viable therapeutic option at this time, but these experiments provide clarity about the specific mechanism by which drugs that look promising in vitro or in flank models fail to show efficacy at tolerated doses in orthotopic brain tumor models.

The disparity between PDX brain tumor response when implanted in the flank versus in the brain is a key reason[52–54] why it is important to conduct experiments in orthotopic models, rather than flank models, before advancing drugs or drug combinations toward human clinical trials. Our laboratory often tests drugs in a small cohort of mice bearing flank tumors first. If the drug fails in that setting, we assume that the drug will not work in orthotopic models and discontinue evaluating that drug. If the drug(s) are effective in flank tumors, we advance the studies to orthotopic PDX models and monitor by MRI with and without contrast.

Vision for the Future

The number of patients within each molecular subclass of brain tumors shrinks as more distinct subclasses are identified. Conducting clinical trials will therefore take more time and financial resources. In many cases, particularly for pediatric brain tumor subclasses, it may only be possible to conduct one definitive study per decade per disease type. In the past, drug candidates were prioritized based on preclinical studies in cohorts of mice that were genetically identical or that carried a xenografted tumor from a single patient. In the future, it may be possible to enroll dozens of mice that represent dozens of patients within a molecular subclass into translational research trials. One would hope that drugs that show a benefit across many patient-derived models would fare better in human trials than those that are active in only one or two models.

SUPPORT

This work was supported by the Seattle Children's Pediatric Brain Tumor Research Fund Guild and NIH R01s CA114567, CA135491, and CA155360.

REFERENCES

1. Lacroix M, Abi-Said D, Fourney DR, Gokaslan ZL, Shi W, DeMonte F, et al. A multivariate analysis of 416 patients with glioblastoma multiforme: prognosis, extent of resection, and survival. *J Neurosurg* 2001;**95**(2):190–8.
2. Sanai N, Berger MS. Glioma extent of resection and its impact on patient outcome. *Neurosurgery* 2008;**62**(4):753–64. discussion 264–266.
3. Shu Q, Wong KK, Su JM, Adesina AM, Yu LT, Tsang YT, et al. Direct orthotopic transplantation of fresh surgical specimen preserves CD133+ tumor cells in clinically relevant mouse models of medulloblastoma and glioma. *Stem Cells* 2008;**26**(6):1414–24.

4. Aoki Y, Hashizume R, Ozawa T, Banerjee A, Prados M, James CD, et al. An experimental xenograft mouse model of diffuse pontine glioma designed for therapeutic testing. *J Neurooncol* 2012;**108**(1):29–35.
5. Candolfi M, Curtin JF, Nichols WS, Muhammad AG, King GD, Pluhar GE, et al. Intracranial glioblastoma models in preclinical neuro-oncology: neuropathological characterization and tumor progression. *J Neurooncol* 2007;**85**(2):133–48.
6. Carlson BL, Pokorny JL, Schroeder MA, Sarkaria JN. Establishment, maintenance and in vitro and in vivo applications of primary human glioblastoma multiforme (GBM) xenograft models for translational biology studies and drug discovery. *Curr Protoc Pharmacol* 2011;52:14.16:14.16.1–14.16.23.
7. Fei XF, Zhang QB, Dong J, Diao Y, Wang ZM, Li RJ, et al. Development of clinically relevant orthotopic xenograft mouse model of metastatic lung cancer and glioblastoma through surgical tumor tissues injection with trocar. *J Exp Clin Cancer Res* 2010;**29**:84.
8. Giannini C, Sarkaria JN, Saito A, Uhm JH, Galanis E, Carlson BL, et al. Patient tumor EGFR and PDGFRA gene amplifications retained in an invasive intracranial xenograft model of glioblastoma multiforme. *Neuro Oncol* 2005;**7**(2):164–76.
9. Girard E, Ditzler S, Lee D, Richards A, Yagle K, Park J, et al. Efficacy of cabazitaxel in mouse models of pediatric brain tumors. *Neuro Oncol* 2015;**17**(1):107–15.
10. Hashizume R, Gupta N, Berger MS, Banerjee A, Prados MD, Ayers-Ringler J, et al. Morphologic and molecular characterization of ATRT xenografts adapted for orthotopic therapeutic testing. *Neuro Oncol* 2010;**12**(4):366–76.
11. Hasselbach LA, Irtenkauf SM, Lemke NW, Nelson KK, Berezovsky AD, Carlton ET, et al. Optimization of high grade glioma cell culture from surgical specimens for use in clinically relevant animal models and 3D immunochemistry. *J Vis Exp* 2014;(83):e51088.
12. Huang X, Sarangi A, Ketova T, Litingtung Y, Cooper MK, Chiang C. Intracranial orthotopic allografting of medulloblastoma cells in immunocompromised mice. *J Vis Exp* 2010;(44).
13. Jeuken JW, Sprenger SH, Wesseling P, Bernsen HJ, Suijkerbuijk RF, Roelofs F, et al. Genetic reflection of glioblastoma biopsy material in xenografts: characterization of 11 glioblastoma xenograft lines by comparative genomic hybridization. *J Neurosurg* 2000;**92**(4):652–8.
14. Joo KM, Kim J, Jin J, Kim M, Seol HJ, Muradov J, et al. Patient-specific orthotopic glioblastoma xenograft models recapitulate the histopathology and biology of human glioblastomas in situ. *Cell Rep* 2013;**3**(1):260–73.
15. Liu Z, Zhao X, Wang Y, Mao H, Huang Y, Kogiso M, et al. A patient tumor-derived orthotopic xenograft mouse model replicating the group 3 supratentorial primitive neuroectodermal tumor in children. *Neuro Oncol* 2014;**16**(6):787–99.
16. Meco D, Servidei T, Lamorte G, Binda E, Arena V, Riccardi R. Ependymoma stem cells are highly sensitive to temozolomide in vitro and in orthotopic models. *Neuro Oncol* 2014;**16**(8):1067–77.
17. Milde T, Kleber S, Korshunov A, Witt H, Hielscher T, Koch P, et al. A novel human high-risk ependymoma stem cell model reveals the differentiation-inducing potential of the histone deacetylase inhibitor Vorinostat. *Acta Neuropathol* 2011;**122**(5):637–50.
18. Milde T, Lodrini M, Savelyeva L, Korshunov A, Kool M, Brueckner LM, et al. HD-MB03 is a novel Group 3 medulloblastoma model demonstrating sensitivity to histone deacetylase inhibitor treatment. *J Neurooncol* 2012;**110**(3):335–48.
19. Misuraca KL, Cordero FJ, Becher OJ. Pre-clinical models of diffuse intrinsic pontine glioma. *Front Oncol* 2015;**5**:172.
20. Oh YT, Cho HJ, Kim J, Lee JH, Rho K, Seo YJ, et al. Translational validation of personalized treatment strategy based on genetic characteristics of glioblastoma. *PLoS One* 2014;**9**(8):e103327.

21. Ozawa T, James CD. Establishing intracranial brain tumor xenografts with subsequent analysis of tumor growth and response to therapy using bioluminescence imaging. *J Vis Exp* 2010;**41**.
22. Pietsch T, Scharmann T, Fonatsch C, Schmidt D, Ockler R, Freihoff D, et al. Characterization of five new cell lines derived from human primitive neuroectodermal tumors of the central nervous system. *Cancer Res* 1994;**54**(12):3278–87.
23. Radaelli E, Ceruti R, Patton V, Russo M, Degrassi A, Croci V, et al. Immunohistopathological and neuroimaging characterization of murine orthotopic xenograft models of glioblastoma multiforme recapitulating the most salient features of human disease. *Histol Histopathol* 2009;**24**(7):879–91.
24. Sterling-Levis K, White L. The role of xenografting in pediatric brain tumor research with specific emphasis on medulloblastoma/primitive neuroectodermal tumors of childhood. *In Vivo* 2003;**17**(4):329–42.
25. Valadez JG, Sarangi A, Lundberg CJ, Cooper MK. Primary orthotopic glioma xenografts recapitulate infiltrative growth and isocitrate dehydrogenase I mutation. *J Vis Exp* 2014;**83**:e50865.
26. Wakimoto H, Mohapatra G, Kanai R, Curry Jr WT, Yip S, Nitta M, et al. Maintenance of primary tumor phenotype and genotype in glioblastoma stem cells. *Neuro Oncol* 2012;**14**(2):132–44.
27. Weingart MF, Roth JJ, Hutt-Cabezas M, Busse TM, Kaur H, Price A, et al. Disrupting LIN28 in atypical teratoid rhabdoid tumors reveals the importance of the mitogen activated protein kinase pathway as a therapeutic target. *Oncotarget* 2015;**6**(5):3165–77.
28. Xie Q, Thompson R, Hardy K, DeCamp L, Berghuis B, Sigler R, et al. A highly invasive human glioblastoma pre-clinical model for testing therapeutics. *J Transl Med* 2008;**6**:77.
29. Xu J, Erdreich-Epstein A, Gonzalez-Gomez I, Melendez EY, Smbatyan G, Moats RA, et al. Novel cell lines established from pediatric brain tumors. *J Neurooncol* 2012;**107**(2):269–80.
30. Yu L, Baxter PA, Voicu H, Gurusiddappa S, Zhao Y, Adesina A, et al. A clinically relevant orthotopic xenograft model of ependymoma that maintains the genomic signature of the primary tumor and preserves cancer stem cells in vivo. *Neuro Oncol* 2010;**12**(6):580–94.
31. Zhao X, Liu Z, Yu L, Zhang Y, Baxter P, Voicu H, et al. Global gene expression profiling confirms the molecular fidelity of primary tumor-based orthotopic xenograft mouse models of medulloblastoma. *Neuro Oncol* 2012;**14**(5):574–83.
32. Staal JA, Lau LS, Zhang H, Ingram WJ, Hallahan AR, Northcott PA, et al. Proteomic profiling of high risk medulloblastoma reveals functional biology. *Oncotarget* 2015;**6**(16):14584–95.
33. Brun SN, Markant SL, Esparza LA, Garcia G, Terry D, Huang JM, et al. Survivin as a therapeutic target in Sonic hedgehog-driven medulloblastoma. *Oncogene* 2015;**34**(29):3770–9.
34. Kool M, Jones DT, Jager N, Northcott PA, Pugh TJ, Hovestadt V, et al. Genome sequencing of SHH medulloblastoma predicts genotype-related response to smoothened inhibition. *Cancer Cell* 2014;**25**(3):393–405.
35. Markant SL, Esparza LA, Sun J, Barton KL, McCoig LM, Grant GA, et al. Targeting sonic hedgehog-associated medulloblastoma through inhibition of Aurora and Polo-like kinases. *Cancer Res* 2013;**73**(20):6310–22.
36. Pierce AM, Keating AK. Creating anatomically accurate and reproducible intracranial xenografts of human brain tumors. *J Vis Exp* 2014;(91):52017.
37. Caretti V, Sewing AC, Lagerweij T, Schellen P, Bugiani M, Jansen MH, et al. Human pontine glioma cells can induce murine tumors. *Acta Neuropathol* 2014;**127**(6):897–909.
38. Louis DN, Ohgaki H, Wiestler OD, Cavenee WK, Burger PC, Jouvet A, et al. The 2007 WHO classification of tumours of the central nervous system. *Acta Neuropathol* 2007;**114**(2):97–109.
39. Comprehensive, integrative genomic analysis of diffuse lower-grade gliomas. *N Engl J Med* 2015;**372**(26):2481–98.

40. Eckel-Passow JE, Lachance DH, Molinaro AM, Walsh KM, Decker PA, Sicotte H, et al. Glioma groups based on 1p/19q, IDH, and TERT promoter mutations in tumors. *N Engl J Med* 2015;**372**(26):2499–508.
41. Ellison DW. Multiple molecular data sets and the classification of adult diffuse gliomas. *N Engl J Med* 2015;**372**(26):2555–7.
42. Huse JT, Rosenblum MK. The emerging molecular foundations of pediatric brain tumors. *J Child Neurol* 2015;**30**(13):1838–50.
43. Korshunov A, Ryzhova M, Hovestadt V, Bender S, Sturm D, Capper D, et al. Integrated analysis of pediatric glioblastoma reveals a subset of biologically favorable tumors with associated molecular prognostic markers. *Acta Neuropathol* 2015;**129**(5):669–78.
44. Chamdine O, Gajjar A. Molecular characteristics of pediatric high-grade gliomas. *CNS Oncol* 2014;**3**(6):433–43.
45. Bender S, Tang Y, Lindroth AM, Hovestadt V, Jones DT, Kool M, et al. Reduced H3K27me3 and DNA hypomethylation are major drivers of gene expression in K27M mutant pediatric high-grade gliomas. *Cancer Cell* 2013;**24**(5):660–72.
46. Yuen BT, Knoepfler PS. Histone H3.3 mutations: a variant path to cancer. *Cancer Cell* 2013;**24**(5):567–74.
47. Wu G, Broniscer A, McEachron TA, Lu C, Paugh BS, Becksfort J, et al. Somatic histone H3 alterations in pediatric diffuse intrinsic pontine gliomas and non-brainstem glioblastomas. *Nat Genet* 2012;**44**(3):251–3.
48. Gajjar A, Bowers DC, Karajannis MA, Leary S, Witt H, Gottardo NG. Pediatric brain tumors: innovative genomic information is transforming the diagnostic and clinical landscape. *J Clin Oncol* 2015;**33**(27):2986–98.
49. Kool M, Jones DT, Jager N, Northcott PA, Pugh TJ, Hovestadt V, et al. Genome sequencing of SHH medulloblastoma predicts genotype-related response to smoothened inhibition. *Cancer Cell* 2014;**25**(3):393–405.
50. Rorke LB, Packer R, Biegel J. Central nervous system atypical teratoid/rhabdoid tumors of infancy and childhood. *J Neurooncol* 1995;**24**(1):21–8.
51. Rao VV, Dahlheimer JL, Bardgett ME, Snyder AZ, Finch RA, Sartorelli AC, et al. Choroid plexus epithelial expression of MDR1 P glycoprotein and multidrug resistance-associated protein contribute to the blood-cerebrospinal-fluid drug-permeability barrier. *Proc Natl Acad Sci USA* 1999;**96**(7):3900–5.
52. Agarwal S, Manchanda P, Vogelbaum MA, Ohlfest JR, Elmquist WF. Function of the blood–brain barrier and restriction of drug delivery to invasive glioma cells: findings in an orthotopic rat xenograft model of glioma. *Drug Metab Dispos* 2013;**41**(1):33–9.
53. Parrish KE, Pokorny J, Mittapalli RK, Bakken K, Sarkaria JN, Elmquist WF. Efflux transporters at the blood–brain barrier limit delivery and efficacy of cyclin-dependent kinase 4/6 inhibitor palbociclib (PD-0332991) in an orthotopic brain tumor model. *J Pharmacol Exp Ther* 2015;**355**(2):264–71.
54. Parrish KE, Cen L, Murray J, Calligaris D, Kizilbash S, Mittapalli RK, et al. Efficacy of PARP inhibitor rucaparib in orthotopic glioblastoma xenografts is limited by ineffective drug penetration into the central nervous system. *Mol Cancer Ther* 2015;**14**(12):2735–43.

Chapter 2

Patient-Derived Xenograft Models of Prostate Tumors

P.J. Russell[1], E.D. Williams[1], R. Taylor[2], M.G. Lawrence[2] and G. Risbridger[2]

[1]Queensland University of Technology at Translational Research Institute, Brisbane, QLD, Australia; [2]Monash University, Clayton, VIC, Australia

BACKGROUND/OVERVIEW

Prostate cancer is one of the most common noncutaneous cancers in the world, with over a million men being diagnosed in 2012 along with over 30,000 deaths annually.[1] Its clinical incidence increases rapidly after age 50 and continues to rise. This, coupled with the long natural history of the disease being in the range of decades, results in a significant burden on the health care system. Currently, the prostate-specific antigen (PSA) test based on the blood levels of PSA, an androgen-responsive gene, is used for the early detection of prostate cancer but PSA can be elevated due to other common nonmalignant conditions of the prostate and the test cannot discriminate indolent from aggressive disease. Both normal prostate and prostate cancers require androgens for growth and cell survival pathways. Prostate cancers are highly heterogeneous and show a complex progression path from organ-confined disease, which may be considered low risk or high risk, to more aggressive locally invasive or disseminated disease. Treatments for localized disease can range from observation alone to radical surgery or radiation. After the failure of local surgery or radiation, the removal of androgens is achieved through androgen deprivation therapy, either alone or together with an androgen receptor antagonist.[2] This treatment initially induces tumor regression and a period of cancer control with exceedingly low PSA levels. Ultimately patients relapse, signaled by a rise in PSA, and develop more aggressive castrate-resistant prostate cancer (CRPC) which is usually accompanied by invasion and metastasis. Several different approaches to therapy are currently under consideration in various clinical trials.[3–6]

It is very difficult to model the different stages of disease, and there are limited options either with mouse or human models. Human tumor–derived cell lines are limited in number and many have been in use for decades. The

Patient Derived Tumor Xenograft Models. http://dx.doi.org/10.1016/B978-0-12-804010-2.00016-3

potential of using patient-derived xenografts (PDXs) from prostate cancer for preclinical research has yet to be fully realized, in contrast to other solid tumors, as it is especially difficult to grow PDX from low-risk organ-confined disease where tumor cell proliferation and the percentage of dividing cells is low.[7] To address these issues tissue recombination (described below) has been used to initiate engraftment. For more advanced stage prostate cancers, there is a predilection to metastasize to the bone and form osteoblastic or mixed lesions rather than the osteolytic lesions which accompany lung and breast cancers.[8,9] Although the use of "rapid autopsy programs" has led to the ability to sample bone and soft tissue metastases for generating PDX, the lack of adequate human/animal models that can recapitulate the many steps of the metastatic cascade has hindered the development of prognostic markers and novel therapeutic strategies.[10,11] The development of PDX mouse models of prostate cancer that recapitulate the unique aspects of this disease is an area of active research.

METHODOLOGY AND MODELS

Three factors that affect the success rate of prostate PDX are the method of preparing fresh prostate tissue, the choice of host mouse strain, and the site of implantation.

Tissue Preparation

Once the fresh tissue has been transported to the laboratory, two different procedures can be used to prepare individual grafts for implantation. Most commonly, a scalpel is used to chop the tissue into small pieces of approximately 4–10 mm^3.[12–14] Alternatively, the tissue can be cut using a tissue slicer into precise pieces of approximately 300 μm thick[15] providing the benefit that the tumor content can be accurately compared between adjacent slices. The thinness of the slices also allows maximum diffusion of oxygen and nutrients into the PDX once they are implanted.

Choice of Mouse Strain

The choice of mouse strain also influences the success of prostate PDXs. Further discussion of types of immune compromised mice strains as well as their advantages is included in Section I, Chapter 5 of this book. It is important to consider the specific background of the mice as this influences the degree of functionality/leakiness of the immune system and propensity to develop thymic lymphomas (and hence reduce lifespan). Early PDX studies used male nude mice for transplanting small segments of tumors, usually derived from prostatectomy, or from transurethral resections of the prostate (TURP) with a relatively low take rate.[16] Subsequently, prostate cancer PDXs were grown in more immunodeficient mice developed through genetic modifications, such as severe combined immunodeficient (SCID) mice homozygous for the *scid* mutation in the protein kinase $Prkdc_{scid}$ which allows limited human hematopoiesis in vivo.[17] However, these mice show limited take rates of prostate cancer PDXs, as mature T and B cells are generated as the mice age, along with strong natural killer (NK) cell function.[18] Nonobese diabetic (NOD-*scid*) mice which have reduced NK cell activity compared with SCID mice[19] but still show a residual innate immune system were used for PDX. These mice have a shortened life span (8.5 months), as they spontaneously develop thymic lymphomas due to the presence of a provirus, Emv-30.[20] While backcrossing of nude mice with NOD-*scid* mice has provided a hairless mouse that lacks the provirus, to the best of our knowledge, this model is currently only available at the laboratory where it was developed.[21] More recent PDX work uses NOD-*scid* gamma (NSG) mice, which lack T and B cells and NK cells[22] and do not develop thymic lymphomas. Despite low initial engraftment and propagation, once PDXs are established as transplantable tumors, take rates are reproducibly high (Table 2.1), providing a robust platform for in vivo investigations.

Site of Implantation

Prostate tissue can be implanted into different sites in immunodeficient mice. Nguyen and Corey[23] have used specific mouse strains for specific sites of injection: C.B-17 SCID mice for subcutaneous, orthotopic, and subrenal implantation; SCID Beige for intratibial and cardiac injections; and Nu/Nu and IL-2 NOD/SCIDS for maintenance of the colonies. To date, most PDXs have been established following either subcutaneous (see Section II, Chapter 3) or orthotopic implantation.[23,24] In addition, some cell lines have been implanted intratibially.[24] The mouse kidney has been used for grafting prostate tissue as several groups have shown that it supports a high take rate,[13,14] possibly due to its high level of vascularization. Wang et al. obtained 94.3% engraftment of prostate cancers under the kidney capsule, compared with 58% for subcutaneous and 71.9% for the orthotopic site.[13] Of particular importance to the prostate cancer field has been the development and adoption of recombination techniques, which involve the use of subrenal capsule implantation, to improve engraftment.

Subrenal grafting is a technique used to improve prostate PDX take rate and growth rate by some laboratories. The method involves exteriorizing each kidney through a small incision in the body wall. Grafts are then carefully inserted under the kidney capsule, a transparent membrane that covers the kidney and holds the grafts in place. Up to four grafts can be placed on each kidney, depending on the size of the tissues. Grafts that are initially established on the kidney can be transferred to other sites for subsequent generations. For example, they can be regrafted subcutaneously where it is easier to perform surgery and monitor the size of tumors, or orthotopically from where some PDXs have been shown to metastasize.[25]

TABLE 2.1 Examples of Established Prostate Cancer PDXs

PDX	Tissue of Origin	Mouse Strain	Implantation Site	Take Rate (Once Established)	First Described
BM18[34]	Bone metastasis	C.B-17 SCID	subcutaneous (s.c.)	100% s.c.	2005
LuCaP23.1/ LuCaP23.12[33,a]	23.1: Lymph node metastasis	BALB/c-*nu/nu*	s.c.	100% s.c.	1996
	23.12: Liver metastasis			67% s.c.	
LuCaP35[b]	Lymph node metastasis	BALB/c-*nu/nu*	s.c.	87% s.c.	2003
LuCaP49[c]	Omental metastasis	Fox Chase C.B-17 SCID	s.c.	100% s.c.	2002
LTL-220N/LTL-220M/ LTL-221[a,d]	Prostate	NOD-SCID	Subrenal capsule	Not specified	2010
MDA PCa 118a/b[e]	Bone metastasis	C.B-17 SCID	s.c.	Not specified	2008
MDA PCa 144 lines[f]	Pelvic exenteration specimen	C.B-17 SCID	s.c.	Not specified	2010
PCSD1[g]	Bone metastasis	*Rag2*$^{-/-}$;γ c$^{-/-}$	s.c. With Matrigel	100% s.c.	2011
				67% Intrafemoral	

[a]*Additional LuCaP*[35] *and LTL*[32] *PDXs have also been previously described.*
[b]*Corey E, Quinn JE, Buhler KR, Nelson PS, Macoska JA, True LD, et al. LuCaP 35: A new model of prostate cancer progression to androgen independence.* Prostate *2003;***55***:239–46.*
[c]*True LD, Buhler K, Quinn J, Williams E, Nelson PS, Clegg N, et al. A neuroendocrine/small cell prostate carcinoma xenograft-LuCaP 49.* Am J Pathol *2002;***161***:705–15.*
[d]*Lin D, Bayani J, Wang Y, Sadar MD, Yoshimoto M, Gout PW, et al. Development of metastatic and non-metastatic tumor lines from a patient's prostate cancer specimen-identification of a small subpopulation with metastatic potential in the primary tumor.* Prostate *2010;***70***:1636–44.*
[e]*Li ZG, Mathew P, Yang J, Starbuck MW, Zurita AJ, Liu J, et al. Androgen receptor-negative human prostate cancer cells induce osteogenesis in mice through FGF9-mediated mechanisms.* J Clin Invest *2008;***118***:2697–710.*
[f]*Aparicio A, Tzelepi V, Araujo JC, Guo CC, Liang S, Troncoso P, et al. Neuroendocrine prostate cancer xenografts with large-cell and small-cell features derived from a single patient's tumor: morphological, immunohistochemical, and gene expression profiles.* Prostate *2011;***71***:846–56.*
[g]*Raheem O, Kulidjian AA, Wu C, Jeong YB, Yamaguchi T, Smith KM, et al. A novel patient-derived intra-femoral xenograft model of bone metastatic prostate cancer that recapitulates mixed osteolytic and osteoblastic lesions.* J Transl Med *2011;***9***:185.*

PDXs are being used to study the localized stage of prostate cancer for which there is a paucity of models. Yet, despite the use of highly immunodeficient mice and subrenal grafting, for specimens of localized prostate cancer, especially of low to moderate Gleason score/Epstein grade,[26] the take rates remain lower compared with more aggressive tumors. Learning from the lessons of tissue recombination, pioneered for the study of mammary and prostate gland development, it became clear that stroma could direct and maintain the differentiation of epithelia.[27,28] Signaling is conserved between the human epithelial cells and mouse stroma.[29] These studies have shown that urogenital mesenchyme directs the development of urogenital epithelium. Tissue recombination studies also showed that cancer-associated fibroblasts promote the tumorigenicity of nonmalignant prostate epithelial cells.[30] Using this background knowledge, urogenital mouse stroma is now used to provide a supporting niche to maximize the survival of the PDX (which already contains cancer-associated fibroblasts)[12,31] (Fig. 2.1A and B). The source of neonatal stroma is usually seminal vesicle mesenchyme obtained from day 0/1 BALB/c or C57/BL/6J male mice. A previous study showed that 66% of grafts of localized prostate cancer contained tumor cells when they were recombined with neonatal mesenchyme compared with 41% of grafts that were implanted alone.[31] Recombination with neonatal mesenchyme also improves the engraftment of sorted prostate cancer cells from enzymatically digested patient tissue, which rarely grow when they are grafted alone.[31]

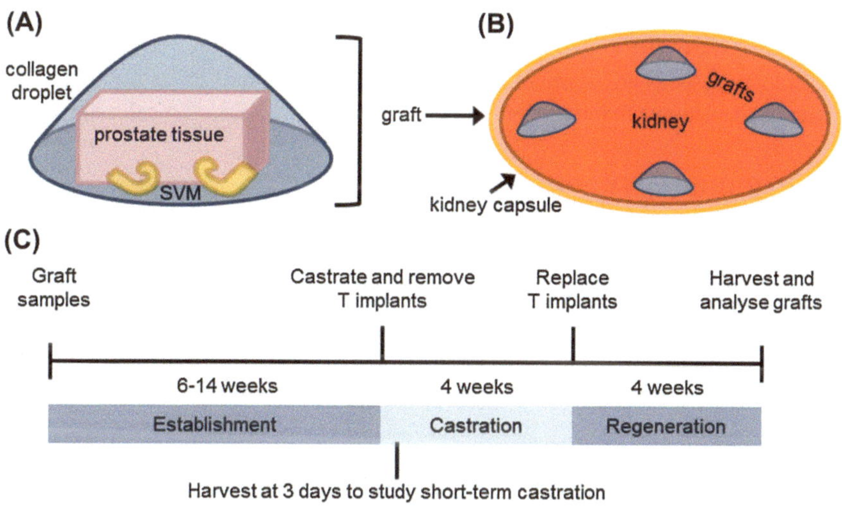

FIGURE 2.1 Overview of the protocol for primary prostate cancer xenografts. (A) Xenografts can be prepared using the tissue recombination method where a piece of prostate tissue is embedded in a gel prepared from rat tail collagen with two pieces of neonatal seminal vesicle mesenchyme (SVM). (B) Multiple recombinant grafts (~4 mm^3) can be implanted under each kidney capsule of immune-deficient host mice. (C) Typical experimental protocol to examine the androgen sensitivity of primary prostate cancer xenografts. After establishing primary xenografts, the effects of androgen deprivation can be examined using castration and testosterone regeneration experiments. *T*, testosterone.[12]

PDXs have also been used to model the advanced stages of prostate cancer. There are various sources of specimens from men with CRPC, for example, from palliative TURP, surgery, and/or rapid autopsy. Each of these specimens present their own complexity and few show good take rates, but they do afford the opportunity to widen the type and source of PDX so that the heterogeneity of disease can be fully examined. The Vancouver group has reported on a panel of prostate cancer PDXs, seven of which were established from needle biopsies from different sites of a primary tumor, to examine tumor heterogeneity;[32] it was shown that different biopsy foci recapitulated the functional heterogeneity of the donor tumors. These tumors were established in NOD/SCID mice supplemented with testosterone.[13] After 3–6 months, tumors were harvested and regrafted into NOD/SCID mice under the kidney capsules and maintained by serial transplantation under the renal capsule. Treatment by androgen withdrawal resulted in the development of CRPC.[32] There was also a recapitulation of key chromosomal alterations, gene architecture, and global gene expression of the donor tumors. Neuroendocrine transdifferentiation was seen in one of the lines postcastration; the similarity of gene expression to neuroendocrine prostate cancers with upregulation of neuronal transcription factors, membrane ion channels receptors, and secreted peptides suggested the evolution of the adenocarcinoma as an adaptive response to androgen withdrawal.

Collection of tissues for PDX from metastatic sites (including lymph nodes and bone) has also been described. These are not easily grown, but several groups have been successful (Table 2.1)[23,24]. Given the propensity of prostate cancer to induce significant bone formation at skeletal metastatic sites, this is a highly sought after property of these PDX. LuCaP23.1[33] and BM18[34] display this phenotype when grown in an osseous environment and thus provide useful models to test novel preclinical interventions that may control this currently intractable clinical issue.

TUMOR BIOLOGY

Metastasis from subcutaneous PDX occurs very infrequently. Following orthotopic implantation, lymph node and lung metastasis have been observed in some models (such as LuCaP23.8, LuCaP35).[35] Incorporation of surgical removal of the primary tumor into the protocol enabled additional time for growth and revealed macroscopic metastasis at both of these sites in the majority of mice in this study. A shortfall in modeling advanced prostate cancer is that PDXs rarely metastasize spontaneously to the bone, even after orthotopic implantation, and if this happens, osteoblastic lesions are not seen, or are not reproducible.[30] To provide a model system to study new therapeutics, bone metastases are "induced" by the use of intracardiac, intravenous, or intratibial injections.[24,34]

PDX models can be divided into two main groups: primary PDX and serially transplantable PDX. There are pros and cons to each model. Primary PDXs are fresh pieces of patient tissue implanted into host mice for one generation, typically 6–14 weeks,[12–14] during which time they can be used for preclinical testing.[36] These primary PDXs can also be transferred into new host mice and some will form serially transplantable xenografts over multiple generations. The major benefit of primary PDXs is their high take rate during the first generation. However, since each specimen is analyzed after a single generation, primary PDX platforms require ongoing sources of patient tissue. In contrast, serially transplantable PDXs provide a continuous source of each tumor specimen, so they can be used for multiple experiments and even shared between laboratories. Unfortunately, only a subset of patient samples have been successfully regrafted for multiple generations. Therefore, one way to maximize the use of tumor tissue, particular for rare patient specimens, is to simultaneously establish grafts for primary PDXs and serially transplantable PDXs. This ensures that a small preclinical study can still be performed with the primary PDX if it fails to survive as serially transplantable PDX.

Importantly, PDXs that are recombined with neonatal mesenchyme recapitulate the histopathological and genomic features of the original tumor specimens.[12,31,36–39] Therefore, notwithstanding the extra effort that is required to recombine PDX with neonatal mesenchyme, it is a useful variation of the protocol for primary grafts of localized prostate cancer specimens which may otherwise be difficult to grow.

Similarly, serially transplantable xenografts have been repeatedly shown to maintain the histopathological and molecular features of the patient donor tumor. For example, the LTL series of PDXs[32] have been shown to preserve the histopathology, including the type of differentiation shown in the donor tumor, along with marker status (eg, expression of *TMPRESS-EFG*, loss of *PTEN* among others) and androgen receptor status. Indeed, only minimal changes were observed in gross genome copy number when early- and late-generation PDXs were compared.

PRECLINICAL/CLINICAL APPLICATIONS

Both primary and established PDXs have been used to model localized castrate-sensitive disease. For example, Risbridger et al. (2015) investigated the characteristics of familial prostate cancer by establishing primary PDXs from radical prostatectomy specimens of patients with pathological germline *BRCA2* mutations, a group of patients known to have poor outcomes.[37] A prominent feature of these PDXs was intraductal cancer of the prostate (IDC-P), an underreported form of prostate cancer that grows within prostatic ducts. This observation prompted a pathology review of the incidence of IDC-P in archived patient specimens, which showed that IDC-P is associated with dramatically decreased overall survival in *BRCA2* carriers with prostate cancer. This study demonstrated the utility and clinical relevance of primary PDXs for studying localized prostate cancer.

PDXs have also been used to examine the response of localized prostate cancer to common clinical therapies. For example, primary PDXs have been subjected to ionizing radiation to model radiation therapy.[40] These experiments showed that prostate cancer cells were more sensitive to radiation than benign cells in control PDXs. In addition, several laboratories have modeled primary androgen deprivation therapy by castrating host mice and removing their testosterone implants (Fig. 2.1C).[13,15,36,41,42] These studies have shown that a subset of prostate cancer cells evade castration and persist in both primary and established PDXs. It is believed that the residual "castrate-tolerant" prostate cancer cells identified in PDXs may subsequently evolve into CRPC and are, therefore, a potential therapeutic target.[43]

It has been shown that the efficacy of treatment of PDX using taxotere, a standard treatment for advanced prostate cancer, differs when used on subcutaneous tumors compared with tumors grown in the bone[44] indicating the need to test treatments for bony metastases in appropriate models.[24]

Studies using a transplantable xenograft of small cell carcinoma of the prostate[16] showed that the neuroendocrine tumors responded to cisplatin therapy, an approach now used in the clinic to treat these types of tumors.

FUTURE/CHALLENGES

The absence of the optimal tumor microenvironment in supporting take rate and model fidelity and the use of immunocompromised rodents as recipients of human tumor grafts are the key limitations of the PDX approach. This is also the case for other types of PDX tumors and is summarized in a 2015 review[45] highlighting the limited inclusion of stromal or immune drivers of malignant progression of other solid tumors. Other limitations include the absence of significant links between the immune system and the skeletal system in cell development, intercellular communication, and signaling, along with effects of an intact immune system on tumor cell growth and spread, none of which can be assessed comprehensively in most PDX models.[46–49] Attempts to overcome this problem include the development of humanized mice; for example, NSG mice, which are commonly used for preparing PDX, lack human-specific cytokines as well as human leukocyte antigen (HLA) expression on stromal cells needed for human cell development and positive selection of T cells, respectively.[50,51] A new strain, NSG-HLA-A2/HHD with homozygous expression of HLA heavy and light chains, injected neonatally with human stem cells has resulted in the establishment of functional HLA-restricted T cells,[52] which might allow engraftment of hematopoietic stem cells to facilitate modeling of bony metastases from prostate and other cancers.[53,54]

Over 80% of novel drug candidates fail to prove their efficacy when tested in humans, or to obtain approval for clinical usage by the US Food and Drug Administration despite positive testing in animal studies.[55] The requirements for good modeling of prostate cancer are described elsewhere, including the need for the appropriate microenvironment.[56] However, these preclinical models may still not fully recapitulate the physiological or pathological processes in humans. It has been suggested that this problem could potentially be overcome by using more humanized models by cotransplanting human immune cells as well as human cancer tissues into appropriately developed mouse strains, to create a "human" niche.[57] Potential methods have been summarized by Holzapfel et al. (2015). The humanized mice better support the ability of PDX to metastasize to bone, and the presence of human immune cells (and hence an immune response) in PDX-bearing mice may allow the efficacy of new therapeutic strategies obtained to more accurately mimic patient responses.

CONCLUSION

Primary PDX have been proved to be very useful for modeling localized prostate cancer and have provided findings that have affected clinical management. Serially transplantable PDXs have been used to model more advanced disease and can be shared between different laboratories to allow new pathway analysis and preclinical studies. There is, however, a need to continue to add to the existing repertoire of PDX, particularly as new treatment regimens come into practice. The use of second- and third-line targeted therapies (including enzalu tamide and abiraterone) result in the emergence of new mechanisms of treatment resistance as the tumors evade these androgen-targeted therapies. Even the variation in the location of the metastases is evolving with the brain and major visceral organs becoming more prevalent metastatic sites in patients treated with abiraterone and enzalutamide, along with an increased incidence of neuroendocrine prostate tumors. Altogether, PDX representing the spectrum of clinical presentations will provide the field with the opportunity to comprehensively define inter- and intrapatient molecular and cellular heterogeneity. The potential use of more humanized mouse models may improve the accuracy for predicting the therapeutic efficacy of novel agents in patients with prostate cancer. The further development and refinement of PDX models will provide understanding and identification of metastatic pathways, new therapeutic targets, and potentially, personalized cancer therapy.

ACKNOWLEDGMENTS

PJR and EDW are supported in part by funding from the Australian Government Department of Health and the Movember Foundation and Prostate Cancer Foundation of Australia through a Movember Revolutionary Team Award.

RAT is supported by an EJ Whitten Fellowship from the Victorian Cancer Agency.

MGL is supported by fellowships from the National Health and Medical Research Council (1035721) and Prostate Cancer Foundation of Australia (Movember Young Investigator Grant).

GPR is supported by a fellowship from the National Health and Medical Research Council (1102752). The Monash Prostate Cancer Research Group is supported by the Peter and Lyndy White Foundation.

REFERENCES

1. Ferlay J, Soerjomataram I, Ervik M, Dikshit R, Eser S, Mathers C, et al. Globocan 2012 v1.0, cancer incidence and mortality worldwide: IARC CancerBase No. 11 [Internet]. *Int Agency Res Cancer* 2013. Available from: http://globocan.iarc.fr. [cited 21/01/2016].
2. Wong YN, Ferraldeschi R, Attard G, de Bono J. Evolution of androgen receptor targeted therapy for advanced prostate cancer. *Nat Rev Clin Oncol* 2014;**11**:365–76.

3. Greasley R, Khabazhaitajer M, Rosario DJ. A profile of enzalutamide for the treatment of advanced castration resistant prostate cancer. *Cancer Manag Res* 2015;**7**:153–64.
4. Mateo J, Carreira S, Sandhu S, Miranda S, Mossop H, Perez-Lopez R, et al. DNA-repair defects and olaparib in metastatic prostate cancer. *N Engl J Med* 2015;**373**:1697–708.
5. Saad F, Fizazi KS. Androgen deprivation therapy and secondary hormone therapy in the management of hormone-sensitive and castration-resistant prostate cancer. *Urology* 2015;**86**: 852–61.
6. Saad F, Miller K. Current and emerging immunotherapies for castration-resistant prostate cancer. *Urology* 2015;**85**:976–86.
7. Berges RR, Vukanovic J, Epstein JI, CarMichel M, Cisek L, Johnson DE, et al. Implication of cell kinetic changes during the progression of human prostatic cancer. *Clin Cancer Res* 1995;**1**:473–80.
8. Mundy GR. Metastasis to bone: causes, consequences and therapeutic opportunities. *Nat Rev Cancer* 2002;**2**:584–93.
9. Roodman GD. Mechanisms of bone metastasis. *N Engl J Med* 2004;**350**:1655–64.
10. Holzapfel BM, Thibaudeau L, Hesami P, Taubenberger A, Holzapfel NP, Mayer-Wagner S, et al. Humanised xenograft models of bone metastasis revisited: novel insights into species-specific mechanisms of cancer cell osteotropism. *Cancer Metastasis Rev* 2013;**32**:129–45.
11. Rosol TJ, Tannehill-Gregg SH, LeRoy BE, Mandl S, Contag CH. Animal models of bone metastasis. *Cancer* 2003;**97**:748–57.
12. Lawrence MG, Taylor RA, Toivanen R, Pedersen J, Norden S, Pook DW, et al. A preclinical xenograft model of prostate cancer using human tumors. *Nat Protoc* 2013;**8**:836–48.
13. Wang Y, Revelo MP, Sudilovsky D, Cao M, Chen WG, Goetz L, et al. Development and characterization of efficient xenograft models for benign and malignant human prostate tissue. *Prostate* 2005;**64**:149–59.
14. Priolo C, Agostini M, Vena N, Ligon AH, Fiorentino M, Shin E, et al. Establishment and genomic characterization of mouse xenografts of human primary prostate tumors. *Am J Pathol* 2010;**176**:1901–13.
15. Zhao H, Nolley R, Chen Z, Peehl DM. Tissue slice grafts: an in vivo model of human prostate androgen signaling. *Am J Pathol* 2010;**177**:229–39.
16. Russell PJ, Russell P, Rudduck C, Tse BW, Williams ED, Raghavan D. Establishing prostate cancer patient derived xenografts: lessons learned from older studies. *Prostate* 2015;**75**: 628–36.
17. Bosma GC, Custer RP, Bosma MJ. A severe combined immunodeficiency mutation in the mouse. *Nature* 1983;**301**:527–30.
18. Greiner DL, Hesselton RA, Shultz LD. Scid mouse models of human stem cell engraftment. *Stem Cells* 1998;**16**:166–77.
19. Shultz LD, Schweitzer PA, Christianson SW, Gott B, Schweitzer IB, Tennent B, et al. Multiple defects in innate and adaptive immunologic function in NOD/LtSz-scid mice. *J Immunol* 1995;**154**:180–91.
20. Prochazka M, Gaskins HR, Shultz LD, Leiter EH. The nonobese diabetic scid mouse: model for spontaneous thymomagenesis associated with immunodeficiency. *Proc Natl Acad Sci USA* 1992;**89**:3290–4.
21. Meyerrose TE, Herrbrich P, Hess DA, Nolta JA. Immune-deficient mouse models for analysis of human stem cells. *Biotechniques* 2003;**35**:1262–72.
22. Shultz LD, Lyons BL, Burzenski LM, Gott B, Chen X, Chaleff S, et al. Human lymphoid and myeloid cell development in NOD/LtSz-scid IL2R gamma null mice engrafted with mobilized human hemopoietic stem cells. *J Immunol* 2005;**174**:6477–89.

23. Nguyen HM, Corey E. Methodology to investigate androgen-sensitive and castration-resistant human prostate cancer xenografts in preclinical setting. *Methods Mol Biol* 2011;**776**:295–312.
24. Saar M, Korbel C, Linxweiler J, Jung V, Kamradt J, Hasenfus A, et al. Orthotopic tumorgrafts in nude mice: a new method to study human prostate cancer. *Prostate* 2015;**75**:1526–37.
25. Wang Y, Xue H, Cutz JC, Bayani J, Mawji NR, Chen WG, et al. An orthotopic metastatic prostate cancer model in scid mice via grafting of a transplantable human prostate tumor line. *Lab Invest* 2005;**85**:1392–404.
26. Egevad L, Srigley JR, Delahunt B. International society of urological pathology (ISUP) consensus conference on handling and staging of radical prostatectomy specimens: rationale and organization. *Mod Pathol* 2011;**24**:1–5.
27. Cunha GR. Tissue recombination techniques for mouse embryonic mammary glands. *J Mammary Gland Biol Neoplasia* 2013;**18**:221–5.
28. Donjacour AA, Cunha GR. Induction of prostatic morphology and secretion in urothelium by seminal vesicle mesenchyme. *Development* 1995;**121**:2199–207.
29. Taylor RA, Cowin PA, Cunha GR, Pera M, Trounson AO, Pedersen J, et al. Formation of human prostate tissue from embryonic stem cells. *Nat Methods* 2006;**3**:179–81.
30. Olumi AF, Grossfeld GD, Hayward SW, Carroll PR, Tlsty TD, Cunha GR. Carcinoma-associated fibroblasts direct tumor progression of initiated human prostatic epithelium. *Cancer Res* 1999;**59**:5002–11.
31. Toivanen R, Berman DM, Wang H, Pedersen J, Frydenberg M, Meeker AK, et al. Brief report: a bioassay to identify primary human prostate cancer repopulating cells. *Stem Cells* 2011;**29**:1310–4.
32. Lin D, Wyatt AW, Xue H, Wang Y, Dong X, Haegert A, et al. High fidelity patient-derived xenografts for accelerating prostate cancer discovery and drug development. *Cancer Res* 2014;**74**:1272–83.
33. Corey E, Quinn JE, Bladou F, Brown LG, Roudier MP, Brown JM, et al. Establishment and characterization of osseous prostate cancer models: intra-tibial injection of human prostate cancer cells. *Prostate* 2002;**52**:20–33.
34. McCulloch DR, Opeskin K, Thompson EW, Williams ED. BM18: a novel androgen-dependent human prostate cancer xenograft model derived from a bone metastasis. *Prostate* 2005;**65**:35–43.
35. Corey E, Vessella R. Xenograft models of human prostate cancer. In: Chung LK, Isaacs W, Simons J, editors. *Prostate cancer*. Contemporary Cancer Research: Humana Press; 2007. p. 3–31.
36. Toivanen R, Frydenberg M, Murphy D, Pedersen J, Ryan A, Pook D, et al. A preclinical xenograft model identifies castration-tolerant cancer-repopulating cells in localized prostate tumors. *Sci Transl Med* 2013;**5**:187–271.
37. Risbridger GP, Taylor RA, Clouston D, Sliwinski A, Thorne H, Hunter S, et al. Patient-derived xenografts reveal that intraductal carcinoma of the prostate is a prominent pathology in BRCA2 mutation carriers with prostate cancer and correlates with poor prognosis. *Eur Urol* 2015;**67**:496–503.
38. Toivanen R, Taylor RA, Pook DW, Ellem SJ, Risbridger GP. Breaking through a roadblock in prostate cancer research: an update on human model systems. *J Steroid Biochem Mol Biol* 2012;**131**:122–31.
39. Lawrence MG, Pook DW, Wang H, Porter LH, Frydenberg M, Kourambas J, et al. Establishment of primary patient-derived xenografts of palliative TURP specimens to study castrate-resistant prostate cancer. *Prostate* 2015;**75**:1475–83.
40. Af Hallstrom TM, Zhao H, Tian J, Rantanen V, Reese SW, Nolley R, et al. A tissue graft model of DNA damage response in the normal and malignant human prostate. *J Urol* 2014;**191**:842–9.

41. Germann M, Wetterwald A, Guzman-Ramirez N, van der Pluijm G, Culig Z, Cecchini MG, et al. Stem-like cells with luminal progenitor phenotype survive castration in human prostate cancer. *Stem Cells* 2012;**30**:1076–86.
42. Zhao H, Thong A, Nolley R, Reese SW, Santos J, Ingels A, et al. Patient-derived tissue slice grafts accurately depict response of high-risk primary prostate cancer to androgen deprivation therapy. *J Transl Med* 2013;**11**:199.
43. Risbridger G, Taylor R. Castrate-tolerant cells: what are the implications for the treatment of localized prostate cancer? *Asian J Androl* 2013;**15**:708.
44. Brubaker KD, Brown LG, Vessella RL, Corey E. Administration of zoledronic acid enhances the effects of docetaxel on growth of prostate cancer in the bone environment. *BMC Cancer* 2006;**6**:15.
45. Cassidy JW, Caldas C, Bruna A. Maintaining tumor heterogeneity in patient-derived tumor xenografts. *Cancer Res* 2015;**75**:2963–8.
46. Rho J, Takami M, Choi Y. Osteoimmunology: interactions of the immune and skeletal systems. *Mol Cells* 2004;**17**:1–9.
47. Richmond A, Su Y. Mouse xenograft models vs GEM models for human cancer therapeutics. *Dis Model Mech* 2008;**1**:78–82.
48. Siegel PM, Massague J. Cytostatic and apoptotic actions of TGF-beta in homeostasis and cancer. *Nat Rev Cancer* 2003;**3**:807–21.
49. Takayanagi H, Ogasawara K, Hida S, Chiba T, Murata S, Sato K, et al. T-cell-mediated regulation of osteoclastogenesis by signalling cross-talk between RANKL and IFN-gamma. *Nature* 2000;**408**:600–5.
50. Ito R, Takahashi T, Katano I, Ito M. Current advances in humanized mouse models. *Cell Mol Immunol* 2012;**9**:208–14.
51. Shultz LD, Ishikawa F, Greiner DL. Humanized mice in translational biomedical research. *Nat Rev Immunol* 2007;**7**:118–30.
52. Shultz LD, Saito Y, Najima Y, Tanaka S, Ochi T, Tomizawa M, et al. Generation of functional human t-cell subsets with HLA-restricted immune responses in HLA class I expressing NOD/SCID/IL2r gamma(null) humanized mice. *Proc Natl Acad Sci USA* 2010;**107**:13022–7.
53. Holzapfel BM, Hutmacher DW, Nowlan B, Barbier V, Thibaudeau L, Theodoropoulos C, et al. Tissue engineered humanized bone supports human hematopoiesis in vivo. *Biomaterials* 2015;**61**:103–14.
54. Holzapfel BM, Wagner F, Loessner D, Holzapfel NP, Thibaudeau L, Crawford R, et al. Species-specific homing mechanisms of human prostate cancer metastasis in tissue engineered bone. *Biomaterials* 2014;**35**:4108–15.
55. Gutman S, Kessler LG. The US Food and Drug Administration perspective on cancer biomarker development. *Nat Rev Cancer* 2006;**6**:565–71.
56. Lin D, Xue H, Wang Y, Wu R, Watahiki A, Dong X,et al. Next generation patient-derived prostate cancer xenograft models. *Asian J Androl* 2014;**16**:407–12.
57. Holzapfel BM, Wagner F, Thibaudeau L, Levesque JP, Hutmacher DW. Concise review: humanized models of tumor immunology in the 21st century: convergence of cancer research and tissue engineering. *Stem Cells* 2015;**33**:1696–704.

Chapter 3

Patient-Derived Xenograft Model of Pancreatic Cancer

M.V. Rios Perez[1,2], J.B. Fleming[1]
[1]The University of Texas MD Anderson Cancer Center, Houston, TX, United States; [2]University of Puerto Rico, San Juan, PR, United States

BACKGROUND AND SIGNIFICANCE

Pancreatic cancer carries a poor prognosis in the majority of patients. This is in part due to the lack of screening tests that could allow an earlier discovery and earlier intervention, which results in advanced stages upon presentation. A patient's tumor is staged according to imaging characteristics as potentially resectable, borderline resectable, and locally advanced or metastatic, and management is followed according to this classification.[4] Neoadjuvant treatment is practiced by several cancer institutions; however, evidence to support this intervention as the standard-of-care is still lacking. Patients with resectable tumors have a better chance of cure from the disease, but tumor recurrence locally or distally is frequently observed. Patients with locally advanced disease lack specific standardized interventions, and unfortunately are enrolled in clinical trials along with patients who have metastasis, which leaves the former group understudied as a separate entity. Patients with metastatic disease are offered two standard-of-care therapies: FOLFIRINOX (a combination of 5-fluorouracil, leucovorin, irinotecan and oxaliplatin) or gemcitabine plus Abraxane, both of which have shown a survival advantage when compared with gemcitabine alone.[5,6] The role of radiotherapy as a single therapy or concurrently with chemotherapy (chemoradiation) is under study. It has been incorporated on a case-by-case basis using a multidisciplinary approach.[1,7] Pancreatic cancer tumors exhibit chemoresistance to the available regimens, even to the standard of care, for which novel therapeutic approaches are warranted. Pancreatic tumor biology (ie, heterogeneity, metabolism, stromal composition, hypoxic environment) may be a strong contributor to chemoresistance, which is best studied using animal models in the preclinical setting.

Defining features of pancreatic adenocarcinoma include a very high rate of activating mutations in KRAS (>90%), progression from distinct types of

Patient Derived Tumor Xenograft Models. http://dx.doi.org/10.1016/B978-0-12-804010-2.00017-5

precursor lesions, a propensity for both local invasion and distant metastasis, an extensive stromal (desmoplastic) reaction as part of the tumor microenvironment, reprogramming of cellular metabolism, and evasion of tumor immunity. This chapter will review the many advantages of PDX as a scaffold for the study of human pancreatic ductal adenocarcinoma (PDAC) and will help researchers to direct efforts toward overcoming the limitations encountered in this model.[1]

Patient-derived xenograft tumors provide an expansion of the surgically resected human malignancy by using the mouse as an intermediary host. The study of tissue obtained from PDX has an important role in understanding both the cancer cell and stroma, the latter being a PDAC-defining characteristic contributing to hypoxia, hypovascularization, and metabolic reprogramming.[1] Development of xenograft tissue banks and their molecular characterization has demonstrated the stability of this model over consecutive generations and its feasibility for clinical translation.[2,8–10]

METHODOLOGY AND MODELS

Tissue Collection and Processing

Pancreas xenografts are established from patients either diagnosed with or suspected to have pancreatic cancer, who undergo potentially curative resection with or without preoperative neoadjuvant treatment (chemotherapy with or without radiation). Xenografts can also be established from patients who undergo diagnostic laparoscopy for staging purposes. The establishment of a tissue bank of pancreatic cancer xenografts allows the study of not only the primary tumor but also the metastasis (ie, liver, bone, lung, ascites, lymph nodes, and peritoneal), which is the most common pathologic presentation of PDAC. Xenografts can be harvested and repassaged in mice to expand the sample or for additional studies. Criteria for the length of time to harvest tissue for passage into more recipient mice is variable and has been based on tumor size or time end points within the range of 1.2–1.5 cm in diameter and up to 3–10.5 months postimplantation for the first generation, respectively.[2,9] For drug testing during in vivo experiments, treatment protocols typically start when the subcutaneous (SQ) tumor reaches a volume of 200 mm^3.[2]

Mouse Strain

The most commonly used immunodeficient mice for xenotransplantation are athymic (nude), NOD/severe combined immunodeficient (SCID), and NOD/SCIDγc null (ie, NSG, NOG) mice. Differences in mouse host are the degrees of immunosuppression, which theoretically correlates with engraftment success. The most immunodeficient strains (ie, NSG, NOG) are often selected as engraftment hosts under the assumption that higher tumor take rates are potentially achieved by using these strains; however, this phenomenon was not observed by Damhofer et al. who used primary and liver metastasis of pancreatic cancer.[15]

Another disadvantage of using highly immunodeficient mouse strains beside the higher cost is that they are more susceptible to infections from environmental contaminants, such as *Corynebacterium bovis*, and strain-related diseases, such as lymphoma, which cause morbidity and mortality, leading to premature death and/or loss of the entire tumor case. The use of NOD/SCID and nude mice has led to acceptable success rates as reported in Table 3.1. A cost-effective recommendation to establish PDX tissue bank of pancreas cancer is to use NOD/SCID for the first murine generation (F1) and nude mice (less expensive) for subsequent generations (>F1). The use of NOG mice has been shown to be useful in the establishment of xenografts; however, lymphoproliferative lesions occurred in 47% of the cases, leading to failure of PDX establishment.[16] On the other hand, the NOG strain has been successfully used for the study of metastasis from cell line implantation (indirect xenograft).[8,18]

Implantation Site

Between 2008 and 2015, MD Anderson's pancreas cancer xenograft program has established approximately 120 out of 180 attempted cases, which represents a 67% engraftment rate, currently the largest tissue bank reported in the literature for this malignancy. It should be noted that an improvement in technique has led to an additional 17% increased success rate since the previous report published in 2012 by Kim et al. for the same research group.[11–13] Success of engraftment for primary pancreatic adenocarcinoma (resected or biopsy derived) is comparable between heterotopic SQ and orthotopic implantation site, 50–80% and 79%, respectively, the latter being understudied due to its labor-intensive requirements.[2] Table 3.1 summarizes a selection of preclinical studies performed to study and characterize this model in the primary and metastatic setting. Fu et al. reported the highest success rate of engraftment (100%) with a selection of five cases implanted orthotopically from undisclosed resection site (primary or metastatic).[14] There are more recent reports by Reyes et al. and Damhofer et al., which include the establishment of metastatic pancreatic cancer xenografts.[12,15] Overall, the engraftment rate for other solid organ malignancies varies depending on the implantation site: breast cancer 13% (SQ) vs 3–27% (orthotopic), non–small cell lung cancer 25% (SQ) vs 90% (renal capsule), and squamous cell carcinoma of the head and neck 85% (SQ, using NSG mice) vs 54% (SQ and oral cavity).[2] One exception is colorectal cancer, which shows similar engraftment rates among variable implantation sites: 64–87% (SQ) vs 89.1% (orthotopic). Pancreatic cancer xenografts have been shown to reconstitute the original tumor not only histologically but also genetically through up to 39 passages, which is advantageous for "murine trials" such as the one described by Rubio-Viqueira et al. using targeted therapy with CI-1040 (ERK inhibitor), temsirolimus (mTOR inhibitor), and erlotinib (EGFR inhibitor), compared with cytotoxic gemcitabine.[13] Similarly, Garrido-Laguna et al. described the use of chemonaive tumors from resected primary pancreatic adenocarcinomas, and

TABLE 3.1 Selection of Preclinical and Translational Models of PDXs of Pancreatic Cancer

Study	*N*	Tumor Origin	Histology	Mice	Implant Site	Success Rate	Engraftment Time (week)	Molecular Annotation	Concordance with Patient	Preclinical or Translational Relevance
Kim et al.[9]	24	Primary	PAC	NOD/ SCID	SQ, Pancreas	50% (12/24)	42	RT-PCR on 9, IHC	Histology recapitulated	Treated tumors had a 2-fold reduction in TGFβ-R2 and a >5-fold increase in IGFBP3 mRNA expression.
Mattie et al.[10]	12	Primary	PAC	ICR SCID	SQ (all), pancreas (3)	67% (8/12)	<12	Gene expression profiling (STR, miRNA, CNV analysis), mutational analysis (SNP)/ whole exome sequencing	Overall genetic stability over passages (up to 39); consistent mutations on KRAS, TP53, KIT, and ATM; SMAD4 and CDKN2 deletion, MYC amplification	Additional *ADME* gene variants identified that could regulate drug metabolism and transport
Garrido-Laguna et al.[11]	69	Primary	PAC	Nude	SQ(all), pancreas (1)	61% (42/69)	NR	Microarray gene expression, IHC	SMAD 4 deletion associated with a more aggressive phenotype (higher rate of engraftment); tumor engraftment is related to a significantly worse patient survival (p=.006)	PDX treatment with gemcitabine corresponds with the one observed with patients in the metastatic setting (n=7) Gemcitabine-resistant tumors exhibited an upregulation of stromal pathway genes Gemcitabine-sensitive tumors showed activated cell cycle and pyrimidine pathways

Reyes et al.[12]	16	Primary (11) Liver Met. (3) Lymph node metastasis (1) Peritoneal metastasis (1)	PAC	Nude	SQ and Pancreas (8), Pancreas only (8)	63% (10/16)	Up to 40	Mutation analysis (PCR)	Dissemination pattern (lymph node or peritoneal metastasis, ascites, or hematogenous seeding)	Genetic stability in orthotopic model; however, KRAS and p53 gene mutations can occur mainly during late disease phase in mouse
Rubio-Viqueira et al.[13]	14	Primary	PAC	Nude	SQ	80%	30.4 ± 18.4 (average)	Mutation analysis, IHC, TMA, Western blot, RT- PCR	Maintain original genotype features and tumor heterogeneity	F3 generation tumor cohorts can be used for drug screening [CI-1040 (ERK inhibitor), temsirolimus (mTOR inhibitor), erlotinib (EGFR inhibitor), and gemcitabine] and biomarker discovery
Fu et al.[14]	5	NR[a]	PAC	Nude	Pancreas	100% (5/5)	NR	IHC	80% (4/5) of the tumors had lymph node and organ metastasis	Similar expression of human tumor–associated antigens (CEA, TAG-72)
Damhofer et al.[15]	38	Primary (7) Liver Met. (5)	PAC	NSG	SQ	32% (12/38)	36	IHC, real-time PCR, flow cytometry, and Hedgehog reporter assay of derived cell lines	Immunohistological and biochemical preservation with original tumor	Matching cell lines derived from xenografts were used for in vitro manipulation for the study of paracrine signaling

Continued

TABLE 3.1 Selection of Preclinical and Translational Models of PDXs of Pancreatic Cancer—cont'd

Study	*N*	Tumor Origin	Histology	Mice	Implant Site	Success Rate	Engraftment Time (week)	Molecular Annotation	Concordance with Patient	Preclinical or Translational Relevance
Chijiwa et al.[16]	19	Primary (16) Lymph node Met. (3)	PDAC (18) Anaplastic (1%)	NOG		53% (10/19)	NR	IHC, RT-PCR	Preservation of histology and genetic alterations LPL described in 47%	LPL associated with EBV infection Proposed personalized cancer therapy
Perez-Torras et al.[17]	14	Primary	PAC	Nude	Pancreas	79% (11/14)	38	TMA, Western blot, IHC, genomic DNA sequencing	Original histology preservation and maintenance of protein expression patterns over passages; similar metastatic pattern (1) peritoneal, (2) mesenteric nodes, (3) liver, (4) lung	Profiling of mucin and cytokeratin markers (ductal differentiation) in concordance with primary tumors strengthens this model MUC1 and MUC4 associated with tumor progression were present in 100% and 80%, respectively, whereas MUC2, associated with a tumor suppressor role only in 20%

ADME, absorption, distribution, metabolism, excretion; *CEA*, carcinoembryonic antigen; *CNV*, copy number variation analysis; *EBV*, Epstein-Barr virus; *ICR SCID*, imprinting control region–severe combined immunodeficient; *IGFB3*, insulinlike growth factor-binding protein-3; *IHC*, immunohistochemistry; *LPL*, lymphoproliferative lesions; *Met.*, metastasis; *miRNA*, microRNA; *NR*, not reported; *PAC*, pancreatic adenocarcinoma; *RT-PCR*, reverse transcription PCR; *SNP*, single nucleotide polymorphism; *STR*, short tandem repeats; *TAG-72*, tumor-associated glycoprotein 72; *TGFβ-R2*, transforming growth factor-β receptor type 2; *TMA*, tissue microarray.
[a]*Pancreatic cancer surgical specimens; unknown if primary or metastatic.*

compared the responses to adjuvant gemcitabine between mouse (PDX) and human, finding matching responses for only seven patients, due to the overall poor response to gemcitabine monotherapy in the metastatic setting.[11]

Engraft Time and Success Rate

Success rate is the engraftment rate or the formation of tumor after implantation from patient's tissue. It is determined by tumors grown divided by tumors implanted in mice. Some studies report success rate or engraftment rate by using a different criteria, such as the presence of the following factors: first-generation growth, greater than 80% tumor take rate at third generation with less than 12 weeks growth rate, stable growth kinetics, and regrowth of the cryopreserved tumor fragment.[10] In some studies, models were passaged beyond the third generation if necessary to reach stable growth kinetics.[10] For the first generation, it has been reported that palpable (approximately 3 mm in size) SQ tumors occur between 4 and 30 weeks postimplantation (average 14 weeks), with a faster tumor formation (less than 10 weeks) in subsequent generations.[8] This information is useful to define failure of tumor engraftment as the absence of tumor growth over a period of 30 weeks postimplantation for the first generation, and 10 weeks for subsequent generations. Following the first mouse generation, the engraftment time is decreased by about a third for the same tumor case, reported by Kim et al. as a 27–30% increase in tumor formation following the first generation.[8] A decision can then be made to terminate and reattempt if cryopreserved tissue is available, which will lower the expenses associated with mice housing.

Engraft Technique

Technical advancements in xenograft mouse surgery have been developed which enhance engraftment success such as the use of matrigel during implantation of xenografts from cell lines.[8,19] Matrigel assists engraftment by providing extracellular matrix proteins (laminin, collagen IV, heparin sulfate, proteoglycans, and entactin) as well as growth factors (transforming growth factor-β, fibroblast growth factor, and tissue plasminogen activator).[8,13,19] Different techniques have been used successfully, including use of different numbers of tumor fragments (1–10), use of different routes of delivery (surgically implanted fragment vs injection of cell suspension), and use of different sites of implantations (heterotopic vs orthotopic).[8,16] Another technical advancement is the use of staples for skin closure. The experience using staples has been superior to the use of suture due a decreased frequency of wound dehiscence, which could cause early postoperative mouse morbidity and mortality. In addition, staple removal by 7–10 days following surgery leads to earlier and easier identification of SQ tumor compared with conventional sutures, due to increased SQ inflammation associated with suture material. These interventions improve mouse survival and allow accurate documentation of the tumor formation time, which has been shown to be important in surveillance for recurrence of disease in patients who underwent curative resection for PDAC.[3]

Two models of xenografting have been described: direct and indirect.[8] Development of an indirect xenograft model is done by manipulation of the tissue which allows cell lines to be derived and transfected with luciferase, resulting in easier tracing of tumor formation in orthotopic models of pancreatic cancer. The most common and cost-effective modality to measure tumor progression is by establishing an SQ model that allows the researcher to construct growth curves by plotting weekly or biweekly tumor size measurements expressed as area or volume. The indirect use of tumor grafts to generate orthotopic and heterotopic mouse models of pancreatic cancer has been reported extensively.[8,15,20] Disease burden and progression can be quantified by tumor bioluminescence imaging, captured by optical imaging after a luciferin fluorophore is injected intraperitoneally in each mouse. Image can be further obtained by using IVIS200 or IVIS Lumina, which allow whole mouse imaging and quantification of luminescence in radiance. Use of orthotopic models of pancreatic cancer allows the detection of metastatic disease as early as five weeks following implantation. Among the pitfalls of this model is the presence of peritoneal leak associated with the cell suspension injection, and not from the natural progression of the disease, which could mislead experimental results. Necropsy findings play an important role for the recording of both primary and metastatic diseases. Similar models using cell lines derived from PDX continue to be developed and show more aggressive and invasive potential than previously established cell lines (ie, MiaPaCa-2).[12,15]

Tumor Biology

Xenografts have been shown to have a direct impact on patient care through the establishment of positive prognostic factors and biomarkers predictive of response, both of which can guide neoadjuvant treatment. Some studies validate the stability of stromal collagen over the first three generations, and show two subsets of PDXs: high and low stromal component.[5] Other studies have shown the relevance of stromal protein lumican (proteoglycan) as a relevant molecular marker that is stable through generations of the same tumor but variable among patient tumors.[21] The presence of lumican has been correlated with prolonged survival in surgically resected PDACs.[21] The study of tumor xenografts allows the researcher to confirm at a tissue level carcinogenesis mechanisms proven at the level of the cell line, and to further relate molecular tumorigenic pathways to patient outcomes. A molecular marker found to predict response to therapy is carboxylesterase 2 (CES2), which has been shown to predict response to Irinotecan and FOLFIRINOX in the neoadjuvant setting using in vitro testing of tumor xenografts from surgically resected PDACs.[22]

Among factors that negatively impact tumor engraftment in PDAC is neoadjuvant treatment.[9] It has been shown that neoadjuvant treatment significantly decreases the engraftment frequency when compared with untreated patients: 33% vs 80%, respectively.[9] This was shown to be related to a twofold decrease in transforming growth factor-β receptor type 2 and a fivefold increase in insulinlike growth factor-binding protein-3 expression among seven treated tumor xenografts when compared with five untreated cases.[9] This phenomena was exhibited with higher frequency in those who underwent preoperative treatment when compared with those untreated (17 vs 2 patients, respectively).[9] One important limitation discussed in this study was the presence of selection bias due to patient cases that were excluded after pathological examination due to inadequate size and/or indiscernible appearance.[9] The establishment of a pancreatic cancer xenograft program allows researchers to study the role of neoadjuvant therapy and mechanisms of resistance for those cases that successfully engraft.[9] Conclusions made from studying PDXs may carry a selection bias important to disclose at the time of experimental results discussion, which could be related to positive pathological response. It will be important to work on the development of methods that could enhance engraftment of those who underwent neoadjuvant treatment to have conclusions more representative of the patients who have an early diagnosis of PDAC and undergo surgical resection with a curative intent.

Ultimately, characterization of xenografts is important to understand the therapeutic challenges such as stromal barrier to drug delivery, tumor metabolomics and mechanism of tumorigenesis, and therapeutic resistance. Characterization of tumor grafts can be accomplished by describing the desmoplastic reaction and stromal composition (ie, collagen staining), determination of the mutation status, and characterization of other histological and genetic factors that could be relevant in tumorigenesis. Determining the frequency of genetic mutations that drive PDAC including KRAS, SMAD4 (DPC4), p16 (CDKN2A), p53, and GNAS, could enhance the development of targeted therapy, which could be validated with both ex vivo and in vivo testing.

Preclinical Applications

Even though it is unlikely that indirect use of PDXs for establishment of cell lines will have a direct impact on the donor patient with pancreatic cancer, it has been an excellent platform to study pancreatic cancer cell biology through in vitro testing of up- or downregulated pathways, genetic mutations, proteomics, metabolomics, migration, invasion, and epithelial and mesenchymal markers, among other tumor characteristics.[20] The use of cell lines derived from PDXs for heterotopic and orthotopic mouse models of pancreatic cancer has been extensively used to show treatment response; however, consensus for a definition of progression vs disease response using these models remains to be established.

Direct xenografts offer certain advantages compared with genetically engineered mouse models (GEMMs) of pancreatic cancer. They not only preserve histological and stromal features comparable with the human tumor of origin but also maintain relevant inter- and intratumor heterogeneity.[9,15] Tumor heterogeneity may decrease rates for tumor engraftment and therefore needs to be taken into consideration when designing a study, since failure of engraftment could lead to an underpowered study. This limitation is overcome by meticulous documentation of engraftment success for each generation and tumor case, the design of larger mouse study groups, and individual mouse monitoring followed by exclusion of those that exhibited tumor regression or failure of engraftment. These measures will ensure reproducibility of experimental results.

Due to the lack of manipulation of the direct heterotopic PDX model from the patient to the mice, these models have several advantages including tumor expansion, preserved human histologic features, stroma-cancer cell interaction, genetic and molecular profiling, rapid in vivo drug testing, and multiplicity of its use indirectly. Among the disadvantages of this model are the limited role of the immune system, lack of understanding of precursor lesions (PanIN), selection bias during tissue collection, differences in mouse host and clonal selection, limited role of tumor microenvironment, and nearly absent metastatic occurrence (heterotopic model). To overcome some of these limitations (tumor microenvironment and metastatic burden) orthotopic immunodeficient mouse models of pancreatic cancer have been developed by using human-derived cell lines, and digested tumor.[8] In contrast with PDXs, GEMM offers the advantage of an immunocompetent host that could help us understand the role of the immune system in tumorigenesis; however, there is little known about the resemblance of mouse tumor biology to that of humans.[23] Some claim to have developed models that resemble human invasive PDAC by using mouse liver metastatic cell lines derived from $KRAS^{G12D/+}$, $Trp53^{R172H/+}$, and Pdx-1-Cre mice.[24] PDX offers a broader understanding of the genetic pool and the heterogeneity that characterizes pancreatic cancer. Moreover, the spontaneous GEMM are time-consuming and require breeding and genotyping efforts for a long time to have the desired set of mutations (ie, KRAS, p53) in a significant group of mice. Nevertheless, it is relevant to mention that the study of carcinogenesis (driving mutations) and preinvasive stages (PanIN) may be better understood with GEMM than with PDXs.

Promising data have been generated by studies such as that by Torphy et al. using subcutaneously implanted PDX (single case) in NOD/SCID mice to demonstrate the treatment effect of BKM120 (PI3K inhibitor) vs vehicle on levels of circulating tumor cell (CTC) quantification, in addition to the conventional tumor volume measurements.[26] In this study a microfluidic chip was used to capture CTC from small volumes of blood collected on day 0 posttreatment and a larger blood volume collected from cardiac puncture at the end of the experiment, on day 28 posttreatment.[26] Results showed not only that CTC can be successfully quantified in tumor-bearing mice when compared with non–tumor-bearing mice with statistical significance but also that both CTC counts and tumor volumes significantly decreased after PI3K inhibitor treatment for the particular tumor case under study, proposing the use of CTC quantification as a reliable indicator of treatment response.[26] More experiments using a similar experimental approach, but a larger number of tumor graft cases, may lead to important conclusions in terms of tumor phenotypes and epithelial to mesenchymal changes.

FUTURE AND CHALLENGES

The majority of patients diagnosed with PDAC are unresectable due to advanced stage of disease at the time of presentation. Metastatic disease is understudied in PDX models. Efforts to establish a liver metastatic model using NOD/SCID and NOG mice via splenic injection followed by splenectomy have been described.[18,25] Patient-derived orthotopic xenograft is a more direct method with the least manipulation. It is a model derived from traditional PDXs that will theoretically maintain tumor microenvironment as well as metastatic pattern that will most resemble the human tumor pathophysiology. This technique requires greater surgical skill and is labor intensive, and has therefore been used less frequently compared with heterotopic methods. However, this approach is worth exploring for the development of more physiologic metastatic models as well as for the study of antimetastatic agents. Transabdominal examination for orthotopic tumors have been described at 12 weeks postimplantation; exploratory laparotomy is another alternative described but is extremely invasive and not feasible for large group animal experiments.[8]

Understanding the stromal composition and the metabolomics of the hypoxic environment under which these tumors grow could help enhance drug delivery. Therefore, characterization of tumor grafts of pancreatic adenocarcinoma requires additional multidisciplinary efforts to understand tumor–stroma interactions and tumor microenvironment metabolism that allows progression of disease even after treatment with therapies that are available today.

ACKNOWLEDGMENTS

This project was supported by T32 NIH research grant T32CA009599 (MV R.P.), Dr. Fleming's laboratory funds including Viragh Family Foundation.

REFERENCES

1. Ryan DP, Hong TS, Bardeesy N. Pancreatic adenocarcinoma. *N Engl J Med* 2014;**371**:1039–49.
2. Hidalgo M, Amant F, Biankin AV, Budinská E, Byrne AT, Caldas C, et al. Patient-derived xenograft models: an emerging platform for translational cancer research. *Cancer Discov* 2014;**4**(9):998–1013.
3. Thomas RM, Truty MJ, Kim M, Kang Y, Zhang R, Chatterjee D, et al. The canary in the coal mine: the growth of patient-derived tumorgrafts in mice predicts clinical recurrence after surgical resection of pancreatic ductal adenocarcinoma. *Ann Surg Oncol* 2015;**22**(6):1884–92.

4. Evans DB. Resectable pancreatic cancer: the role for neoadjuvant/preoperative therapy. *HPB* 2006;**8**:365–8.
5. Conroy T, Desseigne F, Ychou M, et al. Groupe Tumeurs Digestives of Unicancer, PRODIGE Intergroup: FOLFIRINOX versus gemcitabine for metastatic pancreatic cancer. *N Engl J Med* 2011;**364**:1817–25. http://dx.doi.org/10.1056/NEJMoa1011923.
6. Von Hoff DD, Ervin T, Arena FP, et al. Increased survival in pancreatic cancer with nab-paclitaxel plus gemcitabine. *N Engl J Med* 2013;**369**:1691–703. http://dx.doi.org/10.1056/NEJMoa1304369.
7. Rios Perez MV, Dai B, Koay EJ, et al. Regression of stage IV pancreatic cancer to curative surgery and introduction of a novel ex-vivo chemosensitivity assay. *Cureus* 2015;**7**(12):e423. http://dx.doi.org/10.7759/cureus.423.
8. Kim MP, Evans DB, Wang H, Abbruzzese JL, Fleming JB, Gallick GE. Generation of orthotopic and heterotopic human pancreatic cancer xenografts in immunodeficient mice. *Nat Protoc* 2009;**4**(11):1670–80.
9. Kim MP, Truty MJ, Choi W, Kang Y, Chopin-Lally X, Gallick GE, et al. Molecular profiling of direct xenograft tumors established from human pancreatic adenocarcinoma after neoadjuvant therapy. *Ann Surg Oncol* 2012;**19**(Suppl. 3):S395–403.
10. Mattie M, Christensen A, Chang MS, Yeh W, Said S, Shostak Y, et al. Molecular characterization of patient-derived human pancreatic tumor xenograft models for preclinical and translational development of cancer therapeutics. *Neoplasia* 2013;**15**(10):1138–50.
11. Garrido-Laguna I, Uson M, Rajeshkumar NV, Tan AC, de Oliveira E, Karikari C, et al. Tumor engraftment in nude mice and enrichment in stroma-related gene pathways predict poor survival and resistance to gemcitabine in patients with pancreatic cancer. *Clin Cancer Res* 2011;**17**:5793–800.
12. Reyes G, Villanueva A, Garcia C, Sancho FJ, Piulats J, Lluis F, et al. Orthotopic xenografts of human pancreatic carcinomas acquire genetic aberrations during dissemination in nude mice. *Cancer Res* 1996;**56**:5713–9.
13. Rubio-Viqueira B, Jimeno A, Cusatis G, Zhang X, Iacobuzio-Donahue C, Karikari C, et al. An in vivo platform for translational drug development in pancreatic cancer. *Clin Cancer Res* 2006;**12**:4652–61.
14. Fu X, Guadagni F, Hoffman RM. A metastatic nude-mouse model of human pancreatic cancer constructed orthotopically with histologically intact patient specimens. *Proc Natl Acad Sci USA* 1992;**89**:5645–9.
15. Damhofer H, Ebbing EA, Steins A, Welling L, Tol JA, Krishnadath KK, et al. Establishment of patient-derived xenograft models and cell lines for malignancies of the upper gastrointestinal tract. *J Transl Med* 2015;**11**(4):113–5.
16. Chijiwa T, Kawai K, Noguchi A, et al. Establishment of patient-derived cancer xenografts in immunodeficient NOG mice. *Int J Oncol* 2015;**47**(1):61–70. http://dx.doi.org/10.3892/ijo.2015.2997.
17. Pérez-Torras S, Vidal-Pla A, Miquel R, et al. Characterization of human pancreatic orthotopic tumor xenografts suitable for drug screening. *Cell Oncol (Dordr)* 2011;**34**(6):511–21. http://dx.doi.org/10.1007/s13402-011-0049-1.
18. Suemizu H, Monnai M, Ohnishi K, Ito M, Tamaoki N, Nakamura M. Identification of a key molecular regulator of liver metastasis in human pancreatic carcinoma using a novel quantitative model of metastasis in NOD/SCID/γc null (NOG) mice. *Int J Oncol* 2007;**31**:741–51. http://dx.doi.org/10.3892/ijo.31.4.741.
19. Mullen P. The use of Matrigel to facilitate the establishment of human cancer cell lines as xenografts. *Methods Mol Med* 2004;**88**:287–92.

20. Kang Y, Zhang R, Suzuki R, Li SQ, Roife D, Truty MJ, et al. Two-dimensional culture of human pancreatic adenocarcinoma cells results in an irreversible transition from epithelial to mesenchymal phenotype. *Lab Invest* 2015;**95**(2):207–22.
21. Xinqun L, Truty MA, Kang Y, Chopin-Laly X, Zhang R, Roife D, et al. Extracellular lumican inhibits pancreatic cancer cell growth and is associated with prolonged survival after surgery. *Clin Cancer Res* 2014;**20**(24):6529–40.
22. Capello M, Lee M, Wang H, Babel I, Katz MH, Fleming JB, et al. Carboxylesterase 2 as a determinant of response to irinotecan and neoadjuvant FOLFIRINOX therapy in pancreatic ductal adenocarcinoma. *JNCI J Natl Cancer Inst* 2015;**8**:107.
23. Westphalen CB, Olive KP. Genetically engineered mouse models of pancreatic cancer. *Cancer J* 2012;**18**:502–10.
24. Tseng WW, et al. Development of an orthotopic model of invasive pancreatic cancer in an immunocompetent murine host. *Clin Cancer Res* 2010;**16**(14):3684–95.
25. Han H, Grippo P, editors. *Drug discovery in pancreatic cancer models and techniques*. New York: ©Springer; 2010. p. 51–68.
26. Torphy RJ, Tignanelli CJ, Kamande JW, et al. Circulating tumor cells as a biomarker of response to treatment in patient-derived xenograft mouse models of pancreatic adenocarcinoma. *PLoS ONE* 2014;**9**(2):e89474. http://dx.doi.org/10.1371/journal.pone.0089474.

Chapter 4

Modeling Breast Cancer Heterogeneity With Patient-Derived Xenografts

K.W. Evans, N. Paez-Arango, A. Akcakanat, E. Yuca, F. Meric-Bernstam
The University of Texas MD Anderson Cancer Center, Houston, TX, United States

BACKGROUND

Approximately 40,000 women die of breast cancer in the United States every year. Although the overall 5-year survival rate has steadily increased over the past 25 years, metastatic disease still remains incurable. In addition, 10–15% of women diagnosed with breast cancer have a specific type called triple negative (TNBC).[1] Unlike other subtypes, there are no treatment options for these patients if their tumors did not respond to standard cytotoxic agents. Thus, the mortality rate remains higher for these patients.

Breast cancer is known for its pathological and biological heterogeneity, with substantial differences in histology, genetics, and sensitivity to chemo- and targeted therapies. Thus, to improve therapeutics and advance patient selection for current and emerging therapeutics, it is imperative to model the heterogeneity for both identifying broader therapeutics and identifying subgroup-specific therapies.

Established cell lines are used routinely to study breast cancer; they are easy to grow and manipulate and are ideal for examining the intracellular molecular mechanisms of tumor biology. However, they do not represent breast cancer heterogeneity, and there is limited to no clinical information available from the originating patients. On the other hand, genetically modified and spontaneous mouse models of breast cancer have the potential for mimicking the tumor environment and tumor evolution in the innate immune system; however, costs and time have limited the diversity and use of these models. Moreover, their utility is limited by divergent genetics and the questionable ability of forced genetic modifications to mimic spontaneous oncogenic events in some cases. For these reasons, a need has emerged for a heterogeneous patient-based model system that could help identify new therapeutic targets, allow to test sensitivity, and potentially guide the choice of therapy. Patient-derived xenografts (PDXs) model the heterogeneity of breast

Patient Derived Tumor Xenograft Models. http://dx.doi.org/10.1016/B978-0-12-804010-2.00018-7

cancer and have been shown to maintain molecular and phenotypic traits similar to the originating tumor. PDXs are finding synergy with the other models systems, especially fulfilling needs in broader preclinical testing. In this chapter, we review techniques for generating breast cancer PDXs and discuss their current and future uses in assessing therapeutic potentials and identifying predictive biomarkers.

METHODOLOGY AND MODELS

Tumor Source

Breast cancer PDXs are most often developed from solid tumor pieces obtained following surgical resection of primary tumors or local recurrences or affected axillary lymph nodes.[2–6] However, PDXs of the local disease have also been developed from needle biopsies. PDXs have been established from both tumors treated and untreated with neoadjuvant systemic therapies, and some reports have suggested that treatment with neoadjuvant therapy increases the likelihood of engraftment.[7] However, it is plausible that this correlation is not due to therapy-related phenotypic changes, but rather at least in part due to the characteristics of the patients selected to undergo neoadjuvant therapy or inherent inability to collect viable tumor from patients who respond to neoadjuvant therapy.

Breast cancer PDXs have also been developed from distant metastases. Biopsies of cutaneous metastasis and surgically resected metastatic tissues from other sites (eg, brain) have both been successfully engrafted.[2,6] Along with solid metastatic specimens, cells isolated from pleural effusions have been used to generate PDXs.[2–4] The cells are collected from the fluid by centrifugation and injected into mice using a small volume ($<50\,\mu L$). Interestingly, some reports suggest that pleural effusions are an effective means to derive estrogen receptor–positive PDXs,[2,3] which has proven difficult with primary tumors.

Implantation Techniques

Breast cancer PDXs have been generated in athymic nude, NOD-SCID, or NSG mice. There have been limited direct comparisons of receptiveness of strains, but cell line evidence suggests that NSG mice are more receptive to tumor development.[8,9]

Breast cancer PDXs are initiated either orthotopically in the mammary fat pad(s) or heterotopically in subcutaneous space on the mid-dorsal flank(s) of immature female mice. Orthotopic implantation is performed by making a 0.5- to 1.0-cm incision to expose the mammary fat pad—most commonly the inguinal fat pad—and generating a small pocket with a blunt forceps and inserting a small tumor fragment. Alternatively, a suspension of tumor cells is injected into the exposed fat tissue.[2,3,5,6] The cell suspensions are sometimes mixed with tumor fragments coated by Matrigel, an organic substance, prior to implantation. The immature mouse mammary ducts are sometimes surgically removed from the fat pad prior to tumor implantation.

Orthotopic implantation may also be completed following "humanization" of the mouse mammary fat pad. Humanization was originally employed for the establishment of structured human mammary glands in mice.[11] Immature mouse mammary glands are surgically removed and replaced with irradiated and unirradiated immortalized human mammary fibroblasts. Several weeks later, suspensions of human mammary epithelial cells are inoculated into the "humanized" fat pad. The human fibroblasts are thought to provide autologous growth factors and extracellular proteins required for the behavior of the human cells. Heterotopic implantation is typically done by making a small incision on the dorsal flank of the mouse and using blunt forceps to make a pocket down the flank.[7] A tumor fragment is then inserted into the pocket and the wound sealed by suture or metal clips.

The rates of engraftment for orthotopic and heterotopic implants appear to be comparable, but no systematic studies have been performed that illustrate clear advantages or disadvantages between these techniques. Since tumor characteristics can clearly influence the take rate, direct comparisons of techniques with the same tumors would be needed to accurately define the best method in terms of efficiency. Zhang et al. found that humanizing cleared fat pads resulted in a lower take rate in SCID/beige mice.[2] They also found that the take rate was similar between SCID/beige and NSG mice, suggesting that the decreased immunity of NSG mice may not be necessary.[2] Li et al. compared the injection of cell suspensions into humanized fat pads to direct implantation of tumor fragments into unhumanized fat pads. They found that direct implantation had better or equivalent rates of engraftment for primary and metastatic breast tumors. There have been no direct or indirect comparisons of the probability for de novo molecular alterations arising during engraftment. Moreover, such a comparison would require a very large sample size due to the inherit variability in PDX samples and relative molecular stability seen with all techniques. Several comprehensive reviews of engraftment rates with the various techniques have been published,[10,12] and Table 4.1 outlines some relevant studies.

Sample Processing

For surgical specimens and core biopsies, the specimens are commonly cut into small fragments (1–3 mm by 1–8 mm) prior to implantation.[2–4,6,7,13] For single-cell injection of solid tumor specimens, tumors are first dissociated into isolated or small groups of cells by enzymatic and/or mechanical means.[5] The tumors are collected using aseptic conditions and transported in biologic-free media supplemented with antibiotics to a local implantation site. There has been some success in other tumor types with extended transportation times between tumor removal and implantation,[14] but the effectiveness of breast cancer engraftment following extended offsite transportation is unknown.

In the case of tumor cell suspensions, specific subpopulations of the breast cancer cells have been shown to be more adept at generating PDXs. Al-Hajj et al.

TABLE 4.1 Summary of Select Publications Describing Independent Breast Cancer PDXs Collections

References	*N*	Sample Source	Subtype	Strain	Implant Site	Engraft Rate	Molecular Annotation	Concordance with Patient Tumor	Preclinical or Clinical Application
DeRose et al.[3]	42	Primary tumor resections, ascites, pleural fluids	HR+, HER2+, TNBC[a]	NOD SCID	Mammary fat pad[b]	37%	Microarray	HR/HER2 expression, RNA expression, metastatic pattern, morphology	Engraftment correlated with patient survival
Zhang et al.[2]	169	Primary tumor resections, ascites, pleural fluids	HR+, HER2+, TNBC[a]	SCID/beige, NSG	Mammary fat pad[b]	~20%	Microarray, cancer- related SNPs	HR/HER2 expression, morphology	Concordance with patient treatment response
Li et al.[6]	152	Primary tumor resections, metastatic resections, and core biopsies	HR+, HER2+, TNBC[a]	NOD SCID	Mammary fat pad[b,c]	13%	Exome sequencing, RPPA, RNA-Seq	HR/HER2 expression, RNA profile, genomic alterations	Identified genomic alterations promoting hormone-independent growth in PDX/ patient
McAuliffe et al.[7]	55	Primary tumor resections	HR+, HER2+, TNBC[a]	Athymic nude	Dorsal flank	27%	Exome sequencing, RPPA	Genomic alterations	Engraftment correlated with patient survival

[a]*Engraftment rate higher for TNBC.*
[b]*Cleared fat pad.*
[c]*Direct implant.*

showed that breast cancer cells expressing a specific surface marker profile, $CD44^+/CD24^-/lineage^-$, are more efficient at generating tumors in mice compared with the parental populations or the depleted population ($CD44^-/CD24^+$).[4] In addition, $CD44^+/CD24^-$ cells retain the ability to generate tumors in serial passaging while the newly formed $CD44^-/CD24^+$ population does not. The $CD44^+/CD24^-$ cell surface profile was found to also be expressed by normal mammary stem cells, and this fact combined with the apparent hierarchical nature of these subpopulations has given rise to a large body of research linking cancer initiation and stem cells. Based on this finding, numerous marker profiles were developed that identify subpopulations, which were more effective at generating tumors in mice.[15,16] However, in the originating paper, fragment implantation was more efficient for establishing PDXs than cell injections of any subpopulation.

TUMOR BIOLOGY

Model Fidelity

Primary subtyping of breast cancer is based on histological features and expression of a small set of proteins as determined by immunohistochemistry. To date, close similarity between the histological appearance of patient tumors and the resulting PDXs has been widely reported for all techniques.[2,3,5,7]

The protein biomarkers assessed for breast cancer patients at presentation and, if possible at progression, are the hormone receptors (HRs) for estrogen [estrogen receptor (ER)] and progesterone [progesterone receptor (PR)], as well as human epidermal growth factor receptor 2 (HER2). Copy number for the HER2 gene is often also assessed due to the frequency of HER2 amplification in breast cancer patients. Since the expression of these markers dictates the treatment course for the patients, with patients with HR+ tumors receiving endocrine therapy and HER2+ patients receiving anti-HER2 therapy, the concordance of these markers in PDXs is often assessed as a measure of fidelity. The vast majority of PDXs generated to date are from ER-, PR-, and HER2- tumors. However, tumors lacking expression of these markers are more likely to engraft. Furthermore, in one study, the majority of ER+ PDXs, even though still expressing ER at messenger RNA (mRNA) and protein level, were not reliant on estrogen. In most of these PDXs, response to estrogen did not mimic the patients' responses to endocrine therapy. Moreover, only one of these seven ER+ models was derived from a patient who was responding well to endocrine therapy, and this PDX was one of seven that responded positively to estrogen. These findings suggest that HR+ PDXs may often be generated from hormone-independent tumors. Conversely, another team found that tamoxifen decreased the growth rate of ER+ PDXs ($n=3$) but not ER- PDXs ($n=1$), suggesting that ER+ PDXs retain a specific requirement for estrogen.[17] In another study, the ER+ PDXs, although expressing ER, were found to be in subtypes of cancer with gene expression more similar to ER- disease,[2] whereas two other groups found that the majority of their ER+ PDXs exhibited luminal gene expression, which is highly enriched in ER+ patient samples.[2,3]

Genomic Alterations

Several studies have compared somatic alterations in patient tumors with those in the PDXs. Using whole genome deep sequencing, Li et al. found, to a varying extent, that variant allele frequencies in PDXs generated in mammary fat pad correlated with frequencies in the matched patient tumors. They did find that some somatic mutations were unique to the primary tumors and to a greater extent the PDXs, but they also found that most of the unique mutations were in genes not often mutated in breast cancer.[6] Moreover, many of these mutated genes were not expressed as determined by RNA-Seq. McAuliffe et al., using targeted deep sequencing, found that somatic mutation frequencies in cancer-associated genes were relatively stable through 16 PDX generations with increased stability following four generations.[7] However, they did find de novo PTEN deletions in two PDXs, although tumor-associated deletion detection in PDXs may arise due to the enrichment of human tumor DNA versus human normal tissue in mice. Zhang et al. looked at 143 cancer-relevant single nucleotide polymorphisms and found stability at these sites over several PDX generations.[2] Comparative allelic frequencies of cancer-related genes are typically maintained in breast cancer PDXs[2,7]; this argues against drastic clonal evolution on engraftment. In a study in 2015, using >1000 PDXs, Gao et al. found the PDXs better represent the molecular heterogeneity of several types of cancer compared with the available cell lines for those cancers.[18]

Gene Expression

Several studies have compared protein expression between patient tumors and their matched PDX utilizing reverse phase protein arrays (RPPA), which analyze >150 proteins and phosphoproteins, or RNA expression microarrays. There are conflicting reports on the proteomic correlation between patient specimens and the resulting PDXs, but there is agreement that once established, PDXs maintain a unique proteomic profile over generations. Li et al. found, upon unsupervised clustering, that patient samples grouped with their specific PDXs.[6] However, another group found that, upon unsupervised clustering, all patient surgical samples clustered together away from their PDXs, but generations of same PDXs clustered together.[7] This could potentially be linked to differences in time and technique for processing surgical samples versus PDXs. The discordance may also be linked to differences in analysis technique with one team excluding stroma-related proteins, whose expression levels are potentially species specific. Numerous other studies have used mRNA and protein arrays to demonstrate that unique gene expression signatures are maintained in serial passaging of PDXs.[2,3,6,7]

Potential Clonal Evolution

While reports suggest that genomic traits are mostly maintained between patients and generations of PDXs using bulk tumors, technical advancements have enabled gene sequencing at the single cell level, thus enabling more precise analysis of PDXs versus patient. Using these technologies, clones within breast tumors have been found to evolve dynamically.[19,20] In 2015, Eirew et al. used these techniques to show that clonal selection occurs to varying degrees in the establishment and serial passaging of PDXs.[21] They utilized in vitro organoid culture prior to fat pad implantation. They first showed, with bulk tumors, that clusters of single nucleotide alterations are gained and lost during implantation and passaging to varying extents suggesting decreased and increased fitness of specific clones. Interestingly, they found that highly similar clonal changes can occur in parallel grafts of the same PDX. Next, using single cell sequencing and mapping clonal architecture, they were able to track the dynamic evolution of clones within two PDXs over multiple generations. In a similar study, Cheung et al. labeled individual cells from PDXs with unique molecular barcodes prior to engrafting into mice.[22] By determining the representation of the barcodes in proceeding generations of tumors, they found that specific clonal populations expanded to various extents, again suggesting evolution dynamics at play within the PDXs. It has yet to be determined whether clonal evolution in PDXs occurs at a different rate compared with patient tumors over time and treatment, but these findings bring to light a potential need to track the trajectory of clones when utilizing PDXs for therapy testing.

Metastatic Capability of PDXs

The metastatic potential of patient tumors has been shown to be maintained in mice.[2,3] Zhang et al. found that orthotopic PDXs from 12 of the 25 patients had the potential to metastasize to the lungs, whereas none gave rise to detectable liver metastases.[2] Not all the PDXs were generated from patient with known metastatic disease. DeRose et al. found that the majority of their orthotopic PDXs metastasized to distant organs, and the organ-specific metastatic profile of the PDXs resembled that of the patients, including a case that metastasized to the bone in both patient and PDX.[3]

Engraftment Success Linked to Poor Patient Outcome

Studies have found a correlation between patient outcome and PDX engraftment. Derose et al. found that engraftment in NOD-SCID mice correlated with patient survival, and this held true even for patients who were newly diagnosed with breast cancer at the time of PDX implant.[3] McAuliffe et al., using athymic nude mice, found that patients for whom PDX development was successful for the primary tumor had decreased overall survival and decreased time to local or distant recurrence (Fig. 4.1).[7] Tumors which progressed on neoadjuvant chemotherapy were highly likely to engraft in mice with six out seven successful engraftments from these patients.[7] These findings show that pathological characteristics are retained in mice.

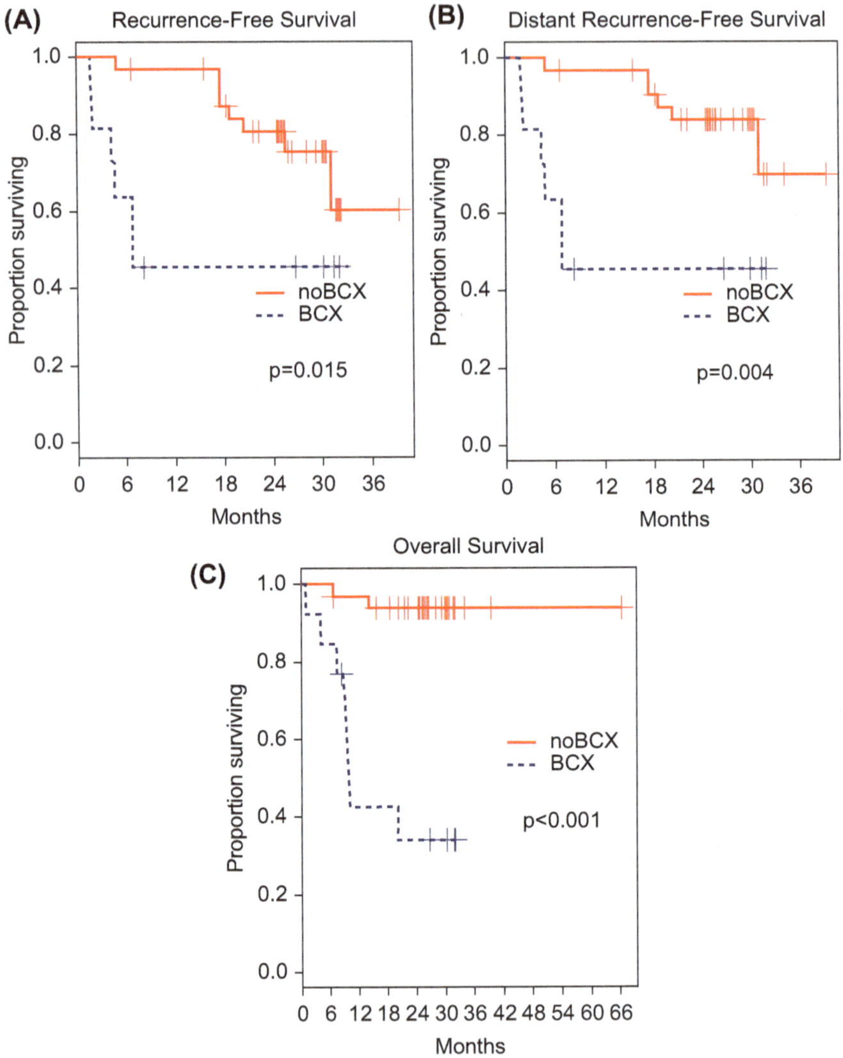

FIGURE 4.1 Successful PDX development linked to poor prognosis. Patients whose tumors developed heterotopic breast cancer xenografts (BCXs) in nude mice had a greater chance developing local (A) and distant (B) recurrence and also had decreased overall survival (C).[7]

PRECLINICAL UTILITY

Over recent years, PDX models have emerged as important tools for translational research. A study evaluated PDXs in six luminal models that all showed different sensitivities to endocrine therapy, thus exhibiting heterogeneity similar to what is observed in the clinic. They tested the sensitivity to hormonal therapies commonly used like ER modulators such as tamoxifen and fulvestrant, as well as suppression of estrogen synthesis by either letrozole or ovariectomy. They also used combined therapies and showed that those models reproduced the heterogeneity of response commonly observed in the clinical setting.[23]

PDX models can also help establish the biological mechanism for new treatments. For example, one study used experimental suppression of PTEN in a PDX model of basal-like breast cancer to show that loss of PTEN expression was sufficient to sensitize the PDX to a novel combination treatment.[24] For this study, PTEN was suppressed in PDX cells in vitro before reimplanting into mice. This approach has the benefit of maintaining an isogenic background but the disadvantage of potential selection and modifications occurring during culture, transduction, and selection.

Oakes et al. demonstrated the use of endogenous gene expression for biomarker identification. Out of five basal-like PDXs, only the three PDXs with high expression of BCL2 responded to a BCL2 inhibitor plus docetaxel.[5] Similarly, Bieniasz et al. found that two breast cancer PDXs with wild-type PIK3CA were sensitive to a Ron kinase inhibitor, whereas two PDXs with mutated PIK3CA were, to a certain degree, less sensitive to the inhibitor.[25] The power and usage of this class of biomarker studies will increase with the increasing size of PDX collections.

In a 2015 study, Gao et al. showed the utility of large PDX collection for preclinical testing. They tested 62 treatments using more than 1000 PDXs from six different cancer types, including breast, implanted to the flank of nude mice.[18] To do this efficiently, they tested only a single animal per PDX–treatment combination. Using stricter clinical response definitions similar to human trials, they found genotype–phenotype relationships suggesting the feasibility of such strategy.

CHALLENGES AND FUTURE DIRECTIONS

Accessible Sample Sources

The majority of breast cancer PDXs have been generated from specimens surgically removed from the primary site. However, breast cancer mortalities are concomitant with the spread of the disease, and genetic and phenotypic changes occur prior to and during the development of metastases. In addition, tumor traits most likely shift during therapy. Thus, PDXs from metastatic and therapy-resistant disease are a necessity. There has been a success with developing models of local disease that are resistant to standard therapy in the neoadjuvant setting, but therapy-resistant disease occurs more often in less accessible locations. Thus more accessible sample sources and alternative collection procedures are being explored.

The ability to generate PDXs from fine-needle aspirates (FNAs) would provide less invasive access to the metastatic site and make serial PDX generation possible. FNA-based PDXs would also enable development prior to neoadjuvant therapy and immediately following progression of metastatic disease. The small mass and low purity could decrease take rates, but if proven feasible, this method would potentially increase the overall number of patients/tumors that could be enrolled on PDX studies compared with surgically resected samples. The ability to generate PDXs from FNAs has been demonstrated in small cell lung cancer.[14]

Some groups have generated breast cancer PDXs utilizing tumor cells circulating in peripheral blood (CTCs). For example, using CTC isolates based on a set of cell surface markers, Zhang et al. generated tumors in mice, following expansion of the tumor cells in vitro, from three breast cancer patients with brain metastasis.[26] However, the three CTC-initiated PDXs displayed a surprising overlap in genetic alterations—all having the same BRAF, KRAS, and TP53 mutation—suggesting that they may not represent unique tumors or that certain genetic alteration in rare clones were selected for. Another group found that CTCs expressing EPCAM, CD47, CD44, and MET, isolated from patients with metastatic luminal breast cancer, were able to establish metastatic tumors in the bone of mice much more efficiently than bulk CTCs.[27] In another study, CTCs were isolated from patients using a microfluidic device. Following expansion in serum-free, nonadherent conditions, they were able to generate tumors in NSG mice from three patients.[28] In this case, the lines developed maintain the genotypic features of the patients' tumors. This technology, if it becomes more widely accessible, can greatly facilitate the ability to noninvasively create PDXs from patients with metastatic disease, and to develop PDXs with serial CTC sampling, capturing molecular changes acquired with tumor progression and selection pressures of targeted therapies.

Molecular Alterations for Target Validation

Currently, PDXs offer a unique opportunity to contrast breast cancers for biomarker studies due to the interminable number of PDXs that can be developed. However, most functional target validation is still done using cell line models due to limited success culturing PDXs or even dissociating PDXs and reimplanting. Cheung et al. were able to successfully grow and transduce PDX cells with lentivirus and reimplant into mice using three-dimensional organoid culture.[22] Two other groups have reported the generation of two-dimensional cell lines from breast cancer PDXs.[7,24] In an alternative approach to gene silencing in PDXs, Chen et al. alleviated difficulties in culturing PDX cells by injecting dissociated PDX cells along with nanoliposomes containing small interfering RNAs (siRNAs) and injecting nanoliposomes containing siRNA into the PDX at continuing intervals.[29] All these methods and others will need to be extended and fine-tuned to determine their general utility, but there is no question that the capacity to systematically alter potential targets in PDX panels would improve current target validation strategies.

Increased Efficiency of Hormone Receptor–Positive PDXs

HR+ tumors, especially from the primary site, are clearly less likely to establish in mice. Although primary ER+ tumors are considered more treatable due to the emergence of endocrine therapies, many women still die following the development of therapy-resistant metastatic disease. Therefore, it is imperative to develop robust techniques for developing PDXs of ER+ disease, especially models of acquired resistance to endocrine therapy. A key component to success appears to be estrogen supplementation, and there are several methods being used to deliver many different doses of estrogen.[12] However, it will take a significant effort to determine if this is the factor affecting the engraftment of ER+ tumors. A possibility to improve take would be to select patients who have failed endocrine therapy as these appear to potentially be more likely to engraft. ER+ PDXs that were moderately inhibited by tamoxifen were found to be sensitized to tamoxifen by combination therapy, whereas an ER- PDX was not.[17] However, the relevance of ER+ models that are no longer reliant on hormone signaling is not clearly established.

Personalized Therapy

Although histological and molecular features identify treatment-relevant groups, there are still inherent and acquired phenotypic variations within these groups. Thus an exciting potential usage of PDXs is personalized therapy testing (as Avatars), and there have been some reports of therapeutic correlation using very small cohorts of patients and mostly retrospective testing.[2,30] To be broadly successful, PDXs would have to engraft and expanded in less time than it takes for the disease to progress to an incurable state, and it has been shown that 77% of breast cancer PDXs reached first passage prior to patient progression.[7] However, several of these were from patients with early-stage disease who had no disease even after >12 months, suggesting ample occasion for significant changes to occur prior to recurrence/progression. To be truly effective, PDXs may have to be tested within the treatment decision windows following recurrence. However, it has not been determined whether primary tumor PDXs can be used for treatment planning of later progression or if it is necessary to generate later PDXs.

Regardless, the most difficult aspect may be developing comparative doses and treatment decision thresholds. Moreover, although PDXs offer the opportunity to concurrently test more than the single therapy that can be used in a patient, it is still not possible, especially from biopsies, to test an infinite number of therapies and combinations in the time often allowed. Barring drastic steps forward, the utility of PDXs in personalized testing may be in distinguishing between a few second-line treatment options. The first step in establishing this process appears to be correlating response in pretreatment biopsy-generated PDXs to response in matched patients in early trials or standard therapies (Fig. 4.2), although the utility in the time frame of neoadjuvant treatment is limited. This initial treatment-specific process would use larger cohorts of animals to

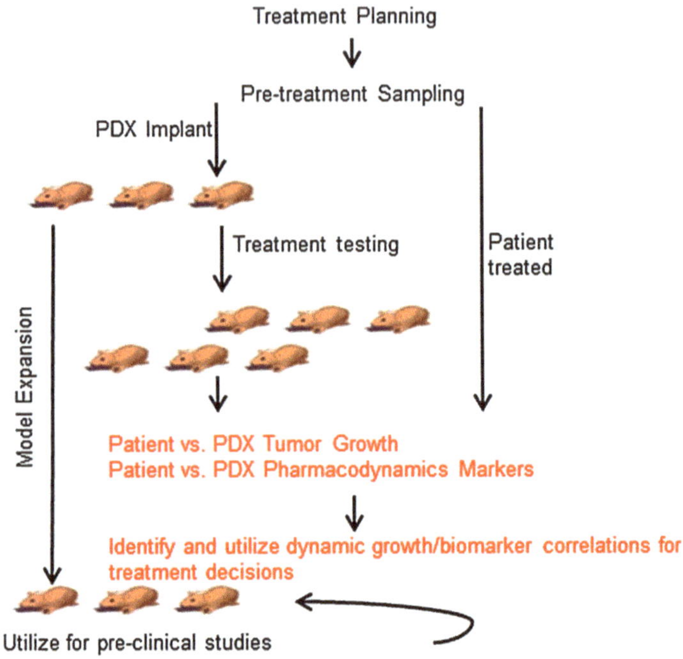

FIGURE 4.2 Utilizing PDXs for personalized medicine. To be effective as Avatars for treatment decisions, correlations must be identified between specific response criteria in mice and responses of matched patient. Subsequently, PDXs can be used to screen second-line agents or dictate earlier treatment changes as well as be used to continue improving criteria for PDX-based decisions.

clearly establish a correlation between detailed human and animal treatments and establish decision-making parameter. Once these metrics are established for a therapy, biopsies would be obtained at times of treatment decisions after recurrence or progression. Alternatively, when it is determined that the patient has significant residual disease after initial neoadjuvant therapy, patients could be treated with additional PDX-directed therapies, either in the neoadjuvant or in the adjuvant setting, after surgical resection if the tumor is operable. Once the PDX expands and any additional biomarker analysis is completed, parallel testing of next-line options can commence to the extent that PDX material is available. Then, with clear guidance from established correlations, PDX results can be made available for future decision making.

CONCLUSION

PDXs appear poised to model the genotypic and phenotypic heterogeneities of breast cancer, especially in the case of HR disease. However, their pre-/coclinical trial utility is only beginning to be established. It will take years to determine whether the use of PDX collections will translate to better therapies entering trials and/or improved patient selection for treatments, and due to the similarity in findings for the various techniques, only future clinical correlations may determine the existence of a best PDX method.

REFERENCES

1. Mo W, Liu Q, Lin CC, Dai H, Peng Y, Liang Y, et al. mTOR inhibitors suppress homologous recombination repair and synergize with PARP inhibitors via regulating SUV39H1 in BRCA-proficient triple-negative breast cancer. *Clin Cancer Res* 2015:1699–712.
2. Zhang X, Claerhout S, Prat A, Dobrolecki LE, Petrovic I, Lai Q, et al. A renewable tissue resource of phenotypically stable, biologically and ethnically diverse, patient-derived human breast cancer xenograft models. *Cancer Res* 2013;**73**(15):4885–97.
3. DeRose YS, Wang G, Lin YC, Bernard PS, Buys SS, Ebbert MT, et al. Tumor grafts derived from women with breast cancer authentically reflect tumor pathology, growth, metastasis and disease outcomes. *NatMed* 2011;**17**(11):1514–20.
4. Al-Hajj M, Wicha MS, Benito-Hernandez A, Morrison SJ, Clarke MF. Prospective identification of tumorigenic breast cancer cells. *Proc Natl Acad Sci USA* 2003;**100**(7):3983–8.
5. Oakes SR, Vaillant F, Lim E, Lee L, Breslin K, Feleppa F, et al. Sensitization of BCL-2-expressing breast tumors to chemotherapy by the BH3 mimetic ABT-737. *Proc Natl Acad Sci USA* 2012;**109**(8):2766–71.
6. Li S, Shen D, Shao J, Crowder R, Liu W, Prat A, et al. Endocrine-therapy-resistant ESR1 variants revealed by genomic characterization of breast-cancer-derived xenografts. *Cell Rep* 2013;**4**(6):1116–30.
7. McAuliffe PF, Evans KW, Akcakanat A, Chen K, Zheng X, Zhao H, et al. Ability to generate patient-derived breast cancer xenografts is enhanced in chemoresistant disease and predicts poor patient outcomes. *PLoS One* 2015;**10**(9):e0136851.
8. Dewan MZ, Terunuma H, Takada M, Tanaka Y, Abe H, Sata T, et al. Role of natural killer cells in hormone-independent rapid tumor formation and spontaneous metastasis of breast cancer cells in vivo. *Breast Cancer Res Treat* 2007;**104**(3):267–75.
9. Milsom CC, Lee CR, Hackl C, Man S, Kerbel RS. Differential post-surgical metastasis and survival in SCID, NOD-SCID and NOD-SCID-IL-2Rgamma(null) mice with parental and subline variants of human breast cancer: implications for host defense mechanisms regulating metastasis. *PLoS One* 2013;**8**(8):e71270.
10. Zhang X, Lewis MT. Establishment of patient-derived xenograft (PDX) models of human breast Cancer. *Curr Protoc Mouse Biol* 2013;**3**(1):21–9.
11. Kuperwasser C, Chavarria T, Wu M, Magrane G, Gray JW, Carey L, et al. Reconstruction of functionally normal and malignant human breast tissues in mice. *Proc Natl Acad Sci USA* 2004;**101**(14):4966–71.
12. Whittle JR, Lewis MT, Lindeman GJ, Visvader JE. Patient-derived xenograft models of breast cancer and their predictive power. *Breast Cancer Res* 2015;**17**:17.
13. Bergamaschi A, Hjortland GO, Triulzi T, Sorlie T, Johnsen H, Ree AH, et al. Molecular profiling and characterization of luminal-like and basal-like in vivo breast cancer xenograft models. *Mol Oncol* 2009;**3**(5–6):469–82.
14. Anderson WC, Boyd MB, Aguilar J, Pickell B, Laysang A, Pysz MA, et al. Initiation and characterization of small cell lung cancer patient-derived xenografts from ultrasound-guided transbronchial needle aspirates. *PLoS One* 2015;**10**(5):e0125255.
15. Ginestier C, Hur MH, Charafe-Jauffret E, Monville F, Dutcher J, Brown M, et al. ALDH1 is a marker of normal and malignant human mammary stem cells and a predictor of poor clinical outcome. *Cell Stem Cell* 2007;**1**(5):555–67.

16. Lim E, Vaillant F, Wu D, Forrest NC, Pal B, Hart AH, et al. Aberrant luminal progenitors as the candidate target population for basal tumor development in BRCA1 mutation carriers. *Nat Med* 2009;**15**(8):907–13.
17. Vaillant F, Merino D, Lee L, Breslin K, Pal B, Ritchie ME, et al. Targeting BCL-2 with the BH3 mimetic ABT-199 in estrogen receptor-positive breast cancer. *Cancer Cell* 2013;**24**(1):120–9.
18. Gao H, Korn JM, Ferretti S, Monahan JE, Wang Y, Singh M, et al. High-throughput screening using patient-derived tumor xenografts to predict clinical trial drug response. *Nat Med* 2015:1318–325.
19. Navin N, Kendall J, Troge J, Andrews P, Rodgers L, McIndoo J, et al. Tumour evolution inferred by single-cell sequencing. *Nature* 2011;**472**(7341):90–4.
20. Wang Y, Waters J, Leung ML, Unruh A, Roh W, Shi X, et al. Clonal evolution in breast cancer revealed by single nucleus genome sequencing. *Nature* 2014;**512**(7513):155–60.
21. Eirew P, Steif A, Khattra J, Ha G, Yap D, Farahani H, et al. Dynamics of genomic clones in breast cancer patient xenografts at single-cell resolution. *Nature* 2015;**518**(7539):422–6.
22. Cheung AM, Nguyen LV, Carles A, Beer P, Miller PH, Knapp DJ, et al. Analysis of the clonal growth and differentiation dynamics of primitive barcoded human cord blood cells in NSG mice. *Blood* 2013;**122**(18):3129–37.
23. Cottu P, Marangoni E, Assayag F, de CP, Vincent-Salomon A, Guyader C, et al. Modeling of response to endocrine therapy in a panel of human luminal breast cancer xenografts. *Breast Cancer Res Treat* 2012;**133**(2):595–606.
24. Xu S, Li S, Guo Z, Luo J, Ellis MJ, Ma CX. Combined targeting of mTOR and AKT is an effective strategy for basal-like breast cancer in patient-derived xenograft models. *Mol Cancer Ther* 2013;**12**(8):1665–75.
25. Bieniasz M, Radhakrishnan P, Faham N, De La OJ, Welm AL. Pre-clinical efficacy of Ron kinase inhibitors alone and in combination with PI3K inhibitors for treatment of sfRon-expressing breast cancer patient-derived xenografts. *Clin Cancer Res* 2015:5588–600.
26. Zhang L, Ridgway LD, Wetzel MD, Ngo J, Yin W, Kumar D, et al. The identification and characterization of breast cancer CTCs competent for brain metastasis. *Sci Transl Med* 2013;**5**(180):180ra48.
27. Baccelli I, Schneeweiss A, Riethdorf S, Stenzinger A, Schillert A, Vogel V, et al. Identification of a population of blood circulating tumor cells from breast cancer patients that initiates metastasis in a xenograft assay. *Nat Biotechnol* 2013;**31**(6):539–44.
28. Yu M, Bardia A, Aceto N, Bersani F, Madden MW, Donaldson MC, et al. Cancer therapy. Ex vivo culture of circulating breast tumor cells for individualized testing of drug susceptibility. *Science* 2014;**345**(6193):216–20.
29. Chen X, Iliopoulos D, Zhang Q, Tang Q, Greenblatt MB, Hatziapostolou M, et al. XBP1 promotes triple-negative breast cancer by controlling the HIF1alpha pathway. *Nature* 2014;**508**(7494):103–7.
30. Stow L, Katz A, Irie H, Port E, Stebbing J, Ciznadija D, et al. Patient-derived xenografts accurately predict patient response in breast cancer patients. *Cancer Res* 2015;**75**(9 Suppl.):Abstract nr P3-06-31.

Chapter 5

Patient-Derived Xenograft Models of Ovarian/Gynecologic Tumors

L. Liang[1,a], I. Mercado-Uribe[1,a], N. Niu[1], Y. Jiang[1,2], W. Cheng[2], J. Zhang[3], G.B. Mills[1], C. Scott[4,b], A.K. Sood[1,b], J. Liu[1,2,b]

[1]The University of Texas MD Anderson Cancer Center, Houston, TX, United States; [2]The First Affiliated Hospital of Nanjing Medical University, Nanjing, People's Republic of China; [3]Fourth Military Medical University, Xi'an, People's Republic of China; [4]Walter and Eliza Hall Institute of Medical Research and Royal Melbourne Hospital, Parkville, VIC, Australia

BACKGROUND

Ovarian cancer is the most lethal gynecological malignancy. The 5-year overall survival rate is approximately 45%.[1,2] The lack of good early screening and diagnostic tests is one of the reasons for the low overall survival rate. Most ovarian cancer patients are diagnosed at an advanced stage of the disease. Moreover, there is no good marker to predict patients' response to chemotherapy.[3]

The majority of ovarian cancers are derived from epithelial cells. The major histotypes of epithelial ovarian cancers are serous (80–85%), endometrioid (~10%), clear cell (~5%), and mucinous (~3%).[4] A two-tier grading system is currently used to classify serous carcinoma as high grade or low grade.[5] Most studies focus on high-grade serous ovarian carcinoma, which comprises approximately 90% of serous carcinoma.[3]

Recent evidence supports the idea that some high-grade serous cancers originate from the fimbriated (distal) end of the fallopian tube, instead of the ovarian surface epithelium or epithelial inclusion glands, as previously believed. In women with *BRCA1* and *BRCA2* mutations undergoing prophylactic salpingo-oophorectomy, the fallopian tube is involved in many early serous carcinomas.[6] Serous tubal intraepithelial carcinoma (STIC), the most common precursor lesion of high-grade serous carcinoma, is characterized by nuclear

a. LL, IM contributed equally to this work and should be considered as co-first authors.

b. SC, AS, JL contributed equally to this work and should be considered as co-corresponding authors.

Patient Derived Tumor Xenograft Models. http://dx.doi.org/10.1016/B978-0-12-804010-2.00019-9

atypia, increased nuclear–cytoplasmic ratio, nuclear stratification, loss of polarity, and loss of ciliated cells. STIC universally demonstrates *TP53* mutation and has a high Ki-67 proliferative index.[7] High-grade serous ovarian carcinoma is believed to develop from STIC cells in the ovary or other tissues of Müllerian origin. The tubal theory is further supported by similar gene expression profiles between STIC and high-grade serous ovarian carcinoma.[8] Furthermore, The Cancer Genome Atlas (TCGA) project has analyzed DNA copy numbers, promoter methylation, gene expression profiles, and microRNA in approximately 500 high-grade serous ovarian carcinomas.[9] TCGA data showed *TP53* mutations in approximately 96% of high-grade serous carcinomas. However, a recent reanalysis demonstrates that many of the *TP53* mutation–negative tumors in the TCGA did not fulfill characteristics for the pathological diagnosis of high-grade serous ovarian cancer with few exceptions making *TP53* mutation a sine qua non of high-grade serous ovarian cancer. However,[10] *BRCA1* and *BRCA2* mutations were identified in 22% of high-grade serous carcinomas (including both germline and somatic mutations), and *NF1*, *RB1*, and *CDK12* mutations in a small percentage of these tumors (less than 6%).[9] In addition, a high degree of genomic instability and copy number aberration were found in high-grade serous carcinoma.[9]

In contrast, low-grade serous carcinoma is generally an indolent tumor arising from serous cystadenoma and borderline tumor. Low-grade serous carcinoma frequently carries *KRAS* and *BRAF* mutations.[11] In addition, clear cell ovarian cancers frequently have *ARID1A* and *PIK3CA* mutations; endometrioid ovarian cancers frequently have *CTNNB1*, *ARID1A*, and *PIK3CA* mutations;[12,13] and mucinous ovarian cancers frequently have *KRAS* mutations.[14]

Ovarian cancer cell lines have played an essential role in studying cancer biology in vitro. However, many previously available ovarian cancer cell lines have been cultured in vitro for a long time under selection pressure and may significantly deviate from the original patient tumor in terms of genetics and biology.[15] Ince and colleagues[16] recently established novel ovarian cancer cell lines using a newly developed culture medium, which retained both the phenotype and molecular characteristics of different subtypes of human ovarian tumors.

Chemoresistance is one of the major clinical issues in ovarian cancer. No good marker is available to predict patients' response to chemotherapy. Many patients whose disease responds to chemotherapy at the beginning have recurrent tumors eventually. As chemosensitive subpopulations of tumor cells are killed by primary chemotherapy, chemoresistant subpopulations drive tumor regrowth. Recent evidence supports the theory that cancer stem-like cells are associated with chemoresistance.[17] The current treatment for advanced-stage ovarian cancer is surgery combined with either neoadjuvant or postoperative platinum- or taxane-based chemotherapy. In addition, novel therapeutics targeting the vascular endothelial growth factor (VEGF) pathway and inhibiting the enzyme poly(ADP-ribose) polymerase have also shown promising results.[18]

Novel therapeutics are being developed to eradicate chemoresistant subpopulations of tumor cells, but these need to be tested in vivo in relevant and informative tumor models.

Patient-derived xenografts (PDXs) are now among the most promising preclinical models for ovarian cancer. In this chapter, we provide an update on the status of gynecologic PDX models with a major emphasis on epithelial ovarian cancers and perspectives on their clinical use.

METHODOLOGY AND MODELS

Tissue Collection and Processing

To generate PDX models of gynecologic malignancies, human tumor cells are procured from biopsy specimens, surgical specimens, or ascitic fluid. The sources can be either primary ovarian and fallopian tumors or metastatic tumors, such as omental implants and peritoneal nodules.[19] Ovarian cancer PDXs have been generated from both therapy-naive and posttherapy tumors.[20–23]

Tissues are prepared by digestion with cell dissociation buffer, mechanical mincing, or slicing into fragments. Chemical digestion may destroy cell surface molecules and decrease the success rate of engraftment. In contrast to tissues prepared via chemical digestion, tissue fragments have a higher engraftment rate.[24] When collecting viable tumor cells from ascites, ascitic fluid is centrifuged at a low speed (eg, 500 g) to preserve cell viability.[23] The time between the collection of human tissue and its implantation into mice is important. Dobbin et al.[19] achieved a high success rate by implanting tumors into mice within 1 h of collection, which required good collaboration between different departments, including surgeons, pathologists, and researchers.

Animals

Several different kinds of immunocompromised mice have been used to develop PDX models of gynecologic malignancies, including thymus-deficient nude mice, severe combined immunodeficient (SCID) mice, and nonobese diabetic (*NOD*)-*SCID IL*-2Rγ^{null} (NSG) mice.[25] Among these host mice, the engrafted rate is lowest in nude mice and highest in NOD-SCID IL-2Rγ^{null} mice.[26,27] Therefore, NOD-SCID IL-2Rγ^{null} mice are considered the best mice to generate PDX models, but they are also the most expensive.[20]

Engraft Time and Success Rate

The engraftment of first-generation ovarian cancer PDXs usually takes 2–6 months (Table 5.1).[28,29] The engraftment time is shorter in successive generations (1–3 months).[29] Success rates for first-generation PDXs range from 25% to 80% depending on many factors, including the time between collection and implanting, type of immunocompromised mice, tumor histotypes, and

TABLE 5.1 Preclinical and Clinical Applications of Patient-Derived Xenograft Models (PDXs) of Ovarian Cancers From Literature

Study	References	*N*	Tumor Origin	Histotypes	Mice	Implant Site	Success Rate	Engraft Time	Molecular Annotation	Concordance With Patient Tumor	Preclinical or Clinical Application
1	Weroha et al.[40]	168	Ovarian, primary peritoneal, or fallopian tube, including both primary and recurrent tumors	Various	SCID	IP	74%	NA	Yes, array CGH on 41 xenografts	Similar morphology, metastatic pattern, and genomic aberrations in low-passage xenografts	Platinum response in PDX models (generated from 9 patients) correlates with patients' response to chemotherapy
2	Ricci et al.[27]	34	Primary ovarian tumors, metastasis, ascites	Various	Nude	SQ, IP, IB	25%	1–15 months (SQ); 1–4 months (IP) to reach 1 g	Yes	Similar morphology and dissemination pattern, but loss of some markers at multiple passages; altered mutation and higher gene copy number in 4 of 34 xenografts	PDXs predicted clinical response to a cisplatin-based therapy in 9 of 11 cases
3	Stewart et al.[45]	31	Solid tumor or ascites	Serous	NOD/SCID or NSG	MFP (mainly), IP, SRC, IB	NA	NA	NA	Similar morphology and immunophenotype (MFP PDXs)	Tumor-initiating cell markers were studied in PDXs
4	Dobbin et al.[19]	NA	Omental metastasis or peritoneal implant	Various	SCID	SQ (mainly), MFP, IP, SRC	85.3% (SQ), 63.6% (MFP), 22.2% (IP), 8.3% (SRC)	17–174 days (SQ), 29–129 days (MFP)	Yes, RT^2 PCR array (4 pairs)	Similar morphology, gene expression profile, except that 5 of 84 genes were downregulated in PDXs	PDXs derived from patients who completely responded to chemotherapy showed more tumor reduction; different genetic profile between treated and untreated PDXs (6 pairs)

5[a]	Xu et al.[49]	13	Both primary and recurrent tumors	Various	SCID	GFP	65%	2–6 months (1–2 cm in diameter)	NA	Similar morphology; human origin confirmed by in situ hybridization; 3 PDXs developed metastasis; 2 PDXs developed ascites	PDXs used in drug testing (IL-12, Flt-3 ligand)[50,51]
6[b]	Kolfschoten et al.[21]	12	Both therapy-naive and posttherapy recurrent tumors	Various	Nude	SQ (flank)	NA	NA	NA	Similar immunophenotype	PDXs used in drug testing (cisplatin, cyclophosphamide, doxorubicin, etc.)
7	Lee et al.[34]	11	Therapy-naive tumors	Various	NOD/SCID	SRC	>95%	30–60 days	NA	Similar morphology; > 90% concordance in immunophenotype; slightly increased Ki67 proliferation index in PDXs	NA
8	Topp et al.[26]	10	Chemo-naive tumors	Serous	NSG	SQ, IB	83%	NA	Yes, *TP53* mutation 100%; 2 *BRCA1* mutation; 3 *BRCA2* mutation; 2 *BRCA1* methylated	Similar morphology and immunophenotype	Platinum sensitivity in PDXs correlates with patients' response to treatment (10 cases)
9	Ghamande et al.[33]	6	NA	Serous	SCID	SQ, GFP	NA	~4 weeks	NA	Similar morphology	PDXs used in drug testing (CD40 ligand, cisplatin, and paclitaxel)
10	Bankert et al.[46]	5	Primary and metastatic solid tumors; ascites	4 serous, 1 NA	NSG	IP	~85%	80–177 days	NA	Similar disease progression pattern; human fibroblasts and lymphocytes retained in first-generation xenografts	NA

N indicates the number of successfully established PDXs; NA indicates not available; NSG indicates NOD-SCID IL-2Rγnull, also called NOD-SCID gamma mice.
BRCA1 and *BRCA2*, breast cancer genes 1 and 2; *CGH*, comparative genomic hybridization; *GFP*, intra-abdominal gonadal fat pad; *Hh*, hedgehog gene; *IB*, intraovarian bursa; *IP*, intraperitoneal; *LOH*, loss of heterogeneity; *MFP*, mammary fat pat; *MLPA*, multiplex ligation-dependent probe amplification; *NOD*, nonobese diabetic; *PARP*, poly(ADP-ribose) polymerase; *SRC*, subrenal capsule; *SQ*, subcutaneous.

[a]*Drug testing was published in two separate publications.*[50,51]

[b]*This study also included three cell line–derived xenograft models.*

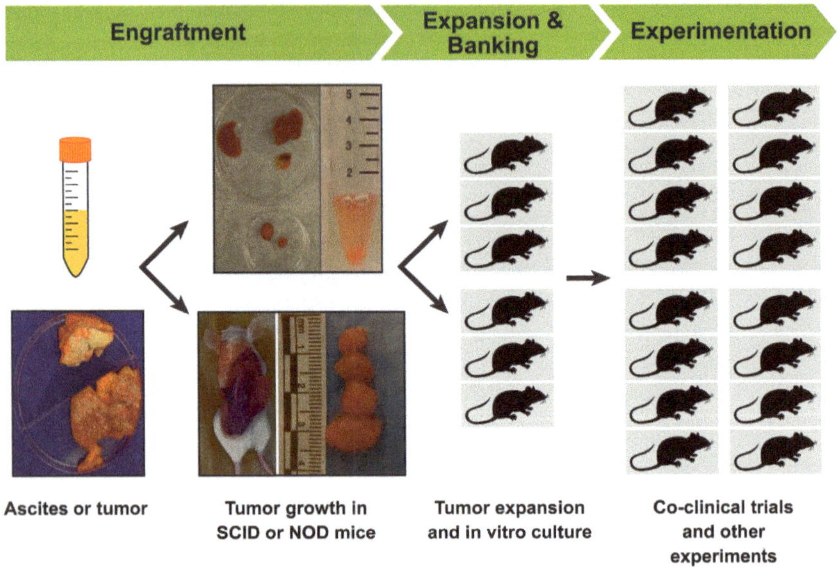

FIGURE 5.1 Schematic of ovarian PDX establishment. Fresh ascites collected from patients is centrifuged and cells are washed with phosphate-buffered saline and antibiotics. Cells are resuspended in 1:1 media and Matrigel and injected intraperitoneally into severe combined immunodeficient (SCID) or nonobese diabetic (NOD) mice (two to three mice). The mice are monitored until abdominal cavity is distended, and then euthanized, and ascites and tumor nodules are collected. Tumor nodules are cut into small pieces of 0.3–0.5 cm^2 implanted subcutaneously into a new group of mice for PDX expansion. Ascites and nodules are placed in freezing media (high content fetal bovine serum plus media and dimethyl sulfoxide) and stored frozen under liquid nitrogen conditions. In our hands, the success rate of the implant depends on the source of tumor type, being the highest from ascites, then ovary, and last omentum. The time frame from implant to expansion and banking is approximately 2–4 months. During this period or after banking commonly used cancer drug or novel therapies can be performed.

implant sites. The schematic of PDX generation is shown in Fig. 5.1. The success rate is histotype specific with a rough correlation with tumor grade: it is highest for high-grade serous carcinoma and lowest for mucinous ovarian carcinoma.[30] Even though the success rate of first-generation PDXs is variable, the success rate of successive generations is quite high (more than 75%).[20] In addition, the histology and immunoprofile of PDXs should be examined and compared with the original tumor from patients (Fig. 5.2). In high-grade serous ovarian carcinoma, we generally used three marker panels, PAX8, WT1, and p53. The first two markers confirm the Müllerian origin of high-grade serous carcinoma. Either intense nuclear positivity for p53 or complete negativity for p53 (null mutation due to deletion in the open reading frame of the gene) supports the diagnosis of high-grade serous carcinoma. Also, as with cell lines, PDXs should be routinely monitored with short tandem repeats, or similar technology to ensure that these PDXs match the original human tumor.

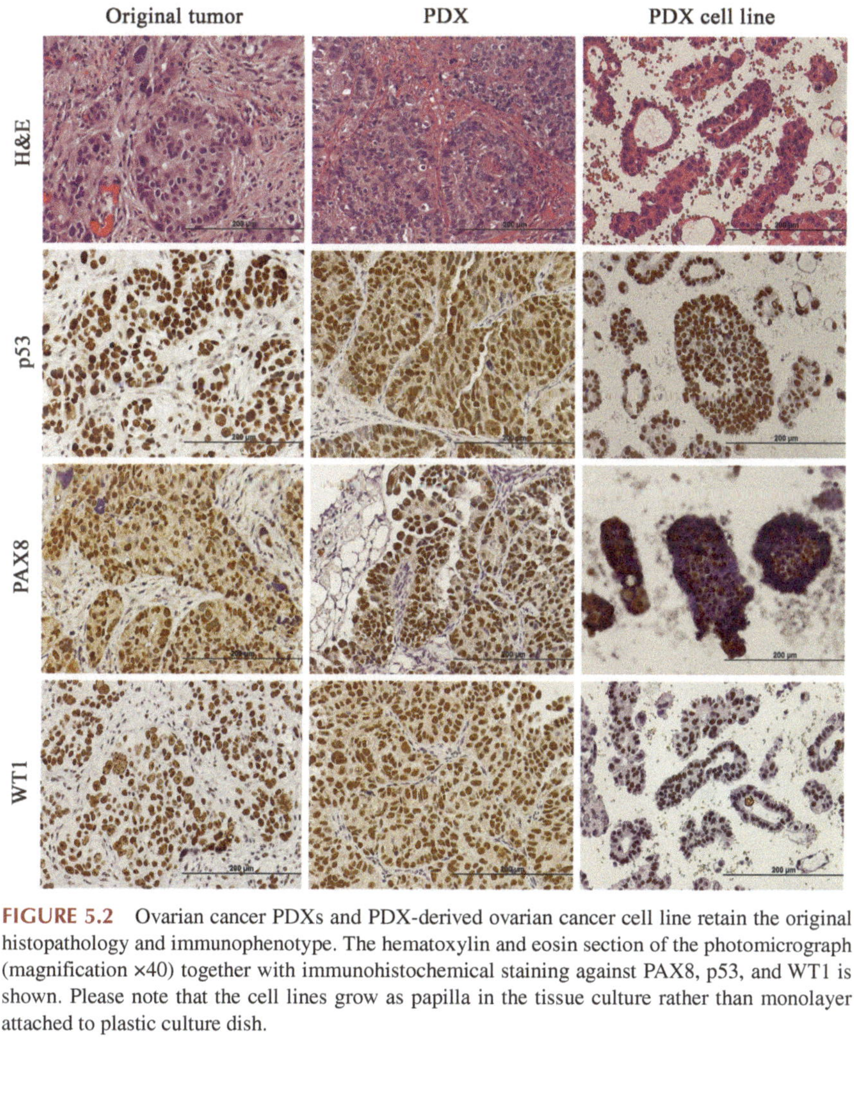

FIGURE 5.2 Ovarian cancer PDXs and PDX-derived ovarian cancer cell line retain the original histopathology and immunophenotype. The hematoxylin and eosin section of the photomicrograph (magnification ×40) together with immunohistochemical staining against PAX8, p53, and WT1 is shown. Please note that the cell lines grow as papilla in the tissue culture rather than monolayer attached to plastic culture dish.

Orthotopic Versus Heterotopic Models

To generate PDX models of ovarian cancer, fresh human tumors have been injected into different sites, including the intraovarian bursa, intraperitoneal cavity, subcutaneous tissue, gonadal fat pad, mammary fat pad, and subrenal capsule. Each implant site has its advantages and disadvantages. Intraovarian bursa implantation has been traditionally considered orthotopic;[31] however, new findings have suggested fallopian tube as the origin of ovarian cancer. The ovarian bursa is a thin membrane that encapsulates the ovary and the distal end of the fallopian tube in rodent species. Ovarian cancer cells can be injected

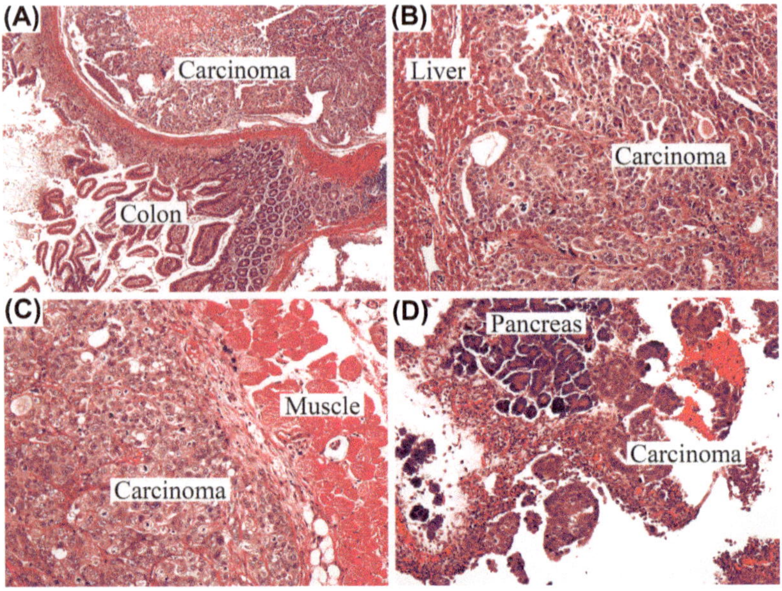

FIGURE 5.3 Ovarian cancer PDXs resemble the mode of clinical ovarian cancer growth and spread in colon (A), liver (B), muscle (C), and pancreas (D) (magnification ×10 in A, B, D; magnification ×20 in C).

into the bursa through the infundibulum of the fallopian tube.[20] Alternatively, tumor fragments can be sutured to the surface of the ovary.[32] Intraperitoneal tumor xenografts frequently undergo peritoneal dissemination to different organs including the colon, pancreas, liver, and muscle as shown in Fig. 5.3 and the development of ascites, similar to tumors in human patients. However, one disadvantage of intraperitoneal xenografts is that the mice may develop large amounts of ascites before a solid tumor can be detected, which makes monitoring tumor growth difficult.[31] Subcutaneous tumor xenografts are the least invasive and easiest to monitor. The subcutaneous site has advantages for drug testing, since it is easy to quantify tumor volume and response to treatment.[19] However, the tumor microenvironment of subcutaneous PDXs is different from that of human ovarian cancer and may influence drug responses. Also, ascites and peritoneal dissemination are rarely found in subcutaneous PDXs. The gonadal fat pad is the adipose tissue encapsulating the ovary or testis.[33] The subrenal capsule lies between the renal capsule, a fibrous layer surrounding the kidney, and the kidney parenchyma. Lee et al. reported that a subrenal capsule xenograft showed a high engraftment for low-grade ovarian cancers[34]; however, their findings have not been confirmed by other authors.[19] Dobbin et al.[19] compared different implant sites and found the highest success rate in subcutaneous sites (85%), followed by the mammary fat pad (64%), intraperitoneal cavity (22%), and subrenal capsule (8.3%).

To monitor tumor load in intraperitoneal cavity, intraovarian bursa, and subrenal capsule xenografts, serial serum cancer antigen 125 (CA125) levels can be useful as a marker for tumor volume.[20] Imaging analysis, including computed tomography, ultrasound, magnetic resonance imaging, positron emission tomography, and single-photon emission computed tomography, can also be used to monitor tumor volume and disease progression. PDXs can be engineered to express fluorescent proteins or either tumor-specific or secreted luciferase as another method to monitor tumor growth. However, not all PDXs are amenable to transfection. Among these techniques, ultrasound is the best to monitor the formation of ascites.[19]

PDX Models of Endometrial and Cervical Cancer

PDX models of both endometrial carcinoma and cervical cancers have been generated at heterotopic sites, such as the subcutaneous or subrenal capsule sites.[31,35,36] PDX models of cervical cancers have also been successfully generated at orthotopic sites. The success rate of orthotopic cervical cancer PDX models is approximately 50%.[37,38]

TUMOR BIOLOGY

Ovarian cancer PDXs have been shown to retain the morphologic, immunophenotypic, and genomic characteristics of original patient tumors. PDX models (up to the sixth generation) and original patient tumors have been reported to share similar histopathologic features.[19] Intratumoral heterogeneity is relatively well preserved in PDX models in contrast with cell line–derived mouse models.[19,39]

In addition, comprehensive genome-wide gene expression analysis has confirmed a high rate of concordance between ovarian cancer PDXs and original patient tumors. Weroha and colleagues[40] performed array comparative genomic hybridization on[41] ovarian cancer PDXs and found genetic changes similar to the findings of TCGA analysis. Dobbin and colleagues[19] analyzed messenger RNA levels of 84 oncogenes using RT^2 PCR array and found excellent correlation between ovarian cancer PDXs and source tumors in 79 genes, whereas only five genes were downregulated in tumor xenografts compared with human tumors: platelet-derived growth factor receptor-α, platelet-derived growth factor receptor-β, and three VEGF receptors (VEGFR1, VEGFR2, and VEGFR3). The authors speculated that these growth factors or growth factor receptors might be produced by the host mice, whereas the primers used in their experiments were specific for human genes. Also, Ricci et al.[27] reported higher gene copy numbers and altered mutations in 4 of 34 ovarian cancer xenografts. Therefore, ideally, all PDX tumors need to be tested by either sequencing or other techniques to confirm their concordance with original patient tumors. Testing only a small percentage of PDX models may not be sufficient.

Ovarian cancer PDXs carrying *BRCA* mutations have also been developed. For example, both Indraccolo et al.[23] and Press et al.[41] generated ovarian cancer PDXs with *BRCA1* mutations. Kortmann et al.[42] generated a *BRCA2*-mutated ovarian cancer PDX and showed that olaparib, a poly(ADP-ribose) polymerase-1 inhibitor, inhibited tumor growth in *BRCA2*-mutated ovarian serous carcinoma. Also, Topp et al. generated ovarian cancer PDXs with *BRCA1* mutations, *BRCA2* mutations, and *BRCA1* promoter methylation.[26]

Of note, immunocompromised mice can develop spontaneous lymphoma.[43] Lymphoma is usually easily differentiated from epithelial ovarian tumors by morphology and immunophenotype; however, this should be constantly evaluated. Lymphoma is typically positive for CD45 and negative for cytokeratin, whereas epithelial ovarian tumor exhibits the opposite immunophenotype.[26]

PRECLINICAL/CLINICAL APPLICATIONS

Previously, there were some concerns about whether ovarian cancer PDXs could predict patients' response to therapy, since tumor xenografts were established in immunocompromised mice. Several recent studies proved that ovarian cancer PDXs are good preclinical models for drug development. Topp et al.[26] demonstrated that cisplatin response in PDX models of high-grade serous ovarian carcinoma correlated well with patient outcome. In their study, all four PDXs sensitive to platinum (no disease progression for at least 100 days) were developed from patients who remained in remission for at least 6 months after first-line, platinum-based chemotherapy. In contrast, six PDXs resistant (disease progression in less than 100 days) or refractory to platinum were developed from patients with unfavorable outcome. Furthermore, three out of four platinum-sensitive PDXs carried DNA repair gene mutations or *BRCA1* methylation, whereas platinum-refractory PDXs overexpressed oncogenes, such as *CCNE1, LIN28B*, and *BCL2*. Weroha et al.[40] have generated 168 PDX models from human ovarian, primary peritoneal, and fallopian tube carcinomas, and so far, this is the largest bank of PDX models. Their study included a variety of histotypes, including serous, clear cell, mucinous, mixed, dedifferentiated, and carcinosarcoma. In keeping with the findings of Topp and colleagues,[26] Weroha et al. showed that ovarian cancer PDXs were able to predict patients' response to platinum chemotherapy. In PDXs developed from four platinum-resistant or refractory patients (disease progression within 6 months), tumor growth was found by ultrasound following platinum chemotherapy. However, in PDXs developed from five platinum-sensitive patients, tumor regression was found following platinum chemotherapy.[40] Moreover, Ricci et al.[27] found that PDXs predicted clinical response to cisplatin-based therapy in nine of 11 cases.

Moreover, PDX models have been used to study ovarian cancer stem cells and/or tumor-initiating cells. Since only a small percentage of cancer cells have stem cell features, they are difficult to identify. Previous functional assays have identified certain markers associated with ovarian cancer stem cells, including aldehyde dehydrogenase family 1 subfamily A1 (ALDH1A1) enzyme activity and cell surface markers CD44 and CD133 (also called prominin-1). None of these markers alone is specific for ovarian cancer stem cells, but the combination of these markers can enrich for a population of cells with tumor-initiating and cancer stem cell-like capabilities.[44] Stewart et al.[45] showed that CD133-expressing tumor-initiating cells in original tumors gave rise to CD133-negative cells in tumor xenografts. Dobbin et al.[19] showed that postchemotherapy tumor xenografts had increased percentage of cancer stem-like cells (ALDH1A1, CD44, and CD133 coexpressing cells) but also retained intratumoral heterogeneity. RNA sequencing analysis further demonstrated that the gene-expressing profile in postchemotherapy tumors was different from that in prechemotherapy tumors.

FUTURE/CHALLENGES

Generating ovarian cancer PDXs are expensive and time consuming, and the option may not be available for every patient at initial diagnosis.[26] The engraftment usually takes weeks to months. We should also keep in mind that the success rate of ovarian cancer PDXs is not 100%. A higher success rate has been reported in patients with more aggressive tumors.[40]

Another caveat is that the gradual loss of human stroma with number of passages may limit studies of therapies designed to target the tumor microenvironment.[22] Bankert et al.[46] reported that tumor-associated human lymphocytes and fibroblasts were functional in tumor xenografts, although it was unclear how long these cells were retained. Functional host immune system is also absent in PDX models, due to the need to use immunocompromised mice for transplantation limiting the utility of the models.[37] New techniques have been developed to study emerging immunotherapies in PDX models. "Super avatars" were developed by cotransplantation of hematopoietic stem cells (eg, $CD34^+$ cord blood cells) and solid tumors providing an opportunity to explore the role of the immune system in the propagation and therapy of the tumor models.[47] Moreover, humanized mouse models, have been developed recently. In these mice, human genes encoding cytokines important for innate immune cell development (ie, human macrophage colony-stimulating factor, human interleukin-3, granulocyte macrophage colony-stimulating factor, and human thrombopoietin) were knocked in to their respective mouse loci.[48] Both super avatars and humanized mice may be good models to study immune response and the tumor microenvironment in ovarian cancer.

Ovarian cancer stem-like cells play an essential role in cancer initiation, progression, and chemoresistance. Cancer stem-like cells are also promising therapeutic targets in gynecologic malignancies. Eradicating cancer stem-like cells may eventually lead to the cure of these cancers. Since tumor heterogeneity is preserved in tumor xenografts,[39] and cancer stem-like cells are enriched in posttherapy xenografts, PDXs may provide models to study cancer stem-like cells.

In the future, a "mouse co-clinical trial" may be possible to test novel therapeutics either prior to or simultaneously with clinical trials. One advantage of mouse co-clinical trials over human clinical trials is that PDXs in both the control and experimental groups can be derived from the same patient and share the same histopathologic and genetic characteristics. This is particularly important in the exploration of the activity of individual components of combination therapy. Furthermore, PDX models can be generated from both therapy-naive and posttreatment tumors, potentially from the same patient. This will help us understand why patients have recurrent disease after originally responding to chemotherapy. Novel therapeutics to eradicate residual or recurrent tumors can also be developed using these PDX models. Furthermore, cell lines can be generated from ovarian cancer PDXs and are used to study molecular mechanisms of drug response.

CONCLUSION

PDX mice are very useful models in cancer biology, tumor biomarker development, and preclinical drug testing. Both intratumoral heterogeneity (within the same tumor) and intertumoral heterogeneity (among tumors of different patients) are preserved in ovarian cancer PDXs, and therefore, PDXs have potential advantages over ovarian cancer cell lines, cell line–derived xenografts, and genetically engineered cancer models. In the era of personalized medicine, PDX models will play a more and more important role in treating gynecologic cancers.

ACKNOWLEDGMENTS

We thank Markeda Wade from the Department of Scientific Publications at the University of Texas MD Anderson Cancer Center for editing the manuscript and Kim-Anh T. Vu from the Department of Pathology for editing the figures. This work is supported by M.D. Anderson Moon Shot Program (AS, JL). This work was also supported in part by grant from the Cancer Prevention and Research Institute of Texas, the MD Anderson Cancer Center SPORE in Ovarian Cancer (National Institutes of Health grant), and a Sister Institution Grant from MD Anderson Cancer Center Global Academic Programs (JL). Dr. Li Liang was supported by the training grant T32CA163185 from NIH/NCI.

REFERENCES

1. DeSantis CE, Lin CC, Mariotto AB, Siegel RL, Stein KD, Kramer JL, et al. Cancer treatment and survivorship statistics, 2014. *CA Cancer J Clin* 2014;**64**:252–71.
2. Siegel R, Ma J, Zou Z, Jemal A. Cancer statistics, 2014. *CA Cancer J Clin* 2014;**64**:9–29.
3. Hasan N, Ohman AW, Dinulescu DM. The promise and challenge of ovarian cancer models. *Transl Cancer Res* 2015;**4**:14–28.
4. Soslow RA. Histologic subtypes of ovarian carcinoma: an overview. *Int J Gynecol Pathol* 2008;**27**:161–74.

5. Malpica A, Deavers MT, Lu K, Bodurka DC, Atkinson EN, Gershenson DM, et al. Grading ovarian serous carcinoma using a two-tier system. *Am J Surg Pathol* 2004;**28**:496–504.
6. Folkins AK, Jarboe EA, Roh MH, Crum CP. Precursors to pelvic serous carcinoma and their clinical implications. *Gynecol Oncol* 2009;**113**:391–6.
7. Vang R, Visvanathan K, Gross A, et al. Validation of an algorithm for the diagnosis of serous tubal intraepithelial carcinoma. *Int J Gynecol Pathol* 2012;**31**:243–53.
8. Tone AA, Begley H, Sharma M, Murphy J, Rosen B, Brown TJ, et al. Gene expression profiles of luteal phase fallopian tube epithelium from BRCA mutation carriers resemble high-grade serous carcinoma. *Clin Cancer Res* 2008;**14**:4067–78.
9. Cancer Genome Atlas Research Network. Integrated genomic analyses of ovarian carcinoma. *Nature* 2011;**474**:609–15.
10. Vang R, Levine DA, Soslow RA, Zaloudek C, Shih IeM, Kurman RJ. Molecular alterations of TP53 are a defining feature of ovarian high-grade serous carcinoma: a review of cases lacking TP53 mutations in the Cancer Genome Atlas Ovarian Study. *Int J Gynecol Pathol* 2016;**35**: 48–55.
11. Della Pepa C, Tonini G, Santini D, Losito S, Pisano C, Di Napoli M, et al. Low Grade Serous Ovarian Carcinoma: from the molecular characterization to the best therapeutic strategy. *Cancer Treat Rev* 2015;**41**:136–43.
12. Wiegand KC, Shah SP, Al-Agha OM, Zhao Y, Tse K, Zeng T, et al. ARID1A mutations in endometriosis-associated ovarian carcinomas. *N Engl J Med* 2010;**363**:1532–43.
13. Kuo KT, Mao TL, Jones S, Veras E, Ayhan A, Wang TL, et al. Frequent activating mutations of PIK3CA in ovarian clear cell carcinoma. *Am J Pathol* 2009;**174**:1597–601.
14. Cuatrecasas M, Villanueva A, Matias-Guiu X, Prat J. K-ras mutations in mucinous ovarian tumors: a clinicopathologic and molecular study of 95 cases. *Cancer* 1997;**79**:1581–6.
15. Domcke S, Sinha R, Levine DA, Sander C, Schultz N. Evaluating cell lines as tumour models by comparison of genomic profiles. *Nat Commun* 2013;**4**:2126.
16. Ince TA, Sousa AD, Jones MA, Harrell JC, Agoston ES, Krohn M, et al. Characterization of twenty-five ovarian tumour cell lines that phenocopy primary tumours. *Nat Commun* 2015;**6**:7419.
17. Steg AD, Bevis KS, Katre AA, Ziebarth A, Dobbin ZC, Alvarez RD, et al. Stem cell pathways contribute to clinical chemoresistance in ovarian cancer. *Clin Cancer Res* 2012;**18**:869–81.
18. Banerjee S, Kaye SB. New strategies in the treatment of ovarian cancer: current clinical perspectives and future potential. *Clin Cancer Res* 2013;**19**:961–8.
19. Dobbin ZC, Katre AA, Steg AD, Erickson BK, Shah MM, Alvarez RD, et al. Using heterogeneity of the patient-derived xenograft model to identify the chemoresistant population in ovarian cancer. *Oncotarget* 2014;**5**:8750–64.
20. Konstantinopoulos PA, Matulonis UA. Current status and evolution of preclinical drug development models of epithelial ovarian cancer. *Front Oncol* 2013;**3**:296.
21. Kolfschoten GM, Pinedo HM, Scheffer PG, Schluper HM, Erkelens CA, Boven E. Development of a panel of 15 human ovarian cancer xenografts for drug screening and determination of the role of the glutathione detoxification system. *Gynecol Oncol* 2000;**76**:362–8.
22. Hylander BL, Punt N, Tang H, Hillman J, Vaughan M, Bshara W, et al. Origin of the vasculature supporting growth of primary patient tumor xenografts. *J Transl Med* 2013;**11**:110.
23. Indraccolo S, Tisato V, Agata S, Moserle L, Ferrari S, Callegaro M, et al. Establishment and characterization of xenografts and cancer cell cultures derived from BRCA1 -/- epithelial ovarian cancers. *Eur J Cancer* 2006;**42**:1475–83.
24. Scott CL, Becker MA, Haluska P, Samimi G. Patient-derived xenograft models to improve targeted therapy in epithelial ovarian cancer treatment. *Front Oncol* 2013;**3**:295.

25. Shultz LD, Lyons BL, Burzenski LM, Gott B, Chen X, Chaleff S, et al. Human lymphoid and myeloid cell development in NOD/LtSz-scid IL2R gamma null mice engrafted with mobilized human hemopoietic stem cells. *J Immunol* 2005;**174**:6477–89.
26. Topp MD, Hartley L, Cook M, Heong V, Boehm E, McShane L, et al. Molecular correlates of platinum response in human high-grade serous ovarian cancer patient-derived xenografts. *Mol Oncol* 2014;**8**:656–68.
27. Ricci F, Bizzaro F, Cesca M, Guffanti F, Ganzinelli M, Decio A, et al. Patient-derived ovarian tumor xenografts recapitulate human clinicopathology and genetic alterations. *Cancer Res* 2014;**74**:6980–90.
28. Morton CL, Houghton PJ. Establishment of human tumor xenografts in immunodeficient mice. *Nat Protoc* 2007;**2**:247–50.
29. Erickson BK, Kinde I, Dobbin ZC, Wang Y, Martin JY, Alvarez RD, et al. Detection of somatic TP53 mutations in tampons of patients with high-grade serous ovarian cancer. *Obstet Gynecol* 2014;**124**:881–5.
30. Kaspari O, Lemmer K, Becker S, Lochau P, Howaldt S, Nattermann H, et al. Decontamination of a BSL3 laboratory by hydrogen peroxide fumigation using three different surrogates for *Bacillus anthracis* spores. *J Appl Microbiol* 2014;**117**:1095–103.
31. Boone JD, Dobbin ZC, Straughn Jr JM, Buchsbaum DJ. Ovarian and cervical cancer patient derived xenografts: the past, present, and future. *Gynecol Oncol* 2015;**138**:486–91.
32. Vidal A, Munoz C, Guillen MJ, Moretó J, Puertas S, Martínez-Iniesta M, et al. Lurbinectedin (PM01183), a new DNA minor groove binder, inhibits growth of orthotopic primary graft of cisplatin-resistant epithelial ovarian cancer. *Clin Cancer Res* 2012;**18**:5399–411.
33. Ghamande S, Hylander BL, Oflazoglu E, Lele S, Fanslow W, Repasky EA. Recombinant CD40 ligand therapy has significant antitumor effects on CD40-positive ovarian tumor xenografts grown in SCID mice and demonstrates an augmented effect with cisplatin. *Cancer Res* 2001;**61**:7556–62.
34. Lee CH, Xue H, Sutcliffe M, Gout PW, Huntsman DG, Miller DM, et al. Establishment of subrenal capsule xenografts of primary human ovarian tumors in SCID mice: potential models. *Gynecol Oncol* 2005;**96**:48–55.
35. Unno K, Ono M, Winder AD, Maniar KP, Paintal AS, Yu Y, et al. Establishment of human patient-derived endometrial cancer xenografts in NOD scid gamma mice for the study of invasion and metastasis. *PLoS One* 2014;**9**:e116064.
36. Groeneweg JW, Hall TR, Zhang L, Kim M, Byron VF, Tambouret R, et al. Inhibition of gamma-secretase activity impedes uterine serous carcinoma growth in a human xenograft model. *Gynecol Oncol* 2014;**133**:607–15.
37. Scott CL, Mackay HJ, Haluska Jr P. Patient-derived xenograft models in gynecologic malignancies. *Am Soc Clin Oncol Educ Book* 2014:e258–66.
38. Chaudary N, Pintilie M, Schwock J, Dhani N, Clarke B, Milosevic M, et al. Characterization of the tumor-microenvironment in patient-derived cervix xenografts (OCICx). *Cancers (Basel)* 2012;**4**:821–45.
39. Cassidy JW, Caldas C, Bruna A. Maintaining tumor heterogeneity in patient-derived tumor xenografts. *Cancer Res* 2015;**75**:2963–8.
40. Weroha SJ, Becker MA, Enderica-Gonzalez S, Harrington SC, Oberg AL, Maurer MJ, et al. Tumorgrafts as in vivo surrogates for women with ovarian cancer. *Clin Cancer Res* 2014;**20**:1288–97.
41. Press JZ, Kenyon JA, Xue H, Miller MA, De Luca A, Miller DM, et al. Xenografts of primary human gynecological tumors grown under the renal capsule of NOD/SCID mice show genetic stability during serial transplantation and respond to cytotoxic chemotherapy. *Gynecol Oncol* 2008;**110**:256–64.

42. Kortmann U, McAlpine JN, Xue H, Guan J, Ha G, Tully S, et al. Tumor growth inhibition by olaparib in BRCA2 germline-mutated patient-derived ovarian cancer tissue xenografts. *Clin Cancer Res* 2011;**17**:783–91.
43. Custer RP, Bosma GC, Bosma MJ. Severe combined immunodeficiency (SCID) in the mouse. Pathology, reconstitution, neoplasms. *Am J Pathol* 1985;**120**:464–77.
44. Shah MM, Landen CN. Ovarian cancer stem cells: are they real and why are they important? *Gynecol Oncol* 2014;**132**:483–9.
45. Stewart JM, Shaw PA, Gedye C, Bernardini MQ, Neel BG, Ailles LE. Phenotypic heterogeneity and instability of human ovarian tumor-initiating cells. *Proc Natl Acad Sci USA* 2011;**108**:6468–73.
46. Bankert RB, Balu-Iyer SV, Odunsi K, Shultz LD, Kelleher Jr RJ, Barnas JL, et al. Humanized mouse model of ovarian cancer recapitulates patient solid tumor progression, ascites formation, and metastasis. *PLoS One* 2011;**6**:e24420.
47. Ishikawa F, Yasukawa M, Lyons B, Yoshida S, Miyamoto T, Yoshimoto G, et al. Development of functional human blood and immune systems in NOD/SCID/IL2 receptor {gamma} chain(null) mice. *Blood* 2005;**106**:1565–73.
48. Rongvaux A, Willinger T, Martinek J, Strowig T, Gearty SV, Teichmann LL, et al. Development and function of human innate immune cells in a humanized mouse model. *Nat Biotechnol* 2014;**32**:364–72.
49. Xu Y, Silver DF, Yang NP, Oflazoglu E, Hempling RE, Piver MS, et al. Characterization of human ovarian carcinomas in a SCID mouse model. *Gynecol Oncol* 1999;**72**:161–70.
50. Silver DF, Hempling RE, Piver MS, Repasky EA. Effects of IL-12 on human ovarian tumors engrafted into SCID mice. *Gynecol Oncol* 1999;**72**:154–60.
51. Silver DF, Hempling RE, Piver MS, Repasky EA. Flt-3 ligand inhibits growth of human ovarian tumors engrafted in severe combined immunodeficient mice. *Gynecol Oncol* 2000;**77**:377–82.

Chapter 6

Patient-Derived Xenografts From Lung Cancer and Their Potential Applications

L. Wang, R. Zhang, B. Fang
The University of Texas MD Anderson Cancer Center, Houston, TX, United States

BACKGROUND

Lung cancer is the second leading cause of death following ischemic heart disease in the United States and in most other high-income countries.[1] Globally, lung cancer's annual incidence is about 1.8 million, and the annual mortality is approximately 1.6 million.[2,3] Approximately 6.6% of men and women may be diagnosed with lung and bronchus cancers at some point during their lifetime. Tobacco smoking and outdoor/indoor air pollution are known to be the major causes of lung cancer.[4–7] Thus, avoiding tobacco smoking and air pollution is regarded as the best way to lower the risk of lung cancer.[8] Early diagnosis is found to be the major factor that improves survival of lung cancer patients,[9] as the 5-year survival rate for patients with stage I non–small cell lung cancer (NSCLC) is approximately 70%, but drops to approximately 5% for stage IV lung cancer patients.[10] Unfortunately, most lung cancers are diagnosed at an advanced stage and thus have a poor prognosis.[4] The overall 5-year survival rate for lung cancer patients in the United States has improved only moderately over the past four decades, from 12.2% in 1975 to 17.4% in 2011,[11–13] despite the use of many therapeutic modalities.

Conventionally, lung cancer patients are treated according to their histopathological diagnoses and clinical stages. Genome-wide gene sequencing analyses have revealed that lung cancers with the same histopathologic diagnoses, and the same clinical stages can be highly heterogeneous in their genetic and epigenetic alterations.[14,15] Advances in molecular profiling and targeted therapy have shown that subgroups of lung cancer patients, particularly adenocarcinomas, are caused by genetic alteration in the genes encoding epidermal growth factor receptor (EGFR) or anaplastic lymphoma kinase (ALK). These cancers are highly sensitive to some small molecule inhibitors targeting EGFR or ALK. These breakthrough discoveries have led to a new paradigm of

Patient Derived Tumor Xenograft Models. http://dx.doi.org/10.1016/B978-0-12-804010-2.00020-5

biomarker-directed precision therapy.[14] It is now clear that mutations in cancer driver genes and alterations in gene expression and/or posttranscriptional modifications can all drastically affect treatment responses or clinical outcomes.[16–18] Moreover, the success of targeted anticancer therapy depends to a large extent on the identification of the patient subgroups that may respond to specific therapeutic agents. Thus, both histological classification and molecular diagnosis for patient stratification will be required for clinical guidance of precision therapy.[19] However, biomarker-directed personalized therapy can benefit only a limited number of patients because most of the currently available predictive biomarkers have low occurrence frequencies[20–22] and because response-predictive biomarkers are not available for most first-line anti–lung cancer drugs. Therefore, an alternative patient-based personalized therapeutic approach will be required to identify optimal treatment regimens for patients in clinics. Furthermore, the development of new anticancer drugs is often hampered by the lack of preclinical tumor models highly predictive for therapeutic effects in humans. In vitro cell line models and in vivo xenograft tumors derived from established human cancer cell lines have limited predictive value for antitumor activity of a drug in clinical trials,[23–25] because anticancer agents that showed promising antitumor activity in those models have often been ineffective for the same type of cancer in clinical trials.[26,27] Together, the challenges encountered in the clinical practice of anticancer therapy and in the development of new anticancer agents highlight the urgency of developing clinically relevant tumor models and/or technologies to improve therapeutic efficacies in clinics and success rates in anticancer drug development.

Evidence from various studies has shown that patient-derived xenografts (PDXs) established directly from patients' primary tumors preserve the histomorphologic features, heterogeneity, gene expression pattern (including cytokine expression by tumor stroma cells), DNA copy number alterations, and gene mutations of the original tumors.[28–30] These features were preserved after a series of passages of the tumorgrafts in mice.[28,30] When PDXs are treated with agents used in a parallel patient population, similar response rates are observed as that reported in human studies, suggesting that the PDX model is a clinically relevant tumor model for efficacy evaluation of anticancer drugs.[28,31–34] A remarkable correlation between drug activity in PDXs and clinical outcome was reported when patients with advanced cancer were treated with selected regimens based on the treatment responses of their PDXs,[35,36] suggesting that the PDX could be a robust model for the identification of effective treatment for cancer patients. Consequently, establishing PDXs from various types of cancers has recently been enthusiastically pursued by several groups. Several recent publications have focused on the generation and characterization of PDXs from lung cancers (Table 6.1).[29,32,34,37,38] Those PDXs are expected to provide useful platforms for translational studies including drug development, molecular characterization of cancer biology, and strategic development of individualized therapy.

TABLE 6.1 Lung Cancer PDXs

Authors	Specimens	Mice/Site of Implant	Engraft Rate (%)	Characterization	References
Perez-Soler et al.	Surgical	Nude/subcutaneous	46	Histology, drug response	34
Fichtner et al.	Surgical	NOD-SCID/subcutaneous	25	Drug response	38
				Mutation/expression	
Dong et al.	Surgical	NOD-SCID/renal capsule	90	Histology, drug response	32
John et al.	Surgical	NOD-SCID/subcutaneous	40	Histology, mutations	29
Lee et al.	Surgical, brain metastasis	NOD-SCID/subcutaneous, subrenal	Brain mets 74, primary 23	Drug response, genomic	67
Leong et al.	SCLC biopsy	NSG/subcutaneous	83	Histology, genomic	68
Hao et al.	Surgical	SCID/subcutaneous	26	Histology, genomic	37
Anderson et al.	SCLC biopsy	NOD-SCID/subcutaneous	67	Biomarkers, drug response	69
Nakajima et al.	Biopsy	NSG/subcutaneous	42	Histology	70
Zhang et al.	Surgical	SCID/subcutaneous	32	Drug response, mutation	65
Ilie et al.	Surgical	SCID/subcutaneous	35	Genomic	64
Stewart et al.	Surgical EGFR mutant	NOD-SCID/subcutaneous	18	Drug response, genomic, expression	66

METHODOLOGIES AND MODELS

The methodologies for generating lung cancer PDXs are the same as those detailed in Section II, Chapter 3. Our own experience suggested that non-obese diabetic-severe combined immunodeficiency (NOD-SCID) with null mutation in the gene encoding the interleukin-2 receptor gamma (NSG) mice have relatively higher engraftment rate than SCID or nude mice, although it was not statistically investigated. Nevertheless, most PDXs established in NSG mice can be successfully passaged in nude mice. Therefore, NSG mice are used for establishing the first generation of PDXs (F1) from primary tumors, whereas nude mice are used for passaging established PDXs in our studies.

PDXs can be established by implanting tumor tissue in the subcutaneous area[29,37,38] or under the renal capsule.[32] Although implanting under renal capsule seemed to have high engraftment,[32] implanting in subcutaneous area is more commonly reported in the literature.[29,37,38] Subcutaneous inoculation of tumor tissues is performed in our studies. The engraftment rate is approximately 25–30%. Squamous cancers seem to have relatively higher engraftment rates compared with adenocarcinomas. Moderate- and poor-differentiated tumors have relatively high engraftment rates compared with well-differentiated tumors.[37] Tumor tissue with substantial viable cancer cells has a high chance of generating PDXs, whereas tumor tissue consisting largely of scar tissues usually failed to grow in mice. Orthotopic PDX models can also be established by percutaneous injection into lung with primary tumor cells obtained through collagenase digestion. Alternatively, needle biopsy–sized samples can be obtained by using 22G needle to collect tumor tissue, which then is inoculated into lung percutaneously. Although direct comparison between PDXs established in subcutaneous and orthotopic sites is not available, accumulating evidence has shown that different anatomical sites affect the tumor microenvironment and response to therapy and that orthotopic tumor models established in the equivalent organs from which cancer originated are more clinically relevant for efficacy evaluation than are subcutaneous tumor models.[39–43]

At our institution, fresh primary tumor tissues are obtained from the pathology department. For generating PDXs, fresh tumor tissues are transported with 10 mL of Roswell Park Memorial Institute (RPMI) medium (serum free, supplemented with 100 μg ampicillin/mL and 100 μg streptomycin/mL). The tumor tissue is usually cut into 1–2 mm in diameters, briefly soaked with Matrigel, and then implanted into the subcutaneous area of NSG mice under anesthesia with isoflurane. If mice are not available, the tissue samples may be stored in cryopreservation medium for later inoculation. We use CryoStor CS10 from StemCell Technologies as the cryopreservation medium. Alternatively, RPMI medium with 10% of dimethyl sulfoxide (DMSO) can be used for cryopreservation. Tumors growing in mice will be harvested when they reach 1.5 cm in diameter and labeled as F1 for the first passage in animals, which will be divided into several portions of about 2 mm^3; each portion will be frozen in cryopreservation medium in liquid nitrogen for future investigation, analyzed for molecular biological characterization, or replanted subcutaneously into nude mice for generating more PDXs (F2, F3, etc., for subsequent passages) to test drug response.

For cryopreservation of tumor tissues, fresh tumor tissues are cut with a surgical blade into 2–3 mm in diameter. Tumor tissues are then transferred to 1.5-mL cryopreservation tube with 1 mL cryopreservation medium (CryoStor CS10 or RPMI medium with 10% DMSO); 2–4 pieces of 2- to 3-mm^2 tissues may be stored in one tube. The tube is placed on ice or at 4°C for 30 min to allow DMSO to penetrate the tissues and then transferred to a freezing box containing isopropanol alcohol that allows the temperature to drop down slowly. The freezing box is placed in a −80°C freezer overnight. The tubes can be kept at −80°C for 1 month, and should be transferred to liquid nitrogen for long-term storage. For thawing tumor tissues from cryopreservation, the cryopreservation tube should be quickly swirled in a 37°C water bath. Tumor tissue is then transferred to a sterile petri dish or a 15-mL centrifuge tube with 10 mL Dulbecco's modified Eagle's medium or RPMI medium containing ampicillin and streptomycin. Incubating the tissue in the medium at 0–4°C for 5–10 min allows DMSO to dilute out of the tissue. The medium is then removed and the tissue is cut into 1- to 2-mm^2 pieces, soaked in Matrigel briefly, and implanted into mice.

TUMOR BIOLOGY

Histologically, lung cancer is classified as small cell lung cancer (SCLC, about 15%) and NSCLC (about 85%), the latter including adenocarcinoma, squamous cell carcinoma, and large cell carcinoma. SCLC is usually sensitive to platinum-based chemotherapy and radiotherapy; however, recurrence and resistance occur inevitably in most SCLC patients, leading to low 5-year overall survival rates.[11] Lung adenocarcinoma usually expresses thyroid transcription factor-1 and napsin A, whereas squamous cell cancer usually expresses truncated p63 (p40) and cytokeratin 5/6.[44,45] Recent genome-wide gene sequencing analyses have found that each lung cancer may have an average of about 150 somatic mutations that are expected to alter their protein products.[14,15] EGFR mutations and ALK gene rearrangement, for which target therapies are available clinically, occur almost exclusively in adenocarcinoma.

Molecular changes in lung adenocarcinoma,[20,21,46,47] squamous cell cancer,[48] SCLC,[49,50] and carcinoids or neuroendocrine tumor[51] have been recently reported by several groups. Based on the data retrieved from The Cancer Genome Atlas (TCGA) databases and publicly available datasets at the website http://www.cbioportal.org,*TP53* is the most frequently mutated cancer driver gene in lung cancers, with frequencies varying from 46% in adenocarcinoma to 86% in SCLC. In addition, *KRAS*, *CDKN2A*, *MLL3*, *STK11*, *KEAP1*, and *EGFR* are the most frequently mutated genes detected in lung adenocarcinomas. *PIK3CA*, *SOX2*, *CDKN2A*, *TP63*, *FGFR1*, and *MLL2* are the most frequently mutated genes in squamous cell cancer, and *RB1*, *EP300*, *MLL2*, *SMO*, and *PIK3CA* are the most common mutant genes in SCLC.[14] It is noteworthy, however, that current TCGA data are derived mostly from patients in Western countries. The mutational status in other ethnic populations can vary greatly.[52,53] For examples, activating *EGFR* mutations are detected in about 10–17% of lung adenocarcinoma patients in the United States and Europe,[20,54–57] but in about 30–65% of lung adenocarcinoma patients in Asia.[58–61] In contrast, *KRAS* mutations were detected in 35–50% of lung adenocarcinomas in Caucasians[47,62] but in less than 5% of Chinese lung adenocarcinomas.[59,60,63]

Generation and characterization of lung PDXs have been reported by several groups. An early study by Dr. Mao's group revealed that squamous cancer had higher engraftment rates than adenocarcinoma.[34] This observation was confirmed by us and others.[29,37,64,65] PDXs were found to be morphologically identical to the original tumors and had a response rate to paclitaxel that is equivalent to that reported in phase 2 studies in patients with advanced NSCLC treated with single-agent paclitaxel.[34] One study found that response to the anti-EGFR therapies did not correlate with mutations in the *EGFR* or *TP53*, but that there was a correlation between *KRAS* mutations and erlotinib resistance.[38] Other studies revealed that *EGFR*-mutant PDXs closely recapitulated their corresponding patient tumor phenotype and clinical course, including response pattern to EGFR tyrosine kinase inhibitors (TKIs).[65,66] Surgical specimens from NSCLC brain metastasis showed a significantly higher successful PDX engraftment rate than primary specimens (74% vs 23%).[67] In contrast, age, sex, smoking status, tumor size, pathologic tumor-node stage, implanted mouse strain (NOD-SCID vs nude), implantation route (subcutaneous vs subrenal), grade of differentiation, neoadjuvant chemotherapy, *KRAS* genotype, and *ALK* genotype showed no significant correlation with in vivo tumor engraftment rate.[67] Nevertheless, one study revealed that subrenal capsule implantation led to an engraftment rate of 90%,[32] whereas another study on lung adenocarcinomas with *EGFR* activating mutations showed an engraftment rate of 18%.[66] PDXs have also been successfully established from biopsy samples from SCLC.[68–70] The SCLC PDXs derived from needle biopsy are similar to matched primary tumors in cancer patients by histology, gene mutations, and chemosensitivity,[68,69] although different gene mutations that were present only in the primary samples or only in the xenografts were detected.[68]

We recently determined gene mutations in 23 lung PDXs and their paired primary tumors by ultradeep exome sequencing of 202 cancer-related genes. Among the PDXs analyzed, 11 were adenocarcinoma, 9 squamous cell cancer, and 3 neuroendocrinal cancer. The primary tumors averaged 13.7 mutations/tumor in the 202 genes, ranging from 2 to 103 mutations. Some tumors were heavily mutated, suggesting genome instability. The numbers of PDXs with potentially deleterious mutations in *TP53*, *KRAS*, *PI3KCA*, *STK11*, *EGFR*, and *ALK* were 10 (43.5%), 5 (21.7%), 4 (17.4%), 3 (13%), 2 (9%), and 3 (13%), respectively.[37] Other genes with potentially deleterious mutations in ≥3 (13%) tumors were *MLL3*, *SETD2*, *HGF*, *KDM6A*, and *ATM*. *MLL3*, *SETD2*, *KDM6A*,

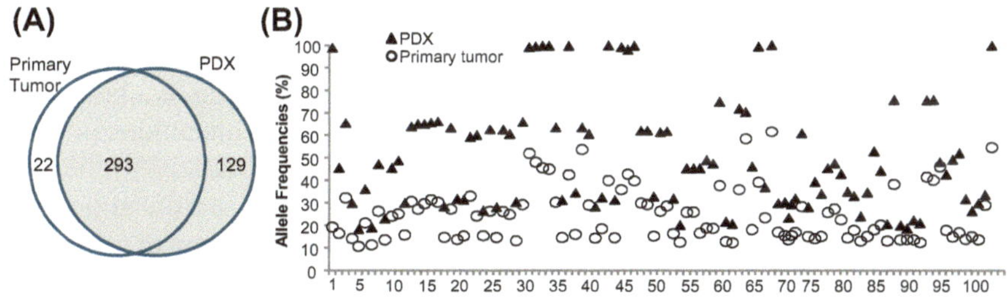

FIGURE 6.1 Comparison of mutations in primary tumors and corresponding PDXs. (A) Mutations identified in 23 pairs of primary tumors and PDXs, showing numbers of unique and common mutations. (B) Allele frequencies of mutations in a pair of primary tumor and its corresponding PDX. The numbers on the X-axis represent individual mutations detected in primary tumor and/or PDX. As shown in the graphs, the allele frequencies in the PDX are often dramatically greater than in the primary tumor.

and *ATM* are involved in regulating DNA repair and genome stability. Ninety-three percent of mutations detected in the primary tumors were also detected in their corresponding PDXs, indicating that PDXs have the capacity to recapitulate the mutations in primary tumors (Fig. 6.1). Nevertheless, a substantial number of mutations had higher allele frequencies in the PDXs than in the primary tumors or were not detectable in the primary tumor, suggesting the possibility of tumor cell enrichment in PDXs or heterogeneity in primary tumors.

APPLICATIONS OF PDXs FOR PRECLINICAL AND CLINICAL STUDIES

PDXs can provide renewable cancer tissue resource for biological studies of cancer, including mechanistic characterization, biomarker discovery, target identification, drug discovery and development, and personalized therapy. Here we discuss a few areas that PDXs may be exploited for preclinical and clinical applications.

Personalized Therapy

EGFR mutations and *ALK* rearrangements are two cancer drivers for which targeted therapies are available clinically. Approximately 10–17% of lung adenocarcinoma patients in the United States and Europe have activation mutations in the *EGFR* gene.[20,54–57] These mutations are more commonly seen in women and nonsmokers.[20,54–57] Lung cancer cells with mutant *EGFR* are highly susceptible to the EGFR inhibitors gefitinib[55,71,72] and erlotinib.[55,73] Both gefitinib and erlotinib have been reported to significantly prolong progression-free survival in patients with *EGFR*-mutant lung cancer.[74–76] Similarly, small molecule inhibitors for hepatocyte growth factor receptor (c-MET) and ALK have been proved to be highly effective for treatment of lung cancers with *ALK* and *ROS1* gene translocations.[77–80] *EML4/ALK* rearrangements are detected in about 4–5% of patients with NSCLC,[81–84] whereas *ROS1* gene rearrangement and activation are detected in about 1–1.5% of NSCLC.[80,85,86] Both *ALK* and *ROS1* gene translocations are predominantly found in adenocarcinoma and in never-smokers. The low frequencies of *EGFR* mutations and *ALK* or *ROS1* gene alterations in lung cancers implicate that the success of anti-EGFR and anti-ALK/ROS1 relies on identifications of responders through biomarker-based patient stratification. For most patients, genetic or biomarker testing may not identify an optimal treatment regimen for them, because response-predictive biomarkers are not available for most first-line anti–lung cancer drugs. The results from a recent Molecular Profiling and Targeted Therapies in Advanced Thoracic Malignancies trials (ClinicTrials.gov identifier:NCT01306045) revealed that in 647 patients enrolled in genomic characterization of oncogenic drivers, 257 patients had mutations and/or amplification in *EGFR*, *KRAS*, *NRAS*, *HRAS*, *BRAF*, *PIK3CA*, *ALT*, *PETN*, *ERBB2*, *KIT*, and *PDGFRA*. However, only 45 patients were enrolled in the biomarker-directed trial.[87] Moreover, despite initial dramatic responses to targeted therapy with EGFR or ALK/ROS1 inhibitors, acquired resistance inevitably occurs in most patients. Thus, an alternative patient-based personalized therapeutic approach will be required to identify optimal treatment regimens as initial anticancer therapy or to overcome the resistance to the genotype-specific target therapy. The studies from Hidalgo et al. have shown that PDXs may provide a powerful investigational platform for treatment decisions or to efficiently guide cancer treatment in clinic.[35,36] In a pilot clinical study with 11 patients receiving 17 prospectively guided treatments based on the responses of PDXs, 15 treatments resulted in durable partial remission, demonstrating a remarkable correlation between drug activity in the PDXs and clinical outcome, both in terms of resistance and sensitivity.[35]

Preclinical Evaluation of Candidate Drugs

Anticancer drug development is often hampered by a lack of preclinical tumor models that are highly predictive of therapeutic effects in humans. Previous studies have shown that in vitro cell line models and in vivo xenograft tumors derived from established human cancer cell lines have limited predictive value for antitumor activity of a drug in clinical trials.[23–25] In fact, only about 5% of anticancer agents evaluated in human studies between 1991 and 2000 were successfully registered.[26,88] Furthermore, 80% of phase 3 failures were caused by a lack of efficacy,[26,88–90] presumably resulting from a lack of clinically relevant models for preclinical efficacy evaluations, or from a lack of biomarkers capable of identifying responders.[26,88] Thus, an innovative drug development approach with clinically relevant cancer models is critical to improving the success rate in clinical trials. Recent studies have shown that PDXs have similar response rates as that observed in human studies for a number of anticancer agents[28,30–34,38] and that PDXs can effectively recapitulate drug response patterns of their corresponding primary tumors, including the response to EGFR TKIs.[65,66] Mice bearing SCLC PDXs were found to respond to a combination therapy of cisplatin plus etoposide similarly to the patients from whom the tumors originated.[69] These results suggested that PDXs are clinically relevant and can be robust preclinical models for predicting efficacies in humans. PDXs have also been used for the assessment of combination therapies, including combination of erlotinib and crizotinib in *EGFR*-mutant and erlotinib-resistant lung cancer PDXs,[91] and the dual PI3K/mTOR small molecule inhibitor PF-04691502 and the pan-ERBB inhibitor dacomitinib in *KRAS*-mutant colorectal PDXs.[92]

Drug Screening and Discovery

In vitro screening for anticancer agents can be performed with molecular target-based biochemical assays or cell-based cytotoxic assays. Molecular target-based assay will be useful for actionable (or druggable) targets. However, most of the commonly identified cancer drivers in lung cancer, such as genetic changes in *TP53*, *STK11*, *RB1*, and *RAS* genes, are either nondruggable or difficult to target using small molecules.[14] Thus, alternative approaches will be required to develop anticancer drugs for cancers caused by those drivers, such as killing cancer cells indirectly through synthetic lethality. Synthetic lethality is a lethal phenotype caused by the combined effects of mutations in two or more genes. This concept has recently been exploited for the development of novel genotype-selective anticancer agents and/or the identification of novel therapeutic targets.[93–96] Most of synthetic lethality screenings were performed by using isogenic cell lines. Nevertheless, previous two-dimensional screening designs that lack critical features of native cancers, such as tumor structures and cancer cells' interactions with tumor microenvironment, may reduce the chance of detecting potential therapeutic targets or agents. Tumor stromal cells (including tumor-associated fibroblasts, mesenchymal-derived smooth muscle cells, endothelial cells, and inflammatory and immune cells), the extracellular matrix (ECM), ECM-degrading enzymes, and growth factors and cytokines produced by tumor and stromal cells are known to be critically involved in cancer initiation and progression. Developments in organotypic (tissue slices)[97] and organoid (dissociated cells embedded in Matrigel)[98–100] cultures derived from primary tumors may provide innovative screening platforms that recapture the possible effects of the tumor microenvironments but overcome the challenges encountered in screening with PDXs, including the cost, time, and large quantities of agents required for in vivo studies. Several studies of organotypic and organoid cultures have demonstrated the feasibility of using culture technologies to test the treatment responses of various drugs in vitro with native tumor microenvironments. For large-scale screening, renewable tumor tissue resources will be required. The ability to expand human tumor tissues in PDXs will provide a constant supply of relatively large amounts of the same tumor tissue for in vitro library screening with organotypic or organoid cultures.

CHALLENGES AND PERSPECTIVES

Although PDXs emerged as promising cancer models that recapture many characteristics of cancers observed in clinics, they also have intrinsic limitations that impose challenges for various studies. One of the noticeable limitations is the cost and time required for generating PDXs and relatively low engraftment rate, which may limit their clinical application in identifying effective regimens for most cancer patients. Although it is feasible to select treatment regimens based on the treatment responses of their PDXs[35,36] to improve the precision therapy, the time required for establishing the first generation of PDXs (usually several months) and the low success rates can be limiting factors for the broad implementation of PDX-based personalized therapy. Moreover, in vivo drug activity studies will require a large quantity of testing agents and a large number of animals, which will drastically increase the testing cost. Some studies have shown that testing on patient-derived cancer tissues and/or cells cultured in vitro may identify effective treatment regimens for cancer patients.[101,102] In comparison with PDXs models, in vitro cultured patient-derived tumor models may provide a quicker and more cost-effective drug sensitivity test. Recently, several groups have shown that patient-derived organoids cultured in vitro may also recapture certain characteristics of primary cancers in vivo, including heterogeneity and genetic alterations, and can be used for drug sensitivity test.[100,103,104] We expect that PDXs and organoids may become complementary platforms of patient-derived tumor models that may change clinical practice in oncology.

Success in immunotherapy with immune checkpoint inhibitors has revolutionized clinical practice in the treatment of lung cancer. The high mutation rates observed in lung cancers[15] make this deadly disease particularly vulnerable to immunotherapy.[105] A recent clinical trial revealed that the risk of death in patients with advanced squamous cell non–small cell lung cancer treated with anti–PD-1 monoclonal antibody nivolumab was 41% lower than those treated with docetaxel.[106] Anti–PD-1 antibodies nivolumab[106–108] and pembrolizumab[105,109] were approved recently for the treatment of NSCLC in the United States. Nevertheless, despite the breakthrough in the immunotherapy with anti–PD-1[105–109] and anti–PD-L1[110–112] antibodies, and the promising results observed in various clinical trials with anti-PD therapy in lung cancer patients, the overall objective response rates in all NSCLC patients receiving anti-PD therapy are approximately 15–20%.[105–107,109–111] Thus, multimodality treatment regimens that may enhance anticancer immunotherapy are expected to be a new area of future studies. Nevertheless, all PDXs are generated in immunocompromised mice, which will limit their applications in evaluating the roles of adaptive and innate immune systems in cancer progression and anticancer therapies. Cotransplantation of human immune system components in PDX-bearing mice may solve some of the limitations. Cotransplantation of human cancer cells and functional human immune cells has been investigated by several groups.[113] Peripheral blood cells, $CD34^+$ human hematopoietic stem cells, and human cord blood cells may be used for this purpose. Possible limitations from these so-called humanized mice models are the development of graft-versus-host disease (GVHD), and/or allogeneic graft versus tumor activity caused by HLA mismatch if the lymphocytes and PDX are not derived from the same person. A recent study revealed that functional loss of Kit receptor increased the receptiveness of NSG mice for human hematopoietic stem cells engraftment, suggesting that GVHD might be ameliorated in immune-deficient mouse strains containing Kit mutations.[114] An alternative approach to evaluate roles of immune system is to induce immune tolerance to human cancer cells/tissues in immunocompetent mice. This may be accomplished by microinjecting human cancer cells or PDX tumor tissue into mouse embryos. Injecting human cancer cell lines into early-stage mouse blastocytes is reported to induce central immune tolerance and produce immunocompetent mice bearing human tumors.[115]

CONCLUSION

The enthusiasm of using PDXs for preclinical studies, particularly for evaluation of in vivo drug efficacy, is growing. The ability to expand human tumor tissues in PDXs will provide a constant supply of relatively large amounts of the same tumor tissue for mechanistic characterization, biomarker discovery, target identification, drug discovery and development, and personalized therapy in clinics. Because of the heterogeneity of human cancers, a large collection or bank of PDXs with comprehensive molecular characterizations is needed for various translational research projects. Nevertheless, generating PDXs is cost and time-consuming. Although many groups have recently reported their success in establishing lung cancer PDXs, access to desirable PDX models for preclinical studies still remains a major barrier for most academic and pharmaceutical industrial investigators. Efforts that promote collaborations and sharing of PDX resources should be encouraged. Lack of immune microenvironment is one of major barrier for using PDXs to assess immunotherapy or roles of immune system in anticancer drug development. Although future technology development in humanized mouse models may solve some of the hurdles, alternative tumor models will be also required for many preclinical and clinical applications.

REFERENCES

1. GBD 2013 Mortality and Causes of Death Collaborators. Global, regional, and national age-sex specific all-cause and cause-specific mortality for 240 causes of death, 1990–2013: a systematic analysis for the Global Burden of Disease Study 2013. *Lancet* 2015;**385**:117–71.
2. Torre LA, Bray F, Siegel RL, Ferlay J, Lortet-Tieulent J, Jemal A. Global cancer statistics, 2012. *CA Cancer J Clin* 2015;**65**:87–108.
3. Ferlay J, Soerjomataram I, Dikshit R, Eser S, Mathers C, Rebelo M, et al. Cancer incidence and mortality worldwide: sources, methods and major patterns in GLOBOCAN 2012. *Int J Cancer* 2015;**136**:E359–86.
4. Herbst RS, Heymach JV, Lippman SM. Lung cancer. *N Engl J Med* 2008;**359**:1367–80.

5. Seow WJ, Hu W, Vermeulen R, Hosgood Iii HD, Downward GS, Chapman RS, et al. Household air pollution and lung cancer in China: a review of studies in Xuanwei. *Chin J Cancer* 2014;**33**:471–5.
6. Hoek G, Raaschou-Nielsen O. Impact of fine particles in ambient air on lung cancer. *Chin J Cancer* 2014;**33**:197–203.
7. Loomis D, Huang W, Chen G. The International Agency for Research on Cancer (IARC) evaluation of the carcinogenicity of outdoor air pollution: focus on China. *Chin J Cancer* 2014;**33**:189–96.
8. Global Burden of Disease Cancer Collaboration, Fitzmaurice C, Dicker D, Pain A, Hamavid H, Moradi-Lakeh M, et al. The global burden of cancer 2013. *JAMA Oncol* 2015;**1**:505–27.
9. Edwards BK, Ward E, Kohler BA, Eheman C, Zauber AG, Anderson RN, et al. Annual report to the nation on the status of cancer, 1975–2006, featuring colorectal cancer trends and impact of interventions (risk factors, screening, and treatment) to reduce future rates. *Cancer* 2010;**116**:544–73.
10. Unger M. A pause, progress, and reassessment in lung cancer screening. *N Engl J Med* 2006;**355**:1822–4.
11. Surveillance Epidemiology and End Results Program. *Cancer of the lung and bronchus*. 2014. http://seer.cancer.gov/csr/1975_2011/results_merged/sect_15_lung_ bronchus.pdf.
12. Edwards BK, Noone AM, Mariotto AB, Simard EP, Boscoe FP, Henley SJ, et al. Annual report to the nation on the status of cancer, 1975–2010, featuring prevalence of comorbidity and impact on survival among persons with lung, colorectal, breast, or prostate cancer. *Cancer* 2014;**120**:1290–314.
13. DeSantis CE, Lin CC, Mariotto AB, Siegel RL, Stein KD, Kramer JL, et al. Cancer treatment and survivorship statistics, 2014. *CA Cancer J Clin* 2014;**64**:252–71.
14. Fang B, Mehran RJ, Heymach JV, Swisher SG. Predictive biomarkers in precision medicine and drug development against lung cancer. *Chin J Cancer* 2015;**34**:26.
15. Vogelstein B, Papadopoulos N, Velculescu VE, Zhou S, Diaz Jr LA, Kinzler KW. Cancer genome landscapes. *Science* 2013;**339**:1546–58.
16. Lu H, Wang L, Gao W, Meng J, Dai B, Wu S, et al. IGFBP2/FAK pathway is causally associated with dasatinib resistance in non-small cell lung cancer cells. *Mol Cancer Ther* 2013;**12**:2864–73.
17. Director's Challenge Consortium for the Molecular Classification of Lung Adenocarcinoma, Shedden K, Taylor JM, Enkemann SA, Tsao MS, Yeatman TJ, et al. Gene expression-based survival prediction in lung adenocarcinoma: a multi-site, blinded validation study. *Nat Med* 2008;**14**:822–7.
18. Cardnell RJ, Feng Y, Diao L, Fan YH, Masrorpour F, Wang J, et al. Proteomic markers of DNA repair and PI3K pathway activation predict response to the PARP inhibitor BMN 673 in small cell lung cancer. *Clin Cancer Res* 2013;**19**:6322–8.
19. Travis WD, Brambilla E, Riely GJ. New pathologic classification of lung cancer: relevance for clinical practice and clinical trials. *J Clin Oncol* 2013;**31**:992–1001.
20. Ding L, Getz G, Wheeler DA, Mardis ER, McLellan MD, Cibulskis K, et al. Somatic mutations affect key pathways in lung adenocarcinoma. *Nature* 2008;**455**:1069–75.
21. Govindan R, Ding L, Griffith M, Subramanian J, Dees ND, Kanchi KL, et al. Genomic landscape of non-small cell lung cancer in smokers and never-smokers. *Cell* 2012;**150**:1121–34.
22. Soda M, Isobe K, Inoue A, Maemondo M, Oizumi S, Fujita Y, et al. A prospective PCR-based screening for the EML4-ALK oncogene in non-small cell lung cancer. *Clin Cancer Res* 2012;**18**:5682–9.
23. Garber K. From human to mouse and back: 'tumorgraft' models surge in popularity. *J Natl Cancer Inst* 2009;**101**:6–8.

24. Johnson JI, Decker S, Zaharevitz D, Rubinstein LV, Venditti JM, Schepartz S, et al. Relationships between drug activity in NCI preclinical in vitro and in vivo models and early clinical trials. *Br J Cancer* 2001;**84**:1424–31.
25. Voskoglou-Nomikos T, Pater JL, Seymour L. Clinical predictive value of the in vitro cell line, human xenograft, and mouse allograft preclinical cancer models. *Clin Cancer Res* 2003;**9**:4227–39.
26. Kola I. The state of innovation in drug development. *Clin Pharmacol Ther* 2008;**83**:227–30.
27. Ellis LM, Fidler IJ. Finding the tumor copycat. Therapy fails, patients don't. *Nat Med* 2010;**16**:974–5.
28. Sivanand S, Pena-Llopis S, Zhao H, Kucejova B, Spence P, Pavia-Jimenez A, et al. A validated tumorgraft model reveals activity of dovitinib against renal cell carcinoma. *Sci Transl Med* 2012;**4**:137ra75.
29. John T, Kohler D, Pintilie M, Yanagawa N, Pham NA, Li M, et al. The ability to form primary tumor xenografts is predictive of increased risk of disease recurrence in early-stage non-small cell lung cancer. *Clin Cancer Res* 2011;**17**:134–41.
30. Rubio-Viqueira B, Jimeno A, Cusatis G, Zhang X, Iacobuzio-Donahue C, Karikari C, et al. An in vivo platform for translational drug development in pancreatic cancer. *Clin Cancer Res* 2006;**12**:4652–61.
31. Julien S, Merino-Trigo A, Lacroix L, Pocard M, Goere D, Mariani P, et al. Characterization of a large panel of patient-derived tumor xenografts representing the clinical heterogeneity of human colorectal cancer. *Clin Cancer Res* 2012;**18**:5314–28.
32. Dong X, Guan J, English JC, Flint J, Yee J, Evans K, et al. Patient-derived first generation xenografts of non-small cell lung cancers: promising tools for predicting drug responses for personalized chemotherapy. *Clin Cancer Res* 2010;**16**:1442–51.
33. Bertotti A, Migliardi G, Galimi F, Sassi F, Torti D, Isella C, et al. A molecularly annotated platform of patient-derived xenografts ("xenopatients") identifies HER2 as an effective therapeutic target in cetuximab-resistant colorectal cancer. *Cancer Discov* 2011;**1**:508–23.
34. Perez-Soler R, Kemp B, Wu QP, Mao L, Gomez J, Zeleniuch-Jacquotte A, et al. Response and determinants of sensitivity to paclitaxel in human non-small cell lung cancer tumors heterotransplanted in nude mice. *Clin Cancer Res* 2000;**6**:4932–8.
35. Hidalgo M, Bruckheimer E, Rajeshkumar NV, Garrido-Laguna I, De OE, Rubio-Viqueira B, et al. A pilot clinical study of treatment guided by personalized tumorgrafts in patients with advanced cancer. *Mol Cancer Ther* 2011;**10**:1311–6.
36. Morelli MP, Calvo E, Ordonez E, Wick MJ, Viqueira BR, Lopez-Casas PP, et al. Prioritizing phase I treatment options through preclinical testing on personalized tumorgraft. *J Clin Oncol* 2012;**30**:e45–8.
37. Hao C, Wang L, Peng S, Cao M, Li H, Hu J, et al. Gene mutations in primary tumors and corresponding patient-derived xenografts derived from non-small cell lung cancer. *Cancer Lett* 2015;**357**:179–85.
38. Fichtner I, Rolff J, Soong R, Hoffmann J, Hammer S, Sommer A, et al. Establishment of patient-derived non-small cell lung cancer xenografts as models for the identification of predictive biomarkers. *Clin Cancer Res* 2008;**14**:6456–68.
39. Devaud C, Westwood JA, John LB, Flynn JK, Paquet-Fifield S, Duong CP, et al. Tissues in different anatomical sites can sculpt and vary the tumor microenvironment to affect responses to therapy. *Mol Ther* 2014;**22**:18–27.
40. Kang Y, Omura M, Suzuki A, Oka T, Nakagami Y, Cheng C, et al. Development of an orthotopic transplantation model in nude mice that simulates the clinical features of human lung cancer. *Cancer Sci* 2006;**97**:996–1001.

41. Killion JJ, Radinsky R, Fidler IJ. Orthotopic models are necessary to predict therapy of transplantable tumors in mice. *Cancer Metastasis Rev* 1998;**17**:279–84.
42. Zhao X, Liu Z, Yu L, Zhang Y, Baxter P, Voicu H, et al. Global gene expression profiling confirms the molecular fidelity of primary tumor-based orthotopic xenograft mouse models of medulloblastoma. *Neuro-Oncology* 2012;**14**:574–83.
43. Onn A, Isobe T, Itasaka S, Wu W, O'Reilly MS, Ki HW, et al. Development of an orthotopic model to study the biology and therapy of primary human lung cancer in nude mice. *Clin Cancer Res* 2003;**9**:5532–9.
44. Ao MH, Zhang H, Sakowski L, Sharma R, Illei PB, Gabrielson E, et al. The utility of a novel triple marker (combination of TTF1, napsin A, and p40) in the subclassification of non-small cell lung cancer. *Hum Pathol* 2014;**45**:926–34.
45. Mukhopadhyay S, Katzenstein AL. Subclassification of non-small cell lung carcinomas lacking morphologic differentiation on biopsy specimens: utility of an immunohistochemical panel containing TTF-1, napsin A, p63, and CK5/6. *Am J Surg Pathol* 2011;**35**:15–25.
46. Imielinski M, Berger AH, Hammerman PS, Hernandez B, Pugh TJ, Hodis E, et al. Mapping the hallmarks of lung adenocarcinoma with massively parallel sequencing. *Cell* 2012;**150**:1107–20.
47. Cancer Genome Atlas Research Network. Comprehensive molecular profiling of lung adenocarcinoma. *Nature* 2014;**511**:543–50.
48. Cancer Genome Atlas Research Network, Hammerman PS, Hayes DN, Wilkerson MD, Schultz N, Bose R, et al. Comprehensive genomic characterization of squamous cell lung cancers. *Nature* 2012;**489**:519–25.
49. Rudin CM, Durinck S, Stawiski EW, Poirier JT, Modrusan Z, Shames DS, et al. Comprehensive genomic analysis identifies SOX2 as a frequently amplified gene in small-cell lung cancer. *Nat Genet* 2012;**44**:1111–6.
50. Peifer M, Fernandez-Cuesta L, Sos ML, George J, Seidel D, Kasper LH, et al. Integrative genome analyses identify key somatic driver mutations of small-cell lung cancer. *Nat Genet* 2012;**44**:1104–10.
51. Fernandez-Cuesta L. Frequent mutations in chromatin-remodelling genes in pulmonary carcinoids. *Nat Commun* 2014;**5**:3518.
52. El-Telbany A, Ma PC. Cancer genes in lung cancer: racial disparities: are there any? *Genes Cancer* 2012;**3**:467–80.
53. Broet P. Genomic profiles specific to patient ethnicity in lung adenocarcinoma. *Clin Cancer Res* 2011;**17**:3542–50.
54. Rosell R, Moran T, Queralt C, Porta R, Cardenal F, Camps C, et al. Screening for epidermal growth factor receptor mutations in lung cancer. *N Engl J Med* 2009;**361**:958–67.
55. Pao W, Miller V, Zakowski M, Doherty J, Politi K, Sarkaria I, et al. EGF receptor gene mutations are common in lung cancers from "never smokers" and are associated with sensitivity of tumors to gefitinib and erlotinib. *Proc Natl Acad Sci USA* 2004;**101**:13306–11.
56. Marchetti A, Martella C, Felicioni L, Barassi F, Salvatore S, Chella A, et al. EGFR mutations in non-small-cell lung cancer: analysis of a large series of cases and development of a rapid and sensitive method for diagnostic screening with potential implications on pharmacologic treatment. *J Clin Oncol* 2005;**23**:857–65.
57. Gahr S, Stoehr R, Geissinger E, Ficker JH, Brueckl WM, Gschwendtner A, et al. EGFR mutational status in a large series of Caucasian European NSCLC patients: data from daily practice. *Br J Cancer* 2013;**109**:1821–8.
58. Choi YL, Sun JM, Cho J, Rampal S, Han J, Parasuraman B, et al. EGFR mutation testing in patients with advanced non-small cell lung cancer: a comprehensive evaluation of real-world practice in an East Asian tertiary hospital. *PLoS One* 2013;**8**:e56011.

59. Li C, Fang R, Sun Y, Han X, Li F, Gao B, et al. Spectrum of oncogenic driver mutations in lung adenocarcinomas from East Asian never smokers. *PLoS One* 2011;**6**:e28204.
60. Gao B, Sun Y, Zhang J, Ren Y, Fang R, Han X, et al. Spectrum of LKB1, EGFR, and KRAS mutations in Chinese lung adenocarcinomas. *J Thorac Oncol* 2010;**5**:1130–5.
61. Tanaka T, Matsuoka M, Sutani A, Gemma A, Maemondo M, Inoue A, et al. Frequency of and variables associated with the EGFR mutation and its subtypes. *Int J Cancer* 2010;**126**:651–5.
62. Mills NE, Fishman CL, Rom WN, Dubin N, Jacobson DR. Increased prevalence of K-ras oncogene mutations in lung adenocarcinoma. *Cancer Res* 1995;**55**:1444–7.
63. Sun Y. Lung adenocarcinoma from East Asian never-smokers is a disease largely defined by targetable oncogenic mutant kinases. *J Clin Oncol* 2010;**28**:4616–20.
64. Ilie M, Nunes M, Blot L, Hofman V, Long-Mira E, Butori C, et al. Setting up a wide panel of patient-derived tumor xenografts of non-small cell lung cancer by improving the preanalytical steps. *Cancer Med* 2015;**4**:201–11.
65. Zhang XC, Zhang J, Li M, Huang XS, Yang XN, Zhong WZ, et al. Establishment of patient-derived non-small cell lung cancer xenograft models with genetic aberrations within EGFR, KRAS and FGFR1: useful tools for preclinical studies of targeted therapies. *J Transl Med* 2013;**11**:168.
66. Stewart EL, Mascaux C, Pham NA, Sakashita S, Sykes J, Kim L, et al. Clinical utility of patient-derived xenografts to determine biomarkers of prognosis and map resistance pathways in EGFR-mutant lung adenocarcinoma. *J Clin Oncol* 2015;**33**:2472–80.
67. Lee HW, Lee JI, Lee SJ, Cho HJ, Song HJ, Jeong da E., et al. Patient-derived xenografts from non-small cell lung cancer brain metastases are valuable translational platforms for the development of personalized targeted therapy. *Clin Cancer Res* 2015;**21**:1172–82.
68. Leong TL, Marini KD, Rossello FJ, Jayasekara SN, Russell PA, Prodanovic Z, et al. Genomic characterisation of small cell lung cancer patient-derived xenografts generated from endobronchial ultrasound-guided transbronchial needle aspiration specimens. *PLoS One* 2014;**9**:e106862.
69. Anderson WC, Boyd MB, Aguilar J, Pickell B, Laysang A, Pysz MA, et al. Initiation and characterization of small cell lung cancer patient-derived xenografts from ultrasound-guided transbronchial needle aspirates. *PLoS One* 2015;**10**:e0125255.
70. Nakajima T, Geddie W, Anayama T, Ko HM, da Cunha SG, Boerner S, et al. Patient-derived tumor xenograft models established from samples obtained by endobronchial ultrasound-guided transbronchial needle aspiration. *Lung Cancer* 2015;**89**:110–4.
71. Lynch TJ, Bell DW, Sordella R, Gurubhagavatula S, Okimoto RA, Brannigan BW, et al. Activating mutations in the epidermal growth factor receptor underlying responsiveness of non-small-cell lung cancer to gefitinib. *N Engl J Med* 2004;**350**:2129–39.
72. Paez JG, Janne PA, Lee JC, Tracy S, Greulich H, Gabriel S, et al. EGFR mutations in lung cancer: correlation with clinical response to gefitinib therapy. *Science* 2004;**304**:1497–500.
73. Shepherd FA, Rodrigues PJ, Ciuleanu T, Tan EH, Hirsh V, Thongprasert S, et al. Erlotinib in previously treated non-small-cell lung cancer. *N Engl J Med* 2005;**353**:123–32.
74. Cappuzzo F, Ciuleanu T, Stelmakh L, Cicenas S, Szczesna A, Juhasz E, et al. Erlotinib as maintenance treatment in advanced non-small-cell lung cancer: a multicentre, randomised, placebo-controlled phase 3 study. *Lancet Oncol* 2010;**11**:521–9.
75. Fukuoka M, Wu YL, Thongprasert S, Sunpaweravong P, Leong SS, Sriuranpong V, et al. Biomarker analyses and final overall survival results from a phase III, randomized, open-label, first-line study of gefitinib versus carboplatin/paclitaxel in clinically selected patients with advanced non-small-cell lung cancer in Asia (IPASS). *J Clin Oncol* 2011;**29**:2866–74.
76. Thatcher N, Chang A, Parikh P, Rodrigues PJ, Ciuleanu T, von PJ, et al. Gefitinib plus best supportive care in previously treated patients with refractory advanced non-small-cell lung cancer: results from a randomised, placebo-controlled, multicentre study (Iressa Survival Evaluation in Lung Cancer). *Lancet* 2005;**366**:1527–37.

77. Shaw AT, Kim DW, Nakagawa K, Seto T, Crino L, Ahn MJ, et al. Crizotinib versus chemotherapy in advanced ALK-positive lung cancer. *N Engl J Med* 2013;**368**:2385–94.
78. Shaw AT, Kim DW, Mehra R, Tan DS, Felip E, Chow LQ, et al. Ceritinib in ALK-rearranged non-small-cell lung cancer. *N Engl J Med* 2014;**370**:1189–97.
79. Davare MA, Saborowski A, Eide CA, Tognon C, Smith RL, Elferich J, et al. Foretinib is a potent inhibitor of oncogenic ROS1 fusion proteins. *Proc Natl Acad Sci USA* 2013;**110**:19519–24.
80. Bergethon K, Shaw AT, Ou SH, Katayama R, Lovly CM, McDonald NT, et al. ROS1 rearrangements define a unique molecular class of lung cancers. *J Clin Oncol* 2012;**30**:863–70.
81. Gainor JF, Varghese AM, Ou SH, Kabraji S, Awad MM, Katayama R, et al. ALK rearrangements are mutually exclusive with mutations in EGFR or KRAS: an analysis of 1,683 patients with non-small cell lung cancer. *Clin Cancer Res* 2013;**19**:4273–81.
82. Solomon B. ALK gene rearrangements: a new therapeutic target in a molecularly defined subset of non-small cell lung cancer. *J Thorac Oncol* 2009;**4**:1450–4.
83. Rodig SJ. Unique clinicopathologic features characterize ALK-rearranged lung adenocarcinoma in the western population. [Erratum appears in *Clin Cancer Res* November 15, 2009;**15**(22):7110] *Clin Cancer Res* 2009;**15**:5216–23.
84. Shaw AT, Yeap BY, Mino-Kenudson M, Digumarthy SR, Costa DB, Heist RS, et al. Clinical features and outcome of patients with non-small-cell lung cancer who harbor EML4-ALK. *J Clin Oncol* 2009;**27**:4247–53.
85. Pan Y, Zhang Y, Li Y, Hu H, Wang L, Li H, et al. ALK, ROS1 and RET fusions in 1139 lung adenocarcinomas: a comprehensive study of common and fusion pattern-specific clinicopathologic, histologic and cytologic features. *Lung Cancer* 2014;**84**:121–6.
86. Davies KD, Le AT, Theodoro MF, Skokan MC, Aisner DL, Berge EM, et al. Identifying and targeting ROS1 gene fusions in non-small cell lung cancer. *Clin Cancer Res* 2012;**18**:4570–9.
87. Lopez-Chavez A, Thomas A, Rajan A, Raffeld M, Morrow B, Kelly R, et al. Molecular profiling and targeted therapy for advanced thoracic malignancies: a biomarker-derived, multiarm, multihistology phase II basket trial. *J Clin Oncol* 2015;**33**:1000–7.
88. Kola I, Landis J. Can the pharmaceutical industry reduce attrition rates? *Nat Rev Drug Discov* 2004;**3**:711–5.
89. Arrowsmith J. Trial watch: phase III and submission failures: 2007–2010. *Nat Rev Drug Discov* 2011;**10**:87.
90. Arrowsmith J. Trial watch: phase II failures: 2008–2010. *Nat Rev Drug Discov* 2011;**10**:328–9.
91. Yang M, Shan B, Li Q, Song X, Cai J, Deng J, et al. Overcoming erlotinib resistance with tailored treatment regimen in patient-derived xenografts from naive Asian NSCLC patients. *Int J Cancer* 2013;**132**:E74–84.
92. Belmont PJ, Jiang P, McKee TD, Xie T, Isaacson J, Baryla NE, et al. Resistance to dual blockade of the kinases PI3K and mTOR in KRAS-mutant colorectal cancer models results in combined sensitivity to inhibition of the receptor tyrosine kinase EGFR. *Sci STKE* 2014;**7**:ra107.
93. Fang B. Genetic interactions in translational research on cancer. *World J Med Genet* 2011;**1**:14–22.
94. Fang B. Development of synthetic lethality anticancer therapeutics. *J Med Chem* 2014;**57**:7859–73.
95. Guo Z, Fang B. Synthetic lethality in anticancer drug discovery and target identification. *Pharmacologia* 2012;**3**:352–61.
96. Fang B. Genetic interactions of STAT3 and anticancer drug development. *Cancers* 2014;**6**:494–525.
97. Vaira V, Fedele G, Pyne S, Fasoli E, Zadra G, Bailey D, et al. Preclinical model of organotypic culture for pharmacodynamic profiling of human tumors. *Proc Natl Acad Sci USA* 2010;**107**:8352–6.

98. Sato T, Stange DE, Ferrante M, Vries RG, van Es JH, Van den Brink S, et al. Long-term expansion of epithelial organoids from human colon, adenoma, adenocarcinoma, and Barrett's epithelium. *Gastroenterology* 2011;**141**:1762–72.
99. Dye BR, Hill DR, Ferguson MA, Tsai YH, Nagy MS, Dyal R, et al. In vitro generation of human pluripotent stem cell derived lung organoids. *eLife* 2015;**4**.
100. Gao D, Vela I, Sboner A, Iaquinta PJ, Karthaus WR, Gopalan A, et al. Organoid cultures derived from patients with advanced prostate cancer. *Cell* 2014;**159**:176–87.
101. Yuan H, Myers S, Wang J, Zhou D, Woo JA, Kallakury B, et al. Use of reprogrammed cells to identify therapy for respiratory papillomatosis. *N Engl J Med* 2012;**367**:1220–7.
102. Crystal AS, Shaw AT, Sequist LV, Friboulet L, Niederst MJ, Lockerman EL, et al. Patient-derived models of acquired resistance can identify effective drug combinations for cancer. *Science* 2014;**346**:1480–6.
103. van de Wetering M, Francies HE, Francis JM, Bounova G, Iorio F, Pronk A, et al. Prospective derivation of a living organoid biobank of colorectal cancer patients. *Cell* 2015;**161**:933–45.
104. Boj SF, Hwang CI, Baker LA, Chio II, Engle DD, Corbo V, et al. Organoid models of human and mouse ductal pancreatic cancer. *Cell* 2015;**160**:324–38.
105. Rizvi NA, Hellmann MD, Snyder A, Kvistborg P, Makarov V, Havel JJ, et al. Cancer immunology. Mutational landscape determines sensitivity to PD-1 blockade in non-small cell lung cancer. *Science* 2015;**348**:124–8.
106. Brahmer J, Reckamp KL, Baas P, Crino L, Eberhardt WE, Poddubskaya E, et al. Nivolumab versus docetaxel in advanced squamous-cell non-small-cell lung cancer. *N Engl J Med* 2015;**373**:123–35.
107. Gettinger SN, Horn L, Gandhi L, Spigel DR, Antonia SJ, Rizvi NA, et al. Overall survival and long-term safety of nivolumab (anti-programmed death 1 antibody, BMS-936558, ONO-4538) in patients with previously treated advanced non-small-cell lung cancer. *J Clin Oncol* 2015;**33**:2004–12.
108. Rizvi NA, Mazieres J, Planchard D, Stinchcombe TE, Dy GK, Antonia SJ, et al. Activity and safety of nivolumab, an anti-PD-1 immune checkpoint inhibitor, for patients with advanced, refractory squamous non-small-cell lung cancer (CheckMate 063): a phase 2, single-arm trial. *Lancet Oncol* 2015;**16**:257–65.
109. Garon EB, Rizvi NA, Hui R, Leighl N, Balmanoukian AS, Eder JP, et al. Pembrolizumab for the treatment of non-small-cell lung cancer. *N Engl J Med* 2015;**372**:2018–28.
110. Brahmer JR, Tykodi SS, Chow LQ, Hwu WJ, Topalian SL, Hwu P, et al. Safety and activity of anti-PD-L1 antibody in patients with advanced cancer. *N Engl J Med* 2012;**366**:2455–65.
111. Herbst RS, Soria JC, Kowanetz M, Fine GD, Hamid O, Gordon MS, et al. Predictive correlates of response to the anti-PD-L1 antibody MPDL3280A in cancer patients. *Nature* 2014;**515**:563–7.
112. Chen L, Han X. Anti-PD-1/PD-L1 therapy of human cancer: past, present, and future. *J Clin Invest* 2015;**125**:3384–91.
113. Holzapfel BM, Wagner F, Thibaudeau L, Levesque JP, Hutmacher DW. Concise review: humanized models of tumor immunology in the 21st century: convergence of cancer research and tissue engineering. *Stem Cells* 2015;**33**:1696–704.
114. Cosgun KN, Rahmig S, Mende N, Reinke S, Hauber I, Schafer C, et al. Kit regulates HSC engraftment across the human-mouse species barrier. *Cell Stem Cell* 2014;**15**:227–38.
115. Chen HJ, Sun J, Huang Z, Hou Jr H, Arcilla M, Rakhilin N, et al. Comprehensive models of human primary and metastatic colorectal tumors in immunodeficient and immunocompetent mice by chemokine targeting. *Nat Biotechnol* 2015;**33**:656–60.

Chapter 7

PDX Models of Colorectal Tumors

J.P. MacKeigan, D.M. Burgenske

Center for Cancer and Cell Biology, Van Andel Research Institute, Grand Rapids, MI, United States

BACKGROUND AND OVERVIEW

Colorectal cancer (CRC) is the second leading cause of cancer-related deaths with 50,310 estimated deaths in the United States alone.[1] An additional 1.2 million patients are living with a history of CRC.[1] Treatment commonly involves surgical resection, chemotherapy, and/or radiation. Although these treatments are a mainstay in the clinical management of CRC, they lack selectivity and cause many adverse side effects.[2] As a result, researchers and physician-scientists are searching for molecularly targeted agents with improved efficacy, potency, and heightened safety profiles. As with many other cancers, CRC patients have the best prognosis when the disease is detected in early stages.[3] Unfortunately, patients with metastatic CRC face 5-year survival rates as low as 10%, roughly 80% lower than patients with localized stage I disease.[3] This unmet medical need, and the quest for more effective therapeutic agents, emphasizes the importance of relevant preclinical CRC models.

METHODOLOGY AND MODELS

Established protocols to create patient-derived xenograft (PDX) models of CRC exist. First, tissue fragments are acquired in collaboration with a skilled colorectal surgeon, pathologist, and health care system. Specimens with corresponding deidentified patient health records are valuable for extracting meaningful clinical data, such as family history, tumor staging, treatments, and survival data. Immediately after surgical resection, patient tumors are engrafted as a tumor fragment or dissociated to prepare single-cell suspensions. Ideally, direct tumor engraftment preserves the three-dimensional structure and maintains cell–cell interactions important in colorectal tumor architecture. In many instances, cell lines can also be established from these tumors. Determining the best PDX method (direct implantation vs cell suspension) depends upon the specific goal of

Patient Derived Tumor Xenograft Models. http://dx.doi.org/10.1016/B978-0-12-804010-2.00021-7

the research. Although direct engraftment of the resected patient tumors maintains the architectural integrity of the specimen, the overall tumor composition (eg, ratio of viable cells to necrotic debris) can vary, particularly if some samples are resected following treatment. Conversely, tumor dissociation provides researchers with a consistent engraftment method, which focuses on delivering an optimal number of viable cells. Moreover, different pieces of the same patient tumor may also possess different genetic or epigenetic features that could affect the course of disease. While the use of isolated cells may address this concern, the loss of tumor architecture could significantly affect subsequent drug studies.

Within the published CRC PDX literature, engrafting the intact tumor fragment is more common, largely due to the preservation of tumor and stromal architectures (Table 7.1). In select instances, researchers use Matrigel matrix, a gelatinous protein mixture composed of laminin, collagen, entactin, and proteoglycans, as a scaffold to mimic the extracellular matrix. This additive provides further sustenance to tumor fragments during engraftment. Additionally, some Matrigel formulations contain growth factors to promote differentiation and proliferation of the various cell types.[4] Within one metastatic CRC PDX model, primary tumors were dissociated and prepared with Matrigel for engraftment into nonobese diabetic-severe combined immunodeficient (NOD-SCID) mice.[5] A comparison of 12 paired samples of primary and xenograft tissues revealed the same mutational pattern, which included CRC-relevant alterations to *KRAS*, *PIK3CA*, *BRAF*, and *APC*.[5] The study authors report that the use of isolated primary cells for PDX models enhances take rate and promotes a higher degree of tumor heterogeneity than those seen using established cell lines. To avoid host immune rejection of patient-derived tumor specimens, immunodeficient mouse strains are commonly used. It is not known if a single mouse strain is superior; however, the majority of CRC PDX models are engrafted onto the *nu/nu* background. Although strain differences do not affect the engraftment efficacy, they can impact the tumor growth rate, at least within the context of solid tumors.[6] Studies have also reported that the engraftment efficacy can be linked to the patient's initial disease severity as cases of advanced disease show better engraftment rates.[5,7,8] As for engraftment location, CRC PDX models have been almost exclusively heterotopic, with the most common site being the subcutaneous flank; while orthotopic engraftment studies allow for metastatic lesions to be analyzed.[5,9,10] Historically, engraftment near the colon results in growth at the primary site and metastatic sites, predominantly to the liver, lung, and lymph nodes.[5,10,11] Successful implementation of orthotopic models requires a higher degree of technical precision, as tumor cells must be carefully embedded into the colon's outer wall.[5]

Upon resection of the xenograft-derived tumors, fragments are commonly flash frozen in liquid nitrogen and stored for later use, or chemically fixed (most often in formalin) for subsequent histological evaluation. Confirming the presence of clinical CRC hallmarks is the next crucial step when establishing and characterizing PDX models (Fig. 7.1). Most often, this is accomplished

TABLE 7.1 Patient-Derived Tumor Xenograft Models of Colorectal Tumors

Samples Implanted (N)	Tumor Origin	Mouse Strain	Implantation Techniques	Success Rate (%)	Tumor Heterogeneity	References
50	Primary	NOD-SCID	Heterotopic	20	Yes	20
48	Primary	NOD-SCID	Heterotopic	74	Yes	35
45	Primary	*nu/nu*	Heterotopic	36	Yes	29
23	Primary	Nude	Heterotopic	n.d.	n.d.	25
21	Primary	*nu/nu*	Heterotopic	14	Yes	36
10	Primary	BALB/c *nu/nu*, NOD-SCID	Heterotopic	100	Yes	7
7	Primary	*nu/nu*	Heterotopic	n.d.	Yes	37
3	Primary	NOD-SCID	Heterotopic	n.d.	n.d.	38
241	Primary, metastasis	BALB/c *nu/nu*	Heterotopic	62	n.d.	39
143	Primary, metastasis	BALB/c *nu/nu*	Heterotopic	67	Yes	40
85	Primary, metastasis	*nu/nu*, SCID	Orthotopic	64	Yes	41,42
48	Primary, metastasis	*nu/nu*	Heterotopic	100	n.d.	28

Continued

TABLE 7.1 Patient-Derived Tumor Xenograft Models of Colorectal Tumors—cont'd

Samples Implanted (N)	Tumor Origin	Mouse Strain	Implantation Techniques	Success Rate (%)	Tumor Heterogeneity	References
40	Primary, metastasis	NOD-SCID	Heterotopic, orthotopic	88	Yes	5
27	Primary, metastasis	NSG	Heterotopic	n.d.	Yes	43
27	Primary, metastasis	NOD-SCID	Heterotopic	n.d.	Yes	44
26	Primary, metastasis	*nu/nu*	Heterotopic	77	Yes	8
18	Primary, metastasis	NOD-SCID, NCR	Heterotopic	n.d.	Yes	45
15	Primary, metastasis	*nu/nu*	Heterotopic	n.d.	Yes	19
150	Metastasis	NOD-SCID	Heterotopic	87	Yes	13,14,46
40	Metastasis	NOD-SCID	Heterotopic	n.d.	n.d.	13

n.d., not determined.

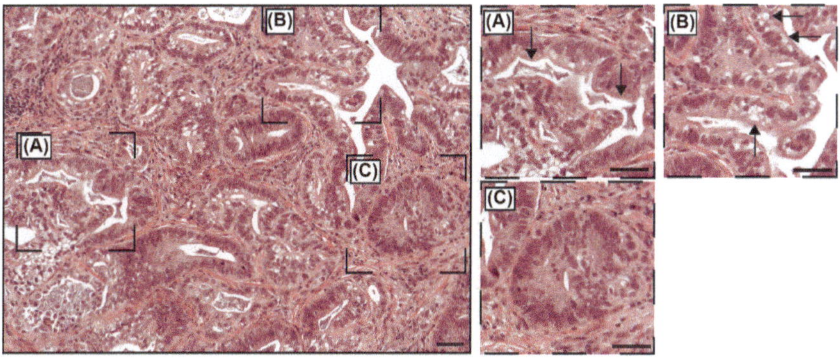

FIGURE 7.1 Hematoxylin and eosin images from CRC PDX model illustrating clinical hallmarks of colorectal cancer. These include evidence of gland formation (arrows in A), mucin-producing cells (arrows in B), and columnar epithelium (C). Scale bars indicate 50 μm.

by histopathological evaluation and mutational analysis comparing the patient specimen to the subsequent xenograft-derived tumors.

TUMOR BIOLOGY

In most CRC diagnoses, an ordered series of genomic alterations promotes disease initiation and progression. As first modeled by Fearon and Vogelstein, the initial steps in colorectal neoplasia are hallmarked by the loss of *APC* with subsequent *KRAS* activation that promotes conversion of the colonic epithelium into advanced polyps.[12] The additional loss of *TP53* is frequently associated with the transition to carcinoma. These principal genetic events are also commonly accompanied by major events in chromosomes 20 and 8.[12] Although this study of tumor progression has clearly defined the initiating steps in CRC pathogenesis, how these molecular changes promote disease progression and affect therapeutic response remains an area of intense investigation. To address this gap in knowledge and inform clinical strategies, the field needs models that mimic the complete CRC landscape.

Alterations in *APC, KRAS, NRAS, BRAF, PIK3CA*, or *p53* occur in a sizeable fraction of CRC cases; as a result, researchers are committed to understanding how these mutational profiles affect disease progression and therapeutic sensitivity. In line with these efforts, PDX models have been informative in uncovering specific driver oncogenes or genomic signatures that promote therapeutic resistance.[13–15] Once the genomic drivers are known, the target itself or downstream signaling pathways can be inhibited through the use of small molecule inhibitors. An example of this pathway approach used CRC PDX models to study targeting RAS effectors, mitogen-activated protein kinase (MEK), and phosphoinositide 3-kinase (PI3K)/mammalian target of rapamycin (mTOR), in a mutant *RAS* setting.[13] This study highlighted the difficulty of targeting oncogenic *RAS* in CRC, as these targeted agents inhibited tumor growth without evidence of disease regression, which is often a requirement of preclinical testing.[13]

It is also worth noting that the phenotypic consequences of genetic point mutations, such as those to *RAS*, may vary even at the same loci, depending on the amino acid substitution.[16–18] For example, 579 CRC patients displayed overall survival and progression-free survival benefits in cases with the *KRAS*^{G13D} mutation when compared with other *KRAS* mutations.[16] Follow-up in vitro and mouse modeling data showed differential sensitivity to cetuximab, with documented resistance in cases with the G12V mutation but not G13D. This underscores the clinical relevance of performing genetic testing in CRC patients to effectively integrate molecularly targeted therapeutics into standard of care. At present, genomic testing within CRC assesses *KRAS* status and microsatellite instability, among others, as these features have informed clinical decision making in the past.

PRECLINICAL AND CLINICAL APPLICATIONS

The strength of PDX models lies in their fidelity to human disease. By maintaining both the tumor bed and the surrounding tumor microenvironment, these models are more readily able to predict tumor response to both chemotherapeutics and targeted agents. The following discussion focuses on the current status of CRC PDX models with respect to therapeutic testing and chemoresistance.

Published reports have emphasized the importance of genetic and molecular markers when assessing cytotoxic drugs.[19] Accordingly, the most relevant treatment strategies require that these mutational profiles be known. Establishing patient-specific PDX models to inform clinical decision making for those individual patients is not realistic given the prolonged engraftment times. However, it is feasible to retrospectively annotate a PDX collection and compare with clinical outcomes to evaluate the actual treatment regimens used for each individual patient. Moreover, these models could then be treated with newer agents, thereby positioning researchers to test novel treatment paradigms. In one such study, 15 PDX models of CRC were treated with one of three cytotoxic regimens [5-flurouracil (5-FU), irinotecan, or oxaliplatin] to test whether these models could have predictive clinical value. The observed patient responses coincided closely with responses from the correlating PDX model.[19] Additionally, tumors were probed for *KRAS* mutations to examine potential correlations with chemosensitivity. Along these lines, mutations to codon 12 exhibited poorer responses to oxaliplatin. This was not recapitulated with codon 13 mutations in the small sample size. Although these retrospective PDX studies may benefit future patients more than those currently enrolled, it is a necessary step in designing effective personalized therapeutic approaches for CRC.

The time to develop PDX models limits their immediate use in a clinically relevant manner. However, PDX models can be a useful source for patient-derived cell lines. This is of particular value when tumor fragments are small. Within these patient-derived cell lines, tumor morphology and mutations can be conserved.[20] In a 2014 colon study, four established lines were used to test preclinical in vitro responses and compare with clinical outcomes. The sensitivity to 5-FU was maintained in a line derived from a patient who responded to 5-FU treatment. The three remaining lines demonstrated more appreciable decreases in proliferation with oxaliplatin treatment than with 5-FU, regardless of the patient's clinical management. Despite a small sample size, this study demonstrates the ability of patient-derived cell lines to mimic therapeutic responses observed in the clinic, while also identifying alternative agents (eg, oxaliplatin) that may be more effective.[20]

In an effort to establish more personalized treatment strategies, the use of preclinical models has undergone a dramatic transformation. What once was a tool for screening lead compounds is now a system for defining targeted agents' therapeutic potential and mechanisms of action. As one of the most intriguing targets, receptor tyrosine kinases (RTKs) quickly became a high priority for PDX model testing. The pharmaceutical industry has prioritized the development of small molecule inhibitors and monoclonal antibodies against RTKs, as activation of these signaling components are common within cancer.[21]

Monoclonal antibodies and small molecules directed against the epidermal growth factor receptor (EGFR) have shown particular promise in the clinical care of CRC. Early studies both in vitro and in vivo with cell line xenografts demonstrated the ability of these agents to stall tumor proliferation.[22,23] Following successful completion of multiple clinical trials, EGFR inhibitors were approved by the Food and Drug Administration (FDA) in 2012 for treatment of metastatic CRC.

Despite the overall success in initial trials, subsequent publication of large randomized trials revealed that genomic complexity, mainly at the level of *KRAS*, greatly influenced the overall efficacy of these inhibitors. In light of these studies, the indications for EGFR-targeted therapies were revised. As a result of inadequate preclinical modeling, some patients are excluded from treatment regimens that could improve their clinical outcomes, whereas others are prescribed an ineffective therapeutic. Conversely, published reports suggest that PDX models would have accurately predicted KRAS-mediated resistance to EGFR inhibition.[24] It has become increasingly clear that CRC's complex genomic nature has important implications in its response to therapy, particularly those that impinge upon specific signaling networks. Thus, PDX models represent an effective system for studying the genomic complexity in human disease, and are an important tool for personalized medicine approaches.

The work discussed earlier touches on an area of immediate focus within the CRC field—novel therapeutic resistance mechanisms. Substantial investment has been made into the genomic characterization of CRC to identify signatures associated with therapeutic resistance. Elucidating these mechanisms will reveal alternative drug targets to resensitize chemoresistant forms of CRC. In one such study, 150 PDX models were established from resected metastatic lesions with the goal of comparing the response of *KRAS* mutant models with their wild-type *KRAS* counterparts after treatment with cetuximab.[14] Neither disease stabilization nor tumor regression occurred within *KRAS* mutant tumors. This cetuximab insensitivity was found in other PDX models of RAS mutant CRC.[25] This finding led to testing additional molecular determinants that may have contributed to therapeutic resistance to anti-EGFR therapies. Previous studies suggested that the upregulation of other RTKs might attenuate the dependence on any one RTK for survival. To that end, Bertotti et al. surveyed all RTKs dysregulated in CRC and found a number of receptors with elevated expression. HER2 was selectively amplified in more than 36% of cetuximab-resistant CRC cases with no alterations in RAS signaling components.[14] Moreover, HER2 was also amplified in patient nonresponders. For these cases, combination therapy that targeted both EGFR and HER2 promoted tumor regression. Consequently, HER2 became a therapeutic target in CRC cases with cetuximab resistance, HER2 amplification, and wild-type RAS.

Another prominent member of the RTK family, vascular endothelial growth factor receptor (VEGFR), has been of focus in CRC. Antiangiogenic drugs have shown efficacy in human trials when combined with conventional chemotherapeutics.[26] Currently, four antiangiogenic therapies have received FDA approval for the treatment of CRC. One such therapy, aflibercept, underwent testing in PDX models. Aflibercept targets the placental growth factor (PGF), a protein with known homology to vascular endothelial growth factor (VEGF). It serves as a ligand for VEGFR and is more highly expressed in CRC tumor tissue than in normal controls. Surprisingly, treatment with anti-VEGF agents increases circulating levels of PGF.[27] Moreover, this elevation occurs prior to metastatic progression, implicating a potential role of PGF in therapeutic resistance.[28] In studying 48 PDX models derived from both primary and metastatic CRC, dual VEGF/PGF inhibition had a more pronounced effect on tumor growth than targeting VEGF alone, in more than 90% of all tested models.[28] This validated observations from other preclinical models that demonstrated heightened potency with aflibercept treatment. Given the robust activity of this drug as a single agent, it shows promise as both a monotherapy and part of a combination treatment strategy for CRC.

In addition to targeting RTKs like HER2 and VEGFR in CRC, inhibition of downstream signaling mechanisms may also be valuable. Three high-priority signaling nodes are the PI3K, mTOR, and the extracellular signal–regulated kinases pathways. In one study, cancer stem cells (CSCs) were isolated from a freshly resected CRC tumor sample and sorted using the expression of CSC markers, CD133 and EpCAM.[15] This population of cells was found to possess heightened tumorigenicity, chemoresistance, and the *PIK3CA*^{H1047R} mutation. Following treatment with the dual PI3K/mTOR inhibitor PF-04691502, the proliferative capability of this model was negatively impacted. These results provided rationale for targeting specific cellular compartments with known genetic mutations for therapeutic benefit in CRC.

In our own studies, we assessed specific targeted compounds in CRC PDX models and observed tumor stasis in most models tested with MEK inhibition alone.[29] However, a *KRAS*^{G12D} CRC PDX model showed resistance to monotherapies directed against MEK, PI3K, mTOR, and PI3K/mTOR; it was the combination of mTOR and MEK inhibition that elicited the best tumor responses. Notably, this tumor response was short-lived as increases in tumor growth were evident 2 weeks after treatment initiation. Reports from an orthotopic PDX model have also shown mixed sensitivity to select treatment strategies, particularly PI3K inhibition within mutant *KRAS* contexts.[5] Taken together, this emphasizes the importance of testing for somatic driver mutations and fully understanding the treatment responses.

While activation of the RAS signaling axis represents one chemoresistant mechanism, other PDX studies have characterized additional mediators of drug resistance. In addition to acquiring somatic mutations within the tumor bed, both primary and acquired resistance mechanisms are a common feature of cancer cells. As such, many scientists have sought to uncover which cell types within the tumor niche are most susceptible. Historically, cytotoxic regimens target cells with high proliferation rates, with the rationale that these cells are responsible for cancer progression. Despite success in some clinical settings, many patients do not respond to these cytotoxic therapies, whereas others relapse after successful initial treatment, suggesting that cytotoxic therapies inadequately target cancer-promoting cell types. Conversely, studies using PDX models and dissociation of patient-derived tumors allow for more specificity, an example of which is described below.

CSCs have long been considered an important source of self-renewal within hematopoietic malignancies and some solid tumors.[30] As a population characterized as relatively quiescent, chemotherapy has little to no effect on the viability of these cell types. In consequence, it has been suggested that this subpopulation of cells is responsible for recurrent disease following initial therapy. Selective targeting of this cell type may promote improved treatment efficacy. A 2013 study investigated this possibility in a PDX model of CRC.[15] A patient-derived sample was propagated into NOD-SCID mice for two generations, at which point CRC tumors were isolated, dissociated, and sorted for CSCs using cell surface markers such as EpCAM, CD133, CD44, and CD26.[15] Mutational analysis uncovered the presence of the activating *PIK3CA*^{H1047R} mutation. This population was then reintroduced in vivo to assess tumor take rates and responses to therapy. Growth was outwardly detected within 6 weeks and persisted at a level that surpassed that of the non-CSC lineage. Treatment with a dual PI3K/mTOR inhibitor reduced AKT phosphorylation and halted tumor growth, thereby suggesting that these pathways are central to the expansion of this population.[15] The benefits of this research were twofold. First, this work illustrated the role that CSCs can play in CRC development within a known genetic background, while also identifying a clinically actionable target to stop cancer cell proliferation. Second, this work demonstrates another avenue of research ideal for PDX models.

This collection of published work illustrates the intense study of therapeutic efficacy and chemoresistance within genetically diverse CRC PDX models.

Implementing clinically relevant models into drug development prevents ineffective investigational agents from advancing past preclinical studies. Further work within PDX models can establish whether this inefficacy is confined to specific patient genotypes, or whether it reflects limitations in targeting a specific signaling pathway and cellular process.

With 89% of preclinical oncology drugs failing to gain FDA approval, models more representative of human disease are desperately needed.[31] In hopes of leveraging existing models, therapeutic agents are now separated based on their mechanisms of action: directly targeting genetic dependencies, critical tumor–stroma interactions, and lastly, the tumor bed.[32] Accurate representation of these components within a preclinical model will ultimately lead to better therapeutic agents. As previously discussed, the homogeneity within cell line xenografts diminishes the value of these models over the course of drug development. Given the significant monetary investment, preclinical testing largely occurs within a select set of tumor models, rather than testing across a broad spectrum of models. Many have proposed this narrow focus to be a driving force behind the high attrition rate of current trials. Efficacy of experimental agents should be tested progressively with the simplest of models (eg, subcutaneous PDX model with limited genomic diversity) being the first "go/no go" end point. Agents shown to be advantageous across multiple studies within this setting would then advance into models of increasing complexity until agents have been tested across a broad range of PDX models. This rigorous approach will allow preclinical outcomes to better align with those observed in clinical trials.

FUTURE AND CHALLENGES

Given the limited success of translating basic research findings into meaningful clinical gains, it has become clear that some approaches commonly implemented by researchers do not adequately mimic the human condition. As a result, tackling some of the most aggressive forms of disease has proven challenging. To gain a more complete understanding of therapeutic failures, researchers must first better understand the mechanisms behind these false starts. It has been shown that long-term study of tumor-derived cell lines in culture dramatically alters their properties and tendencies. Furthermore, the data derived from their experimental use does not always align with the clinical evidence.

With the growing advances and implementation of next-generation sequencing, it has been revealed that patient tumors possess a vast spectrum of mutations that are not always shared across patient populations. This mutational diversity likely drives the divergent behavior of some CRC subsets. Until experimental approaches evolve to encompass this mutational diversity, therapeutic development will remain inefficient. As this chapter has highlighted, CRC PDX models preserve the cellular and genetic hallmarks that are lacking in other preclinical models. While the time to create these models (>6 months) prohibits their use in clinical decision making, PDX models of CRC will continue to be a valuable asset to oncologists in evaluating therapeutic efficacy and uncovering new genetic targets for the disease.

The research community has rallied behind initiatives to create PDX consortiums to make these models available to both academia and industry.[33] Establishing this global resource will introduce well-characterized models, detailed methodology, and standard operating procedures into preclinical cancer research. These tools will be highly valuable for drug discovery, and also for biomarker development, patient stratification, and consistent preclinical modeling practices. Within the United States, the large network of National Cancer Institute (NCI)-sponsored cancer centers and clinical trial sites, together with the biotechnology industry, plays an important role in the initiation and development of this publicly available repository. In 2015, the Repository of Patient-Derived Models featured hundreds of PDX models in development, including CRC and many more expected. The ultimate starting goal of this program is the full annotation of over 1000 models across multiple tumor types. Similar initiatives are underway in Europe.[33] In addition to these government-sanctioned programs, private companies and pharmaceutical companies are testing PDX collections.

Despite meeting many preclinical development needs, some challenges remain before the benefit of CRC PDX models can be fully realized. Although the CRC PDX approach has much to offer, it does require a substantial time and monetary investment. Some CRC models may require over a year of expansion before subsequent studies can be initiated, whereas other CRC tumors may never successfully engraft. For example, breast cancer PDX models have proven difficult to establish with take rates as low as 27%.[6] Conversely, in other malignancies such as lung, melanoma, and colorectal, nearly half of all engraftment attempts are successful. These engraftment challenges may arise as a consequence of human stroma depletion during the expansion process,[6] and upon replacement with murine stroma, necessary cell types and/or microenvironment cues may be lost, thereby negatively impacting engraftment.

In addition to requiring substantial investment of time and resources, CRC PDX models are conducted using immunodeficient mice thereby preventing the study of potentially relevant immunotherapies and the role of immunity in disease; however, efforts are underway to address these limitations. One such example involves the transplant of cells with enriched hematopoietic lineage to spur human innate and adaptive immune response in mice.[34] The transplant of human thymus or bone marrow may precede the transplant of these hematopoietic cells so as to provide a human stromal environment. It will be exciting to see whether these models will enable the study of interactions between human stroma and patient-derived colorectal tumor fragments. Until more work has been completed to validate these immune-competent models, their promise in drug discovery remains an exciting avenue of future research and impact.

CONCLUSIONS

The aggressiveness of advanced CRC is a significant clinical challenge. The 5-year survival rate for metastatic CRC reiterates the growing need for better therapeutic agents and better preclinical models. CRC PDX models retain clinically relevant features and are central to developing more personalized therapeutic strategies. The genomic landscape of each tumor in each patient must be treated as unique. With more genomic medicine finding its way into the clinic, therapeutic approaches have transitioned from an exclusive reliance on cytotoxic drugs to precision treatment strategies encompassing both chemotherapeutics and targeted therapies best suited for the patient. It is within this capacity that CRC PDX models show their promise, potential, and practice in oncology drug development.

REFERENCES

1. Meester RG, Doubeni CA, Lansdorp-Vogelaar I, Goede SL, Levin TR, Quinn VP, et al. Colorectal cancer deaths attributable to nonuse of screening in the United States. *Ann Epidemiol* 2015;**25**(3):208–13.
2. DeVita Jr VT, Chu E. A history of cancer chemotherapy. *Cancer Res* 2008;**68**(21):8643–53.
3. Haggar FA, Boushey RP. Colorectal cancer epidemiology: incidence, mortality, survival, and risk factors. *Clin Colon Rectal Surg* 2009;**22**(4):191–7.
4. Kleinman HK, Martin GR. Matrigel: basement membrane matrix with biological activity. *Semin Cancer Biol* 2005;**15**(5):378–86.
5. Puig I, Chicote I, Tenbaum SP, Arques O, Herance JR, Gispert JD, et al. A personalized preclinical model to evaluate the metastatic potential of patient-derived colon cancer initiating cells. *Clin Cancer Res* 2013;**19**(24):6787–801.
6. Williams SA, Anderson WC, Santaguida MT, Dylla SJ. Patient-derived xenografts, the cancer stem cell paradigm, and cancer pathobiology in the 21st century. *Lab Invest* 2013;**93**(9):970–82.
7. Lee WS, Kim HY, Seok JY, Jang HH, Park YH, Kim SY, et al. Genomic profiling of patient-derived colon cancer xenograft models. *Medicine* 2014;**93**(28):e298.
8. Dangles-Marie V, Pocard M, Richon S, Weiswald LB, Assayag F, Saulnier P, et al. Establishment of human colon cancer cell lines from fresh tumors versus xenografts: comparison of success rate and cell line features. *Cancer Res* 2007;**67**(1):398–407.
9. Fu XY, Besterman JM, Monosov A, Hoffman RM. Models of human metastatic colon cancer in nude mice orthotopically constructed by using histologically intact patient specimens. *Proc Natl Acad Sci USA* 1991;**88**(20):9345–9.
10. Furukawa T, Kubota T, Watanabe M, Kuo TH, Nishibori H, Kase S, et al. A metastatic model of human colon cancer constructed using cecal implantation of cancer tissue in nude mice. *Surg Today* 1993;**23**(5):420–3.
11. Fu X, Herrera H, Kubota T, Hoffman RM. Extensive liver metastasis from human colon cancer in nude and scid mice after orthotopic onplantation of histologically-intact human colon carcinoma tissue. *Anticancer Res* 1992;**12**(5):1395–7.
12. Fearon ER, Vogelstein B. A genetic model for colorectal tumorigenesis. *Cell* 1990;**61**(5):759–67.
13. Migliardi G, Sassi F, Torti D, Galimi F, Zanella ER, Buscarino M, et al. Inhibition of MEK and PI3K/mTOR suppresses tumor growth but does not cause tumor regression in patient-derived xenografts of RAS-mutant colorectal carcinomas. *Clin Cancer Res* 2012;**18**(9):2515–25.

14. Bertotti A, Migliardi G, Galimi F, Sassi F, Torti D, Isella C, et al. A molecularly annotated platform of patient-derived xenografts ("xenopatients") identifies HER2 as an effective therapeutic target in cetuximab-resistant colorectal cancer. *Cancer Discov* 2011;**1**(6):508–23.
15. Fang DD, Zhang CC, Gu Y, Jani JP, Cao J, Tsaparikos K, et al. Antitumor efficacy of the dual PI3K/mTOR inhibitor PF-04691502 in a human xenograft tumor model derived from colorectal cancer stem cells harboring a mutation. *PLoS One* 2013;**8**(6):e67258.
16. De Roock W, Jonker DJ, Di Nicolantonio F, Sartore-Bianchi A, Tu D, Siena S, et al. Association of KRAS p.G13D mutation with outcome in patients with chemotherapy-refractory metastatic colorectal cancer treated with cetuximab. *JAMA* 2010;**304**(16):1812–20.
17. Tejpar S, Celik I, Schlichting M, Sartorius U, Bokemeyer C, Van Cutsem E. Association of KRAS G13D tumor mutations with outcome in patients with metastatic colorectal cancer treated with first-line chemotherapy with or without cetuximab. *J Clin Oncol* 2012;**30**(29):3570–7.
18. Tan C, Du X. KRAS mutation testing in metastatic colorectal cancer. *World J Gastroenterol* 2012;**18**(37):5171–80.
19. Fichtner I, Slisow W, Gill J, Becker M, Elbe B, Hillebrand T, et al. Anticancer drug response and expression of molecular markers in early-passage xenotransplanted colon carcinomas. *Eur J Cancer* 2004;**40**(2):298–307.
20. Seol HS, Kang HJ, Lee SI, Kim NE, Kim TI, Chun SM, et al. Development and characterization of a colon PDX model that reproduces drug responsiveness and the mutation profiles of its original tumor. *Cancer Lett* 2014;**345**(1):56–64.
21. Zhang J, Yang PL, Gray NS. Targeting cancer with small molecule kinase inhibitors. *Nat Rev Cancer* 2009;**9**(1):28–39.
22. Wakeling AE, Guy SP, Woodburn JR, Ashton SE, Curry BJ, Barker AJ, et al. ZD1839 (Iressa): an orally active inhibitor of epidermal growth factor signaling with potential for cancer therapy. *Cancer Res* 2002;**62**(20):5749–54.
23. Prewett MC, Hooper AT, Bassi R, Ellis LM, Waksal HW, Hicklin DJ. Enhanced antitumor activity of anti-epidermal growth factor receptor monoclonal antibody IMC-C225 in combination with irinotecan (CPT-11) against human colorectal tumor xenografts. *Clin Cancer Res* 2002;**8**(5):994–1003.
24. Lieu CH, Tan AC, Leong S, Diamond JR, Eckhardt SG. From bench to bedside: lessons learned in translating preclinical studies in cancer drug development. *J Natl Cancer Inst* 2013;**105**(19):1441–56.
25. Krumbach R, Schuler J, Hofmann M, Giesemann T, Fiebig HH, Beckers T. Primary resistance to cetuximab in a panel of patient-derived tumour xenograft models: activation of MET as one mechanism for drug resistance. *Eur J Cancer* 2011;**47**(8):1231–43.
26. Grothey A, Galanis E. Targeting angiogenesis: progress with anti-VEGF treatment with large molecules. *Nat Rev Clin Oncol* 2009;**6**(9):507–18.
27. Fischer C, Jonckx B, Mazzone M, Zacchigna S, Loges S, Pattarini L, et al. Anti-PlGF inhibits growth of VEGF(R)-inhibitor-resistant tumors without affecting healthy vessels. *Cell* 2007;**131**(3):463–75.
28. Chiron M, Bagley RG, Pollard J, Mankoo PK, Henry C, Vincent L, et al. Differential antitumor activity of aflibercept and bevacizumab in patient-derived xenograft models of colorectal cancer. *Mol Cancer Ther* 2014;**13**(6):1636–44.
29. Burgenske DM, Monsma DJ, Dylewski D, Scott SB, Sayfie AD, Kim DG, et al. Establishment of genetically diverse patient-derived xenografts of colorectal cancer. *Am J Cancer Res* 2014;**4**(6):824–37.
30. Dean M, Fojo T, Bates S. Tumour stem cells and drug resistance. *Nat Rev Cancer* 2005;**5**(4):275–84.

31. Sharpless NE, Depinho RA. The mighty mouse: genetically engineered mouse models in cancer drug development. *Nat Rev Drug Discov* 2006;**5**(9):741–54.
32. Caponigro G, Sellers WR. Advances in the preclinical testing of cancer therapeutic hypotheses. *Nat Rev Drug Discov* 2011;**10**(3):179–87.
33. Siolas D, Hannon GJ. Patient-derived tumor xenografts: transforming clinical samples into mouse models. *Cancer Res* 2013;**73**(17):5315–9.
34. Talmadge JE, Singh RK, Fidler IJ, Raz A. Murine models to evaluate novel and conventional therapeutic strategies for cancer. *Am J Pathol* 2007;**170**(3):793–804.
35. Linnebacher M, Maletzki C, Ostwald C, et al. Cryopreservation of human colorectal carcinomas prior to xenografting. *BMC Cancer* 2010;**10**:362.
36. Zhou W, Zhu H, Chen W, et al. Treatment of patient tumor-derived colon cancer xenografts by a TRAIL gene-armed oncolytic adenovirus. *Cancer Gene Ther* 2011;**18**:336–45.
37. Guenot D, Guerin E, Aguillon-Romain S, et al. Primary tumour genetic alterations and intratumoral heterogeneity are maintained in xenografts of human colon cancers showing chromosome instability. *J Pathol* 2006;**208**:643–52.
38. Neijzen R, Wong MQ, Gill N, et al. Irinophore C, a lipid nanoparticulate formulation of irinotecan, improves vascular function, increases the delivery of sequentially administered 5-FU in HT-29 tumors, and controls tumor growth in patient derived xenografts of colon cancer. *J Control Release* 2015;**199**:72–83.
39. Oh BY, Lee WY, Jung S, et al. Correlation between tumor engraftment in patient-derived xenograft models and clinical outcomes in colorectal cancer patients. *Oncotarget* 2015;**6**:16059–68.
40. Cho YB, Hong HK, Choi YL, et al. Colorectal cancer patient-derived xenografted tumors maintain characteristic features of the original tumors. *J Surg Res* 2014;**187**:502–9.
41. Julien S, Merino-Trigo A, Lacroix L, et al. Characterization of a large panel of patient-derived tumor xenografts representing the clinical heterogeneity of human colorectal cancer. *Clin Cancer Res* 2012;**18**:5314–28.
42. Nunes M, Vrignaud P, Vacher S, et al. Evaluating patient-derived colorectal cancer xenografts as preclinical models by comparison with patient clinical data. *Cancer Res* 2015;**75**:1560–6.
43. Chou J, Fitzgibbon MP, Mortales CL, et al. Phenotypic and transcriptional fidelity of patient-derived colon cancer xenografts in immune-deficient mice. *PLoS One* 2013;**8**:e79874.
44. Uronis JM, Osada T, McCall S, et al. Histological and molecular evaluation of patient-derived colorectal cancer explants. *PLoS One* 2012;**7**:e38422.
45. Ziemke EK, Dosch JS, Maust JD, et al. Sensitivity of KRAS Mutant Colorectal Cancers to Combination Therapy that Co-Targets MEK and CDK4/6. *Clin Cancer Res* 2015.
46. Kavuri SM, Jain N, Galimi F, et al. HER2 Activating Mutations Are Targets for Colorectal Cancer Treatment. *Cancer Discov* 2015;**5**:832–41.

Chapter 8

Patient-Derived Tumor Xenografts in Hematologic Disorders

M. Pizzi[1], G. Inghirami[2,3,4]
[1]*University of Padova, Padova, Italy;* [2]*Weill Cornell Medical College, New York, NY, United States;* [3]*University of Torino, Torino, Italy;* [4]*New York University School of Medicine, New York, NY, United States*

Hematologic disorders represent ~10% of all the newly diagnosed neoplasms in the United States, with an estimated number of ~50,000 deaths in 2015. These neoplasms are currently classified according to clinical, morphological, immunophenotypic, and molecular parameters, which reflect biological differences in terms of lineage and cell of origin.[1]

The clinical and scientific progress in the arena of hematologic disorders has fostered the development and delivery of "Precision Medicine" programs. The application of new technologies/platforms (ie, whole genome sequencing, global transcriptomics) has pointed out the complexity and heterogeneity of tumor pathobiology. Individual entities differ in terms of tumorigenic events, natural evolution, and response to the selective pressure of conventional and targeted therapies. It is now well established that the clinicobiologic features of these disorders depend on the balance between host and cancer cells.

These new perspectives have led to the formulation of a number of questions, whose solution requires new models and innovative approaches. This is epitomized by the poor efficacy of the current drug discovery programs and by the enormous costs sustained to perform obsolete clinical trials. Toward this end, we anticipate that innovative mouse models will play a critical role. Here we will review the state-of-the-art hematologic mouse models, focusing on patient-derived tumor xenografts (PDXs).

OVERVIEW AND CLASSIFICATION OF HEMATOPOIETIC AND LYMPHOID TISSUE TUMORS

The classification of these tumors has been a matter of debate for decades, and many uncertainties still remain on the true biological nature of some entities.

Patient Derived Tumor Xenograft Models. http://dx.doi.org/10.1016/B978-0-12-804010-2.00022-9

The current classification has been proposed by the World Health Organization (WHO) in 2008,[1] and an update is going to be published in 2016.

A thorough analysis of the several entities included in the 2008 WHO classification is beyond the scopes of this chapter. In this section, we will present the major diagnostic categories, to provide a general frame for the subsequent analysis of PDXs in hematologic tumors. According to the 2008 WHO classification, hematopoietic and lymphoid tumors can be broadly classified based on their cell lineage in (1) myeloid neoplasms, (2) lymphoid neoplasms, and (3) histiocytic and dendritic cell neoplasms.

Myeloid tumors are a very large group of neoplasms, spanning from chronic and relatively indolent disorders to extremely aggressive and fatal ones. The current classification includes:

- Myeloproliferative neoplasms (MPNs), which are driven by fully maturing neoplastic cells and are usually characterized by a prolonged and relatively indolent clinical course (Table 8.1). The most important entities are (1) chronic myeloid leukemia (CML), driven by the recurrent chromosomal translocation t(9; 22)(q34; q11) (ie, Philadelphia chromosome, juxtaposing the *BCR* to the *ABL1* gene); (2) primary myelofibrosis (PMF); (3) essential thrombocythemia (ET); and (4) polycythemia vera (PV). Of note, PMF, ET, and PV are never associated with the t(9; 22)(q34; q11), but are driven by recurrent *JAK2*, *CALR*, or *Mpl* gene mutations.
- Myelodysplastic syndromes (MDSs), which are biologically characterized by the defective maturation of neoplastic hematopoietic stem cells (HSCs); MDSs clinically present with variable cytopenias and normal to increased CD34-positive blasts. Based on such clinical and laboratory findings, MDSs are further subclassified into different subtypes, bearing the variable risk of evolving to acute myeloid leukemia (AML).
- MPNs/MDSs, a group of hematologic neoplasms with clinical and pathologic features intermediate between MPN and MDS; MPNs/MDSs indeed present with both cytopenias and/or dysplasia (MDS-like features) and with increased numbers of different myeloid cells (MPN-like features); definite and provisional entities are currently included in the MPN/MDS category (Table 8.1).
- AMLs are characterized by a maturation arrest at the blast phase. AMLs are aggressive neoplasms, bearing a poorer prognosis compared with MPNs or MDSs. Based on recurrent cytogenetic/molecular derangements, AMLs are currently classified into six subgroups, namely, (1) AML with recurrent genetic abnormalities (characterized by variable outcome, depending on the specific genomic defect); (2) AML with myelodysplasia-related changes; (3) therapy-related myeloid neoplasms (a heterogeneous group of neoplasms, encompassing AML-like, MDS-like, and MDS/MPN-like forms); (4) AML, not otherwise specified; (5) myeloid sarcoma (ie, a tumor mass consisting of myeloid blasts, arising outside the bone marrow); and (6) myeloid proliferations

TABLE 8.1 2008 WHO Classification of Myeloid Neoplasms

Myeloproliferative neoplasms
Chronic myelogenous leukemia, BCR-ABL1 positive Polycythemia vera Primary myelofibrosis Essential thrombocythemia Chronic eosinophilic leukemia Mastocytosis Myeloproliferative neoplasm, unclassifiable
Myeloid and lymphoid neoplasms with eosinophilia and abnormalities of PDGFRA, PDGFRB, or FGFR1
Myeloid and lymphoid neoplasms with PDGFRA rearrangement Myeloid and lymphoid neoplasms with PDGFRB rearrangement Myeloid and lymphoid neoplasms with FGFR1 abnormalities
Myelodysplastic/myeloproliferative neoplasms
Chronic myelomonocytic leukemia Atypical chronic myelogenous leukemia BCR-ABL1 negative Juvenile myelomonocytic leukemia Myelodysplastic/myeloproliferative neoplasm, unclassifiable Refractory anemia with ring sideroblasts associated with marked thrombocytosis[a]
Myelodysplastic syndromes (MDS)
Refractory cytopenias with unilineage dysplasia Refractory anemia with ring sideroblasts Refractory cytopenia with multilineage dysplasia Refractory Anemia with Excess blasts MDS associated with isolated del(5q) MDS, unclassifiable Childhood MDS
Acute myeloid leukemia (AML)
AML with recurrent genetic abnormalities AML with MDS-related changes Therapy-related myeloid neoplasms AML, NOS (FAB categories M0, M1, M2, M3, M4, M5, M6, M7) Myeloid sarcoma Myeloid proliferations related to Down syndrome
Blastic plasmacytoid dendritic cell neoplasm
Acute leukemias of ambiguous lineage

[a]*Provisional entity.*

related to Down syndrome (DS). Within the group of blastic tumors of myeloid lineage, the WHO classification also considers blastic plasmacytoid dendritic cell neoplasm, a hematopoietic tumor arising from myeloid precursors of plasmacytoid dendritic cells. Several excellent studies have shed light on the molecular biology and pathobiology of this very rare entity.[2–4,5a]

- Myeloid/lymphoid neoplasms with eosinophilia and abnormalities of PDGFRA, PDGFRB, or FGFR1, a group of rare hematopoietic disorders whose unifying features are (1) the presence of peripheral blood eosinophilia and (2) the presence of genetic imbalances (usually chromosomal translocations) involving one of the aforementioned tyrosine kinases (TK). Although the majority of such tumors are of myeloid origin, a consistent subset of cases is of lymphoid nature. The discovery that specific TK inhibitors (ie, imatinib) can prove curative at least for cases with PDGFRA/PDGFRB alterations has revolutionized the treatment of these entities.[5b]

Lymphoproliferative disorders constitute a second, large group of hematopoietic tumors, traditionally classified into two major branches: Hodgkin lymphomas (HLs) and non-Hodgkin leukemias/lymphomas (Table 8.2). HLs have peculiar clinical and pathologic features. Histologic examination typically reveals a low number of neoplastic cells, scattered within a reactive inflammatory background. Neoplastic cells are large, with polylobated nuclei and evident nucleoli. Based on specific cytological and histologic features, HLs are further divided into (1) classical HL (cHL), with its four variants (nodular sclerosis, mixed cellularity, lymphocyte rich, and lymphocyte depleted) and (2) nodular lymphocyte predominance HL (NLPHL). Both cHL and NLPHL seem to arise from B lymphocytes passed through the germinal center (GC).[1]

Non-Hodgkin lymphomas constitute a broad and more complex group of tumors, with different clinical and biological features. The 2008 WHO classification distinguishes neoplasms arising from lymphoid precursors (ie, B and T lymphoblasts) and tumors originating from more mature cells (ie, B and T lymphocytes). The first group encompasses B-cell and T-cell acute lymphoblastic leukemias/lymphomas (B-ALL and T-ALL), a subset of lymphoid malignancies characterized by an immature phenotype, very high proliferation index, and poor prognosis. The second group includes the majority of non-Hodgkin lymphomas. Non-Hodgkin B-cell lymphomas are much more common than their T-cell counterpart, and encompass a broad spectrum of both indolent and aggressive tumors. Their classification is based on the putative cell of origin (ie. pre-GC, GC, and post-GC lymphocytes) and relies on specific histological, cytological, and immunophenotypic features (Table 8.2). Indolent B-cell lymphomas usually experience a protracted clinical course and can hardly be cured by conventional chemotherapy. Conversely, aggressive B-cell tumors [eg, diffuse large B-cell lymphoma (DLBCL) and Burkitt lymphoma] respond to medical therapies and can undergo durable remission.

TABLE 8.2 2008 WHO Classification of Lymphoid Neoplasms

Precursor lymphoid neoplasms
B-lymphoblastic leukemia/lymphoma
-not otherwise specified
-with recurrent genetic abnormalities
T-lymphoblastic leukemia/lymphoma
Mature B-cell neoplasms
Chronic lymphocytic leukemia/small lymphocytic lymphoma
Follicular lymphoma
Mantle cell lymphoma
Marginal zone lymphoma
-nodal type
-splenic type
-extranodal type
Lymphoplasmacytic lymphoma
Hairy cell leukemia
B-cell prolymphocytic leukemia
Diffuse large B-cell lymphoma (DLBCL), not otherwise specified and variants
Burkitt lymphoma (BL)
B-cell lymphoma, unclassifiable, with intermediate features between DLBCL and BL
B-cell lymphoma, unclassifiable, with intermediate features between DLBCL and Hodgkin lymphoma
Plasma cell neoplasms
Mature T-cell and NK cell neoplasms
Angioimmunoblastic T-cell lymphoma
Anaplastic large cell lymphoma (ALCL)
-ALCL, ALK-positive
-ALCL, ALK-negative[a]
Enteropathy-associated T-cell lymphoma
Hepatosplenic T-cell lymphoma
T-cell prolymphocytic leukemia
T-cell Large granular lymphocytic leukemia
Adult T-cell leukemia/lymphoma
Mycosis fungoides and other cutaneous T-cell neoplasms (CD30-positive and CD30-negative)
Peripheral T-cell lymphomas, not otherwise specified
Extranodal NK/T-cell lymphoma, nasal type
Aggressive NK cell leukemia
Chronic lymphoproliferative disorder of NK cells[a]
EBV-positive systemic lymphoproliferative disorders of childhood

Continued

TABLE 8.2 2008 WHO Classification of Lymphoid Neoplasms—cont'd

Hodgkin lymphoma
Nodular lymphocyte predominant Hodgkin lymphoma
Classical Hodgkin lymphoma (cHL)
-nodular sclerosis cHL
-lymphocyte-rich cHL
-mixed cellularity cHL
-lymphocyte-depleted cHL
Posttransplant lymphoproliferative disorders (PTLDs)
Early lesions
-Plasmacytic hyperplasia
-Infectious mononucleosis-like PTLD
Polymorphic PTLD
Monomorphic PTLD (B- and T/NK-cell type)
cHL-type PTLD

[a]*Provisional entity.*

Within T-cell lymphomas many entities have been thoroughly characterized [eg, anaplastic large cell lymphoma (ALCL), angioimmunoblastic T-cell lymphoma (AITL), enteropathy-associated T-cell lymphoma, adult T-cell leukemia/lymphoma (ATLL)], meanwhile others cannot be precisely assigned to any specific subtype and are currently referred to as "peripheral T-cell lymphomas, not otherwise specified" (PTCL, NOS) (Table 8.2). Overall, PTCLs are aggressive neoplasms with a poor prognosis. Therapeutic strategies are still poorly defined, and several ongoing trials are testing different chemotherapeutic regimens.

Finally, histiocytic and dendritic cell neoplasms are a small but definite group of hematopoietic tumors, encompassing (1) histiocytic sarcoma, (2) tumors derived from Langerhans cells (formerly known as Langerhans cell histiocytosis), (3) interdigitating dendritic cell sarcoma, (4) follicular dendritic cell sarcoma, and (4) other rare neoplasms (fibroblastic reticular cell and indeterminate dendritic cell tumor). Their differential diagnosis mainly relies on the clinical presentation, histologic findings (ie, growth pattern, cytology, background infiltrate), and immunohistochemical features (ie, variable positivity for S100, CD68-PGM1, Langerin, CD1a, Clusterin, CD23, CD21, and CD35).[1]

IN VIVO MODELS OF HEMATOLOGIC DISORDERS

PDXs have emerged as novel and powerful systems to study both solid and hematologic neoplasms.[6–15] The general advantages and limitations of these models have been extensively described in other chapters of this book; here, we will focus on studying the role of PDXs in human hematopoietic malignancies. Unlike solid tumors, the generation of hematologic PDXs has focused on a limited group of disorders. This is due to (1) the relative low frequency of such malignancies, (2) the very large number of different entities, (3) the frequent occurrence of malignancies with only low to intermediate malignant potential, and (4) the complex pathogenesis of these diseases, which frequently rely on protumorigenic signals from the microenvironment.[16,17]

Indeed, the host microenvironment plays a pivotal role in the development of hematologic tumors. Myeloid and lymphoid malignancies require the engagement of specialized receptors on tumor and microenvironmental host cells and the production of chemokines and lymphokines. Host–tumor interactions also regulate the homing of tumor cells in specialized tissue compartments[18] and provide protumorigenic niches, protecting tumor cells from stress and genotoxic insults.[19] This is epitomized by the survival signals provided by CXCR4 on T-lymphoblastic leukemia cells upon interaction with endothelial-derived CXCL12.[20,21] The same holds true for peripheral T-cell lymphomas, whose microenvironment dictates the successful growth and survival of the neoplastic cells.[22] In particular, GATA3-positive neoplastic T-cells produce large amounts of interleukin (IL)-4, IL-10, and IL-13, which favor the M2 polarization of nonneoplastic macrophages.[23] These, in turn, influence antitumor immune responses and stimulate tumor angiogenesis via VEGF and other cytokines. Similar observations have been reported in AITL[24] and in several myeloid neoplasms.[25,26]

The Role of Patient-Derived Tumor Xenografts in the Study of Myeloid Disorders

Human myeloid tumors are a broad spectrum of disorders with unique clinicopathologic features. Their characterization in PDX models has mainly focused on AML, but a number of studies have reported very interesting results also in MDSs and MPNs.

The Role of Patient-Derived Tumor Xenografts in the Study of CML

CML is a clonal multilineage myeloproliferative disorder, derived from a common myeloid precursor bearing translocations of the *c-abl* and *bcr-1* genes. The most frequent translocation produces the p210 BCR-ABL fusion protein, whereas the p190 BCR-ABL (most common in Philadelphia-positive ALL) or the p230 BCR-ABL chimera (mu-bcr breakpoint) are less frequent.

In 1998, Wang and colleagues implanted human CML cells into irradiated NOD/SCID mice using peripheral blood and/or CD34-positive enriched cells of CML patients.[27] This original work demonstrated that human cells could successfully engraft and persist up to 7 months in mice. Using a colony-forming assay, the authors could then demonstrate the presence of long-term culture-initiating cells, bearing the t(9; 22) translocation. The highest engraftment rates were obtained with the CD34-positive enriched cells.

Similar studies were performed with peripheral blood cells from chronic-phase CML patients.[28] Early marrow engraftment of human CML cells was slightly higher in NOD-*Prkdc*^{scid}-*Il2rg*^{null} (NSG) than in NOD/SCID mice, but this difference was lost over time. Interestingly, sorted $CD34^{+}CD38^{+}$ CML cells produced an early transient population that disappeared after 6 weeks. Conversely, the injection of more primitive $CD34^{+}CD38^{-}$ cells led to a persistent engraftment. Of note, 3 weeks after transplantation, the largest BCR-ABL^{+} population was of erythroid lineage; later on (6 weeks), BCR-ABL^{+} cells were mainly of granulocytic and, to a lesser extent, lymphoid origin. Verstegen and colleagues obtained similar data, demonstrating that SCID or NOD/SCID mice can sustain the production of myeloid, B-lymphoid, erythroid, and CD34-positive cells from normal and CML donor cells.[29] Of note, long-term engraftment of erythroid and myeloid clonogenic cells from Philadelphia-positive cells was lower compared with those from Philadelphia-negative elements. This deficiency was in part overcome by the injection of purified CD34-positive CML cells, which induced the persistence of leukemic precursors even 20 weeks after transplantation. These cells could produce high levels of IL-3 and G-CSF and survived even without the administration of exogenous growth factors.

Taken together, these studies demonstrate different requirements for Philadelphia-positive and Philadelphia-negative CD34-positive cells. The murine microenvironment may indeed support normal hematopoietic elements better than their neoplastic counterpart. These observations are in keeping with the "bad niche" theory, which sustains that alterations in the nonneoplastic microenvironment contribute to tumor cell overgrowth.[30,31] This idea is further confirmed by bone niche–remodeling studies, demonstrating a reduction of CML engraftment in mice treated with bone-remodeling agents (eg, parathyroid hormone)[32]

The Role of Patient-Derived Tumor Xenografts in the Study of Philadelphia-Negative MPNs

In the setting of Philadelphia-negative MPNs, most PDX-based studies have focused on the biology and treatment of PMF. PMF derives from hematopoietic progenitor cells (HPCs), undergoing uncontrolled proliferation and anomalous maturation. One of the most striking morphologic features in the bone marrow of patients with PMF is the presence of large clusters of atypical megakaryocytes. These cells play a pivotal role in the pathogenesis of the disease, as they mediate bone marrow fibrosis and progression to AML.[33,34]

The mechanisms of acute myeloid transformation in PMF have thoroughly been investigated. Several models suggest the progressive accumulation of gene mutations within PMF clones, which ultimately undergo a leukemic transformation.[35,36] This hypothesis is, however, challenged by the occurrence of post-PMF AML cases, lacking MPN-associated mutations. These AMLs probably arise from normal hematopoietic cells, whose leukemic transformation is triggered by paracrine signals from PMF cells. This fascinating theory has been confirmed for the first time on a PDX model.[37]

In this study, NSG mice engrafted with human PMF cells were noted to develop AML at significantly higher rates than control mice. Notably, all such AMLs were of mouse origin; moreover, the risk of leukemic transformation correlated with specific patient samples, as demonstrated by different AML incidence in independent mouse cohorts.[37] Taken together, these results unequivocally demonstrate a role for PMF in inducing the leukemic transformation of the surrounding (nonneoplastic) myeloid cells.[37] More recently, the nature of PMF-derived leukemogenic signals has been characterized by in vitro and in vivo studies, highlighting the synthesis of lipocalin-2 (LCN2) by human PMF cells. LCN2 is an inflammatory cytokine, involved in the production of reactive oxygen species and in DNA strand breaks, which induce genomic instability of both neoplastic and nonneoplastic hematopoietic cells.[38]

In the setting of MPNs, PDXs were also used to characterize the in vivo effects of new therapies. Human xenograft models can indeed integrate in to in vitro results, as they can more reliably reproduce the complex interplay between neoplastic cells and the host organism. This integrated approach was first used to assess the response of PMF to 5-aza-2-deoxycytidine (5azaD) and trichostatin A (TSA), two chromatin-modifying agents (CMAs).[39] The authors first demonstrated the in vitro efficacy of 5azaD and TSA to induce PMF-derived HPCs apoptosis. They subsequently tested the efficacy of these drugs on an in vivo PDX model, by transplanting NSG mice with primary PMF cells treated with either cytokines alone or cytokines *plus* CMAs. In line with the in vitro experiments, the number of PMF short- and long-term repopulating cells was markedly reduced in mice treated with cytokines *plus* 5azaD/TSA.[39] Using a similar approach, they also demonstrated the efficacy of a MDM2 antagonist (RG7112) and pegylated interferon-α 2a (pegIFNα-2a) for the treatment of PMF and PV.[40] RG7112 and pegIFNα-2a increased the apoptosis of patient-derived HPCs and impaired their capacity to repopulate the bone marrow (BM) and spleen of mice.[40] Taken together, these results indicate CMAs and MDM2 antagonists as novel therapeutic options for the treatment of MPNs.[33]

In myeloid neoplasms, PDXs have finally been used to better characterize the effects of a standard-of-practice therapy (ie, the JAK1/2 inhibitor, ruxolitinib). Two multiinstitutional trials have indeed reported the efficacy of ruxolitinib in reducing PMF-related splenomegaly and constitutional symptoms (COMFORT I and COMFORT II clinical trials).[41,42] Treatment with this drug has also been associated with prolonged 5-year overall survival of PMF patients.[43] These results have, however, been questioned by a Cochrane review, reporting insufficient evidence on the efficacy and safety of ruxolitinib in PMF.[44] Based on these data, a PDX study addressed the many still open issues concerning ruxolitinib in MPNs and characterized the biological effects of JAK inhibitors in such disorders. This study first tested the effects of a JAK1/2/3 inhibitor (AZD1480) on an in vitro model of PMF and disclosed its limited efficacy to eliminate patient-derived neoplastic cells. To further characterize the effects of AZD1480, PMF-derived splenic HPCs were treated with AZD1480 and subsequently injected in NSG mice. Exposure to AZD180 did not affect the degree of human cell chimerism and the proportion of malignant HPCs in the bone marrow and spleen of transplanted mice. These results demonstrate the limited effect of JAK inhibitors against splenic PMF stem cells and provide a biological explanation to the rapid relapse of splenomegaly in patients who discontinue ruxolitinib therapy.[45]

Patient-Derived Tumor Xenografts and MDS

Myelodysplastic syndromes are a broad group of hematologic disorders, characterized by the impaired maturation of progenitor cells, variable expansion of the myeloid lineages and increased risk of AML transformation.[1] The unique features of MDS make their biological characterization a true challenge. The development of in vitro and in vivo models has indeed been hampered by the low percentage of MDS-propagating cells, the variety of cytogenetic/molecular derangements, and the large spectrum of clinicopathologic presentations.

PDX models have been used mainly to define the nature and biology of MDS HSCs. No PDX studies have as yet been performed on the effects of MDS-specific therapies. Several technical and theoretical issues have indeed delayed the development of PDX models of MDS, including (1) the choice of the appropriate mouse model; (2) the identification of human accessory cells, sustaining the engraftment of MDS; and (3) the definition of MDS-propagating cells.

Seminal studies from Nilsson and colleagues reported low engraftment rates for MDS cells in NOD/SCID mice.[46,47] These results were in keeping with in vitro long-term culture assays and suggested the defective maturation of MDS HSCs. The same data were later reported by a study demonstrating the total absence of clonal MDS precursors in NOD/SCID transplanted mice.[48] Of note, the only detectable human cells in these animals were residual nonneoplastic hematopoietic cells, whose in vitro and in vivo expansion is markedly increased compared with MDS.[46–48] Significantly higher engraftment rates have been subsequently obtained with other mouse models, including NOD/SCID-β2 microglobulin null mice, NSG mice, and NSG mice constitutively expressing IL3, GM-CSF, and SCF (NSGS mice).[49–53]

The engraftment of patient-derived MDS cells can also be influenced by the presence of accessory cells, promoting the survival and expansion of the neoplastic clones. This is for instance the case of human mesenchymal stromal cells (MSCs), whose coinjection in NSG mice increases the engraftment of MDS cells.[50–52] This view is supported by the observation that MSCs from MDS patients have an intrinsically altered gene expression profile, supporting the growth of neoplastic cells in secondary hosts. This abnormal gene signature is likely induced by the neoplastic cells themselves.[52]

Finally, the engraftment of MDS cells in nude mice is greatly influenced by the differentiation stage of the transplanted cells. Early studies on NOD/SCID-β2 microglobulin-null mice have reported inconsistent and/or transient reconstitution rates with unselected MDS cells.[49] Conversely, good results were obtained with the injection of purified MDS cells with HSC-like features ($Lin^-CD34^+CD38^-CD90^+CD45RA^-$ cells).[51,53,54] In mouse xenografts, these cells reproduces the aberrant hematopoiesis observed in MDS patients, with increased differentiation toward the myeloid lineages and marked reduction of B-cell lymphopoiesis.[51] The key role of MDS HSCs is further confirmed by the low reconstitution rates obtained with more committed progenitors.[53] PDX have also helped highlight the maturation pattern of MDS stem cells. Mouse xenografts were indeed characterized by an increase of common myeloid precursor (CMP) frequency, with a paralleled reduction of granulocyte monocyte precursors (GMPs). Erythroid and megakaryocytic differentiation at the MEP level was apparently unaffected.[51] The functional bases of this skewed maturation were elegantly demonstrated by in vitro experiments, showing increased apoptosis of MDS progenitors. GMPs (but not CMPs and MEPs) also expressed the phagocytic marker calreticulin, which prompted the in vitro elimination of GMPs by human macrophages. Taken together, these studies unequivocally demonstrate (1) the existence of MDS stem cells, capable of maintaining and propagating neoplastic clones in xenograft models; (2) the impaired differentiation of MDS hematopoietic progenitors; and (3) the importance of accessory cells (eg, MSCs) to sustain the growth and survival of MDS clones.

Patient-Derived Tumor Xenografts and AML

The first attempt to establish a PDX of AML can be traced back to the mid-1970s, when Franks and colleagues subcutaneously implanted immunocompromised CBA mice with fresh and frozen blood cells from AML patients.[55] Even though mice were also pretreated with antithymocyte serum, the engraftment of leukemic cells was unsatisfactory with a success of only 22.5% three weeks after inoculation. The engraftment of frozen leukemic cells was even poorer (3.2%).[55] Soon after, Palù and colleagues obtained similar results using thymectomized CBA mice, treated with cytosine arabinoside and total body irradiation.[56] The authors injected cultured AML cells at different stages of maturation and they demonstrated that immature AML cells had better engraftment rates than the mature counterpart. Notably, immature cells formed stable and growing tumors (40%).[56]

These attempts paved the way to other studies, which have demonstrated that the development of AML xenografts is influenced by (1) the mouse model, (2) the route of injection, (3) the AML subtype, and (4) the clinical features of donor patients.

Overall, poor results have been obtained with nude mice even after heavy immune suppression (eg, whole body radiation, antibody treatment, and/or splenectomy)[57,58] and only slightly better results were achieved with beige and X-linked immunodeficient mice.[59,60] Conversely, the SCID animal models marked a turning point.[61] In these mice, the AML engraftment could be improved by the exogenous administration of growth factors (eg, IL-3, IL-6, GM-CSF, and erythropoietin) or by reducing natural killer (NK)-mediated immune responses with radiation and/or antibodies (antisialo-GM antibody).[62]

Further improvements were gained using NOD/SCID[63] and, ultimately, with NOG- and NSG-based mice.[64] The latter are currently considered the best models to establish AML PDXs,[62] which have allowed the serial transplantation of AML cells, thus providing clues on the hierarchical structure of neoplastic subclones.[65] The stability of AML PDX models has also led to the genetic engineering of transplanted cells and to the development of in vivo bioluminescence models for cell tracking and quantification.[65]

The engraftment of AML is also strongly influenced by the route of administration with the intravenous injection being definitively superior.[66,67]

Moreover, the AML engraftment depends on the biological features of the original tumor. Rombouts and others have reported higher engraftment rates in FAB M0 compared with more differentiated (ie, M2, M3, M4, M5) subtypes.[63,68] More recently, the predictive role of the FAB subclassification for AML engraftment has been questioned,[69] and further studies are needed to clarify this issue.

Beside the degree of differentiation, AML engraftment seems to correlate with other clinicobiologic parameters, including (1) high white blood cell counts in the donor patient, (2) high CD34 expression, (3) presence of the FLT3-ITD mutation, (4) presence of adverse cytogenetic features, (5) history of relapse after first-line therapy.[63,67–69]

PDX models have also contributed to the understanding of AML biology and treatment. Several studies have shown that neoplastic stem cells can vary according to the AML subtype and that the universal CD34 marker of stemness does not predict engraftment. This is particularly true for *NPM*-mutated AMLs, whose CD34-negative and CD34-positive HPCs can engraft equally.[70] Xenograft models of *NPM*-mutated AML have also disclosed the existence of preleukemic myeloid populations, whose biological features are close (but not equal) to AML. Preleukemic clones are indeed characterized by mutations of proleukemic genes (eg, *DNMT3A*), which confer a survival advantage in mouse xenografts. The acquisition of further genomic aberrances (ie, mutation of *NPM1*) induces the overt transformation of such clones to *DNMT3A*- and *NPM*-mutated AML.[71]

PDX models have also highlighted the peculiar biological features of rare AML subtypes, such as those associated with DS.[72] Myeloid proliferations related to DS encompass a spectrum of clinicobiologic entities, ranging from transient abnormal myelopoiesis (TAM) to overt DS-associated AML (Table 8.3).[1] Using a PDX model, Saida and colleagues have demonstrated the biological continuum between these entities, as serial transplantation of TAM-derived cells led to the emergence of subclones with molecular and biological features of overt AML. Of note, these subclones were already present in the bone marrow of TAM patients, where they constituted a minor population.[72]

From a more clinical perspective, PDX of AML have been widely used for (1) the discovery and characterization of novel anti-AML therapies and (2) the study of AML resistance mechanisms against standard therapies. The rationale for using PDX models is provided by the observation of similar response rates and toxicity patterns in AML patients and engrafted mice.[73]

TABLE 8.3 AML-Specific Therapies Tested in PDX Models

Compound/Immunotherapy	Notes and Mechanisms of Action	References
(–)BI97D6	Pan-BCL2 inhibitor blocking Mcl-1	Pan et al., 2015
5-Azacytidine	Overexpression of SOX7, inhibition of AML proliferation and reduced engraftment in immunocompromised mice	Man et al., 2015
A2-32-01	Inhibitor of the mitochondrial protease ClpP; altered metabolism and increased apoptosis of AML cells	Cole et al., 2015
ABT-199	Selective BCL2 inhibitor	Pan et al., 2014
ABT-737	BCL2 inhibitor effective in combination therapy with 5-azacytidine	Tsao et al., 2012
ADI-PEG 20	Depletion of arginine for AML metabolism	Miraki-Moud et al., 2015
Anti-CD123 CAR	T-cells with CAR directed against the myeloid antigen CD123; eradication of neoplastic and nonneoplastic myeloid cells (high toxicity)	Gill et al., 2014
Anti-CD33 CAR	T-cells with CAR directed against the myeloid antigen CD33; eradication of neoplastic and nonneoplastic myeloid cells (high toxicity)	Kenderai et al., 2015
Anti-CD44v6 CAR	T cells with CAR directed against the myeloid antigen CD44v6; effective against AML and multiple myeloma cells	Casucci et al., 2013
Anti-HMW-MAA antibodies	Monoclonal antibodies targeting the HMW-MAA antigen on 11p23-positive AML cells; no effects on AML proliferation and survival in vivo	Drake et al., 2009
Anti-human TIM3 antibody	Human antibody targeting TIM3 on AML cells; no effects on normal hematopoiesis	Kikushige et al., 2013
Anti-IL1RAP antibodies	Inhibition of IL-1 signaling and antibody-mediated cellular cytotoxicity against AML cells	Ågerstam et al., 2015

Continued

TABLE 8.3 AML-Specific Therapies Tested in PDX Models—cont'd

Compound/Immunotherapy	Notes and Mechanisms of Action	References
Anti-IREM1 antibodies	Monoclonal antibodies targeting IREM1 on AML cells; complement-dependent and antibody-dependent cytotoxicity against neoplastic cells	Korver et al., 2009
AS101	Redox modulation of the adhesion molecule VLA-4; decreased PI3K/Akt/BCL2 signaling	Layani-Bazar et al., 2014
Avocatin B	Inhibition of mitochondrial fatty acid oxidation, decrease of NADH levels, and increase of ROS production	Lee et al., 2015
BC2059	β-Catenin antagonist; combined therapy with panobinostat (pan-HDAC inhibitor) improves survival of mice engrafted with human AML	Fiskus et al., 2015
Calicheamicin immunoconjugate	Calicheamicin conjugated with an anti-CD33 antibody (gemtuzumab ozogamicin); inhibition of AML cell growth	Boghaert et al., 2006
CD4+ Vα24NKT-cells	T cells effective against M4 AML; no effects on M0 and M1 AML	Nieda et al., 2001
CSL362	Monoclonal antibody directed against CD123; reduction of AML cells in mouse xenograft models	Busfield et al., 2014
Darinaparsin	Organic arsenical effective against AML with inv(3)	Nielsen et al., 2013
Decitabine *plus* cytarabine	Combination therapy more effective in reducing tumor burden than cytarabine alone	Leonard et al., 2014
$DT_{388}IL3$	Diphtheria toxin-IL-3 fusion protein, effective against AML progenitor cells	Feuring-Buske et al., 2002
F14512	Inhibitor of topoisomerase II, inducing AML cell death	Kruczynski et al., 2013
Hu5F9-G4	Monoclonal antibody targeting CD47 on AML cells; enhanced phagocytosis of neoplastic cells	Liu et al., 2015

I-BET151	Inhibitor of the BET family of epigenetic readers, effective against *NPM*-mutated AML	Dawson et al., 2014
IDH1 mutant inhibitors	Decrease of 2-hydroxyglutarate and induction of granulocytic differentiation	Okoye-Okafor et al., 2015
IL27	Immunomodulatory cytokine blocking AML proliferation and dissemination	Zorzoli et al., 2012
Interferon-β	Stable interferon-β expression has antileukemic activity	Benjamin et al., 2007
LY2510924	CXCR4 antagonist, inducing AML cell mobilization and death	Cho et al.[121]
MK-2206, rapamycin and BEZ-235	Inhibition of the PI3K/mTOR pathway; antileukemic activity against *MLL*-rearranged AML	Sandhöfer et al., 2015
Nimesulide	COX-2 selective inhibitor, effective against AML of various karyotypes	Zhang et al.[137]
Oxi4503	Vascular disrupting agent inducing AML cell apoptosis	Madlambayan et al.[78]
Parthenolide	Induction of apoptosis in AML cells	Guzman et al., 2015
PIK-75	Tyrosine kinase inhibitor targeting Cdk7/9 and PI3K signaling	Thomas et al., 2013
PR1 cytotoxic T cells	T cells directed against the AML-specific antigen PR1; effective in eradicating neoplastic cells in engrafted mice	Ma et al., 2010
Rucaparib	PARP inhibitor effective against AML	Verga Falzacappa et al., 2015
SALL4-inhibitor peptide	Activation of PTEN through epigenetic modifications	Gao et al., 2012
SP2509	Inhibition of the histone demethylase LSD1 and induction of AML differentiation; combined therapy with panobinostat (pan-HDAC inhibitor) improves survival of mice engrafted with human AML cells	Fiskus et al., 2014
TH-302	Hypoxia-activated prodrug, effective against AML stem cells	Benito et al., 2015

Several studies have employed AML xenografts to test proapoptotic drugs, inhibitors of leukemogenic signals, inhibitors of cell metabolism and immune-mediated strategies [ie, chimeric antigen receptors (CARs), monoclonal antibodies (mAbs) against AML antigens, AML-targeting T cells]. A thorough presentation of all such therapies is beyond the scope of the present chapter and has been summarized in Table 8.3. AML xenograft models have also been used to test the biological effects of palliative therapies. This is the case of eltrombopag, a thrombopoietin receptor agonist commonly used in patients with severe/refractory immune thrombocytopenia.[74] Eltombopag may prove beneficial also against AML-related thrombocytopenia, provided that it does not stimulate malignant hematopoiesis. A study by Will and colleagues specifically addressed this issue and showed that Eltrombopag treatment neither increased in vitro proliferation of neoplastic cells nor enhanced their engraftment in NOG mice.[75]

Finally, PDX models have been used to study the mechanisms of AML resistance against conventional therapies. Saito and colleagues have demonstrated that AML HPCs homing to the endosteal surface of trabecular bones are quiescent and resistant to systemic chemotherapy. They also noticed that GM-CSF administration promotes the proliferation of these HPCs, rendering them susceptible to conventional chemotherapy.[76] These observations are in line with the work of Cogle and collaborators, who demonstrated a survival advantage for AML cells interacting with nonneoplastic endothelial cells.[77] In particular, xenotransplanted AML cells may interact (and even fuse) with murine endothelial cells, thus reducing their proliferative activity. This allows them to enter a dormant state that may provide resistance to conventional chemotherapy. The leukemogenic potential of such endothelial-like cells is demonstrated by their induction of AML in secondary recipient mice.[77] The importance of such leukemia–endothelial interaction is also demonstrated by the efficacy of vascular disrupting agents (eg, Oxi4503) for the treatment of AML.[78]

THE ROLE OF PATIENT-DERIVED TUMOR XENOGRAFTS IN THE STUDY OF LYMPHOPROLIFERATIVE DISORDERS

In 2015, non-Hodgkin leukemias/lymphomas have been responsible for approximately 25,500 deaths in the United States. In the past 30 years, the incidence of such neoplasms has indeed slowly and steadily increased: B-cell neoplasms dominate in Western countries, whereas T-cell lymphomas are more frequent in Asia and South America. Based on the current WHO classification, B- and T-cell neoplasms are classified into two major subgroups: (1) precursor lymphoproliferative disorders (B-ALL and T-ALL) and (2) mature B-cell leukemias/lymphomas (Table 8.2).

Patient-Derived Tumor Xenografts and B-ALL/T-ALL

B-ALL and T-ALL are aggressive hematologic disorders that frequently affect children and young adults of Caucasian and Hispanic origin (estimated incidence of 30 cases per million). B-ALL accounts for approximately 80–85% of all precursor lymphoid neoplasms and typically presents in a leukemic phase. T-ALL is less frequent and usually manifests with bulky mediastinal masses.[79] The prognosis of ALL depends on several clinical and molecular features: durable responses are achieved in 80–90% of pediatric cases, whereas lower survival rates have been reported in adults (35–40% of cases). Several recurrent genomic defects (ie, gene fusions, chromosomal deletions, DNA gains, and de novo somatic mutations) influence ALL prognosis.[79]

Many studies have proved the value of PDX for the molecular and biological characterization of ALL. In line with other hematologic neoplasms, several factors may influence the engraftment of ALL in immunocompromised mice. These include (1) the mouse model, (2) the route of primary cell injection, (3) the source and properties of the donor samples (fresh versus cryopreserved cells), (4) the percentage of cotransplanted nonneoplastic donor cells, and (5) the preconditioning of recipient mice (Fig. 8.1).

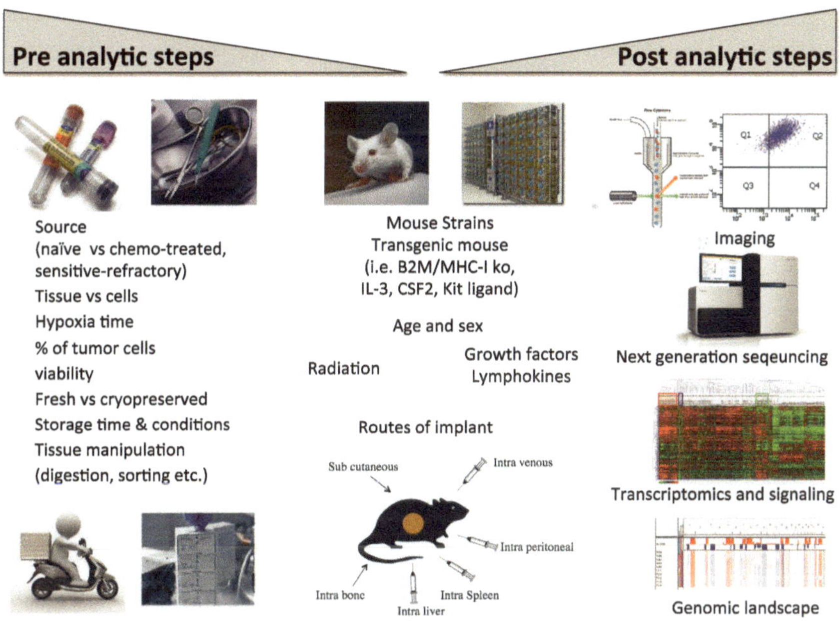

FIGURE 8.1 **Rate and successful implant of human hematopoietic tumors are conditioned by multiple factors.** Several preanalytic factors can influence cancer implants; these include samples' properties, surgical procedures, and tissue processing. Animals' strains have also a role, so do the animal sex and age. Since the microenvironment and the host protumorigenic signals critically influence the survival and growth of human cancer cells, transgenic and/or humanized mice have been used to facilitate tumor growth. There are multiple routes of implantation, which can be selected based on the mouse models and the nature of the disease (ie, leukemia versus lymphoma). The PDX success, the percentage of tumor cells, and their tissue distribution can be assessed using different procedures. Genomic fingerprints are ultimately defining the genomic and transcriptomic profile of tumor cells and the relatively contribution of mouse versus human elements.

The best engraftment rates have been reported in NSG mice,[11] with limited success in nude, SCID, and NOD/SCID mice.[80–82] Of interest, Notta and colleagues have shown that subsets of Philadelphia-positive ALLs are characterized by shorter time to leukemia in NOD/SCID mice.[83] Apart from the murine immunologic background, other features of the recipient mice may influence the engraftment of ALL. These include the gender and (at least for SCID and NOD/SCID mice) the age at inoculation. Young SCID and NOD/SCID mice show higher engraftment rates, as a direct consequence of their peculiar immunologic status (lower levels of NK cells, which recognize and eliminate the human neoplastic lymphocytes).[84]

As for the route of primary cell administration, intrabone and intrahepatic injection have been associated with high engraftment rates (Di Giacomo F et al., personal communication). By contrast, intraperitoneal administration is characterized by poor success in both NSG, NSB, and NOD/SCID mice.[11] Even lower engraftment rates have been reported with subcutaneous implantation[83] (Di Giacomo F. et al, personal communication).

The cell viability of ALL also determines the rate of implantation. Of note, neoplastic cell enrichment (via cell sorter and/or magnetic bead enrichment) negatively influences cell viability and significantly reduces ALL engraftment. The percentage of viable cells is also influenced by cell processing and storage procedures. In cryopreserved samples, the percentage of viable cells correlates with several technical issues, including (1) the time elapsed between sample collection and freezing, (2) the freezing modalities, (3) the time and modalities of cell storage, and (4) the defrosting procedures.

The cotransplantation of nonneoplastic donor cells can further influence the engraftment of ALL. The coinjection of MSCs can favor ALL growth and survival (similarly to what is observed in MDS). By contrast, ALL engraftment is impaired by the clonal expansion of Epstein-Barr virus (EBV)+ human lymphoblastoid cells or by donor T cells, mediating graft-versus-host disease (GVHD) against murine tissues.

Finally, preconditioning of mouse recipients (ie, sublethal irradiation, lymphokine conditioning, and/or support) facilitates the engraftment and homing of tumor cells in the vast majority of cases. A negative influence has, however, been reported in rare cases.[85]

Conversely, the engraftment of ALL in immunocompromised mice seems to be marginally influenced by the biological features of the leukemic cells (eg, ALL subtype or specific clinical risk subgroups). Shorter time to leukemia has, however, been associated with worse clinical outcome[81,86] and with the presence of efficient antiapoptotic mechanisms in tumor cells.[87] Moreover, T-ALL engraftment in SCID models identifies a subset of patients at higher risk of relapse after early response to induction chemotherapy.[88] Taken together, these data indicate that ALL engraftment in NOD/SCID mice cannot per se predict the patients' prognosis, but may be used to study the biology of the disease.[81]

A major issue concerning PDX models of ALL regards the clonal selection of leukemic cells in recipient animals. Of note, we have seen a decrease of time to leukemia after serial implants of B-ALL, which suggests clonal selection and/or increased clonal fitness of leukemic cells in immunocompromised mice. In T-ALL PDXs, xenografts were more similar to relapsed diseases than first diagnostic samples, suggesting the selection of specific clones during engraftment and the expansion of refractory-like best-fitted clones which genetically resemble those emerging in refractory patients.[89] These findings should be taken into consideration by any drug development program using PDX of ALL.

The clonal selection of ALL grafts strictly depends on the presence of different populations of leukemia HPCs. Leukemia stem cell activity has indeed been described in both early progenitor cells and more mature hematopoietic elements. These populations variably influence ALL engraftment in immunocompromised mice. In particular, early precursors (ie, $CD34^{+}CD38^{-}$ cells) expand more efficiently in NGS compared with NOD/SCID mice.[90–94] Similarly, $CD7^{+}CD1a^{-}$ T-ALL cells show higher engraftment rates and increased therapy resistance compared to $CD7^{+}CD1a^{+}$ cells.[95] In addition, leukemia stem cells with specific genomic defects may only grow under unique biological conditions. This is the case of non-t(4; 11) B-ALL, whose expansion needs the preconditioning with total body irradiation and the induction of SDF-1/CXCR4 signaling pathway.[96] Of note, the treatment of B-ALL with IL-27 significantly impairs cell growth and expansion in vitro and in vivo.[97]

In the past 5–10 years, many studies have taken advantage of PDX models to investigate anti-ALL therapeutic approaches. Toward this end, Ong and colleagues have used a PDX model to show that the equilibrium between polymerized and unpolymerized tubulin within leukemic cells reflects the sensitivity of childhood ALL to vincristine.[98] Moreover, PDX models have nicely been used to characterize the mechanisms of resistance to corticosteroid therapy. The resistance to glucocorticoid agonists is a hallmark of relapsed ALL and represents a strong predictor of poor outcome. Jones and colleagues have used a genome-scale short hairpin RNA to demonstrate that MEK2 and MEK4 (two members of the MAPK pathway) mediate the resistance of ALL to prednisolone and used a PDX model to demonstrate that treatment with the MAPK inhibitor, trametinib, could lead to a significant reduction of the leukemic burden.[99]

This research has been further expanded by a study, defining new mechanisms of glucocorticoid resistance in ALL. Using PDXs of ALL variably sensitive to glucocorticoids, Jing and colleagues have demonstrated that changes in *KLF13* and *MYB* expression are significantly associated with the response to dexamethasone treatment. *MYB* expression could be repressed by *KLF13* only in dexamethasone-sensitive PDXs and this, in turn, favored ALL cell apoptosis through the downmodulation of BCL2 and the overexpression of the proapoptotic protein BIM. These events were consistently absent in dexamethasone-resistant PDXs.[100]

Many other studies have addressed the molecular and biological mechanisms of ALL resistance to chemotherapy. Such mechanisms include recurrent translocations and several genomic defects,[101–105] whose identification has fostered the implementation of novel and more effective anti-ALL therapies.[106] In ALL, somatic mutations of the Ras pathway (NRAS, KRAS, FLT3, and PTPN11) are associated with early relapse, chemoresistance, central nervous system (CNS) involvement, and reduced overall survival. Ras-mutated subclones are present at very early stages, and their emergence is thought to mediate chemotherapy resistance. Evaluation of the MAPK1/2 inhibitor, selumetinib, in PTDXs has demonstrated stronger preclinical activity against Ras pathway–mutated ALL compared with unmutated ALL. These data demonstrate the key role of MEK inhibitors for the treatment of relapsed ALL, bearing mutations of the Ras pathway. These compounds may also be used in frontline therapies to counteract the emergence of refractory ALL phenotypes.[107]

Similar studies have been performed on Early T-cell precursor (ETP) ALL. This leukemia has a high rate of induction failure and harbors frequent defects of cytokine receptors (ie, IL-7R) and of the JAK/STAT pathway, leading to the aberrant activation of STAT5 upon IL-7 stimulation. This molecular background has led to test the efficacy of the JAK1/2 inhibitor, ruxolitinib, in a xenograft model of ETP ALL. Treatment with ruxolitinib significantly decreased peripheral and splenic blast counts. Of note, ruxolitinib had similar effects in ALL lacking JAK/STAT mutations, which suggests a potential efficacy of JAK/STAT inhibitors, irrespective of the JAK mutational status.[108]

These studies were in part confirmed using the JAK1/2 inhibitor AZD1480 in coadministration with selumetinib: combined therapy synergistically induced leukemia cell death in vitro, but did not lead to a substantial control of the disease in PDX models. Such discrepancy may be related to the limited drug bioavailability and to the need of prolonged target inhibition in vivo.[109]

Beside the characterization of standard therapies, ALL PDX models have also been used (1) to test new compounds targeting XIAP, thus overcoming leukemic resistance to apoptosis[110]; (2) to prove the efficacy of bortezomib *plus* histone deacetylase inhibitors against ALL progenitors[111]; (3) to demonstrate the proapoptotic effects of various drugs and plant derivatives (eg, the thalidomide analog, CC-4047[112]; the kava extract, flavokawain B[113]; the serine/threonine kinase inhibitor, AZD1775[114]); and (4) to test the efficacy of immune-based therapies.

Immune therapy has indeed become one of the most promising approaches for the treatment of hematologic diseases, including ALL. Although the host mice of PDX models are immunologically impaired, they still represent invaluable tools for the thorough characterization of this therapeutic approach in many leukemia/lymphoma models. In particular, PDXs of ALL have been used to prove that immune-stimulatory CpG oligonucleotides elicit anti-ALL immune responses through the production of IL-12p70, IFNα, and IFNγ and the activation of NK cells.[115] They also helped characterize the proleukemia effects of various chemokines, including CXCL12. Several studies have indeed demonstrated the key role of the CXCL12/CXCR4 axis to control T-ALL cell growth, bone localization, and resistance to chemotherapy.[116–118] PDXs have also indicated this pathway as a possible target for anti-ALL therapies,[119] fostering the discovery of several CXCR4 inhibitors, including lerixafor (a bicyclam derivative),[120] LY2510924,[121,122] KRH-1636,[123] and POL5551.[124] The last of these has been tested in breast cancer and ALL models, showing potent antitumor activity.[125,126]

Immunotherapy strategies can also take advantage of the nearly invariable expression of specific surface antigens by B and T cells. CD19 represents one of the most studied antigens, given its key role in (benign and malignant) B-cell biology. A number of anti-CD19 agents have been developed, including (1) naked or conjugated mAbs; (2) bispecific T-cell engagers (BiTEs); and (3) CARs. While results with naked mAbs are controversial, BiTEs and CARs have been associated with relevant clinical responses.[127]

BiTEs are synthetic proteins composed of two single-chain antibodies (scFvs), connected by a short linker sequence.[128] One of such scFvs recognizes the tumor antigen (eg, CD19), whereas the other binds to invariable antigens of immune system cells (eg, CD3). A CD19-CD3 BiTE (blinatumomab) has demonstrated strong antileukemic activity in adult B-ALL patients with minimal residual disease[127,129] and in relapsing/refractory B-ALL.[128] Our group has tested the efficacy of novel CD19/CD3 antibodies in a NGS model of primary B-ALL and DLBCL. In these mice, GVHD was prevented by the coinjection of expanded cytokine-induced killer cells [a subset of major histocompatibility complex (MHC)-unrestricted cytotoxic cells expressing the TCR-CD3 complex, but incapable of mediating clinically relevant GVHD[130,131]]. The engraftment of $CD19^+CD34^+$ leukemic cells led to a rapid and massive infiltration of lymphoid and parenchymal organs (liver, kidneys, lungs, etc.), with rapid mouse demise. Conversely, the combination of CIK cells and BiTEs efficiently controlled the growth of leukemic cells and led to prolonged mouse survival (Circosta P. et al., personal communication).

CARs represent another valuable resource for anti-ALL immune therapies. CARs are produced by the fusion of T-cell receptor intracellular domains with extracellular antibody fragments, recognizing specific tumor antigens (eg, CD19). The expression of these constructs is forced into autologous T cells, which are then expanded and reinfused into the donor patient.[128] CAR technology has been used to develop T cells targeting the thymic stromal lymphopoietin receptor (TSLPR), whose overexpression has been reported in a subset of high-risk B-ALLs. Adoptive transfer of TSLPR-targeting T cells was associated with encouraging results in a PDX model of ALL.[132] CARs have also been tested for the treatment of T-ALL. In this case, T cells have been engineered to recognize the panT-cell antigen CD5 and have been injected in xenograft mouse models of T-ALL.[133a]

These studies clearly illustrate the potential usefulness of PDXs for the characterization of both standard and innovative antileukemic therapies. Major drawbacks may, however, affect their use, namely, (1) the still limited number of available PDXs models, (2) the relatively high costs and technically demanding procedures to establish a PDX facility, and (3) the lack of genomic fingerprints to assess clonal evolution at the first implant and after multiple passages. The development of the Public Repository of Xenografts (PRoXe; https://proxesite.wordpress.com/) marks a step toward this end. This project has also shown that large academic repositories of hematologic PDXs can be created within integrated institutional networks and that this collaboration may constitute a powerful tool for both academic and industrial initiatives (Townsend et al.[133b]; http://weinstock.dfci.harvard.edu/index.php/projects/6-pd).

Patient-Derived Tumor Xenografts and Mature B-Cell Lymphomas

Many cell lines derived from mature B- and T-cell lymphoproliferative disorders have been used in the past two to three decades. These correspond to both low/intermediate processes [eg, chronic lymphocytic leukemia (CLL), mantle cell lymphoma (MCL), hairy cell leukemia (HCL)] and highly aggressive disorders (eg, DLBCL and ALCL). Although these lines have been instrumental for the biological characterization of non-Hodgkin lymphomas, many of them are associated with significant limitations. For example, the most commonly used CLL lines (Mec-1 and Mec-2) are EBV-infected,[134] despite the fact that primary CLLs are never driven by EBV viral infection. Moreover, many HCL lines do not carry the HCL-pathogenic mutation BRAF-V600E.[135,136] Among aggressive lymphoproliferative disorders, very few DLBCL cell lines bear gene mutations commonly observed in primary samples[137] and the majority of T-cell lymphoma cell lines have been derived from a limited number of patients and histotypes (ie, ATLL, ALCL).[138–140]

Engineered mouse models have also greatly contributed to the biological and molecular characterization of lymphoid tumors.[141–143] However, although several B-cell lymphoma models have been developed, transgenic mice of specific mature T-cell neoplasms are lacking.[144–146]

In this context, PDXs have emerged as valuable alternatives, and an increasing number of models have been generated.[147] Their number is, however, limited and the engraftment success rates is often unsatisfactory.[148] The reasons for this can be traced back to (1) the relative low frequency of lymphoma; (2) the limited amount of implantable fresh tissue (several cases are indeed diagnosed by fine needle biopsy); (3) the low rates of excisional biopsy in refractory/relapsed patients; (4) the biological features of these tumors, which require host/microenvironment interactions usually not available in mouse models; and (5) the lack of through molecular, biological, and clonal characterization of the engrafted tumors.

Patient-Derived Tumor Xenografts and B-Cell Chronic Lymphocytic Leukemia

Among low-grade lymphomas, PDX models of B-CLL were first described by Bagnara and colleagues.[149] The authors demonstrated that primary B-CLL cells could be transferred into NSG mice under the influence of B-CLL-derived activated T cells and the critical role of CD4-positive T lymphocytes for the expansion of B-CLL. They also highlighted a direct link between T-cell activation and CD38 expression on leukemic cells. Of note, the activation of autologous T lymphocytes was apparently induced by allogeneic antigen-presenting cells, irrespective of their origin. This B-CLL PDX model closely mimicked primary tumor biology, as neoplastic cells retain their specific immunophenotype (eg, expression of CD38) and localize the organs commonly involved in humans. These features are at least partly due to a specific microenvironmental relationship between multiple host elements and B-CLL cells (Serra S et al., personal communication).

This model also proved the existence of a relatively short window to study B-CLL in vivo, as all mice died as the result of GVHD or autologous antitumor reactions soon after implantation. Such a limitation might be overcome by the use of NSG mice (which lack β2-microglobulin or MHC antigens)[150,151] or by the injection of engineered CLL cells without accompanying T-cells.

Last, the generation of these CLL PDXs has fostered the design of novel therapies. In particular, interesting data have been reported with novel bifunctional CD20/CD3 antibodies,[152] and with a potent antagonist of PPARα.[153]

Patient-Derived Tumor Xenografts and Other Small B-Cell Lymphomas

We and others have generated PDX models of follicular lymphoma (FL), marginal zone[154] and mantle cell (MCL) lymphoma. Some of these models are now available from private commercial enterprise or academic PDX repositories (PRoXe; https://proxesite.wordpress.com/).

In a seminal study by Klanova and colleagues, 12 samples of MCL have been implanted into NGS mice via tail injection.[155] Successful engraftment was observed in the majority of these tumors, irrespective of the MCL variant (ie, classical, pleomorphic, and blastoid). Localization of cyclin D1-positive cells was more frequent in the spleen than in the liver and/or BM. In some cases, EBV-infected neoplastic cells were also present. However, re-implantation was carried out in a single case, with successful re-engraftment into secondary recipients. Secondary implants were associated with a shorter engraftment time when compared with primary samples.[155]

Similar data were obtained with MCL cells from a single donor patient (ie, CCMCL1 cell line).[156] In this PDX, engrafted cells displayed blastoid morphology and a phenotype compatible with a highly proliferative MCL (Ki67>95%). Neoplastic cells conserved their complex karyotype and lacked deletions of the *ATM* and *TP53* genes.

Patient-Derived Tumor Xenografts and Aggressive B-Cell Lymphomas

Among high-grade B-cell lymphomas, PDX models of DLBCL have been produced (PRoXe; https://proxesite.wordpress.com/; https://globenewswire.com/news-release/2015/06/22/746147/10139172/en/Karyopharm-Presents-Hematologic-Cancer-Data-on-Lead-Drug-Candidate-Selinexor-at-International-Conference-on-Malignant-Lymphoma.html[157]).

In particular, Chapuy and colleagues have established eight PDX lines of DLBCL, reflecting the immunophenotypic, genetic, and functional heterogeneity of primary tumors: six lines display activated B-cell (ABC) features, and two lines have a germinal center B-cell (GCB) phenotype. An additional line features plasmablastic differentiation. Lymphoma cells harbor gene mutations associated with either ABC or GCB DLBCL, two lines show inactivating mutations of *TP53*, whereas six lines exhibit copy number alterations of *TP53* or *CDKN2A*.[158] According to whole transcriptome sequencing and consensus clustering classification criteria, six PDXs exhibit selective surface immunoglobulin expression and sensitivity to the SYK inhibitor, entospletinib.

In similar experiments, Sugimoto and colleagues generated four DLBCL lines (three conventional DLBCLs and one intravascular large cell lymphoma) with gene expression profiling (GEP) resembling those of primary tumor samples.[159] PDX cells have shown better resistance to multiple drug therapies compared with lymphoma cell lines and have been used to screen more than 2000 putative antitumor compounds. This search led to the discovery of pyrvinium pamoate as a potent antitumor agent: its administration as single therapy could indeed induce the eradication of the engrafted lymphoma cells.[159]

Beside DLBCL, PDXs have been used to establish mouse models of B-cell lymphomas, unclassifiable, with intermediate features between DLBCL and BL[154] (Table 8.2). These xenografts carry the t(8; 14)(q24; q32) translocation, feature high c-myc expression, and show high rates of BM and CNS dissemination. Analogous models have been generated by our group, including (1) FL-derived secondary DLBCLs; (2) double-hit lymphomas of both GCB and ABC subtype; and (3) triple-hit lymphomas (even in leukemic phase), carrying XPO1 gene amplification. This third line was used for in vitro experiments, which demonstrated the efficacy of an XPO1 inhibitor (selinexor) to control neoplastic cell growth (Cerchietti L and Inghirami G, personal communication).

Patient-Derived Tumor Xenografts and Plasma Cell Neoplasms

Plasma cell neoplasms are a heterogeneous group of hematologic disorders, characterized by peculiar clinical and biological features. Multiple myeloma (MM) is the most frequent plasma cell malignancy and presents with a broad variety of clinical and laboratory manifestations. From a biological perspective, MM is characterized by remarkable genomic instability, with complex karyotypes and chromosomal translocations involving the immunoglobulin heavy chain genes.[160]

The first in vivo models of MM were developed in athymic mice more than 50 years ago. Since then, several attempts have been made to improve the engraftment of neoplastic cells. In 1992, Feo-Zuppardi reported the engraftment of primary MM cells after peritoneal injection in SCID mice.[161] Human MM cell lines[162,163] and primary MM plasma cells were later engrafted in SCID mice, subcutaneously cotransplanted with human fetal bone fragments.[164] Neoplastic cell growth was indeed favored by the presence of human BM niches in recipient mice. More recently, several studies have demonstrated widespread dissemination of MM cells after intravenous injection in variably conditioned immunocompromised mice.[165–167] All such xenograft models have contributed optimizing the clinical management of patients. Their relatively low clinical predictive power on new chemical entities represents, however, a major limitation.[167]

Patient-Derived Tumor Xenografts and Mature T-Cell Lymphomas

T-cell neoplasms are significantly less frequent than their B-cell counterpart. Their low incidence and complex biology have significantly prevented the development of reproducible models.[168]

Early PDXs have been generated for very selected T-cell lymphomas, such as Sézary syndrome (ie, the leukemic manifestation of cutaneous T-cell tumors). Even in these cases, however, the clonal relationship between primary and engrafted cells has not been clarified and few data are available on disease engraftment rates.[169] Under the auspices of the multi-institution *Translational Discovery in Peripheral T-Cell Lymphomas* project (LLS Score grant 2015), we have developed multiple PDXs from other primary human T-cell lymphomas, including (1) ALCL (both ALK-positive and ALK-negative variants); (2) AITL; (3) PTCL, NOS; (4) T-cell prolymphocytic leukemia (T-PLL); and (5) cutaneous T-cell lymphomas.

In general, we have observed that the subcutaneous route of implantation is associated with the local growth of tumor cells, which can eventually localize to distant organs (eg, lung, liver, and spleen). This feature is usually observed in slowly growing and/or large subcutaneous tumors. Exceptions are represented by cutaneous T-cell lymphomas (CTCLs) and AITL: CTCLs remain strictly localized to the site of injection, whereas AITL displays distant dissemination with frequent absence of skin lesions. The timeframe of neoplastic cell growth is highly variable (from 3 weeks to more than 9 months).

In line with what observed in other xenograft models, uncontrolled proliferation of EBV+ nonneoplastic lymphoid cells has been reported in some cases. This phenomenon is usually associated with rapid mice demise.

The immunophenotype of the engrafted tumors usually corresponds to that of primary samples, with no significant changes even after serial passages. In the case of AITL, we observed the concomitant presence of EBV+ B cells. Low percentages of circulating lymphoma cells are commonly detected. In such cases, flow cytometry represents a valuable tool to define engraftment and to monitor disease evolution/response to therapies.

PDXs have greatly contributed to the biological characterization of ALCL (both ALK-positive and ALK-negative cases). GEP analysis has indeed shown that ALCL PDX lines have backbone genomic features, defining their biological origin. Beside these common expression profiles, each line displays unique gene signatures, which may predict clinical outcomes and response to therapies.

Using a PDX model of ALCL, we could test the efficacy of antitumor compounds[170–172] and the existence of putative molecular predictors of therapy response.[173] These studies confirmed the power of PDXs, but also highlighted problems concerning their use for the screening of large drug libraries. It thus seems more reasonable to test compounds in in vitro cultures from PDX or primary lymphoma cells. Complex in vivo models could be used only for second-line studies on the most promising compounds.

Like PDXs of Sézary syndrome, the clonal evolution and rate of genomic defects in serially transplanted ALCLs has never been investigated. To address these issues, we applied whole exome and RNA sequencing to serially transplanted ALCLs (>15 passages). This analysis has shown remarkable genomic stability, although additional mutations were detected in virtually all cases.

CONCLUSIONS

PDXs represents invaluable tools for the study of both myeloid and lymphoid tumors. They have indeed contributed to better understand the biological and clinical features of such malignancies, also highlighting the possibility of new therapeutic approaches.

Although several hematologic PDXs are already accessible and additional models will be soon developed, many questions on mouse xenografts remain to be answered. We believe that many pitfalls concerning their use will be eventually overcome by the creation of large and representative multiinstitutional libraries. This is definitively critical for hematologic tumors, which constitute a large and heterogeneous group of biologically unrelated entities.

REFERENCES

1. Swerdlow SH, International Agency for Research on Cancer, Organization, WH. In: *WHO classification of tumours of haematopoietic and lymphoid tissues*. 4th ed. Lyon, France: International Agency for Research on Cancer; 2008.
2. Martin-Martin L, Lopez A, Vidriales B, et al. Classification and clinical behavior of blastic plasmacytoid dendritic cell neoplasms according to their maturation-associated immunophenotypic profile. *Oncotarget* 2015;**6**(22):19204–16.
3. Yu H, Zhang P, Yin X, et al. Human BDCA2+CD123+CD56+ dendritic cells (DCs) related to blastic plasmacytoid dendritic cell neoplasm represent a unique myeloid DC subset. *Protein Cell* 2015;**6**(4):297–306.

4. Sapienza MR, Fuligni F, Agostinelli C, et al. Molecular profiling of blastic plasmacytoid dendritic cell neoplasm reveals a unique pattern and suggests selective sensitivity to NF-kB pathway inhibition. *Leukemia* 2014;**28**(8):1606–16.
5. (a) Stenzinger A, Endris V, Pfarr N, et al. Targeted ultra-deep sequencing reveals recurrent and mutually exclusive mutations of cancer genes in blastic plasmacytoid dendritic cell neoplasm. *Oncotarget* 2014;**5**(15):6404–13.
   (b) Tabbò F, Pizzi M, Kyriakides PW, et al. Oncogenic kinase fusions: an evolving arena with innovative clinical opportunities. *Oncotarget* March 2, 2016; http://dx.doi.org/10.18632/oncotarget.7853. [Epub ahead of print].
6. Malaney P, Nicosia SV, Dave V. One mouse, one patient paradigm: new avatars of personalized cancer therapy. *Cancer Lett* 2014;**344**(1):1–12.
7. Hidalgo M, Amant F, Biankin AV, et al. Patient-derived xenograft models: an emerging platform for translational cancer research. *Cancer Discov* 2014;**4**(9):998–1013.
8. Scott CL, Becker MA, Haluska P, Samimi G. Patient-derived xenograft models to improve targeted therapy in epithelial ovarian cancer treatment. *Front Oncol* 2013;**3**:295.
9. Bhadri VA, Cowley MJ, Kaplan W, Trahair TN, Lock RB. Evaluation of the NOD/SCID xenograft model for glucocorticoid-regulated gene expression in childhood B-cell precursor acute lymphoblastic leukemia. *BMC Genomics* 2011;**12**:565.
10. Agnusdei V, Minuzzo S, Frasson C, et al. Therapeutic antibody targeting of Notch1 in T-acute lymphoblastic leukemia xenografts. *Leukemia* 2014;**28**(2):278–88.
11. Agliano A, Martin-Padura I, Mancuso P, et al. Human acute leukemia cells injected in NOD/LtSz-scid/IL-2Rgamma null mice generate a faster and more efficient disease compared to other NOD/scid-related strains. *Int J Cancer* 2008;**123**(9):2222–7.
12. Saito Y, Yuki H, Kuratani M, et al. A pyrrolo-pyrimidine derivative targets human primary AML stem cells in vivo. *Sci Transl Med* 2013;**5**(181):181ra152.
13. Tentler JJ, Tan AC, Weekes CD, et al. Patient-derived tumour xenografts as models for oncology drug development. *Nat Rev Clin Oncol* 2012;**9**(6):338–50.
14. Jin K, Teng L, Shen Y, He K, Xu Z, Li G. Patient-derived human tumour tissue xenografts in immunodeficient mice: a systematic review. *Clin Transl Oncol* 2010;**12**(7):473–80.
15. Decaudin D. Primary human tumor xenografted models ('tumorgrafts') for good management of patients with cancer. *Anticancer Drugs* 2011;**22**(9):827–41.
16. Ghia P, Caligaris-Cappio F. The indispensable role of microenvironment in the natural history of low-grade B-cell neoplasms. *Adv Cancer Res* 2000;**79**:157–73.
17. McMillin DW, Negri JM, Mitsiades CS. The role of tumour-stromal interactions in modifying drug response: challenges and opportunities. *Nat Rev Drug Discov* 2013;**12**(3):217–28.
18. Ghobrial IM, Zhang Y, Liu Y, et al. Targeting the bone marrow in Waldenstrom macroglobulinemia. *Clin Lymphoma Myeloma Leuk* 2011;**11**(Suppl. 1):S65–9.
19. Duan CW, Shi J, Chen J, et al. Leukemia propagating cells rebuild an evolving niche in response to therapy. *Cancer Cell* 2014;**25**(6):778–93.
20. Passaro D, Irigoyen M, Catherinet C, et al. CXCR4 is required for leukemia-initiating cell activity in T Cell acute lymphoblastic leukemia. *Cancer Cell* 2015;**27**(6):769–79.
21. Pitt LA, Tikhonova AN, Hu H, et al. CXCL12-Producing vascular endothelial niches control acute T cell leukemia maintenance. *Cancer Cell* 2015;**27**(6):755–68.
22. Tse E, Kwong YL. T-cell lymphoma: microenvironment-related biomarkers. *Semin Cancer Biol* 2015;**34**:46–51.
23. Wang T, Feldman AL, Wada DA, et al. GATA-3 expression identifies a high-risk subset of PTCL, NOS with distinct molecular and clinical features. *Blood* 2014;**123**(19):3007–15.

24. Ohshima KS, Suzumiya J, Kawasaki C, Kanda M, Kikuchi M. Cytoplasmic cytokines in lymphoproliferative disorders: multiple cytokine production in angioimmunoblastic lymphadenopathy with dysproteinemia. *Leuk Lymphoma* 2000;**38**(5–6):541–5.
25. Cogle CR, Saki N, Khodadi E, Li J, Shahjahani M, Azizidoost S. Bone marrow niche in the myelodysplastic syndromes. *Leuk Res* 2015;**39**(10):1020–7.
26. Seke Etet PF, Vecchio L, Nwabo Kamdje AH. Signaling pathways in chronic myeloid leukemia and leukemic stem cell maintenance: key role of stromal microenvironment. *Cell Signal* 2012;**24**(9):1883–8.
27. Wang JC, Lapidot T, Cashman JD, et al. High level engraftment of NOD/SCID mice by primitive normal and leukemic hematopoietic cells from patients with chronic myeloid leukemia in chronic phase. *Blood* 1998;**91**(7):2406–14.
28. Eisterer W, Jiang X, Christ O, et al. Different subsets of primary chronic myeloid leukemia stem cells engraft immunodeficient mice and produce a model of the human disease. *Leukemia* 2005;**19**(3):435–41.
29. Verstegen MM, Cornelissen JJ, Terpstra W, Wagemaker G, Wognum AW. Multilineage outgrowth of both malignant and normal hemopoietic progenitor cells from individual chronic myeloid leukemia patients in immunodeficient mice. *Leukemia* 1999;**13**(4):618–28.
30. Wu S, Powers S, Zhu W, Hannun YA. Substantial contribution of extrinsic risk factors to cancer development. *Nature* 2016;**529**(7584):43–7.
31. Rafii S, Butler JM, Ding BS. Angiocrine functions of organ-specific endothelial cells. *Nature* 2016;**529**(7586):316–25.
32. Krause DS, Fulzele K, Catic A, et al. Differential regulation of myeloid leukemias by the bone marrow microenvironment. *Nat Med* 2013;**19**(11):1513–7.
33. Pizzi M, Silver RT, Barel A, Orazi A. Recombinant interferon-alpha in myelofibrosis reduces bone marrow fibrosis, improves its morphology and is associated with clinical response. *Mod Pathol* 2015;**28**(10):1315–23.
34. Schmitt A, Jouault H, Guichard J, Wendling F, Drouin A, Cramer EM. Pathologic interaction between megakaryocytes and polymorphonuclear leukocytes in myelofibrosis. *Blood* 2000;**96**(4):1342–7.
35. Sloma I, Jiang X, Eaves AC, Eaves CJ. Insights into the stem cells of chronic myeloid leukemia. *Leukemia* 2010;**24**(11):1823–33.
36. Engle EK, Fisher DA, Miller CA, et al. Clonal evolution revealed by whole genome sequencing in a case of primary myelofibrosis transformed to secondary acute myeloid leukemia. *Leukemia* 2015;**29**(4):869–76.
37. Triviai I, Ziegler M, Bergholz U, et al. Endogenous retrovirus induces leukemia in a xenograft mouse model for primary myelofibrosis. *Proc Natl Acad Sci USA* 2014;**111**(23):8595–600.
38. Kagoya Y, Yoshimi A, Tsuruta-Kishino T, et al. JAK2V617F+ myeloproliferative neoplasm clones evoke paracrine DNA damage to adjacent normal cells through secretion of lipocalin-2. *Blood* 2014;**124**(19):2996–3006.
39. Wang X, Zhang W, Tripodi J, et al. Sequential treatment of CD34+ cells from patients with primary myelofibrosis with chromatin-modifying agents eliminate JAK2V617F-positive NOD/SCID marrow repopulating cells. *Blood* 2010;**116**(26):5972–82.
40. Lu M, Xia L, Li Y, Wang X, Hoffman R. The orally bioavailable MDM2 antagonist RG7112 and pegylated interferon alpha 2a target JAK2V617F-positive progenitor and stem cells. *Blood* 2014;**124**(5):771–9.
41. Mesa RA, Kiladjian JJ, Verstovsek S, et al. Comparison of placebo and best available therapy for the treatment of myelofibrosis in the phase 3 COMFORT studies. *Haematologica* 2014;**99**(2):292–8.

42. Verstovsek S, Mesa RA, Gotlib J, et al. A double-blind, placebo-controlled trial of ruxolitinib for myelofibrosis. *N Engl J Med* 2012;**366**(9):799–807.
43. Passamonti F, Maffioli M, Cervantes F, et al. Impact of ruxolitinib on the natural history of primary myelofibrosis: a comparison of the DIPSS and the COMFORT-2 cohorts. *Blood* 2014;**123**(12):1833–5.
44. Marti-Carvajal AJ, Anand V, Sola I. Janus kinase-1 and Janus kinase-2 inhibitors for treating myelofibrosis. *Cochrane Database Syst Rev* 2015;**4**:CD010298.
45. Tefferi A, Pardanani A. Serious adverse events during ruxolitinib treatment discontinuation in patients with myelofibrosis. *Mayo Clin Proc* 2011;**86**(12):1188–91.
46. Nilsson L, Astrand-Grundstrom I, Anderson K, et al. Involvement and functional impairment of the CD34(+)CD38(-)Thy-1(+) hematopoietic stem cell pool in myelodysplastic syndromes with trisomy 8. *Blood* 2002;**100**(1):259–67.
47. Nilsson L, Astrand-Grundstrom I, Arvidsson I, et al. Isolation and characterization of hematopoietic progenitor/stem cells in 5q-deleted myelodysplastic syndromes: evidence for involvement at the hematopoietic stem cell level. *Blood* 2000;**96**(6):2012–21.
48. Benito AI, Bryant E, Loken MR, et al. NOD/SCID mice transplanted with marrow from patients with myelodysplastic syndrome (MDS) show long-term propagation of normal but not clonal human precursors. *Leuk Res* 2003;**27**(5):425–36.
49. Thanopoulou E, Cashman J, Kakagianne T, Eaves A, Zoumbos N, Eaves C. Engraftment of NOD/SCID-beta2 microglobulin null mice with multilineage neoplastic cells from patients with myelodysplastic syndrome. *Blood* 2004;**103**(11):4285–93.
50. Muguruma Y, Matsushita H, Yahata T, et al. Establishment of a xenograft model of human myelodysplastic syndromes. *Haematologica* 2011;**96**(4):543–51.
51. Pang WW, Pluvinage JV, Price EA, et al. Hematopoietic stem cell and progenitor cell mechanisms in myelodysplastic syndromes. *Proc Natl Acad Sci USA* 2013;**110**(8):3011–6.
52. Medyouf H, Mossner M, Jann JC, et al. Myelodysplastic cells in patients reprogram mesenchymal stromal cells to establish a transplantable stem cell niche disease unit. *Cell Stem Cell* 2014;**14**(6):824–37.
53. Woll PS, Kjallquist U, Chowdhury O, et al. Myelodysplastic syndromes are propagated by rare and distinct human cancer stem cells in vivo. *Cancer Cell* 2014;**25**(6):794–808.
54. Ryan JL, Kaufmann WK, Raab-Traub N, Oglesbee SE, Carey LA, Gulley ML. Clonal evolution of lymphoblastoid cell lines. *Lab Invest* 2006;**86**(11):1193–200.
55. Franks CR, Bishop D, Balkwill FR, Oliver RT, Spector WG. Growth of acute myeloid leukaemia as discrete subcutaneous tumours in immune-deprived mice. *Br J Cancer* 1977;**35**(5):697–700.
56. Palu G, Selby P, Powles R, Alexander P. Spontaneous regression of human acute myeloid leukaemia xenografts and phenotypic evidence for maturation. *Br J Cancer* 1979;**40**(5):731–5.
57. Nara N, Miyamoto T. Direct and serial transplantation of human acute myeloid leukaemia into nude mice. *Br J Cancer* 1982;**45**(5):778–82.
58. Caretto P, Forni M, d'Orazi G, et al. Xenotransplantation in immunosuppressed nude mice of human solid tumors and acute leukemias directly from patients or in vitro cell lines. *Ric Clin Lab* 1989;**19**(3):231–43.
59. Kamel-Reid S, Dick JE. Engraftment of immune-deficient mice with human hematopoietic stem cells. *Science* 1988;**242**(4886):1706–9.
60. Dick JE, Kamel-Reid S, Murdoch B, Doedens M. Gene transfer into normal human hematopoietic cells using in vitro and in vivo assays. *Blood* 1991;**78**(3):624–34.
61. De Lord C, Clutterbuck R, Titley J, et al. Growth of primary human acute leukemia in severe combined immunodeficient mice. *Exp Hematol* 1991;**19**(9):991–3.

62. Shang Y, Zhu T, Lenz AG, et al. Reduced in vitro toxicity of fine particulate matter collected during the 2008 Summer Olympic Games in Beijing: the roles of chemical and biological components. *Toxicol Vitro* 2013;**27**(7):2084–93.
63. Rombouts WJ, Martens AC, Ploemacher RE. Identification of variables determining the engraftment potential of human acute myeloid leukemia in the immunodeficient NOD/SCID human chimera model. *Leukemia* 2000;**14**(5):889–97.
64. Woiterski J, Ebinger M, Witte KE, et al. Engraftment of low numbers of pediatric acute lymphoid and myeloid leukemias into NOD/SCID/IL2Rcgammanull mice reflects individual leukemogenecity and highly correlates with clinical outcome. *Int J Cancer* 2013;**133**(7):1547–56.
65. Vick B, Rothenberg M, Sandhofer N, et al. An advanced preclinical mouse model for acute myeloid leukemia using patients' cells of various genetic subgroups and in vivo bioluminescence imaging. *PLoS One* 2015;**10**(3):e0120925.
66. Terpstra W, Prins A, Visser T, et al. Conditions for engraftment of human acute myeloid leukemia (AML) in SCID mice. *Leukemia* 1995;**9**(9):1573–7.
67. Lumkul R, Gorin NC, Malehorn MT, et al. Human AML cells in NOD/SCID mice: engraftment potential and gene expression. *Leukemia* 2002;**16**(9):1818–26.
68. Ailles LE, Gerhard B, Kawagoe H, Hogge DE. Growth characteristics of acute myelogenous leukemia progenitors that initiate malignant hematopoiesis in nonobese diabetic/severe combined immunodeficient mice. *Blood* 1999;**94**(5):1761–72.
69. Sanchez PV, Perry RL, Sarry JE, et al. A robust xenotransplantation model for acute myeloid leukemia. *Leukemia* 2009;**23**(11):2109–17.
70. Taussig DC, Vargaftig J, Miraki-Moud F, et al. Leukemia-initiating cells from some acute myeloid leukemia patients with mutated nucleophosmin reside in the CD34(-) fraction. *Blood* 2010;**115**(10):1976–84.
71. Shlush LI, Zandi S, Mitchell A, et al. Identification of pre-leukaemic haematopoietic stem cells in acute leukaemia. *Nature* 2014;**506**(7488):328–33.
72. Saida S, Watanabe K, Sato-Otsubo A, et al. Clonal selection in xenografted TAM recapitulates the evolutionary process of myeloid leukemia in Down syndrome. *Blood* 2013;**121**(21):4377–87.
73. Wunderlich M, Mizukawa B, Chou FS, et al. AML cells are differentially sensitive to chemotherapy treatment in a human xenograft model. *Blood* 2013;**121**(12):e90–7.
74. Saleh MN, Bussel JB, Cheng G, et al. Safety and efficacy of eltrombopag for treatment of chronic immune thrombocytopenia: results of the long-term, open-label EXTEND study. *Blood* 2013;**121**(3):537–45.
75. Will B, Kawahara M, Luciano JP, et al. Effect of the nonpeptide thrombopoietin receptor agonist Eltrombopag on bone marrow cells from patients with acute myeloid leukemia and myelodysplastic syndrome. *Blood* 2009;**114**(18):3899–908.
76. Saito Y, Uchida N, Tanaka S, et al. Induction of cell cycle entry eliminates human leukemia stem cells in a mouse model of AML. *Nat Biotechnol* 2010;**28**(3):275–80.
77. Cogle CR, Goldman DC, Madlambayan GJ, et al. Functional integration of acute myeloid leukemia into the vascular niche. *Leukemia* 2014;**28**(10):1978–87.
78. Madlambayan GJ, Meacham AM, Hosaka K, et al. Leukemia regression by vascular disruption and antiangiogenic therapy. *Blood* 2010;**116**(9):1539–47.
79. Hunger SP, Mullighan CG. Acute lymphoblastic leukemia in children. *N Engl J Med* 2015;**373**(16):1541–52.
80. Kawata A, Yoshida M, Okazaki M, Yokota S, Barcos M, Seon BK. Establishment of new SCID and nude mouse models of human B leukemia/lymphoma and effective therapy of the tumors with immunotoxin and monoclonal antibody: marked difference between the SCID and nude mouse models in the antitumor efficacy of monoclonal antibody. *Cancer Res* 1994;**54**(10):2688–94.

81. Steele JP, Clutterbuck RD, Powles RL, et al. Growth of human T-cell lineage acute leukemia in severe combined immunodeficiency (SCID) mice and non-obese diabetic SCID mice. *Blood* 1997;**90**(5):2015–9.
82. Diamanti P, Cox CV, Blair A. Comparison of childhood leukemia initiating cell populations in NOD/SCID and NSG mice. *Leukemia* 2012;**26**(2):376–80.
83. Notta F, Mullighan CG, Wang JC, et al. Evolution of human BCR-ABL1 lymphoblastic leukaemia-initiating cells. *Nature* 2011;**469**(7330):362–7.
84. Dewan MZ, Terunuma H, Ahmed S, et al. Natural killer cells in breast cancer cell growth and metastasis in SCID mice. *Biomed Pharmacother* 2005;**59**(Suppl. 2):S375–9.
85. Spiegel A, Kollet O, Peled A, et al. Unique SDF-1-induced activation of human precursor-B ALL cells as a result of altered CXCR4 expression and signaling. *Blood* 2004;**103**(8):2900–7.
86. Meyer LH, Eckhoff SM, Queudeville M, et al. Early relapse in ALL is identified by time to leukemia in NOD/SCID mice and is characterized by a gene signature involving survival pathways. *Cancer Cell* 2011;**19**(2):206–17.
87. Queudeville M, Seyfried F, Eckhoff SM, et al. Rapid engraftment of human ALL in NOD/SCID mice involves deficient apoptosis signaling. *Cell Death Dis* 2012;**3**:e364.
88. Uckun FM, Waurzyniak BJ, Sather HN, et al. Prognostic significance of T-lineage leukemic cell growth in SCID mice: a Children's Cancer Group study. *Leuk Lymphoma* 1999;**32**(5–6):475–87.
89. Clappier E, Gerby B, Sigaux F, et al. Clonal selection in xenografted human T cell acute lymphoblastic leukemia recapitulates gain of malignancy at relapse. *J Exp Med* 2011;**208**(4):653–61.
90. Kong Y, Yoshida S, Saito Y, et al. CD34+CD38+CD19+ as well as CD34+CD38-CD19+ cells are leukemia-initiating cells with self-renewal capacity in human B-precursor ALL. *Leukemia* 2008;**22**(6):1207–13.
91. Cox CV, Evely RS, Oakhill A, Pamphilon DH, Goulden NJ, Blair A. Characterization of acute lymphoblastic leukemia progenitor cells. *Blood* 2004;**104**(9):2919–25.
92. Cobaleda C, Gutierrez-Cianca N, Perez-Losada J, et al. A primitive hematopoietic cell is the target for the leukemic transformation in human philadelphia-positive acute lymphoblastic leukemia. *Blood* 2000;**95**(3):1007–13.
93. le Viseur C, Hotfilder M, Bomken S, et al. In childhood acute lymphoblastic leukemia, blasts at different stages of immunophenotypic maturation have stem cell properties. *Cancer Cell* 2008;**14**(1):47–58.
94. Heidenreich O, Vormoor J. Malignant stem cells in childhood ALL: the debate continues!. *Blood* 2009;**113**(18):4476–7. author reply 4477.
95. Chiu PP, Jiang H, Dick JE. Leukemia-initiating cells in human T-lymphoblastic leukemia exhibit glucocorticoid resistance. *Blood* 2010;**116**(24):5268–79.
96. Patel B, Dey A, Castleton AZ, et al. Mouse xenograft modeling of human adult acute lymphoblastic leukemia provides mechanistic insights into adult LIC biology. *Blood* 2014;**124**(1):96–105.
97. Canale S, Cocco C, Frasson C, et al. Interleukin-27 inhibits pediatric B-acute lymphoblastic leukemia cell spreading in a preclinical model. *Leukemia* 2011;**25**(12):1815–24.
98. Ong V, Liem NL, Schmid MA, et al. A role for altered microtubule polymer levels in vincristine resistance of childhood acute lymphoblastic leukemia xenografts. *J Pharmacol Exp Ther* 2008;**324**(2):434–42.
99. Jones CL, Gearheart CM, Fosmire S, et al. MAPK signaling cascades mediate distinct glucocorticoid resistance mechanisms in pediatric leukemia. *Blood* 2015;**126**(19):2202–12.
100. Jing D, Bhadri VA, Beck D, et al. Opposing regulation of BIM and BCL2 controls glucocorticoid-induced apoptosis of pediatric acute lymphoblastic leukemia cells. *Blood* 2015;**125**(2):273–83.

101. Mullighan CG, Goorha S, Radtke I, et al. Genome-wide analysis of genetic alterations in acute lymphoblastic leukaemia. *Nature* 2007;**446**(7137):758–64.
102. Kuiper RP, Schoenmakers EF, van Reijmersdal SV, et al. High-resolution genomic profiling of childhood ALL reveals novel recurrent genetic lesions affecting pathways involved in lymphocyte differentiation and cell cycle progression. *Leukemia* 2007;**21**(6):1258–66.
103. Mullighan CG, Miller CB, Radtke I, et al. BCR-ABL1 lymphoblastic leukaemia is characterized by the deletion of Ikaros. *Nature* 2008;**453**(7191):110–4.
104. Kawamata N, Ogawa S, Zimmermann M, et al. Molecular allelokaryotyping of pediatric acute lymphoblastic leukemias by high-resolution single nucleotide polymorphism oligonucleotide genomic microarray. *Blood* 2008;**111**(2):776–84.
105. Mullighan CG, Su X, Zhang J, et al. Deletion of IKZF1 and prognosis in acute lymphoblastic leukemia. *N Engl J Med* 2009;**360**(5):470–80.
106. Pui CH, Jeha S. New therapeutic strategies for the treatment of acute lymphoblastic leukaemia. *Nat Rev Drug Discov* 2007;**6**(2):149–65.
107. Irving J, Matheson E, Minto L, et al. Ras pathway mutations are prevalent in relapsed childhood acute lymphoblastic leukemia and confer sensitivity to MEK inhibition. *Blood* 2014;**124**(23):3420–30.
108. Maude SL, Dolai S, Delgado-Martin C, et al. Efficacy of JAK/STAT pathway inhibition in murine xenograft models of early T-cell precursor (ETP) acute lymphoblastic leukemia. *Blood* 2015;**125**(11):1759–67.
109. Suryani S, Bracken LS, Harvey RC, et al. Evaluation of the in vitro and in vivo efficacy of the JAK inhibitor AZD1480 against JAK-mutated acute lymphoblastic leukemia. *Mol Cancer Ther* 2015;**14**(2):364–74.
110. Fakler M, Loeder S, Vogler M, et al. Small molecule XIAP inhibitors cooperate with TRAIL to induce apoptosis in childhood acute leukemia cells and overcome Bcl-2-mediated resistance. *Blood* 2009;**113**(8):1710–22.
111. Bastian L, Hof J, Pfau M, et al. Synergistic activity of bortezomib and HDACi in preclinical models of B-cell precursor acute lymphoblastic leukemia via modulation of p53, PI3K/AKT, and NF-kappaB. *Clin Cancer Res* 2013;**19**(6):1445–57.
112. Shalapour S, Zelmer A, Pfau M, et al. The thalidomide analogue, CC-4047, induces apoptosis signaling and growth arrest in childhood acute lymphoblastic leukemia cells in vitro and in vivo. *Clin Cancer Res* 2006;**12**(18):5526–32.
113. Tang YL, Huang LB, Tian Y, et al. Flavokawain B inhibits the growth of acute lymphoblastic leukemia cells via p53 and caspase-dependent mechanisms. *Leuk Lymphoma* 2015;**56**(8):2398–407.
114. Ford JB, Baturin D, Burleson TM, Van Linden AA, Kim YM, Porter CC. AZD1775 sensitizes T cell acute lymphoblastic leukemia cells to cytarabine by promoting apoptosis over DNA repair. *Oncotarget* 2015;**6**(29):28001–10.
115. Fujii H, Trudeau JD, Teachey DT, et al. In vivo control of acute lymphoblastic leukemia by immunostimulatory CpG oligonucleotides. *Blood* 2007;**109**(5):2008–13.
116. Kato I, Niwa A, Heike T, et al. Identification of hepatic niche harboring human acute lymphoblastic leukemic cells via the SDF-1/CXCR4 axis. *PLoS One* 2011;**6**(11):e27042.
117. Konoplev S, Jorgensen JL, Thomas DA, et al. Phosphorylated CXCR4 is associated with poor survival in adults with B-acute lymphoblastic leukemia. *Cancer* 2011;**117**(20):4689–95.
118. Juarez JG, Thien M, Dela Pena A, Baraz R, Bradstock KF, Bendall LJ. CXCR4 mediates the homing of B cell progenitor acute lymphoblastic leukaemia cells to the bone marrow via activation of p38MAPK. *Br J Haematol* 2009;**145**(4):491–9.

119. de Lourdes Perim A, Amarante MK, Guembarovski RL, de Oliveira CE, Watanabe MA. CXCL12/CXCR4 axis in the pathogenesis of acute lymphoblastic leukemia (ALL): a possible therapeutic target. *Cell Mol Life Sci* 2015;**72**(9):1715–23.
120. Uy GL, Rettig MP, Cashen AF. Plerixafor, a CXCR4 antagonist for the mobilization of hematopoietic stem cells. *Expert Opin Biol Ther* 2008;**8**(11):1797–804.
121. Cho BS, Zeng Z, Mu H, et al. Antileukemia activity of the novel peptidic CXCR4 antagonist LY2510924 as monotherapy and in combination with chemotherapy. *Blood* 2015;**126**(2):222–32.
122. Galsky MD, Vogelzang NJ, Conkling P, et al. A phase I trial of LY2510924, a CXCR4 peptide antagonist, in patients with advanced cancer. *Clin Cancer Res* 2014;**20**(13):3581–8.
123. Murakami T, Kumakura S, Yamazaki T, et al. The novel CXCR4 antagonist KRH-3955 is an orally bioavailable and extremely potent inhibitor of human immunodeficiency virus type 1 infection: comparative studies with AMD3100. *Antimicrob Agents Chemother* 2009;**53**(7):2940–8.
124. Karpova D, Dauber K, Spohn G, et al. The novel CXCR4 antagonist POL5551 mobilizes hematopoietic stem and progenitor cells with greater efficiency than Plerixafor. *Leukemia* 2013;**27**(12):2322–31.
125. Xiang J, Hurchla MA, Fontana F, et al. CXCR4 protein epitope mimetic antagonist POL5551 disrupts metastasis and enhances chemotherapy effect in triple-negative breast cancer. *Mol Cancer Ther* 2015;**14**(11):2473–85.
126. Sison EA, Magoon D, Li L, et al. POL5551, a novel and potent CXCR4 antagonist, enhances sensitivity to chemotherapy in pediatric ALL. *Oncotarget* 2015;**6**(31):30902–18.
127. Topp MS, Gokbuget N, Zugmaier G, et al. Long-term follow-up of hematologic relapse-free survival in a phase 2 study of blinatumomab in patients with MRD in B-lineage ALL. *Blood* 2012;**120**(26):5185–7.
128. Ruella M, Gill S. How to train your T cell: genetically engineered chimeric antigen receptor T cells versus bispecific T-cell engagers to target CD19 in B acute lymphoblastic leukemia. *Expert Opin Biol Ther* 2015;**15**(6):761–6.
129. Topp MS, Gokbuget N, Zugmaier G, et al. Phase II trial of the anti-CD19 bispecific T cell-engager blinatumomab shows hematologic and molecular remissions in patients with relapsed or refractory B-precursor acute lymphoblastic leukemia. *J Clin Oncol* 2014;**32**(36):4134–40.
130. Schmidt-Wolf IG, Lefterova P, Mehta BA, et al. Phenotypic characterization and identification of effector cells involved in tumor cell recognition of cytokine-induced killer cells. *Exp Hematol* 1993;**21**(13):1673–9.
131. Baker J, Verneris MR, Ito M, Shizuru JA, Negrin RS. Expansion of cytolytic CD8(+) natural killer T cells with limited capacity for graft-versus-host disease induction due to interferon gamma production. *Blood* 2001;**97**(10):2923–31.
132. Qin H, Cho M, Haso W, et al. Eradication of B-ALL using chimeric antigen receptor-expressing T cells targeting the TSLPR oncoprotein. *Blood* 2015;**126**(5):629–39.
133. (a) Mamonkin M, Rouce RH, Tashiro H, Brenner MKA. T-cell-directed chimeric antigen receptor for the selective treatment of T-cell malignancies. *Blood* 2015;**126**(8):983–92.
(b) Townsend EC, Murakami MA, Christodoulou A, et al. The Public Repository of Xenografts Enables Discovery and Randomized Phase II-like Trials in Mice. *Cancer Cell* April 11, 2016;**29**(4): 574–86.
134. Rasul E, Salamon D, Nagy N, et al. The MEC1 and MEC2 lines represent two CLL subclones in different stages of progression towards prolymphocytic leukemia. *PLoS One* 2014;**9**(8):e106008.
135. Tiacci E, Pucciarini A, Bigerna B, et al. Absence of BRAF-V600E in the human cell lines BONNA-12, ESKOL, HAIR-M, and HC-1 questions their origin from hairy cell leukemia. *Blood* 2012;**119**(22):5332–3.

136. Tiacci E, Trifonov V, Schiavoni G, et al. BRAF mutations in hairy-cell leukemia. *N Engl J Med* 2011;**364**(24):2305–15.
137. Zhang J, Grubor V, Love CL, et al. Genetic heterogeneity of diffuse large B-cell lymphoma. *Proc Natl Acad Sci USA* 2013;**110**(4):1398–403.
138. Drexler HG, MacLeod RA. Leukemia-lymphoma cell lines as model systems for hematopoietic research. *Ann Med* 2003;**35**(6):404–12.
139. Matsuo Y, Drexler HG. Immunoprofiling of cell lines derived from natural killer-cell and natural killer-like T-cell leukemia-lymphoma. *Leuk Res* 2003;**27**(10):935–45.
140. Drexler HG, MacLeod RA. Malignant hematopoietic cell lines: in vitro models for the study of anaplastic large-cell lymphoma. *Leukemia* 2004;**18**(10):1569–71.
141. Simonetti G, Bertilaccio MT, Ghia P, Klein U. Mouse models in the study of chronic lymphocytic leukemia pathogenesis and therapy. *Blood* 2014;**124**(7):1010–9.
142. Donnou S, Galand C, Touitou V, Sautes-Fridman C, Fabry Z, Fisson S. Murine models of B-cell lymphomas: promising tools for designing cancer therapies. *Adv Hematol* 2012;**2012**:701704.
143. Yu D, Thomas-Tikhonenko A. A non-transgenic mouse model for B-cell lymphoma: in vivo infection of p53-null bone marrow progenitors by a Myc retrovirus is sufficient for tumorigenesis. *Oncogene* 2002;**21**(12):1922–7.
144. Panfil AR, Al-Saleem JJ, Green PL. Animal models utilized in HTLV-1 research. *Virol Auckl* 2013;**4**:49–59.
145. Warner K, Crispatzu G, Al-Ghaili N, et al. Models for mature T-cell lymphomas–a critical appraisal of experimental systems and their contribution to current T-cell tumorigenic concepts. *Crit Rev Oncol Hematol* 2013;**88**(3):680–95.
146. Tesio M, Trinquand A, Macintyre E, Asnafi V. Oncogenic PTEN functions and models in T-cell malignancies. *Oncogene* 2015.
147. Herter-Sprie GS, Kung AL, Wong KK. New cast for a new era: preclinical cancer drug development revisited. *J Clin Invest* 2013;**123**(9):3639–45.
148. Monsma DJ, Monks NR, Cherba DM, et al. Genomic characterization of explant tumorgraft models derived from fresh patient tumor tissue. *J Transl Med* 2012;**10**:125.
149. Bagnara D, Kaufman MS, Calissano C, et al. A novel adoptive transfer model of chronic lymphocytic leukemia suggests a key role for T lymphocytes in the disease. *Blood* 2011;**117**(20):5463–72.
150. King MA, Covassin L, Brehm MA, et al. Human peripheral blood leucocyte non-obese diabetic-severe combined immunodeficiency interleukin-2 receptor gamma chain gene mouse model of xenogeneic graft-versus-host-like disease and the role of host major histocompatibility complex. *Clin Exp Immunol* 2009;**157**(1):104–18.
151. Shultz LD, Brehm MA, Garcia-Martinez JV, Greiner DL. Humanized mice for immune system investigation: progress, promise and challenges. *Nat Rev Immunol* 2012;**12**(11):786–98.
152. Sun LL, Ellerman D, Mathieu M, et al. Anti-CD20/CD3 T cell-dependent bispecific antibody for the treatment of B cell malignancies. *Sci Transl Med* 2015;**7**(287):287ra270.
153. Messmer D, Lorrain K, Stebbins K, et al. A selective novel peroxisome proliferator-activated receptor (PPAR)-alpha antagonist induces apoptosis and inhibits proliferation of CLL cells in vitro and in vivo. *Mol Med* 2015;**21**:410–9.
154. Ghosn EE, Waters J, Phillips M, et al. Fetal hematopoietic stem cell transplantation fails to fully regenerate the B-Lymphocyte compartment. *Stem Cell Rep* 2016;**6**(1):137–49.
155. Klanova M, Soukup T, Jaksa R, et al. Mouse models of mantle cell lymphoma, complex changes in gene expression and phenotype of engrafted MCL cells: implications for preclinical research. *Lab Invest* 2014;**94**(7):806–17.

156. Zhao X, Chen-Kiang S, Shetty S, et al. CCMCL1: a new model of aggressive mantle cell lymphoma. *Blood* 2015;**125**(17):2730–2.
157. Kuruvilla J, Cerchietti L, Wagner-Johnston N, et al. The oral selective inhibitor of nuclear export (SINE) selinexor (KTP-330) activity in double hit diffuse large B cell lymphomas (DLBCL) in preclinical models & clinical activity in patients with DLBCL. In: *Poster presented at the 13th International Conference on malignant lymphoma*. June 17–20, 2015 (Lugano, Switzerland).
158. Chapuy B, Cheng H, Watahiki A, et al. Diffuse large B-cell lymphoma patient-derived xenograft models capture the molecular and biologic heterogeneity of the disease. *Blood* 2016;**127**(18).
159. Sugimoto K, Hayakawa F, Shimada S, et al. Discovery of a drug targeting microenvironmental support for lymphoma cells by screening using patient-derived xenograft cells. *Sci Rep* 2015;**5**:13054.
160. Agnelli L, Tassone P, Neri A. Molecular profiling of multiple myeloma: from gene expression analysis to next-generation sequencing. *Expert Opin Biol Ther* 2013;**13**(Suppl. 1):S55–68.
161. Feo-Zuppardi FJ, Taylor CW, Iwato K, et al. Long-term engraftment of fresh human myeloma cells in SCID mice. *Blood* 1992;**80**(11):2843–50.
162. Urashima M, Chen BP, Chen S, et al. The development of a model for the homing of multiple myeloma cells to human bone marrow. *Blood* 1997;**90**(2):754–65.
163. Tassone P, Neri P, Carrasco DR, et al. A clinically relevant SCID-hu in vivo model of human multiple myeloma. *Blood* 2005;**106**(2):713–6.
164. Yaccoby S, Barlogie B, Epstein J. Primary myeloma cells growing in SCID-hu mice: a model for studying the biology and treatment of myeloma and its manifestations. *Blood* 1998;**92**(8):2908–13.
165. Lemaire M, Fristedt C, Agarwal P, et al. The HDAC inhibitor LBH589 enhances the antimyeloma effects of the IGF-1RTK inhibitor picropodophyllin. *Clin Cancer Res* 2012;**18**(8):2230–9.
166. Caers J, Menu E, De Raeve H, et al. Antitumour and antiangiogenic effects of Aplidin in the 5TMM syngeneic models of multiple myeloma. *Br J Cancer* 2008;**98**(12):1966–74.
167. Sanchez E, Chen H, Berenson JR. In vivo models of multiple myeloma (MM). *Biochem Pharmacol* 2014;**89**(3):313–20.
168. O'Brien S, Jeha S, Kantarjian H, et al. Engraftment of chronic prolymphocytic and T cell leukemia in SCID mice. *Leukemia* 1996;**10**(2):338–44.
169. van der Fits L, Rebel HG, Out-Luiting JJ, et al. A novel mouse model for Sézary syndrome using xenotransplantation of Sézary cells into immunodeficient RAG2(-/-) gammac(-/-) mice. *Exp Dermatol* 2012;**21**(9):706–9.
170. Cheng M, Quail MR, Gingrich DE, et al. CEP-28122, a highly potent and selective orally active inhibitor of anaplastic lymphoma kinase with antitumor activity in experimental models of human cancers. *Mol Cancer Ther* 2011;**11**(3):670–9.
171. Crescenzo R, Abate F, Lasorsa E, et al. Convergent mutations and kinase fusions lead to oncogenic STAT3 activation in anaplastic large cell lymphoma. *Cancer Cell* 2015;**27**(4):516–32.
172. Scarfo I, Pellegrino E, Mereu E, et al. Identification of a new subclass of ALK-negative ALCL expressing aberrant levels of ERBB4 transcripts. *Blood* 2016;**127**(2):221–32.
173. Abate F, Todaro M, van der Krogt J, et al. A novel patient-derived tumorgraft model with TRAF1-ALK anaplastic large cell lymphoma translocation. *Leukemia* 2014;**29**(6).

Chapter 9

Patient-Derived Xenografting of Human Melanoma

S.E. Boyle[1,2], C.G. Fedele[1], M. Shackleton[1,2]
[1]*Peter MacCallum Cancer Centre, East Melbourne, VIC, Australia;* [2]*University of Melbourne, Parkville, VIC, Australia*

BACKGROUND AND OVERVIEW

Melanoma is a cancer of melanocytes, which are pigment-producing cells normally located in the skin and also less abundantly in the eye and the respiratory, gastrointestinal, and urogenital tracts. Although melanoma accounted for 3% of cancer diagnoses and 0.7% of cancer-related deaths across the world in 2012, it is a far more substantial health and socioeconomic problem in locations with large proportions of fair-skinned people and high levels of exposure to environmental ultraviolet (UV) radiation from the sun, such as southern United States, Australia, and New Zealand.[1] Patients with cutaneous melanoma are staged pathologically according to the degree of invasion and spread of disease. Early stage or primary melanomas (stages 1 and 2) are confined to the skin, whereas metastatic melanomas include disease that has spread to regional lymphatics (stage 3) or to distant sites (stage 4).

Although most primary melanomas are cured by surgery, metastatic disease was traditionally associated with a poor prognosis.[2] However, advances in the systemic treatment of melanoma have dramatically changed the outcomes of some patients with metastatic disease.[3] Immunotherapy with agents that promote antitumor effector T cells by targeting inhibitory signaling axes, such as B7–CTLA4[4,5] and PD-1L–PD-1[6] interactions, has extended median survival in patients with metastatic disease.[7,8] Targeted therapies, particularly with agents that target components of the mitogen-activated protein kinase (MAPK) molecular signaling pathway, have also changed the face of melanoma treatment. These therapies have dominantly focused on patients with mutations in the *BRAF* gene, the constitutive activation of which drives disease progression in 40–50% of patients.[9,10]

Although these advances in systemic therapy have been quantum, the majority of patients with advanced melanoma still die because of their cancer. Accordingly, work to understand biological features of the disease, and their molecular drivers, is as important as ever. While high-throughput discovery in

Patient Derived Tumor Xenograft Models. http://dx.doi.org/10.1016/B978-0-12-804010-2.00023-0

cancer genomics has revealed numerous prospective therapy targets in melanoma, such as mutant BRAF, deciphering a functional role for these remains essential. The ability to model experimentally key aspects of cancer biology and response to therapy in a manner that is relevant to patients remains pivotal in improving patient outcomes.

In melanoma, there are major limitations to most current experimental modeling approaches. In vitro culture of passaged cell lines[11] is the most convenient, simple, and cost-effective approach, with over 5000 melanoma cell lines available[12] and numerous important discoveries based on their use. Cell lines are particularly useful for biochemical studies. However, their usefulness in revealing fundamental and clinically relevant aspects of disease biology and in predicting the effectiveness of therapies in patients has been questioned.[13–15]

Genetically engineered mouse models (GEMMs) are also used to model melanoma,[16] providing critical in vivo contexts for studying disease biology. GEMMs have enabled in vivo study of specific molecular pathways in melanocytes and melanoma, such as the MAPK pathway. For example, GEMMs have been developed to model melanomas driven in vivo by *BRAF* or *NRAS* mutations,[10,17] which are mutually exclusive driver events in patients.[18] However, there remain questions about the ability of mouse models to faithfully recapitulate human melanomagenesis. Mice largely lack melanocytes in the interfollicular epidermis, the cellular compartment in which most human melanomas are thought to arise. To address this, models have been developed in which melanocytes migrate to the interfollicular region, where they can be UV irradiated to drive melanomagenesis.[16] However, the relevance of this approach to human melanoma initiation remains to be confirmed.[19] Moreover, GEMMs in which tumor formation is driven by powerful oncogenes may lack key features of human cancer, such as genomic instability, and thus do not model well the inter- and intrapatient disease heterogeneity that frequently confounds therapy in patients.

In some contexts, patient-derived xenograft (PDX) models, in which freshly isolated cancers from patients are grown in immunocompromised host mice, are considered to be superior models of human cancer because they recapitulate disease heterogeneity better than other approaches.[14,15,20] Furthermore, although the requirement for immunocompromised mice currently precludes the use of PDX for testing immunotherapies, PDX models may improve prediction of response to therapies that target cancer cell–intrinsic mechanisms of disease in patients.[21] Aspects of melanoma PDX establishment, as well as uses and limitations of PDX melanoma modeling, will be discussed in this chapter.

METHODOLOGY AND MODELS

Sources of Fresh Human Melanoma Cells

Cutaneous melanomas are on average among the smallest tumors surgically removed from patients. This is because they are usually distinctly pigmented and arise in locations on the skin that are easily visible, facilitating relatively early detection and treatment. The small size of most primary melanomas presents challenges in the establishment of PDX from them, as tumor tissue in excess of diagnostic requirements is rarely available. Furthermore, it is not always apparent clinically that lesions being removed are in fact melanomas, and complete excision biopsies are usually recommended for histopathological diagnosis (via formalin fixation). For these reasons, most primary cutaneous melanomas for which fresh tissue is available are relatively large, have been previously biopsied to establish the diagnosis, and are not representative of the spectrum of primary stage disease. Of the 18 published studies reporting the generation of PDX melanomas, only four have included PDXs generated from primary cutaneous melanomas (Table 9.1).

Most PDX melanomas are derived from metastatic disease (usually stage 3 disease involving regional lymph nodes or in-transit lymphatic structures), for which the diagnosis is typically known prior to surgery. With supportive clinicians and tissue banking staff to obtain patient consent, alert pathology services, and prompt processing of samples, fresh tumor tissue can be delivered to laboratories as soon as 20–30 min after resection for the generation of PDXs. It is also possible to establish PDXs from melanoma tumors removed at rapid autopsy, although substantial logistic issues must be overcome to minimize the time from patient death to provision of tumor material, which is typically at least 4 h.

Processing of Fresh Human Melanomas for PDX

A strength of PDX is its potential to model the tumor cell–intrinsic heterogeneity of cancers in patients. However, the only way to ensure maximal recapitulation of cancer cell heterogeneity is to implant entire patient tumors, which is rarely feasible. To represent in PDX tumors as much of the cellular diversity that is present in patients, it is important to consider methods of tumor processing.

Time From Tumor Procurement to In Vivo Implantation

Although no data exist to indicate the effect of time between tumor procurement and in vivo implantation of melanoma cells on the efficiency of initial PDX engraftment, it is assumed that shorter times increase efficiency. Consistent with this, establishment of PDX melanomas from tumors obtained at rapid autopsy, whose viability may be compromised by hypoperfusion during the immediate premortem period as well as the time of absolute ischemia postmortem, is ~50% less efficient than from tumors obtained freshly from otherwise well patients (unpublished data). For the latter, with prompt processing after surgical removal, almost every melanoma and even very small pieces from the primary cutaneous disease can be established as a PDX. Prolonged times between tumor removal and implantation would be expected to reduce the efficiency of PDX engraftment, although it is unknown if there is a threshold beyond which cell viability diminishes more rapidly. Without prompt processing of tumors, selection of cells specifically adapted to resist ischemia might be expected in PDX tumors.

TABLE 9.1 Studies That Have Used PDX Melanomas to Investigate Melanoma Biology

Publication (Author/Year)	Samples Implanted (*n*)	Tumor Origin	Implantation Technique	Average Latency (weeks)	Experimental End Point (weeks)	Patient Melanomas Engrafted (%)	Mouse Strain	Comparison of PDX and Original Patient Tumors
Schatton et al.[31]	4	Metastatic	Single-cell suspension/ heterotopic	n/a	8	75	NOD/SCID	Marker expression via flow cytometry and IHC
Quintana et al.[26]	19	Metastatic	Single-cell suspension/ heterotopic	11.4–14.3	32	89	NOD/SCID, NSG	n/a
Quintana et al.[37]	16	Primary and metastatic	Single-cell suspension/ heterotopic	n/a	n/a	100	NSG	Marker expression via flow cytometry
Boiko et al.[32]	5 (2 with prior in vitro expansion)	Primary and metastatic	Tumor pieces and single-cell suspension/ orthotopic	n/a	32	n/a	$Rag2^{-/-}\gamma c^{-/-}$	n/a
Boonyaratanakornkit et al.[33]	13	Metastastic	Single-cell suspension/ heterotopic	7.8	24–36	n/a	NOD/SCID	n/a
Civenni et al.[34]	19	Metastatic	Single-cell suspension/ heterotopic	n/a	6–8	100	BALB/C nude, NOD/SCID, NSG	IF of CD271, Sox10, S100, HBM45, MelanA, and MITF

Luo et al.[35]	6	Primary and metastatic	Single-cell suspension/ orthotopic	4.3–8.6	24	n/a	NOD/SCID, NSG	Marker expression via flow cytometry ($n=1$)
Quintana et al.[38]	27 (From 25 patients)	Metastatic	Single-cell suspension/ heterotopic	n/a	n/a	n/a	NSG	Presence or absence of overall metastasis and brain metastasis
Guerreschi et al.[48]	3 (From the same patient)	Metastatic	Tumor pieces/ heterotopic	n/a	n/a	n/a	SCID	Therapy response
Das Thakur et al.[46]	3	Primary and metastatic	Tumor pieces/ heterotopic	n/a	n/a	n/a	Athymic nu/nu	n/a
Einarsdottir et al.[79]	26	Metastatic	Single-cell suspension/ heterotopic	n/a	n/a	88	NSG	IHC staining (S100, Melan-A, HMB45) and exome sequencing and RNAseq comparison
Kobelt et al.[50]	1	n/a	Tumor pieces/ heterotopic	n/a	n/a	n/a	NMRI nu/nu	n/a
Girotti et al.[47]	6	Metastatic	Tumor pieces/ heterotopic	n/a	n/a	n/a	NSG	n/a
Kemper et al.[49]	6 (From the same patient)	Metastatic	Tumor pieces/ heterotopic	n/a	n/a	n/a	NSG	IHC staining (BRAFV600E)

Continued

TABLE 9.1 Studies That Have Used PDX Melanomas to Investigate Melanoma Biology—cont'd

Publication (Author/Year)	Samples Implanted (*n*)	Tumor Origin	Implantation Technique	Average Latency (weeks)	Experimental End Point (weeks)	Patient Melanomas Engrafted (%)	Mouse Strain	Comparison of PDX and Original Patient Tumors
Monsma et al.[51]	5	Metastatic	Tumor pieces/ heterotopic	n/a	n/a	n/a	Athymic nu/nu	n/a
Krepler et al.[78]	12 (From 10 patients	Metastatic	Tumor slurry/ heterotopic	5.75	n/a	100	NSG	Histological comparison
Dewaele et al.[94]	4	Metastatic	Tumor pieces/ heterotopic	n/a	n/a	n/a	NOD. Cg-Prkdcscid Il2rgtm1Sug/ JicTac	n/a
Girotti et al.[84]	118 Cutaneous, 7 acral, 1 uveal	Metastatic	Tumor pieces/ heterotopic	7	n/a	72%	NSG	Histological, genomic, and therapy response

IF, immunofluorescence; *IHC*, immunohistochemistry; *n/a*, not reported.

Effect of Cryopreservation

The complex logistic requirements of PDX establishment sometimes require that freshly isolated tumor pieces or cells need to be stored prior to implantation into mice. This is commonly performed via cryopreservation in 5–10% (v/v) dimethyl sulfoxide and controlled-rate passive freezing.[22] However, low cell recovery rates may be observed following cryopreservation.[23–25] We observe that purified and cryopreserved melanoma cells that survive freeze-thaw have a two- to threefold decreased efficiency of PDX tumor engraftment (unpublished data). Through cell loss during the freeze-thaw process and through reduced tumorigenic potential in thawed but viable cells, PDX melanomas established from cryopreserved cells will contain cells selected for the ability to form tumors after cryopreservation.

The Nature of Implanted Tumor Material Pieces or Cells

PDX melanomas can be established either by implantation (usually subcutaneous, but numerous other sites—intramuscular, intracranial, renal subcapsular—are feasible) of small tumor pieces or via injection of tumor cell suspensions derived following mechanical and enzymatic dissociation. Engraftment of PDX melanomas from highly necrotic patient samples is far less efficient following injection of dissociated cell suspensions than from subcutaneous transplantation of small pieces of the same tumor (unpublished data). However, for most patient melanomas, PDX establishment from cell suspensions can be very efficient[26] and is preferred because it enables PDX tumor formation from representative cell populations rather than from geographically separated regions within tumors that may be enriched for genetically distinct subclones.[27] Furthermore, transplantation of tumor pieces is more traumatic to mice and may increase the complications of PDX tumor generation.[28,29] Implantation of tumor pieces usually results in cotransplantation of nonmalignant cells, which may include lymphocytes infected with Epstein-Barr virus that can transform to lymphomas in immunocompromised mice.[28–30]

Obtaining Melanoma Cell Suspensions From Solid Tumors

Various methods are described for deriving cell suspensions from patient melanomas (Table 9.2). If in vitro culture is planned, all dissociation steps should be performed in a laminar flow hood. However, this is not necessary prior to injection of cells into immunocompromised mice, which only rarely develop infective complications. Each method begins with a mechanical dissociation step in which tumors are macroscopically cleared of obvious normal and necrotic tissue, and then chopped to a fine slurry. Several groups have used relatively long (>30 min) tumor dissociation times in buffer containing enzymes (eg, collagenase) that break down extracellular matrix components.[31–35] Others use more rapid dissociation that additionally involves tissue grinders[36] or enzymatic treatment with dilute trypsin to disrupt cell–cell adhesion complexes.[36,37] Cells

TABLE 9.2 Differences in Experimental Methods Used to Dissociate Melanoma Cells in Published Studies

	Studies						
Method	**Schatton et al.**[31]	**Quintana et al.**[26]	**Boiko et al.**[32]	**Boonyaratanakornkit et al.**[33]	**Civenni et al.**[34]	**Luo et al.**[35]	**Krepler et al.**[78]
Enzymatic dissociation	$CaCl_2$, C	C4, DNAse, $CaCl_2$	Liberase blendzyme 2 and 4	C, hyaluronidase, DNAse	C3, dispase	C1, hyaluronidase	C4
Dissociation time	180 min	20 min	100 min	90–120 min	60 min	120 min	20 min
Trypsin	–	0.05%	–	–	–	–	0.05%
Matrigel	–	25% High concentration	30% Standard	Standard	30% Standard	50% Standard	Standard
Mice	NOD/SCID	NOD/SCID, NSG	$Rag2^{-/-}$ $\gamma c^{-/-}$, NSG	NOD/SCID, NSG	Nude, NOD/SCID, NSG	NOD/SCID, NSG	NSG
Injection type	SQ	SQ	Interdermal	SQ	SQ	Interdermal	SQ

C, collagenase; *C1/3/4*, collagenase 1/3/4; *SQ*, subcutaneous.

dissociated from patient melanomas may be cryopreserved as mentioned earlier for future use, injected directly into mice, or labeled with antibodies to enable immunoselection of enriched melanoma cell populations that can then be injected, cultured, or even transduced with virus-packaged DNA expression vectors.[38]

Animals for Xenotransplantation

An important goal in establishing PDX is to generate tumors that are maximally representative of patient tumors. Thus, using mice that reveal tumorigenic potential in as many transplanted cells as possible is essential. Until recently, nude and nonobese diabetic severe combined immunodeficiency (NOD/SCID) mice were commonly used as immunocompromised recipients of implanted melanoma cells.[26,31] However, studies of side-by-side transplantation of freshly isolated melanoma cells into NOD/SCID mice versus NOD/SCID mice that were additionally modified to lack the interleukin-2 gamma receptor (IL2γR) (NSG mice) revealed approximately 50,000-fold increased efficiency of PDX tumor formation in NSG mice.[26] Deletion of IL2γR in NSG mice results in loss of natural killer cell function and further impairs innate immunity.[39] This apparently dramatically suppresses the xenogeneic immune response that otherwise occurs, even in NOD/SCID mice, against transplanted human cells. Consequently, NSG mice have become preferred animal recipients in most PDX melanoma studies.

In some human cancers, approaches to establish PDX lines require the coinjection of noncancer cells or other material to support PDX tumor engraftment.[40–42] For melanoma, the use of coinjected Matrigel, which is an extracellular matrix formulation derived from the Engelbreth–Holm–Swarm mouse sarcoma cell line,[43,44] improves by several fold the efficiency of PDX tumor formation from injected cells.[26] Matrigel is mainly composed of basement membrane and extracellular matrix proteins such as laminin, collagen, entactin, and proteoglycans, as well as a range of cell growth factors.[43,44] Although it is possible that growth factors in Matrigel confer tumorigenicity on transplanted cells that lack tumorigenic potential in patients; this is unlikely as we find that use of modified, growth factor–reduced Matrigel does not reduce the efficiency of PDX melanoma formation in NSG mice (unpublished data). Rather, it is more likely that Matrigel components, such as laminin and collagen, provide survival signals to prevent cellular anoikis until, once implanted into mice, tumor cells can generate a suitable extracellular environment.[45] In limiting dilution assays of cells derived from a range of melanomas, with the use of comixed Matrigel and injection of cells into NSG mice, an average of 25% of injected cells was capable of PDX melanoma formation.[26]

The effect of the site of transplantation on PDX melanoma engraftment may also be considered. Although orthotopic transplantation via intradermal injection has been suggested to provide a more physiologically relevant context for PDX melanoma growth,[32] this is not necessarily the case. In patients, most cancer cells reside within a microenvironment composed of other cancer cells and the factors they produce, interacting relatively minimally with the normal tissues in which they arose. Regardless, as melanomas used to establish PDX lines are most readily available from metastases in lymph nodes or subcutaneous lymphatics of patients, transplantation into nondermal sites is appropriate.

For implantation of tumor pieces, subcutaneous, intramuscular or renal subcapsular sites may be used. Although most groups generate PDX melanomas through subcutaneous implantation (Table 9.1),[46–51] there are little data to compare different sites. In our experience, the intramuscular route is superior to subcutaneous implantation for engrafting PDX melanomas from pieces of highly necrotic patient tumor material, consistent with published data in esophageal cancer.[30] However, subcutaneous implantation is usually adequate for implanting pieces of healthy melanoma tissue. For injection of cell suspensions, the subcutaneous route of injection is simple, rapid, nontraumatic to mice, and offers very efficient PDX engraftment.[26]

Engraft Time and Success Rate

Despite the notorious aggressiveness of melanomas in patients, the formation of PDX tumors from melanoma cell implantation usually takes several months, although injections of larger numbers of cells generally and unsurprisingly result in shorter tumor latencies. Tumor initiation in our laboratory can occur as early as 5 weeks after injection but has been delayed by as much as 58 weeks, with an average tumor latency of 15 ± 10 weeks, consistent with previous reports.[26] This is important for experimental end points that rely on tumor formation, which will be reduced if insufficient time is allowed for PDX tumor formation. This effect may be compounded if more than one injection is performed per mouse (eg, into either flank), whereupon the growth of one tumor to a size that ethically requires euthanasia of the mouse may occur before the other tumor has formed.

Propagation of PDX Lines

Once an initial PDX melanoma has formed, its maintenance and propagation are straightforward. PDX melanomas may be removed and tumors either stored or processed as mentioned earlier for serial transplantation. Tumor removal may be performed at necropsy, or via survival surgeries from which mice typically recover well. This approach is useful for facilitating studies of spontaneous metastasis (see later). The latency of PDX tumor formation in NSG mice from injected cells obtained from PDX melanomas is on average approximately 50% shorter than when cells derived directly from patient samples are used.[26] This presumably reflects the adaptation of human melanoma cells from PDX tumors to growth in the murine environment. Alternatively, shorter tumor latencies in

PDX-to-PDX tumor propagation might reflect enrichment of cells with tumorigenic potential in PDX melanomas. Against this, increases in empirically determined proportions of tumorigenic cells are not consistently observed during passaging of PDX melanomas in NSG mice.[37]

TUMOR BIOLOGY

Although PDX models are not applicable to studying melanoma initiation from normal melanocytes, they are very useful in modeling the progression of established invasive and metastatic disease. A striking biological feature of many cancers, including melanoma, is extensive intratumoral cellular heterogeneity.[52–56] One mechanism that contributes to intratumoral cellular heterogeneity in some cancers is the generation by irreversible epigenetic mechanisms of features of cellular differentiation, including reduced proliferative/tumorigenic potential, in some progeny of highly tumorigenic cells. Cancers that generate subpopulations of phenotypically distinct and less tumorigenic cells in this manner are said to follow a "cancer stem cell" (CSC) model, as their hierarchical cellular structure is akin to classical stem cell–based ontogenies of normal organ development.[57] Another source of tumor heterogeneity is cancer cell plasticity, in which reversible epigenetic mechanisms drive transient changes in subpopulations of cells that are defined by distinct phenotypic and functional states.[58] Genomic instability and the selection by clonal evolution of genetically distinct subclones also contribute to intratumoral cellular heterogeneity,[54] potentially concurrently with the aforementioned epigenetically driven mechanisms. Each of these mechanisms has been evaluated in PDX melanomas.

PDX Melanoma Modeling of the Cancer Stem Cell Model

Along with in vivo lineage tracing,[59–61] in vivo tumorigenesis using uncultured cells is considered a gold-standard method for testing whether a particular cancer follows a CSC model.[62,63] PDX assays have been pivotal to exploration in this field by facilitating efficient in vivo engraftment of tumors from purified cells derived freshly from the vast majority of donating patients. The general experimental approach is to identify differences in marker expression among subpopulations of cells within a tumor, separate cells according to these differences (eg, using flow cytometry and cell sorting), inject phenotypically distinct cells into mice, and monitor for tumor formation. In cancers that follow a CSC model linked to the expression of a particular marker, tumor formation will be more efficient from one marker-defined subpopulation than the other, and marker reexpression in transplanted tumors will be consistent with hierarchical relationships between marker-defined subpopulations.[64] Such experiments may be performed syngeneically, using mouse-to-mouse transplants, or xenogeneically by transplanting human cancer cells into immunocompromised mice to form PDX tumors.

Testing of the CSC model in melanoma using PDX has provided contrasting data. Although several groups found enrichment of tumorigenicity in subpopulations of melanoma cells defined by increased expression of markers such as ABCB5,[31,33,35] Aldefluor activity which is a marker of aldehyde dehydrogenase activity,[31,33,35] and CD271,[32,34] these data have not always been reproducible.[26,37] PDX assay variations among groups have been proposed to explain discordant data in the field.[34,37,65–67]

One contributing factor is the use of different strains of immunocompromised mice as recipients of transplanted melanoma cells. Although $ABCB5^+$ and $CD271^+$ melanoma cells are far more tumorigenic than marker-negative counterpart cells in NOD/SCID mice, differences in tumorigenicity are substantially reduced when the same experiments are performed in NSG mice.[34,68] These data also suggest that some melanoma cells might be more antigenic than others in NOD/SCID mice, in which the xenogeneic immune response is stronger compared with NSG mice. Of course, this may not reflect differences in antigenicity in syngeneic cell–host interactions, or in tumorigenic potential among marker-positive and marker-negative melanoma cells in patients. These data highlight the potential of differences in PDX assay methodologies to influence the nature and interpretations of data in cancer biology studies.

PDX Modeling of Melanoma Cell Plasticity

Plasticity is a key mechanism through which cancer cells adapt to changing environmental contexts in tumors. In most cancers, plasticity has been studied mainly using highly passaged cell lines. For example, cells in the B16 mouse melanoma line interconvert between more and less pigmented phenotypes, driven by reciprocally increased expression of microphthalmia-associated transcription factor (MITF) and Brn2, and linked to proliferative and invasive phenotypes, respectively.[52,69,70] Although these observations have not yet been confirmed in uncultured melanoma cells in PDX melanomas (or in patient melanomas), extensive plasticity of other markers is observed in PDX passaging experiments. In transplantations of cells purified according to the expression of each of the 22 melanoma cell surface markers, resultant PDX tumors derived from marker-negative or marker-positive cells showed similarly heterogeneous expression of markers to one another and to parental tumors.[26,37] This suggests plastic equilibration in melanomas of the expression of at least some markers, as was proposed from in vitro studies of cell lines.[58] However, the stability of this phenomenon has not been examined across multiple sibling PDX melanomas. Furthermore, plasticity of functional states has yet to be formally demonstrated in uncultured cells in PDX melanomas.

PDX Modeling of Clonal Evolution in Melanoma

Melanoma is one of the most highly mutated human cancers, largely due to the acquisition of UV light–induced mutations in precursor melanocytes.[71] In addition to this, increasing evidence indicates that new mutations continue to be acquired after a melanoma has formed,[72] seeding new and genetically distinct intratumoral clones that may be favorably selected via clonal evolution[54] in specific environmental contexts. For example, resistance to treatment of BRAF-mutant melanomas with BRAF-targeted therapy often results in the emergence of tumors with genetic mutations that confer resistance to therapy but were not detectable before treatment.[73–77]

PDX modeling has proved to be a powerful approach for identifying mutational mechanisms of acquired resistance to targeted therapy with BRAF inhibitors[51,78] that evolve during therapy.[49] BRAF inhibitor–resistant tumors sampled from patients have been established as PDX lines, which have been used to study and overcome resistance mechanisms.[47] In addition, dynamics of acquired resistance can be modeled and characterized using PDX by treating tumor-bearing mice with BRAF inhibitors and inducing spontaneous drug resistance.[46,51] A notable example was the generation of PDX tumors that became resistant to BRAF inhibition as a result of amplified mutant BRAF. Although this amplification drove resistance, upon removal of drug, PDX melanoma cells were intolerant of the high degree of BRAF amplification.[46] This introduced the concept of intermittent dosing with targeted therapies to maintain drug-sensitive clones that compete with and impede drug-resistant cells.

Without therapy, the degree to which melanomas in patients evolve to generate intratumoral genetic and biological diversity, and the nature of this diversity, are largely unknown. Evaluating serially transplanted passages of therapy-naive PDX melanomas, which might spontaneously acquire new mutations, offers a potentially clinically relevant approach for this. PDX and patient melanomas were found to cluster based on gene expression data and mutational status.[79] In another study, different mutations in different metastatic lesions within a patient were represented in matching PDX melanomas, suggesting a correlation between PDX and patient tumors.[49] Although it is unknown to what degree the selective pressures for tumor growth that drive evolutionary change in PDX melanomas might also exist in patients, the demonstration of genomic instability in PDX melanomas provides the opportunity to study tumor cell–intrinsic mechanisms that generate this fuel of clonal evolution.

PDX Modeling of Circulating Melanoma Cells

Circulating tumor cells arise from shedding into the blood malignant cells from a solid tumor.[80] Thus, they are proposed to be mediators and early predictors of metastasis formation.[81] Unlike other cancers, the study of circulating melanoma cells has been confounded by a lack of reliable markers to enable their identification, isolation, and quantitation. Despite these challenges, circulating melanoma cells have been detected in patients[6,82–84] and in PDX melanoma models.[36,38]

PDX modeling of circulating melanoma cells has been greatly facilitated by the use of cell tagging. PDX melanomas may be grown from cells freshly isolated from patients and rapidly transduced with lentiviral vectors carrying expression plasmids that encode for reporter fluorescence proteins such as green fluorescence protein (GFP)[38] (Fig. 9.1). Cells shed from GFP-tagged PDX tumors cells are able to be detected as GFP^+ cells in the mouse circulation and isolated by flow cytometry for further analysis. This approach was used to identify the important role of oxidative stress in regulating the efficiency of melanoma metastasis.[36]

PDX Modeling of Melanoma Metastasis

An advantage of PDX melanoma modeling in NSG mice is its ability to generate spontaneous metastasis in mice from implanted subcutaneous tumors. This was first described in the observation of macrometastases involving a range of mouse organs from some, but not all, transplanted patient melanomas.[37] Interestingly, the number and range of mouse organs with metastases varies according to the melanoma of origin, indicating that the propensities to metastasize per se, and to metastasize to specific organs, are determined by melanoma cell–intrinsic mechanisms. The sensitivity of metastasis detection is improved by using luciferase tagging of transplanted melanoma cells and bioluminescence imaging,[38] which may reveal spontaneous seeding to sites of particular clinical importance, such as the brain and leptomeninges, that have been notoriously difficult to phenocopy experimentally (Fig. 9.1). The ability to model spontaneous metastasis formation from subcutaneous tumors grown from uncultured melanoma cells provides an advance over other approaches, such as direct intravascular or end-organ injection of cancer cells, as it incorporates important steps in the metastatic cascade such as tumor cell shedding and intravasation.

PRECLINICAL APPLICATIONS: USE OF PDX MELANOMAS TO MODEL PATIENT OUTCOMES

All cancer models aim to replicate at least some aspects of human disease, and PDX models are proposed to be particularly useful for this. However, relatively few studies[38,41,84–87] have attempted to correlate directly biological and molecular features and therapy responsiveness of the same cancers growing in patients and in immunocompromised mice. Such studies are challenging and resource intensive, as they require integration of patient cohorts, including careful annotation of patient management and tumor outcomes, with extensively characterized PDX lines. In melanoma, some groups have achieved this, although more development of such infrastructure is needed.

Modeling Metastasis Outcomes

As discussed earlier, a major advantage of PDX melanoma modeling is the ability of subcutaneous PDX melanomas in NSG mice to seed spontaneous

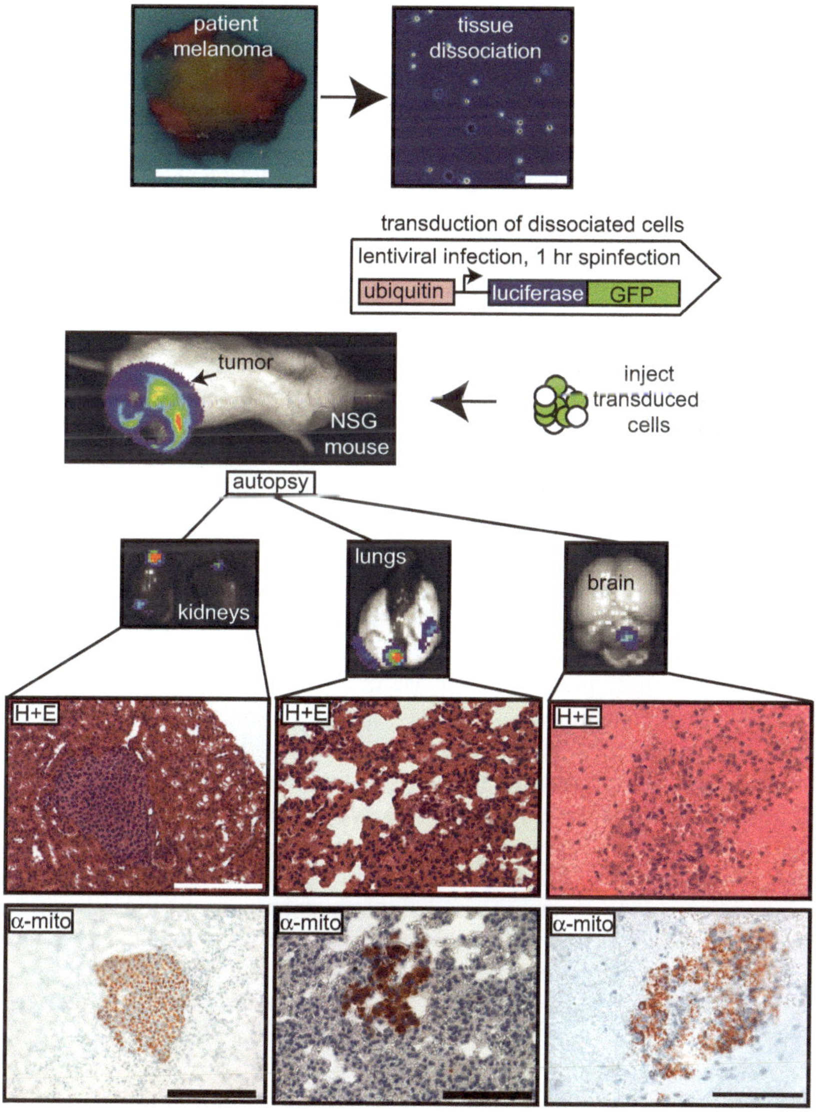

FIGURE 9.1 Melanoma metastasis detection using bioluminescent (BLI) imaging. Patient melanomas (top left, bar: 1 cm) are mechanically and enzymatically dissociated, generating single-cell suspensions of live melanoma cells (top right, bar: 100 μm). Cells are transduced with a lentivirus containing a tandem luciferase–GFP construct driven by a ubiquitin promoter, prior to subcutaneous transplantation into NSG mice. When tumors reach up to 20 mm diameter, mice are analyzed using bioluminescence imaging, which provides a luminescent signal (image of mouse shows a luminescent tumor in the right flank). Organs may need to be removed at autopsy to perform separate and organ-specific BLI, as luminescence signals from subcutaneous tumors can be very strong and overwhelm weaker signals from internal organs. The presence of metastases in organs can be confirmed in sections, here using hematoxylin and eosin (H+E) and anti–human mitochondrial staining (α-mito) (bottom images, bars: 100 μm).

metastases to distant organs. Adding strength to this is the observation that melanomas that are more likely to metastasize in patients are also more likely to metastasize in NSG mice. In a study of 22 patient melanomas (mostly from patients with regionally metastatic stage 3 disease) established as PDX lines in NSG mice, 16 melanomas that recurred in patients also formed overt metastases in mice. In contrast, of the six melanomas that did not recur in patients, only one metastasized substantially in mice, such that patient survival in the cohort was predicted by the ability of PDX melanomas to spontaneously metastasize.[38] Interestingly, brain metastases were also more likely observed in the mice if they developed in patients, suggesting the possibility that metastasis organotropism occurs in melanoma patients and may be predicted in PDX assays.

Modeling Responses to Therapy

Despite the spectacular advances in antimelanoma therapies, including targeted therapies such as *BRAF* and *MEK* inhibitors[88–90] and immune therapies such as anti–CTLA-4 and anti–PD-1 antibodies,[7,91] the majority of patients with metastatic melanoma still die of their disease. This compels the efficient development of new and improved therapies, including via improved preclinical modeling.[92]

Although in some cancers correlations in response to therapy exist between patient and matched PDX tumors,[86,87,93] formal testing of this in melanoma is limited. One study predicted response in a patient with relapsed disease to rechallenge with vemurafenib, a BRAF inhibitor, by testing the sensitivity of PDX tumors generated from the patient's resistant disease.[48] Another study similarly used PDX melanomas to predict patient responses to targeted therapy and also showed that the time needed to perform such testing could feasibly guide patient therapy.[79] A third study suggested that PDX melanoma responses could be used to predict durations of response in patients.[84]

Increasingly, PDX melanoma modeling is being used in preclinical research, particularly in studies of targeted therapy resistance[51] and the testing of novel treatments or new combinations to overcome it.[47,50,78,94] If PDX melanoma responses to targeted therapies reliably predict patient response, then early phase clinical development of new drugs should be more efficient as the proportion of agents with strong efficacy signals would increase. This would benefit patients and reduce the costs of bringing new drugs to the market.

FUTURE/CHALLENGES

Modern PDX melanoma assays in NSG mice are more efficient than PDX assays described for most other cancers, as tumor formation can be generated from very high proportions (25–30% on average) of transplanted cells. This means that only small numbers of cells are necessary to first establish a PDX line, and that only very few patient melanomas cannot be established as PDX tumors.

Moreover, there is a relatively low degree of selection in PDX melanomas of cells with tumor-forming potential in patients, meaning that the heterogeneity of patient tumors is well represented. This heterogeneity can be maintained or even increased during propagation of PDX lines due to continued genomic instability, as is seen in patients. These properties encourage use of PDX melanomas for examining mechanisms through which melanomas adapt and evolve during disease progression and in the face of therapy. Indeed, a major advantage of using PDX melanomas is their facilitation of study of cell-intrinsic determinants of disease biology and therapy response/resistance, which in immunocompromised mice may be substantially uncoupled from cell-extrinsic effects such as immune regulation of disease.

However, this strength is also a limitation in light of the increasingly recognized importance of cell-extrinsic mechanisms, such as antitumor immunity, in determining patient outcomes—even outcomes to treatment with agents that target cell intrinsic disease drivers (ie, mutated BRAF[95]). Immunotherapy, which has rapidly become a cornerstone of melanoma treatment, cannot be modeled with current PDX melanoma approaches. Work is underway to develop PDX-recipient mice with "humanized" hematopoietic and immune systems, which might provide more clinically relevant tumor cell–extrinsic contexts in which to evaluate both targeted and immune therapies.[13,96,97] However, considerable innovation will be required based on the current status of this field, and clinical correlations will be essential where possible.

As PDX melanomas are increasingly used, additional work is also required to improve understanding of the degree to which they recapitulate human disease. This should include extending studies to correlate metastatic patterns in mice and patients. For example, metastasis of PDX melanomas to mouse kidneys is often seen, even though renal involvement is rarely observed in patients, at least outside of autopsy series.[98] Further correlative studies of responses to targeted therapies are also needed as, thus far, these have mostly focused on positive correlations. It is just as important to ascertain negative correlations (ie, test whether nonresponses in PDX melanomas predict nonresponse in patients). This would provide a compelling rationale for use of PDX melanomas as patient "avatars" to test therapies that might be offered to individual patients in the clinic.

ACKNOWLEDGMENTS

This work was supported by the Peter MacCallum Cancer Centre, the Australian National Health and Medical Research Council (NHMRC), the Victorian Cancer Agency (VCA), and the Melbourne Melanoma Project. Mark Shackleton was supported by the NHMRC, Pfizer Australia, and the Victorian Endowment for Science, Knowledge and Innovation. Samantha Boyle was supported by the Cancer Council of Victoria. Clare Fedele was supported by the VCA and the NHMRC.

REFERENCES

1. Ferlay J, Soerjomataram I, Dikshit R, Eser S, Mathers C, Rebelo M, et al. Cancer incidence and mortality worldwide: sources, methods and major patterns in GLOBOCAN 2012. *Int J Cancer* 2015;**136**(5):E359–86.
2. Balch CM, Gershenwald JE, Soong SJ, Thompson JF, Atkins MB, Byrd DR, et al. Final version of 2009 AJCC melanoma staging and classification. *J Clin Oncol* December 20, 2009;**27**(36):6199–206. PMID:19917835, PMCID: 2793035. Epub 2009/11/18.
3. Chapman PB, Hauschild A, Robert C, Haanen JB, Ascierto P, Larkin J, et al. Improved survival with vemurafenib in melanoma with BRAF V600E mutation. *N Engl J Med* June 30, 2011;**364**(26):2507–16. PMID:21639808, PMCID:3549296. Epub 2011/06/07.
4. Linsley PS, Brady W, Urnes M, Grosmaire LS, Damle NK, Ledbetter JA. CTLA-4 is a second receptor for the B cell activation antigen B7. *J Exp Med* September 1, 1991;**174**(3):561–9. PMID:1714933, PMCID:2118936.
5. Linsley PS, Greene JL, Brady W, Bajorath J, Ledbetter JA, Peach R. Human B7-1 (CD80) and B7-2 (CD86) bind with similar avidities but distinct kinetics to CD28 and CTLA-4 receptors. *Immunity* December 1994;**1**(9):793–801. PMID:7534620.
6. Freeman GJ, Long AJ, Iwai Y, Bourque K, Chernova T, Nishimura H, et al. Engagement of the PD-1 immunoinhibitory receptor by a novel B7 family member leads to negative regulation of lymphocyte activation. *J Exp Med* October 2, 2000;**192**(7):1027–34. PMID:11015443, PMCID:2193311.
7. Hodi FS, O'Day SJ, McDermott DF, Weber RW, Sosman JA, Haanen JB, et al. Improved survival with ipilimumab in patients with metastatic melanoma. *N Engl J Med* August 19, 2010;**363**(8):711–23. PMID:20525992, PMCID:3549297. Epub 2010/06/08.
8. Robert C, Thomas L, Bondarenko I, O'Day S, Weber J, Garbe C, et al. Ipilimumab plus dacarbazine for previously untreated metastatic melanoma. *N Engl J Med* June 30, 2011;**364**(26): 2517–26. PMID:21639810, Epub 2011/06/07.
9. Conde-Perez A, Larue L. Human relevance of NRAS/BRAF mouse melanoma models. *Eur J Cell Biol* January–February 2014;**93**(1–2):82–6. PMID:24342721, Epub 2013/12/18.
10. Davies H, Bignell GR, Cox C, Stephens P, Edkins S, Clegg S, et al. Mutations of the BRAF gene in human cancer. *Nature* June 27, 2002;**417**(6892):949–54. PMID:12068308, Epub 2002/06/18.
11. Beaumont KA, Mohana-Kumaran N, Haass NK, editors. Modeling melanoma in vitro and in vivo. *Healthcare* 2013. Multidisciplinary Digital Publishing Institute.
12. Herlyn M, Fukunaga-Kalabis M. What is a good model for melanoma?. *J Invest Dermatol* April 2010;**130**(4):911–2. PMID:20231823. Epub 2010/03/17.
13. Merlino G, Flaherty K, Acquavella N, Day CP, Aplin A, Holmen S, et al. Meeting report: the future of preclinical mouse models in melanoma treatment is now. *Pigment Cell Melanoma Res* July 2013;**26**(4):E8–14. PMID:23531109, PMCID:4109982. Epub 2013/03/28.
14. Siolas D, Hannon GJ. Patient-derived tumor xenografts: transforming clinical samples into mouse models. *Cancer Res* September 1, 2013;**73**(17):5315–9. PMID:23733750, PMCID:3766500. Epub 2013/06/05.
15. Tentler JJ, Tan AC, Weekes CD, Jimeno A, Leong S, Pitts TM, et al. Patient-derived tumour xenografts as models for oncology drug development. *Nat Rev Clin Oncol* June 2012;**9**(6):338–50. PMID:22508028, PMCID:3928688. Epub 2012/04/18.
16. Walker G. P-REX1, a Rac guanine exchange factor, links melanocyte development and melanoma progression. *Pigment Cell Melanoma Res* December 2011;**24**(6):1086–7. PMID:22216451. Epub 2012/01/05.

17. Ackermann J, Frutschi M, Kaloulis K, McKee T, Trumpp A, Beermann F. Metastasizing melanoma formation caused by expression of activated N-RasQ61K on an INK4a-deficient background. *Cancer Res* May 15, 2005;**65**(10):4005–11. PMID:15899789. Epub 2005/05/19.
18. Hodis E, Watson IR, Kryukov GV, Arold ST, Imielinski M, Theurillat JP, et al. A landscape of driver mutations in melanoma. *Cell* July 20, 2012;**150**(2):251–63. PMID:22817889, PMCID:3600117. Epub 2012/07/24.
19. Kunisada T, Lu SZ, Yoshida H, Nishikawa S, Nishikawa S, Mizoguchi M, et al. Murine cutaneous mastocytosis and epidermal melanocytosis induced by keratinocyte expression of transgenic stem cell factor. *J Exp Med* May 18, 1998;**187**(10):1565–73. PMID:9584135, PMCID:2212288.
20. Dobbin ZC, Katre AA, Steg AD, Erickson BK, Shah MM, Alvarez RD, et al. Using heterogeneity of the patient-derived xenograft model to identify the chemoresistant population in ovarian cancer. *Oncotarget* August 19, 2014. PMID:25209969. Epub 2014/09/12.
21. Becker JC, Houben R, Schrama D, Voigt H, Ugurel S, Reisfeld RA. Mouse models for melanoma: a personal perspective. *Exp Dermatol* February 2010;**19**(2):157–64. PMID:19849715. Epub 2009/10/24.
22. Paynter SJ. Principles and practical issues for cryopreservation of nerve cells. *Brain Res Bull* January 31, 2008;**75**(1):1–14. PMID:18158089. Epub 2007/12/26.
23. Baust JM, Van B, Baust JG. Cell viability improves following inhibition of cryopreservation-induced apoptosis. *In Vitro Cell Dev Biol Anim* April 2000;**36**(4):262–70. PMID:10852352. Epub 2000/06/14.
24. Chesne C, Guyomard C, Fautrel A, Poullain MG, Fremond B, De Jong H, et al. Viability and function in primary culture of adult hepatocytes from various animal species and human beings after cryopreservation. *Hepatology* August 1993;**18**(2):406–14. PubMed PMID:8340070. Epub 1993/08/01.
25. Izadyar F, Matthijs-Rijsenbilt JJ, den Ouden K, Creemers LB, Woelders H, de Rooij DG. Development of a cryopreservation protocol for type A spermatogonia. *J Androl* July–August 2002;**23**(4):537–45. PMID:12065461. Epub 2002/06/18.
26. Quintana E, Shackleton M, Sabel MS, Fullen DR, Johnson TM, Morrison SJ. Efficient tumour formation by single human melanoma cells. *Nature* 2008;**456**(7222):593–8.
27. Gerlinger M, Rowan AJ, Horswell S, Larkin J, Endesfelder D, Gronroos E, et al. Intratumor heterogeneity and branched evolution revealed by multiregion sequencing. *N Engl J Med* March 8, 2012;**366**(10):883–92. PMID:22397650. Epub 2012/03/09.
28. Chen K, Ahmed S, Adeyi O, Dick JE, Ghanekar A. Human solid tumor xenografts in immunodeficient mice are vulnerable to lymphomagenesis associated with Epstein-Barr virus. *PLoS One* 2012;**7**(6):e39294. PMID:22723990, PMCID:3377749.
29. John T, Yanagawa N, Kohler D, Craddock KJ, Bandarchi-Chamkhaleh B, Pintilie M, et al. Characterization of lymphomas developing in immunodeficient mice implanted with primary human non-small cell lung cancer. *J Thorac Oncol* July 2012;**7**(7):1101–8. PMID:22617243.
30. Read M, Liu D, Duong CP, Cullinane C, Murray WK, Fennell CM, et al. Intramuscular transplantation improves engraftment rates for esophageal patient-derived tumor xenografts. *Ann Surg Oncol* February 18, 2015. PMID:25691278.
31. Schatton T, Murphy GF, Frank NY, Yamaura K, Waaga-Gasser AM, Gasser M, et al. Identification of cells initiating human melanomas. *Nature* January 17, 2008;**451**(7176):345–9. PMID:18202660, PMCID:3660705. Epub 2008/01/19.
32. Boiko AD, Razorenova OV, van de Rijn M, Swetter SM, Johnson DL, Ly DP, et al. Human melanoma-initiating cells express neural crest nerve growth factor receptor CD271. *Nature* July 1, 2010;**466**(7302):133–7. PMID:20596026, PMCID:2898751. Epub 2010/07/03.

33. Boonyaratanakornkit JB, Yue L, Strachan LR, Scalapino KJ, LeBoit PE, Lu Y, et al. Selection of tumorigenic melanoma cells using ALDH. *J Invest Dermatol* December 2010;**130**(12):2799–808. PMID:20739950. Epub 2010/08/27.
34. Civenni G, Walter A, Kobert N, Mihic-Probst D, Zipser M, Belloni B, et al. Human CD271-positive melanoma stem cells associated with metastasis establish tumor heterogeneity and long-term growth. *Cancer Res* April 15, 2011;**71**(8):3098–109. PMID:21393506. Epub 2011/03/12.
35. Luo Y, Dallaglio K, Chen Y, Robinson WA, Robinson SE, McCarter MD, et al. ALDH1A isozymes are markers of human melanoma stem cells and potential therapeutic targets. *Stem Cells* October 2012;**30**(10):2100–13. PMID:22887839, PMCID:3448863. Epub 2012/08/14.
36. Piskounova E, Agathocleous M, Murphy MM, Hu Z, Huddlestun SE, Zhao Z, et al. Oxidative stress inhibits distant metastasis by human melanoma cells. *Nature* October 14, 2015. PMID:26466563.
37. Quintana E, Shackleton M, Foster HR, Fullen DR, Sabel MS, Johnson TM, et al. Phenotypic heterogeneity among tumorigenic melanoma cells from patients that is reversible and not hierarchically organized. *Cancer Cell* November 16, 2010;**18**(5):510–23. PMID:21075313, PMCID:3031091. Epub 2010/11/16.
38. Quintana E, Piskounova E, Shackleton M, Weinberg D, Eskiocak U, Fullen DR, et al. Human melanoma metastasis in NSG mice correlates with clinical outcome in patients. *Sci Transl Med* November 7, 2012;**4**(159):159ra49. PMID:23136044, Epub 2012/11/09.
39. Shultz LD, Lyons BL, Burzenski LM, Gott B, Chen X, Chaleff S, et al. Human lymphoid and myeloid cell development in NOD/LtSz-scid IL2Rγ^{null} mice engrafted with mobilized human hemopoietic stem cells. *J Immunol* May 15, 2005;**174**(10):6477–89. PMID:15879151. Epub 2005/05/10.
40. Bao L, Matsumura Y, Baban D, Sun Y, Tarin D. Effects of inoculation site and Matrigel on growth and metastasis of human breast cancer cells. *Br J Cancer* August 1994;**70**(2):228–32. PMID:8054270, PMCID:2033496.
41. DeRose YS, Wang G, Lin YC, Bernard PS, Buys SS, Ebbert MT, et al. Tumor grafts derived from women with breast cancer authentically reflect tumor pathology, growth, metastasis and disease outcomes. *Nat Med* 2011;**17**(11):1514–20. PMID:22019887, PMCID:3553601. Epub 2011/10/25.
42. Fridman R, Benton G, Aranoutova I, Kleinman HK, Bonfil RD. Increased initiation and growth of tumor cell lines, cancer stem cells and biopsy material in mice using basement membrane matrix protein (Cultrex or Matrigel) co-injection. *Nat Protoc* June 2012;**7**(6):1138–44. PMID:22596226.
43. Kleinman HK, McGarvey ML, Hassell JR, Star VL, Cannon FB, Laurie GW, et al. Basement membrane complexes with biological activity. *Biochemistry* January 28, 1986;**25**(2):312–8. PMID:2937447. Epub 1986/01/28.
44. Kleinman HK, McGarvey ML, Liotta LA, Robey PG, Tryggvason K, Martin GR. Isolation and characterization of type IV procollagen, laminin, and heparan sulfate proteoglycan from the EHS sarcoma. *Biochemistry* November 23, 1982;**21**(24):6188–93. PMID:6217835, Epub 1982/11/23.
45. Oikawa Y, Hansson J, Sasaki T, Rousselle P, Domogatskaya A, Rodin S, et al. Melanoma cells produce multiple laminin isoforms and strongly migrate on alpha5 laminin(s) via several integrin receptors. *Exp Cell Res* May 1, 2011;**317**(8):1119–33. PMID:21195710.
46. Das Thakur M, Salangsang F, Landman AS, Sellers WR, Pryer NK, Levesque MP, et al. Modelling vemurafenib resistance in melanoma reveals a strategy to forestall drug resistance. *Nature* February 14, 2013;**494**(7436):251–5. PMID:23302800, PMCID:3930354. Epub 2013/01/11.

47. Girotti MR, Lopes F, Preece N, Niculescu-Duvaz D, Zambon A, Davies L, et al. Paradox-breaking RAF inhibitors that also target SRC are effective in drug-resistant BRAF mutant melanoma. *Cancer Cell* January 12, 2015;**27**(1):85–96. PMID:25500121, PMCID:4297292.
48. Guerreschi P, Scalbert C, Qassemyar A, Kluza J, Ravasi L, Huglo D, et al. Patient-derived tumor xenograft model to guide the use of BRAF inhibitors in metastatic melanoma. *Melanoma Res* October 2013;**23**(5):373–80. PMID:23852164.
49. Kemper K, Krijgsman O, Cornelissen-Steijger P, Shahrabi A, Weeber F, Song JY, et al. Intra- and inter-tumor heterogeneity in a vemurafenib-resistant melanoma patient and derived xenografts. *EMBO Mol Med* 2015;**7**(9):1104–18. PMID:26105199.
50. Kobelt D, Aumann J, Schmidt M, Wittig B, Fichtner I, Behrens D, et al. Preclinical study on combined chemo- and nonviral gene therapy for sensitization of melanoma using a human TNF-alpha expressing MIDGE DNA vector. *Mol Oncol* May 2014;**8**(3):609–19. PMID:24503218.
51. Monsma DJ, Cherba DM, Eugster EE, Dylewski DL, Davidson PT, Peterson CA, et al. Melanoma patient derived xenografts acquire distinct vemurafenib resistance mechanisms. *Am J Cancer Res* 2015;**5**(4):1507–18. PMID:26101714, PMCID:4473327.
52. Hoek KS, Goding CR. Cancer stem cells versus phenotype switching in melanoma. *Pigment Cell Melanoma Res* December 2010;**23**(6):746–59. PMID:20726948. Epub 2010/08/24.
53. Magee JA, Piskounova E, Morrison SJ. Cancer stem cells: impact, heterogeneity, and uncertainty. *Cancer Cell* March 20, 2012;**21**(3):283–96. PMID:22439924. Epub 2012/03/24.
54. Nowell PC. The clonal evolution of tumor cell populations. *Science* October 1, 1976;**194**(4260):23–8. PMID:959840, Epub 1976/10/01.
55. Polyak K, Haviv I, Campbell IG. Co-evolution of tumor cells and their microenvironment. *Trends Genet* January 2009;**25**(1):30–8. PMID:19054589, Epub 2008/12/05.
56. Shackleton M. Normal stem cells and cancer stem cells: similar and different. *Semin Cancer Biol* April 2010;**20**(2):85–92. PMID:20435143. Epub 2010/05/04.
57. Reya T, Morrison SJ, Clarke MF, Weissman IL. Stem cells, cancer, and cancer stem cells. *Nature* November 1, 2001;**414**(6859):105–11. PMID:11689955. Epub 2001/11/02.
58. Gupta PB, Fillmore CM, Jiang G, Shapira SD, Tao K, Kuperwasser C, et al. Stochastic state transitions give rise to phenotypic equilibrium in populations of cancer cells. *Cell* August 19, 2011;**146**(4):633–44. PMID:21854987. Epub 2011/08/23.
59. Chen J, Li Y, Yu TS, McKay RM, Burns DK, Kernie SG, et al. A restricted cell population propagates glioblastoma growth after chemotherapy. *Nature* August 23, 2012;**488**(7412):522–6. PMID:22854781, PMCID:3427400.
60. Driessens G, Beck B, Caauwe A, Simons BD, Blanpain C. Defining the mode of tumour growth by clonal analysis. *Nature* August 23, 2012;**488**(7412):527–30. PMID:22854777.
61. Schepers AG, Snippert HJ, Stange DE, van den Born M, van Es JH, van de Wetering M, et al. Lineage tracing reveals Lgr5$^+$ stem cell activity in mouse intestinal adenomas. *Science* August 10, 2012;**337**(6095):730–5. PMID:22855427.
62. Clarke MF, Dick JE, Dirks PB, Eaves CJ, Jamieson CH, Jones DL, et al. Cancer stem cells – perspectives on current status and future directions: AACR Workshop on cancer stem cells. *Cancer Res* October 1, 2006;**66**(19):9339–44. PMID:16990346. Epub 2006/09/23.
63. Kreso A, Dick JE. Evolution of the cancer stem cell model. *Cell Stem Cell* March 6, 2014;**14**(3):275–91. PMID:24607403. Epub 2014/03/13.
64. Shackleton M. Moving targets that drive cancer progression. *N Engl J Med* August 26, 2010;**363**(9):885–6. PMID:20818851.
65. Nguyen N, Couts KL, Luo Y, Fujita M. Understanding melanoma stem cells. *Melanoma Manag* 2015;**2**(2):179–88.

66. Villani V, Sabbatino F, Ferrone CR, Ferrone S. Melanoma initiating cells: where do we stand? *Melanoma Manag* 2015;**2**(2):109–14.
67. Visvader JE, Lindeman GJ. Cancer stem cells: current status and evolving complexities. *Cell Stem Cell* June 14, 2012;**10**(6):717–28. PMID:22704512. Epub 2012/06/19.
68. Frank NY, Schatton T, Kim S, Zhan Q, Wilson BJ, Ma J, et al. VEGFR-1 expressed by malignant melanoma-initiating cells is required for tumor growth. *Cancer Res* February 15, 2011;**71**(4):1474–85. PMID:21212411, PMCID:3083845.
69. Carreira S, Goodall J, Denat L, Rodriguez M, Nuciforo P, Hoek KS, et al. MITF regulation of Dia1 controls melanoma proliferation and invasiveness. *Genes Dev* December 15, 2006;**20**(24):3426–39. PMID:17182868, PMCID:1698449. Epub 2006/12/22.
70. Pinner S, Jordan P, Sharrock K, Bazley L, Collinson L, Marais R, et al. Intravital imaging reveals transient changes in pigment production and Brn2 expression during metastatic melanoma dissemination. *Cancer Res* October 15, 2009;**69**(20):7969–77. PMID:19826052, PMCID:2763120.
71. Alexandrov LB, Nik-Zainal S, Wedge DC, Aparicio SA, Behjati S, Biankin AV, et al. Signatures of mutational processes in human cancer. *Nature* August 22, 2013;**500**(7463):415–21. PMID:23945592, PMCID:3776390. Epub 2013/08/16.
72. Shain AH, Yeh I, Kovalyshyn I, Sriharan A, Talevich E, Gagnon A, et al. The genetic evolution of melanoma from precursor lesions. *N Engl J Med* November 12, 2015;**373**(20):1926–36. PMID:26559571.
73. Shi H, Hugo W, Kong X, Hong A, Koya RC, Moriceau G, et al. Acquired resistance and clonal evolution in melanoma during BRAF inhibitor therapy. *Cancer Discov* January 2014;**4**(1):80–93. PMID:24265155, PMCID:3936420. Epub 2013/11/23.
74. Shi H, Moriceau G, Kong X, Lee MK, Lee H, Koya RC, et al. Melanoma whole-exome sequencing identifies (V600E)B-RAF amplification-mediated acquired B-RAF inhibitor resistance. *Nat Commun* 2012;**3**:724. PMID:22395615, PMCID:3530385.
75. Van Allen EM, Wagle N, Sucker A, Treacy DJ, Johannessen CM, Goetz EM, et al. The genetic landscape of clinical resistance to RAF inhibition in metastatic melanoma. *Cancer Discov* January 2014;**4**(1):94–109. PMID:24265153, PMCID:3947264.
76. Wagle N, Emery C, Berger MF, Davis MJ, Sawyer A, Pochanard P, et al. Dissecting therapeutic resistance to RAF inhibition in melanoma by tumor genomic profiling. *J Clin Oncol* August 1, 2011;**29**(22):3085–96. PMID:21383288, PMCID:3157968.
77. Wagle N, Van Allen EM, Treacy DJ, Frederick DT, Cooper ZA, Taylor-Weiner A, et al. MAP kinase pathway alterations in BRAF-mutant melanoma patients with acquired resistance to combined RAF/MEK inhibition. *Cancer Discov* January 2014;**4**(1):61–8. PMID:24265154, PMCID:3947296.
78. Krepler C, Xiao M, Spoesser K, Brafford PA, Shannan B, Beqiri M, et al. Personalized preclinical trials in BRAF inhibitor resistant patient derived xenograft models identify second line combination therapies. *Clin Cancer Res* December 16, 2015. PMID:26673799. Epub 2015/12/18.
79. Einarsdottir BO, Bagge RO, Bhadury J, Jespersen H, Mattsson J, Nilsson LM, et al. Melanoma patient-derived xenografts accurately model the disease and develop fast enough to guide treatment decisions. *Oncotarget* October 30, 2014;**5**(20):9609–18. PMID:25228592, PPMCID:4259423. Epub 2014/09/18.
80. Torphy RJ, Tignanelli CJ, Kamande JW, Moffitt RA, Herrera Loeza SG, Soper SA, et al. Circulating tumor cells as a biomarker of response to treatment in patient-derived xenograft mouse models of pancreatic adenocarcinoma. *PLoS One* 2014;**9**(2):e89474. PMID:24586805, PMCID:3929698.
81. Giuliano M, Giordano A, Jackson S, De Giorgi U, Mego M, Cohen EN, et al. Circulating tumor cells as early predictors of metastatic spread in breast cancer patients with limited metastatic dissemination. *Breast Cancer Res* 2014;**16**(5):440. PMID:25223629, PMCID:4303121.

82. Nagrath S, Sequist LV, Maheswaran S, Bell DW, Irimia D, Ulkus L, et al. Isolation of rare circulating tumour cells in cancer patients by microchip technology. *Nature* December 20, 2007;**450**(7173):1235–9. PMID:18097410, PMCID:3090667.
83. Roland CL, Ross MI, Hall CS, Laubacher B, Upshaw J, Anderson AE, et al. Detection of circulating melanoma cells in the blood of melanoma patients: a preliminary study. *Melanoma Res* August 2015;**25**(4):335–41. PMID:26011119.
84. Girotti MR, Gremel G, Lee R, Galvani E, Rothwell D, Viros A, et al. Application of sequencing, liquid biopsies, and patient-derived xenografts for personalized medicine in melanoma. *Cancer Discov* March 2016;**6**(3):286–99. PMID:26715644.
85. Cottu P, Marangoni E, Assayag F, de Cremoux P, Vincent-Salomon A, Guyader C, et al. Modeling of response to endocrine therapy in a panel of human luminal breast cancer xenografts. *Breast Cancer Res Treat* June 2012;**133**(2):595–606. PMID:22002565.
86. Fichtner I, Slisow W, Gill J, Becker M, Elbe B, Hillebrand T, et al. Anticancer drug response and expression of molecular markers in early-passage xenotransplanted colon carcinomas. *Eur J Cancer* January 2004;**40**(2):298–307. PMID:14728946. Epub 2004/01/20.
87. Fiebig HH, Maier A, Burger AM. Clonogenic assay with established human tumour xenografts: correlation of in vitro to in vivo activity as a basis for anticancer drug discovery. *Eur J Cancer* April 2004;**40**(6):802–20. PMID:15120036. Epub 2004/05/04.
88. Larkin J, Ascierto PA, Dreno B, Atkinson V, Liszkay G, Maio M, et al. Combined vemurafenib and cobimetinib in BRAF-mutated melanoma. *N Engl J Med* November 13, 2014;**371**(20):1867–76. PMID:25265494. Epub 2014/09/30.
89. Long GV, Stroyakovskiy D, Gogas H, Levchenko E, de Braud F, Larkin J, et al. Combined BRAF and MEK inhibition versus BRAF inhibition alone in melanoma. *N Engl J Med* November 13, 2014;**371**(20):1877–88. PMID:25265492. Epub 2014/09/30.
90. Robert C, Karaszewska B, Schachter J, Rutkowski P, Mackiewicz A, Stroiakovski D, et al. Improved overall survival in melanoma with combined dabrafenib and trametinib. *N Engl J Med* January 2015;**372**(1):30–9. PMID:25399551. Epub 2014/11/18.
91. Johnson DB, Peng C, Sosman JA. Nivolumab in melanoma: latest evidence and clinical potential. *Ther Adv Med Oncol* March 2015;**7**(2):97–106. PMID:25755682, PMCID:4346215. Epub 2015/03/11.
92. Weinstein JN. Drug discovery: cell lines battle cancer. *Nature* March 29, 2012;**483**(7391):544–5. PMID:22460893. Epub 2012/03/31.
93. Waddell N, Pajic M, Patch AM, Chang DK, Kassahn KS, Bailey P, et al. Whole genomes redefine the mutational landscape of pancreatic cancer. *Nature* February 26, 2015;**518**(7540):495–501. PMID:25719666, PMCID:4523082.
94. Dewaele M, Tabaglio T, Willekens K, Bezzi M, Teo SX, Low DH, et al. Antisense oligonucleotide-mediated MDM4 exon 6 skipping impairs tumor growth. *J Clin Invest* January 4, 2016;**126**(1):68–84. PMID:26595814, PMCID:4701541.
95. de Andrade LF, Ngiow SF, Stannard K, Rusakiewicz S, Kalimutho M, Khanna KK, et al. Natural killer cells are essential for the ability of BRAF inhibitors to control BRAFV600E mutant metastatic melanoma. *Cancer Res* October 28, 2014. PMID:25351955. Epub 2014/10/30.
96. Seitz G, Pfeiffer M, Fuchs J, Warmann SW, Leuschner I, Vokuhl C, et al. Establishment of a rhabdomyosarcoma xenograft model in human-adapted mice. *Oncol Rep* October 2010;**24**(4):1067–72. PMID:20811690. Epub 2010/09/03.
97. Shultz LD, Brehm MA, Bavari S, Greiner DL. Humanized mice as a preclinical tool for infectious disease and biomedical research. *Ann N Y Acad Sci* December 2011;**1245**:50–4. PMID:22211979, PMCID:3514446. Epub 2012/01/04.
98. Patel JK, Didolkar MS, Pickren JW, Moore RH. Metastatic pattern of malignant melanoma. A study of 216 autopsy cases. *Am J Surg* June 1978;**135**(6):807–10. PMID:665907.

Chapter 10

Advances in Organoid Culturing of Patient-Derived Tumors

S.D. Kaffenberger[1], Y. Chen[1,2,3]
[1]Memorial Sloan Kettering Cancer Center, New York, NY, United States; [2]Weill Cornell Medical College, New York, NY, United States; [3]New York-Presbyterian Hospital, New York, NY, United States

BACKGROUND

The heterogeneous nature of adult solid tumors has been demonstrated through advances in genomics technology and large-scale genomic studies of multiple human tumor types.[1–7] Preclinical models of human cancer, necessary to elucidate biological mechanisms involved in oncogenesis, progression, metastasis, and treatment response, are important for clinically relevant advances, such as drug response prediction biomarkers and for the development of novel therapeutics. These preclinical models ideally are easily manipulatable in vitro, efficiently produced from human tumors, representative of the heterogeneity of human cancer, stable across serial passages, and suitable for high-throughput drug screening. The primary biologic models to date have been cancer cell lines and patient-derived xenografts (PDXs). Although these have been instrumental in the exploration of cancer biology and drug response, there are a number of limitations associated with each modeling system.

Cancer cell lines have been invaluable to cancer research ever since the HeLa line, derived from an aggressive cervical cancer, was first developed. Cell lines have been critical in the discovery and validation of targeted therapy, such as the roles of BRAF V600E mutations in sensitivity to MAP kinase pathway inhibition, epidermal growth factor receptor (EGFR) mutations in sensitivity to EGFR inhibitors, KIT mutation in sensitivity to imatinib, DNA repair mutations to PARP inhibitors, etc. They have also had utility in the discovery of drug resistance mechanisms after challenge with drug either in vitro or as xenografts in vivo.[8–14] Although they have a number of clear advantages including rapid and indefinite growth, ease of maintenance, suitability toward high-throughput drug screening, and ease of genomic manipulation, a number of problems related to adaptation to culture conditions and poor efficiency of cell line development exist, particularly within certain subsets of human cancers. For instance,

Patient Derived Tumor Xenograft Models. http://dx.doi.org/10.1016/B978-0-12-804010-2.00024-2

prostate cancer has an extremely low efficiency of cancer cell line development. Prior to the development of organoid culturing, there were only seven commercially available cell lines.[15] The selection pressures involved in adapting in vivo tumors to two-dimensional (2D) culture have resulted in a compendium of lines which are specifically selected toward growth in these conditions, and which broadly speaking, do not accurately convey the complexity and diversity of human cancer. This selection toward in vitro growth occurs in populations of clones within a given tumor as well as across tumors of a given cancer type. A further loss of diversity occurs during serial passaging over time as continued adaptation toward the culture conditions occurs.[16] These selection alterations occur rapidly, often after several passages, via genetic or epigenetic mechanisms.[17] This incomplete representation of the heterogeneity and behavior of human cancers may explain the discrepancy between preclinical performance and clinical trial performance for numerous drug candidates which show good response in cell line models, but which fail in clinical trials.

In part to overcome some of the inadequacies of cancer cell line modeling, PDX models were developed to allow tumor growth in an environment simulating in vivo conditions. PDX models are discussed in detail in other chapters. The absence of 2D culturing selection pressures is thought to allow PDX models to maintain physiologic heterogeneity, even across serial passages.[18–20] This may allow for more accurate and clinically relevant drug response prediction. In addition, aspects such as drug delivery and pharmacokinetics and the influence of these factors on tumoral drug response may be investigated. However, the establishment of PDX models is inefficient, time- and resource-intensive, and requires a large quantity of tumor tissue at initiation. The process of establishing and performing drug treatment on a given tumor is a lengthy process with high engraftment failure rates, making the translatability to the clinical realm on a patient-by-patient basis impractical and high-throughput drug screening is generally not possible.[21,22] Furthermore, genomic manipulation for the purpose of mechanistic discovery and cancer biology research is much more challenging in PDX models.

More recently, two culturing strategies using appropriate stem cell factors have been developed to overcome some of the limitations of PDX and cancer cell line models, termed "conditional reprogrammed cells" (CRCs) and "organoids."[23,24] Both these systems, described in detail below, arise from studies of detailed mechanisms of stem cell regeneration to derive culture conditions that can propagate normal stem cells indefinitely in vitro. These systems have challenged our previous assumptions of in vitro culture systems: it has been long observed that normal cells can only propagate a finite number of cell divisions before entering irreversible cellular senescence, known as the Hayflick limit.[25] This senescence is mediated by multiple mechanisms including telomere shortening and activation of the p53 and retinoblastoma tumor suppressors,[26] but is likely bypassed in vivo in the stem cell niche. Both CRCs and organoids recreate elements of this niche. Although originally discovered to culture normal cells, these technologies also significantly improve the efficiency of generating in vitro cultures from patient-derived cancers of epithelial origin. These organoid models have great potential for biomarker development and have been developed with excellent clinical and genomic annotation. Efforts to establish a large repertoire of in vitro organoid models which can provide an accurate representation of the heterogeneity of human cancers and can thereby provide an invaluable resource for drug screening and cancer biology research are underway. Thus, organoid culturing technologies may represent a promising strategy for novel therapeutic development and clinically relevant precision medicine.

THE HISTORY OF ORGANOID CANCER MODELS

In order to study the stem cell compartment of intestinal epithelium, a culturing system was required which allowed for the maintenance, stability, and division of the intestinal crypt including all differentiated cell types.[24] Using laminin-rich Matrigel as a scaffold, and various growth and signaling factors known to be required for growth, differentiation, and division of the intestinal epithelium, optimized serum-free culturing conditions were created for the growth of benign intestinal structures with crypt–villus architecture comparable to in vivo intestinal epithelium.[24] These ex vivo three-dimensional (3D) recapitulations of the histology of intestinal epithelium including the appropriate component differentiated and undifferentiated cell types were termed organoids. Organoids contain several cell types generated from stem cells or organ progenitors and contain spatially restricted lineage commitment and are further characterized by indefinite propagation without senescence, similar to cancer cell lines.[27] They are self-organized, undergo cell sorting, and have since been generated to model benign and malignant colon, prostate, stomach, liver, thyroid, and pancreas tissues.[28–32] While providing a more complex and physiologic model than cancer cell lines, organoids are also able to be genetically manipulated and are amenable to high-throughput drug screening. The ability to create and sustain organoids has directly resulted from crucial advances in culture conditions.

CONDITIONAL REPROGRAMMED CELLS

Serum-free conditions using irradiated fibroblast feeder cells and Y-27632, the Rho kinase inhibitor, have been recently developed and have allowed for indefinite and stable propagation of keratinocytes; breast, prostate, and lung cells; and other epithelial cell types via the activation of endogenous telomerase.[23,33] In vitro, these cell types maintain a stemlike phenotype, but since they retain the capacity to differentiate, they were called CRCs. The clinical relevance and potential of these CRCs was highlighted in several experiments in which cancer cells were isolated and tested for drug sensitivities.[34] Direct clinical utility of CRCs was demonstrated in a patient with respiratory papillomatosis in which surgically removed tumor cells were cultured in medium containing Y-27632 and irradiated fibroblasts, expanded, and tested for response to several drugs, of which one elicited a clinical response.[33] The attributes of these culture conditions were translated to the organoid experience to allow for indefinite propagation without genetic alterations.

BENIGN ORGANOID CULTURES

While the laminin-rich Matrigel provided an extracellular scaffold for the 3D intestinal organoids, the breakthrough for organoid creation came through the culture media conditions.[24] It had been observed that intestinal stem cells expressed the LGR5 receptor, and furthermore, that they required active Wnt pathway signaling for survival. Using the CRC serum-free media supplemented with R-spondin—the ligand of the LGR5 receptor—and WNT3a, dissociated single LGR5-positive stem cells were able to form 3D structures with the proper component cell types and crypt–villus histology in the Matrigel scaffold. Cell division within these organoids occurred in the crypt with more differentiated cells migrating distally up the villi, and eventually sloughing off, in a manner analogous to normal intestinal epithelium.[24,27] Furthermore, similarly to cancer cell lines, these organoids were able to grow indefinitely and undergo genomic manipulation. For instance, using the CRISPR/Cas9 system, the wild-type CFTR gene was able to be reinserted in intestinal organoids with mutant CFTR genes from a patient with cystic fibrosis.[35] These same organoid culturing conditions with minor alterations specific to the tissue type can be used to develop organoids from numerous epithelial tissues, including prostate,[32] brain,[36] kidney,[37–39] stomach,[29] thyroid,[31] inner ear,[40] retina,[41] pituitary gland,[42] colon,[28] and liver.[30] Organoids have also provided insight into lineage plasticity and the identification of epithelial stem cell compartments.[32] Normal human prostate epithelium is composed of a basal and a luminal layer, with human prostate cancer characteristically displaying a luminal phenotype. The location and lineage of the progenitor cells for each layer have been controversial with some data showing independent stem cells for each compartment, and other data suggesting basal layer stem cells which then differentiate to populate both basal and luminal compartments.[43–45] In 2014, it has been shown that prostate epithelial organoids can be derived from both basal and luminal stem cells, a novel finding.[32]

CANCER ORGANOID CULTURES

The unlimited propagation of epithelial cell types afforded by the recent CRC and organoid culturing technologies has led to great interest in the development of patient-derived in vitro organoid cancer models. Capitalizing on the ease of genetic manipulation of organoid models, benign intestinal organoids were engineered with the $KRAS^{G12V}$ mutation as a model of human tumorigenesis, with additional deletions of APC, SMAD4, and p53.[46] The engineered benign-derived organoids resembled the phenotype of human colorectal cancer.

Beyond the exploration of tumorigenesis, patient-derived cancer organoids of numerous cancer types have been developed from cancer specimens obtained through surgery, biopsies, and even circulating tumor cells (CTCs).[15,24,47] Several recent studies have reported disease-specific repositories of nascent organoid lines, including in colorectal, pancreas, and prostate cancer.[15,24,47] These lines are all clinically and genomically annotated, with multiple integrated levels of genomic information, and information on treatment response and other clinical characteristics. Furthermore, these cancer organoid models have been stable over multiple passages, broadly reflect the molecular alterations common to each cancer type, and are also representative of the heterogeneity of each cancer. In addition to these reports, numerous unpublished efforts are taking place in other cancer types. Herein, we highlight recent progress in prostate cancer organoid culturing technology given the notoriously scant success in establishing cancer cell lines in prostate cancer prior to the inception of organoid culturing.

PROSTATE CANCER ORGANOIDS

Prostate cancer is the most common solid tumor in Western men, and despite tremendous resources devoted to developing preclinical models, prior to organoid culturing, there were only seven publicly available cancer cell lines. These cancer cell lines were further limited by lack of heterogeneity and long-term adaptation to culture conditions, and based upon large whole exome sequencing prostate cancer cohorts, were poorly representative of human prostate cancer.[48–50] Many canonical genomic alterations in prostate cancer (and rare in other malignancies), such as CHD1 deletion, SPOP mutations, and FOXA1 mutations were not represented within the cancer cell lines. The recent development of seven novel well-annotated prostate cancer organoid lines utilizing organoid culturing technology with prostate-specific modifications doubled the existing number of cancer cell lines within the time period of approximately 1 year.[15,32,51] Interestingly, the prostate cancer organoid lines were derived from a number of metastatic sources, including CTCs. Unfortunately, due to overgrowth of benign prostate epithelial cells, no primary prostate cancer has been able to reliably establish an organoid line. These novel organoid lines included detailed patient information including castration status, prostate-specific antigen level, treatment course and drug response, and clinicopathologic information. They also included comprehensive genomic characterization, including whole exome sequencing to identify somatic mutations, array comparative genomic hybridization to determine copy number aberrations, and paired-end RNA sequencing to detect fusion events and characterize the transcriptional landscape.[15] A broad array of recurrently altered genomic events in prostate cancer, such as *TMPRSS2-ERG* fusion and PTEN loss, were represented and the organoids were found to be amenable to engrafting as well (Fig. 10.1B). Consistent with findings of the Cancer Genome Atlas and other large-scale

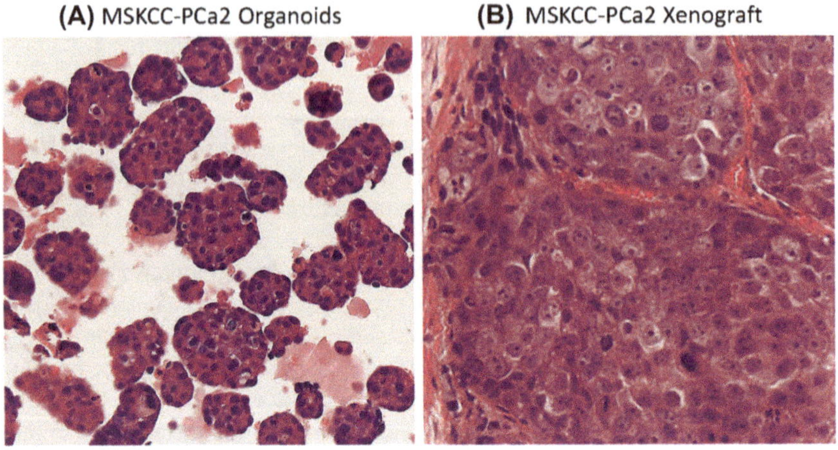

FIGURE 10.1 A morphologic comparison of prostate cancer organoid line, MSKCC-PCa2 (A) forming organoids in three-dimensional culture and (B) engrafted subcutaneously as a patient-derived xenograft; hematoxylin and eosin stain.

genomic cohorts, the prostate cancer organoid models harbored a low rate of somatic mutations with a mean of 45 nonsynonymous single nucleotide variations per sample, and a range of 29–74 on whole exome sequencing.[15,48,49,52,53] A large number of copy number variations were, however, present, and analysis of RNA sequencing data confirmed the phenotypic diversity of the prostate cancer organoid lines.[53] As can be seen in Fig. 10.1, the 3D histology of the prostate cancer organoids is similar to that of the tumor xenograft. Indeed, in several of the lines, whole exome and whole transcriptome sequencing of the originating metastatic tumor specimens was performed, which confirmed the genomic stability of the organoid lines over time. Although incredibly useful to prostate cancer basic research already, the translational aspects require validation and work is continuing. Drug screening on the organoid lines with drugs targeted at androgen receptor, phosphoinositide-3-kinase, cyclin-dependent kinase 4/6, and polo-like kinase 4 along with many others are ongoing, and already highly differential sensitivities have emerged, which appear to correlate with actual clinical responses in some instances. Certainly, a large repository of diverse cancer organoids suitable for high-throughput drug screening and genomic manipulation would be invaluable.

PANCREAS CANCER ORGANOIDS

Pancreatic adenocarcinoma is a highly lethal cancer with few in vitro models. Using organoid conditions, Tuveson and colleagues derived organoids from normal and malignant pancreas cells from both mouse and humans.[47] Pancreas organoids derived from normal and malignant ducts recapitulate benign and malignant ductal features in 3D culture. When the organoids are grafted in vivo, they generate a morphology that recapitulates the patient tumor, with dense desmoplastic reaction from stromal components. The unique ability to culture genetically engineered mouse models of prostate cancer using organoid technology also allowed the investigators to query specific transcriptomic and proteomic changes associated with common genetic alterations, such as KRAS mutation.

COLORECTAL CANCER ORGANOIDS

Since organoid technology was initially optimized for growth of intestinal epithelial cells, they were readily adapted to culture of colorectal cancer. A series of the first 20 tumor and normal adjacent colon epithelial organoid characterization has been published.[54] Using optimized organoid conditions, normal cells actually proliferate faster than cancer cells from the same patients. However, due to ubiquitous activating mutations in the Wnt pathway in colorectal cancer, removal of R-spondin from the media can be used to selectively propagate cancer organoids. The organoids span the genetic spectrum of colorectal cancer. There is a group of hypermutated cancers that have fewer copy number alterations and nonhypermutated cancers with increased number of copy number alterations. The mutations in the cultures were highly concordant with the tumor specimen.

These 20 colorectal cancer organoids were used for proof-of-concept screening of therapeutic agents. One sample was particularly sensitive to a porcupine inhibitor that inhibits the production of Wnt ligands. This sample was found to lack mutations in APC and β-catenin, but harbored a mutation in RNF43. RNF43 degrades Lgr5 and these tumors are hypothesized to still depend on Wnt ligands for pathway activation.[55] In addition, tumors with mutations in KRAS or BRAF were resistant to the EGFR antibody cetuximab, whereas those with mutations in TP53 were resistant to nutlin-3 that inhibits HDM2 to stabilize wild-type p53 protein.

LUNG CANCER CONDITIONAL REPROGRAMMED CELLS

Although EGFR and ALK inhibitors have revolutionized the therapy of EGFR mutant and ALK translocated lung cancers, respectively, acquired resistance invariably develops. To understand the mechanisms of acquired resistance, Engelman and colleagues developed lung cancer CRCs from patients with acquired resistance. Using in vitro drug screening to add a panel of drugs to EGFR inhibitors and ALK inhibitors in EGFR mutant and ALK translocated tumors, respectively, they identified a subset of patients with MET amplification, SRC activation, and MEK activation that are sensitive to the addition of MET, SRC, and MEK inhibitors respectively. These types of studies open a window to the possibility of truly personalized treatment in the future guided by patients' own tumor samples studied in vitro.

FUTURE DIRECTIONS

There is increasing realization of the profound heterogeneity of human cancers which is poorly represented by current 2D cancer cell lines and PDX models. This likely underlies a large number of failed human clinical trials at great societal and individual cost. To minimize the harm to patients on trial and maximize the chance of clinical benefit, improved preclinical models are of great importance. Organoid culturing technologies offer an intriguing compromise between the ease of manipulation and drug screening of cancer cell lines, and the more complex and physiologic but cumbersome PDX models. They are able to be established at increased efficiency, even in difficult-to-culture cancers such as prostate cancer; can be stably propagated; and have excellent clinical and genomic annotation. However, continued refinement of culturing conditions on a cancer-by-cancer basis is necessary to improve the efficiency of establishment, better recapitulate the in vivo local environment, and provide accurate drug response data. For instance, although initial drug response data in prostate cancer organoid lines correlate with the clinical response of matching patients, it will be important to continue to determine the accuracy of in vitro predictions to real-world patient drug response data.[15] Furthermore, for drug screening programs to be successful, large numbers of organoid lines will need to be generated for each cancer type to cover the spectrum of alterations for any given tumor. Currently, there are several large-scale efforts to generate genetically well-defined organoids and CRCs from multiple tumor types at the Broad and Sanger institutes. With continued advancements in precision medicine, newly discovered targetable pathways, and predictive biomarkers, there is great opportunity to better study and develop therapeutic strategies based on these next-generation patient-derived organoid cancer models. Eventually, if in vitro response can be shown to be highly representative of patient response, these technologies may be used as personalized models to guide therapy selection.

ACKNOWLEDGMENTS

Supported by the Sidney Kimmel Center for Prostate and Urologic Cancers. Dr. Kaffenberger received support from the Ruth L. Kirschstein National Research Service Award T32CA082088.

REFERENCES

1. Ceccarelli M, Barthel FP, Malta TM, et al. Molecular profiling reveals biologically discrete subsets and pathways of progression in diffuse glioma. *Cell* 2016;**164**:550–63.
2. Cancer Genome Atlas N. Genomic classification of cutaneous melanoma. *Cell* 2015;**161**:1681–96.
3. Cancer Genome Atlas N. Comprehensive genomic characterization of head and neck squamous cell carcinomas. *Nature* 2015;**517**:576–82.
4. Cancer Genome Atlas Research N. Integrated genomic characterization of papillary thyroid carcinoma. *Cell* 2014;**159**:676–90.

5. Davis CF, Ricketts CJ, Wang M, et al. The somatic genomic landscape of chromophobe renal cell carcinoma. *Cancer Cell* 2014;**26**:319–30.
6. Cancer Genome Atlas Research N. Comprehensive molecular profiling of lung adenocarcinoma. *Nature* 2014;**511**:543–50.
7. Cancer Genome Atlas Research N. Comprehensive molecular characterization of urothelial bladder carcinoma. *Nature* 2014;**507**:315–22.
8. Solit DB, Garraway LA, Pratilas CA, et al. BRAF mutation predicts sensitivity to MEK inhibition. *Nature* 2006;**439**:358–62.
9. Rubin BP, Singer S, Tsao C, et al. KIT activation is a ubiquitous feature of gastrointestinal stromal tumors. *Cancer Res* 2001;**61**:8118–21.
10. Garnett MJ, Edelman EJ, Heidorn SJ, et al. Systematic identification of genomic markers of drug sensitivity in cancer cells. *Nature* 2012;**483**:570–5.
11. Barretina J, Caponigro G, Stransky N, et al. The Cancer Cell Line Encyclopedia enables predictive modelling of anticancer drug sensitivity. *Nature* 2012,**483**:603–7.
12. Farmer H, McCabe N, Lord CJ, et al. Targeting the DNA repair defect in BRCA mutant cells as a therapeutic strategy. *Nature* 2005;**434**:917–21.
13. Lynch TJ, Bell DW, Sordella R, et al. Activating mutations in the epidermal growth factor receptor underlying responsiveness of non-small-cell lung cancer to gefitinib. *N Engl J Med* 2004;**350**:2129–39.
14. Paez JG, Janne PA, Lee JC, et al. EGFR mutations in lung cancer: correlation with clinical response to gefitinib therapy. *Science* 2004;**304**:1497–500.
15. Gao D, Vela I, Sboner A, et al. Organoid cultures derived from patients with advanced prostate cancer. *Cell* 2014;**159**:176–87.
16. Olivotto M, Dello Sbarba P. Environmental restrictions within tumor ecosystems select for a convergent, hypoxia-resistant phenotype of cancer stem cells. *Cell Cycle* 2008;**7**:176–87.
17. O'Driscoll L, Gammell P, McKiernan E, et al. Phenotypic and global gene expression profile changes between low passage and high passage MIN-6 cells. *J Endocrinol* 2006;**191**:665–76.
18. Hidalgo M, Amant F, Biankin AV, et al. Patient-derived xenograft models: an emerging platform for translational cancer research. *Cancer Discov* 2014;**4**:998–1013.
19. Tentler JJ, Tan AC, Weekes CD, et al. Patient-derived tumour xenografts as models for oncology drug development. *Nat Rev Clin Oncol* 2012;**9**:338–50.
20. Hidalgo M, Bruckheimer E, Rajeshkumar NV, et al. A pilot clinical study of treatment guided by personalized tumorgrafts in patients with advanced cancer. *Mol Cancer Ther* 2011;**10**:1311–6.
21. Lawrence MG, Taylor RA, Toivanen R, et al. A preclinical xenograft model of prostate cancer using human tumors. *Nat Protoc* 2013;**8**:836–48.
22. DeRose YS, Wang G, Lin YC, et al. Tumor grafts derived from women with breast cancer authentically reflect tumor pathology, growth, metastasis and disease outcomes. *Nat Med* 2011;**17**:1514–20.
23. Liu X, Ory V, Chapman S, et al. ROCK inhibitor and feeder cells induce the conditional reprogramming of epithelial cells. *Am J Pathol* 2012;**180**:599–607.
24. Sato T, Vries RG, Snippert HJ, et al. Single Lgr5 stem cells build crypt-villus structures in vitro without a mesenchymal niche. *Nature* 2009;**459**:262–5.
25. Hayflick L, Moorhead PS. The serial cultivation of human diploid cell strains. *Exp Cell Res* 1961;**25**:585–621.
26. Hahn WC, Counter CM, Lundberg AS, Beijersbergen RL, Brooks MW, Weinberg RA. Creation of human tumour cells with defined genetic elements. *Nature* 1999;**400**:464–8.
27. Lancaster MA, Knoblich JA. Organogenesis in a dish: modeling development and disease using organoid technologies. *Science* 2014;**345**:1247125.

28. Sato T, Stange DE, Ferrante M, et al. Long-term expansion of epithelial organoids from human colon, adenoma, adenocarcinoma, and Barrett's epithelium. *Gastroenterology* 2011;**141**:1762–72.
29. Barker N, Huch M, Kujala P, et al. Lgr5(+ve) stem cells drive self-renewal in the stomach and build long-lived gastric units in vitro. *Cell Stem Cell* 2010;**6**:25–36.
30. Huch M, Dorrell C, Boj SF, et al. In vitro expansion of single Lgr5+ liver stem cells induced by Wnt-driven regeneration. *Nature* 2013;**494**:247–50.
31. Antonica F, Kasprzyk DF, Opitz R, et al. Generation of functional thyroid from embryonic stem cells. *Nature* 2012;**491**:66–71.
32. Karthaus WR, Iaquinta PJ, Drost J, et al. Identification of multipotent luminal progenitor cells in human prostate organoid cultures. *Cell* 2014;**159**:163–75.
33. Chapman S, Liu X, Meyers C, Schlegel R, McBride AA. Human keratinocytes are efficiently immortalized by a Rho kinase inhibitor. *J Clin Invest* 2010;**120**:2619–26.
34. Yuan H, Myers S, Wang J, et al. Use of reprogrammed cells to identify therapy for respiratory papillomatosis. *N Engl J Med* 2012;**367**:1220–7.
35. Schwank G, Koo BK, Sasselli V, et al. Functional repair of CFTR by CRISPR/Cas9 in intestinal stem cell organoids of cystic fibrosis patients. *Cell Stem Cell* 2013;**13**:653–8.
36. Lancaster MA, Renner M, Martin CA, et al. Cerebral organoids model human brain development and microcephaly. *Nature* 2013;**501**:373–9.
37. Taguchi A, Kaku Y, Ohmori T, et al. Redefining the in vivo origin of metanephric nephron progenitors enables generation of complex kidney structures from pluripotent stem cells. *Cell Stem Cell* 2014;**14**:53–67.
38. Xia Y, Nivet E, Sancho-Martinez I, et al. Directed differentiation of human pluripotent cells to ureteric bud kidney progenitor-like cells. *Nat Cell Biol* 2013;**15**:1507–15.
39. Takasato M, Er PX, Becroft M, et al. Directing human embryonic stem cell differentiation towards a renal lineage generates a self-organizing kidney. *Nat Cell Biol* 2014;**16**:118–26.
40. Koehler KR, Mikosz AM, Molosh AI, Patel D, Hashino E. Generation of inner ear sensory epithelia from pluripotent stem cells in 3D culture. *Nature* 2013;**500**:217–21.
41. Eiraku M, Takata N, Ishibashi H, et al. Self-organizing optic-cup morphogenesis in three-dimensional culture. *Nature* 2011;**472**:51–6.
42. Suga H, Kadoshima T, Minaguchi M, et al. Self-formation of functional adenohypophysis in three-dimensional culture. *Nature* 2011;**480**:57–62.
43. Goldstein AS, Huang J, Guo C, Garraway IP, Witte ON. Identification of a cell of origin for human prostate cancer. *Science* 2010;**329**:568–71.
44. Wang X, Kruithof-de Julio M, Economides KD, et al. A luminal epithelial stem cell that is a cell of origin for prostate cancer. *Nature* 2009;**461**:495–500.
45. Choi N, Zhang B, Zhang L, Ittmann M, Xin L. Adult murine prostate basal and luminal cells are self-sustained lineages that can both serve as targets for prostate cancer initiation. *Cancer Cell* 2012;**21**:253–65.
46. Matano M, Date S, Shimokawa M, et al. Modeling colorectal cancer using CRISPR-Cas9-mediated engineering of human intestinal organoids. *Nat Med* 2015;**21**:256–62.
47. Boj SF, Hwang CI, Baker LA, et al. Organoid models of human and mouse ductal pancreatic cancer. *Cell* 2015;**160**:324–38.
48. Cancer Genome Atlas Research Network. Electronic address S.C.M.O. and Cancer Genome Atlas research N. The molecular taxonomy of primary prostate cancer. *Cell* 2015;**163**:1011–25.
49. Barbieri CE, Baca SC, Lawrence MS, et al. Exome sequencing identifies recurrent SPOP, FOXA1 and MED12 mutations in prostate cancer. *Nat Genet* 2012;**44**:685–9.
50. Taylor BS, Schultz N, Hieronymus H, et al. Integrative genomic profiling of human prostate cancer. *Cancer Cell* 2010;**18**:11–22.

51. Drost J, Karthaus WR, Gao D, et al. Organoid culture systems for prostate epithelial and cancer tissue. *Nat Protoc* 2016;**11**:347–58.
52. Baca SC, Prandi D, Lawrence MS, et al. Punctuated evolution of prostate cancer genomes. *Cell* 2013;**153**:666–77.
53. Grasso CS, Wu YM, Robinson DR, et al. The mutational landscape of lethal castration-resistant prostate cancer. *Nature* 2012;**487**:239–43.
54. van de Wetering M, Francies HE, Francis JM, et al. Prospective derivation of a living organoid biobank of colorectal cancer patients. *Cell* 2015;**161**:933–45.
55. Koo BK, Spit M, Jordens I, et al. Tumour suppressor RNF43 is a stem-cell E3 ligase that induces endocytosis of Wnt receptors. *Nature* 2012;**488**:665–9.

Section IV

PDX Models in Cancer Research and Therapy Around the World

Chapter 1

Global Practices in PDX Programs

G.Y. Ho[1,2,3], C.L. Scott[1,2,4,a], K. Pham[1,2,a]
[1]*The Walter and Eliza Hall Institute of Medical Research, Parkville, VIC, Australia;* [2]*The University of Melbourne, Parkville, VIC, Australia;* [3]*The Royal Women's Hospital, Parkville, VIC, Australia;* [4]*Royal Melbourne Hospital, Parkville, VIC, Australia*

THE SURVEY

We conducted a survey of 64 academic patient-derived xenograft (PDX) programs over December 2015. The main areas covered by the survey centered on:

- Demographics of the responders including information on location of institute, lead researcher, size and type of institute, and tumor subtype coverage;
- Modes of PDX generation and characterization, and the use of molecular characterization such as next generation sequencing, gene expression analysis, and epigenomics;
- Outcomes of the PDX program with regard to scientific and clinical achievements, licensing, and maintaining funding for current and future PDX model development;
- Expenditure on PDX programs;
- Governance and occupational health and safety (OHS) aspects related to using viable human tissues in animal models.

This survey was designed to capture important key performance indices of successful PDX programs. Respondents refer to individual programs, and responders refer to number of responses for a particular survey question. We aimed to characterize each individual PDX program and identify key strengths and areas for improvement of these programs overall.

[a] These authors contributed equally to this work.

Patient Derived Tumor Xenograft Models. http://dx.doi.org/10.1016/B978-0-12-804010-2.00025-4

PDX PROGRAMS: A GLOBAL SNAPSHOT

The Countries Involved in PDX Programs

PDX academic programs occur globally but center on developed and economically stable countries, such as North America (including Canada), Europe, and Asia Pacific countries, in particular Australia, Singapore, Japan, and China. We received 64 respondents to our survey with the majority of respondents being from North America (30), followed by Europe (22). The Asia Pacific region was mainly represented by Australian programs (10) and then Singapore (1). One respondent declined to comment on the country of origin.

The Laboratories

Most academic-based PDX programs are run within well-established research institutes, with access to the necessary infrastructure required, such as animal research facilities and bioservice support. These institutes can be broadly subcategorized as medical research institutes, university-based laboratories, or consortia in partnership based on general platform facilities. These institutes are led by various types of investigators including basic scientists, clinician scientists, facility managers, consortium managers, or translational scientists.

These research institutes are of various sizes with differing levels of associations to medical facilities or niche research industries. The types of association with surrounding facilities would inevitably drive the research directions of each institute type. From this survey, the majority of the PDX programs are run within medical research institutes and 50% (32/64 respondents) are from large institutes of more than 500 staff, whereas less than 16% (10/64 respondents) are from medical institutes with less than 500 staff (Fig. 1.1A). About 28% (18/64 respondents) of these laboratories are based within universities with medical research capacity. A minority of PDX programs operates from independent research institutes, cancer hospitals, and consortia (4/64 respondents).

There are significant regional differences in terms of the organizations involved in PDX programs. The PDX programs in North America are predominantly run within larger medical research institutes (63%, 19/30 responders) unlike in Europe where these comprise only 18% of PDX programs (4/22, responders). The majority of European programs are run in smaller medical institutes (36%, 8/22 responders). All the respondents from Australia (10 respondents) are from large medical research institutes or universities. There are likely to be fundamental differences in how these programs operate and the objectives of the research.

Overall, 31% (20/64 respondents) of PDX programs are led by clinician scientists. The North American PDX programs (47%, 14/30 respondents) have a higher proportion of clinician-scientist-led PDX programs compared with those in Europe (25%, 5/22 respondents) (Fig. 1.1B). The majority of lead investigators for PDX programs in Europe are basic scientists (55%, 12/22 respondents), whereas in North America, there are almost equivalent proportions of clinician-scientists (47%, 14/30 respondents) and basic scientists (40%, 12/30 respondents). Of the Australian PDX programs, 70% (7/10 respondents) were run by basic scientists and 30% (3/10

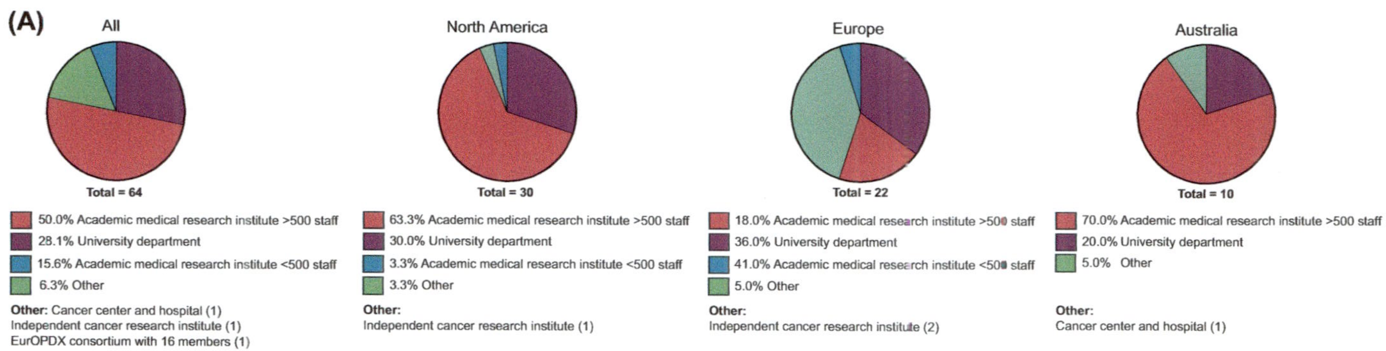

FIGURE 1.1 A breakdown of (A) laboratory types and (B) type of lead investigator in academic PDX programs by overall respondents and by country. The number of respondents are underneath each graph and the percentages shown in the legend key.

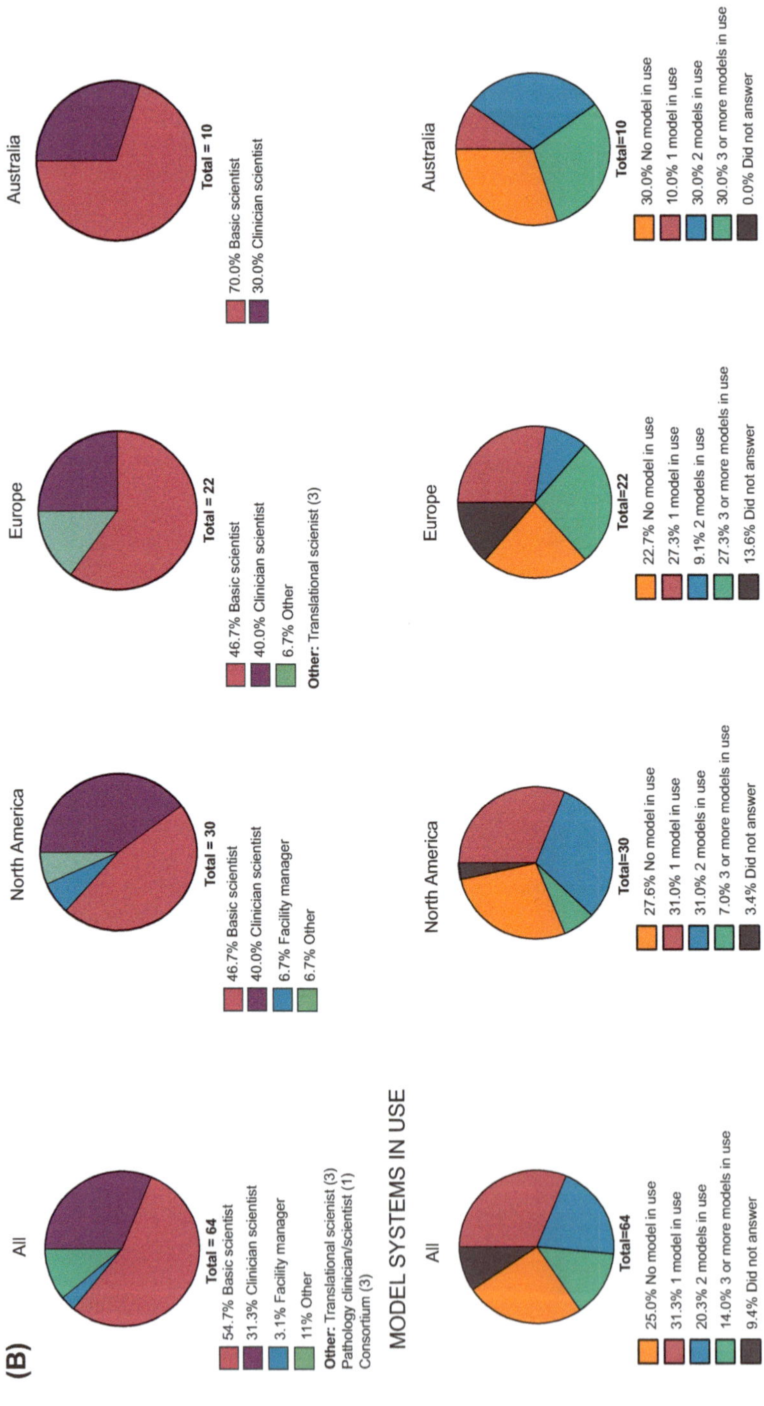

FIGURE 1.1 Cont'd

respondents) by clinician-scientists. Although we did not collect data on the collaborative structure of each program where clinician scientists might be working with basic scientists, the results show that in the field of PDX there is significant collaborative participation of both groups, underscoring the translational nature of this field. Clinicians including oncologists, pathologists, and hematologists bring in clinical links to patients, clinical perspectives, as well as data, while basic scientists may play a major role in asking more fundamental questions on tumor biology. Interaction/collaboration between these two groups can contribute positively to PDX programs. Consortia is one method for providing fertile ground for these collaborations, an example being the EurOPDX consortium and its role in linking not only researchers but also institutes and industry together.[1] The role of research facility managers was noted only for institutes in North America, suggesting a potential need for dedicated managerial staff elsewhere to oversee PDX programs.

Tumor Coverage by PDX Programs

Globally, PDX programs cover more than 20 different tumor subtypes from the common solid tumor subtypes, such as breast cancer, lung cancer, and colorectal cancer to the less common tumor subtypes, such as ovarian and pancreatic cancers (Fig. 1.2). These tumor subtypes were the top five cancer types featured

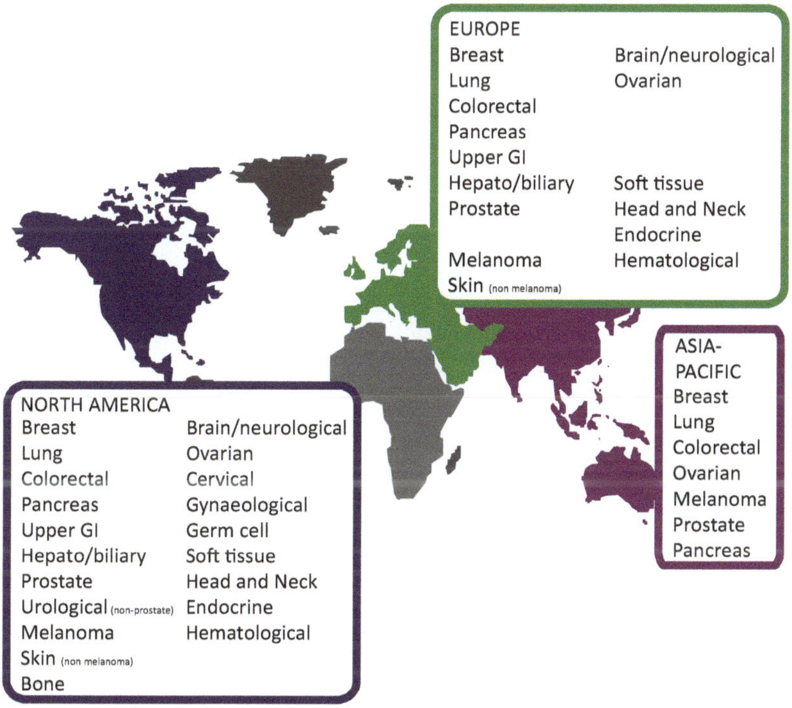

FIGURE 1.2 A global atlas of PDX programs. *GI*, gastrointestinal.

in this survey, with significant international study coverage. Other tumor subtypes displayed are covered by 5–15 PDX programs (except nonmelanoma skin cancer and rare endocrine tumors).

North American PDX programs provide more comprehensive coverage with broad representation of all cancer subtypes, including some rare cancers, such as uveal melanoma (other skin cancers, nonmelanoma) and endocrine cancers. In contrast, the European and Australian PDX programs focus more on the common cancer types, with some niche cancers, such as melanoma in Australia and pancreatic cancer in Europe (Fig. 1.2).

PDX programs based on the more common cancer types generate higher transplantability success rates (between 75% and 100%) and these include colorectal cancer, breast cancer, and melanoma, as well as less common types including, upper gastrointestinal, pancreatic, and ovarian cancers and some rare types, such as cervical, brain, and hematological malignancies (Fig. 1.3).

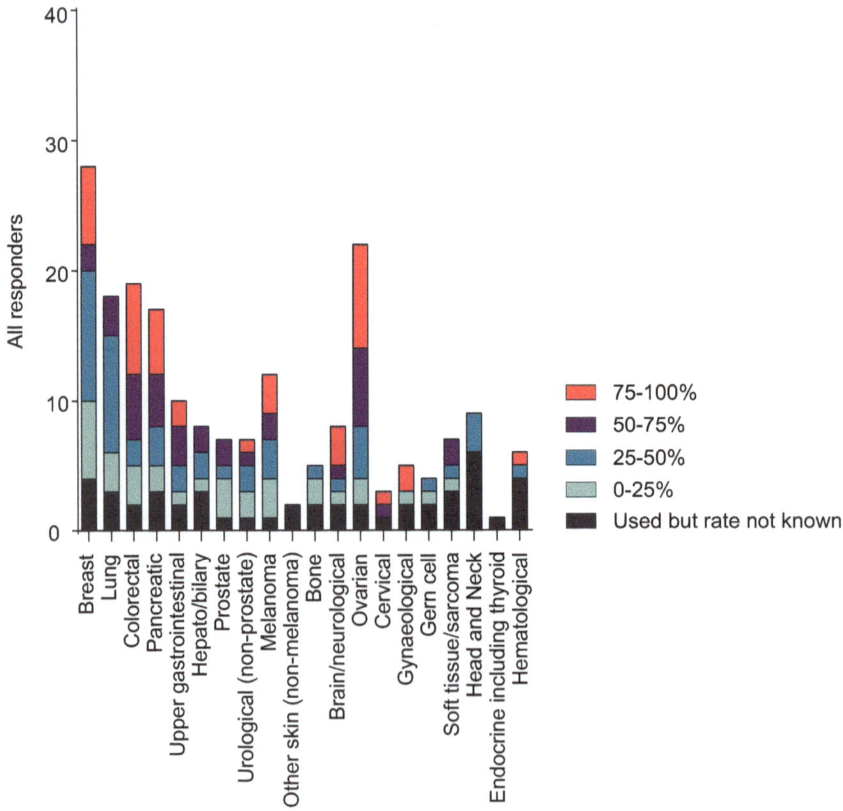

FIGURE 1.3 Tumor subtypes and take rates in PDX programs globally. Legend for take rates: pink (75–100%), purple (50–75%), dark blue (25–50%), light blue (0–25%), gray (used but rate not known).

The success rates for transplantability of a subtumor type may be reflected by the underlying biology. Despite one-third of PDX programs reporting working with lung cancer PDX, tansplantability was poor at only 25–50%. This suggests that some tumor types are more difficult to generate into a PDX model. This is also reflected in groups working on prostate cancer, bone cancer, and germ cell cancer in which poor transplantability rates are reported (up to 50%). For this reason we have not identified the take rate of PDX as a key performer indicator of a successful PDX program.

CURRENT PRACTICES IN ACADEMIC PDX PROGRAMS

PDX Model Generation: Human Tissue Source and PDX Techniques

Globally, 70% (42/60 respondents) of PDX programs source their tumor material through collaboration with an academic (or public) hospital and a smaller proportion (10%, 6/60 respondents) source their tumor material internationally from other academic hospitals. A significant proportion of responders report obtaining tumor material from private hospitals, directly from patients, or from a biobank (27%, 16/60 respondents). Seven responders received materials from consortia, and of these, four were from international consortia.

From this survey the most common source of tissue appears to be linked to the availability of collaborative opportunities with hospitals. This can involve taking advantage of established clinician networks and direct access to patients, and using preexisting sample collection protocols. A small number of respondents sourced their materials from private hospitals (16 respondents), directly from patients (17 respondents) and biobanks (15 respondents).

Biobanks are platforms set up to collect, verify, and store biological samples from patients. Most tissues that are banked are used for genomic and molecular analysis as frozen samples, although biobanks can also collect and supply fresh tumors from patients. A fee applies to cover the administrative and recovery costs of each sample. Biobanks are usually set up by researchers to aid ethical collection of human tissue samples and are often attached to academic hospitals. Biobanks provide an invaluable source of material for PDX generation and appear to be currently underutilized in global PDX programs, perhaps due to their lack of availability, lack of awareness, research expenditure constraints, or incentives provided by other arrangements, such as service agreements with industry.

Following the choice of tissue source, one of the most important decisions is the choice of immune-deficient mouse strain chosen by various PDX programs. The genetic makeup of the recipient mouse can affect the uptake rate,[1,2] and different competencies of the mouse strain immune systems may aid the optimal balance for successful transplantation. Perhaps to a lesser extent, the cost incurred for each mouse strain may also play a part in strain choice. Some institutes may have in-house animal breeding facilities that provide access to particular mouse strains at a cheaper cost.

In this survey, the most common mouse strains (see Lodhia et al.[2]) used for generating and passaging PDX was the NOD.Cg-Prkdc^{scid} Il2rg$^{tm1Wjl/SzJ}$ (NSG) mouse strain (45 respondents), followed by severe combined immune deficiency (SCID) mice (15 respondents) and nude (nu/nu) mice (14 respondents). Five respondents reported using recipient mice of different transgenic combinations, such as *Rag2* mice and only three respondents had tried a humanized hematopoietic system in mouse model.

A more immunodeficient mouse strain, such as *Rag2* mice or NSG mice may improve the success rate of tumor uptake.[3–5] However, these mice are more expensive and prone to illness. Interestingly, for the top three tumor subtypes studied within PDX programs (breast, colorectal, and lung), those with better take rates between 75% and 100%, such as breast (25% 6/24 responders) and colorectal cancers (37%, 7/19 responders) were more likely to have been generated using NSG mice or humanized mice compared with the overall survey average (11%, 23/203 responders for all subtypes and take rates). In contrast, lung cancer PDX programs tended to favor the use of *nu/nu* mice and had lower take rates, the median take rate being 25–50% (9/15 responders) (Fig. 1.3 and data not shown). It is possible that the choice of mouse stain from this survey merely reflected historical experience. Standardizing the recipient mouse strain and the experimental design (such as staging of tumors) may allow a better comparison of take rates and tumor responses across different PDX programs.

67% (41/61 respondents) of programs used orthotopic sites for at least some of their transplants, which highlights the increased understanding of the importance of microenvironment and tumor biology for many cancer types.[2] 84% percent (51/61 respondents) of programs described using unmanipulated tissue fragments. 31% percent (19/61 respondents) of programs reported using tissue which had been manipulated by digestion, with or without flow sorting, prior to initial transplant. While implanting tissue fragments reduces damage and preserves stromal architecture, physical or chemical dissociation and flow sorting before implantation may allow a better representation of tumor heterogeneity in some cases, as shown previously for colon cancer.[6]

Cellular and Passage Characterization of PDX Tumor Models

Basic information regarding each PDX tumor, such as morphology, xenograft tumor growth rate, and in vivo cancer-specific treatment sensitivity are important basic aspects of PDX characterization. At least 85–96% of all academic PDX programs reported routinely validating their PDX using microscopy-based techniques by histology or immunohistochemistry as well as acquiring data related to the PDX tumor dynamics, such as measurement of tumor volume and identification of clonal selection based on change in growth rate and morphology in response to standard treatment.

It is widely accepted that passaging a PDX tumor in mice for up to 8–10 passages can be performed with maintenance of critical features of that tumor, provided that revalidation of each passage by reassessing the tumor dynamics has confirmed lack of drift.[7,8] Globally, the median number of passages utilized for treatment studies and cohort maintenance was five (from survey, data not shown). In rarer PDX tumor subtypes, such as renal cell carcinoma, hematological malignancies, and endocrine cancer, respondents reported using up to 20 passages or more (from survey, data not shown). It is therefore possible to extend the passage number of each PDX model with careful curation of each passage, including monitoring of each tumor for aberrant tumor behavior.

Molecular Characterization

The appropriate use of molecular characterization forms the crux of a well-annotated and informative PDX program. Detailed data on the genotypic, phenotypic, gene expression, and protein expression features of each PDX will soon be a fundamental component required for personalizing the direction of each PDX model for drug development and biomarker discovery.

This survey detailed specific use of various techniques as listed below:

- Next generation sequencing: on-target panels of genes (<100, 100–1000, or >1000 genes), whole exome sequencing (<100 or entire exome), and whole genome sequencing (light, moderate, and deep).
- Gene expression array: RNA sequencing, single nucleotide polymorphism array, microarray, and nanostring analysis.
- Protein expression array: Western blotting, reverse-phase protein lysate array, whole proteasome analysis, and enzyme-linked immunosorbent assay.
- Epigenomics: gene methylation analysis, chromatin immunoprecipitation (ChIP) sequencing, methyl chip analysis, and whole methylome analysis.

About 47% (28/60 respondents) reported using at least one form of next generation sequencing analysis routinely, apart from five respondents who would perform gene sequencing only when necessary to characterize their PDX model. Similarly, with gene expression array, 44% (26/60 respondents) reported routinely using one or more method(s) of gene expression analysis and only two responders did not use any form of gene expression analysis. With regard to protein analysis, a high proportion of PDX programs reported using Western blotting (51%, 31/60 respondents) routinely for protein expression analysis and only three respondents (5%, 3/60 respondents) reported using the reverse-phase protein array technique. From this survey, it appears that molecular characterization such as protein, gene expression, or next generation sequencing are emerging techniques. In contrast, most PDX programs underutilize epigenomic analysis with only four PDX programs (7%, 4/54 respondents) routinely performing one or more form of epigenetic analysis on their PDX models. Almost

84% (47/56 respondents) of PDX programs reported no use of any form of epigenomics.

Despite financial constraints, it is clear that all PDX programs are striving to molecularly annotate their models. Most will select relevant PDX to be tested to maximize their limited resources. However, PDX programs could shift their characterization by refocusing on newer more effective analytic techniques, such as those for protein analysis and also the emerging role of epigenomics. When we reviewed published literature regarding PDX models in the past 15 years (Table 1.1 and Fig. 1.4), our analysis revealed a trend of a shift from microscopy-based characterization of PDX models to more sophisticated molecular characterization. Access to cheaper sequencing methodologies may allow a dramatic acceleration of this shift.

PDX Model Development

One of the biggest challenges in any PDX program is to diversify from the current PDX model to develop and generate new and improved PDX models. A major trend in successful PDX programs involves extending the primary PDX via PDX-derived cell lines or PDX-derived organoids (such as through silencing RNA/CRISPR, drug library screening, CHIPseq), which can provide additional functionality to downstream pathway and biomarker identification.[2,9] Depending on the tumor subtype the generation of cell lines may be challenging, requiring the assessment and incorporation of new culture media and extensive reanalysis of derivative cell lines to ensure that they recapitulate the primary tumor and PDX. Thus far, more than 50% of respondents (34/64 respondents) surveyed from academic PDX programs were routinely generating PDX-derived cell lines. The more complex model of organoid generation was less commonly performed, and only 15–19% and 10% of respondents reported success in PDX-derived organoid and patient tumor–derived organoid generation, respectively. Nevertheless, close to 50% (31/64 respondents) intend to develop their PDX models in this direction and one-fifth (20%, 15/64) of PDX programs have already developed and use new generation culture media within their laboratory.

Of all responding PDX programs involving common tumor types (breast, colorectal, and lung), 78–82% have described developing or using one or more new PDX model derivatives. In contrast, only 14% (4/28 respondents) of breast PDX programs, 26% (4/19 respondents) of colorectal PDX programs, and 22% (4/18 respondents) of lung PDX programs reported successfully developing and using three or more new PDX model derivatives. Rates of derivative use were lower for the less common cancer types.

In terms of regional differences, the European academic PDX programs appear to lead in PDX model development with 27% (five respondents) of programs having developed three or more new PDX model derivatives, followed by the Australian PDX programs (two respondents) and the North American programs (only one respondent) (Fig. 1.5).

TABLE 1.1 A Review of PDX Papers in the Years pre-2005, 2005–10, 2010–15, and Currently Describing Their Molecular Characterization

Year	Tumor Subtype	Microscopy-Based Analysis	Next Generation Sequencing	Gene Expression Analysis	Protein Expression Analysis	Epigenomics
2001[10]	Prostate	Yes (IHC, H&E)	Nil	Nil	Nil	Nil
2000[11]	Merkel cell carcinoma	Yes (IHC, H&E)	Nil	Yes (qRT-PCR)	Yes (Western blotting)	Nil
2002[12]	Neuroblastoma	Yes (IHC, H&E)	Nil	Yes (FISH and Southern blotting)	Nil	Nil
2003[13]	Prostate	Yes (IHC, H&E)	Nil	Nil	Nil	Nil
2003[14]	Gynaeological	Yes (IHC, H&E)	Nil	Nil	Nil	Nil
2004[15]	Various tumor subtypes	Yes (IHC, H&E)	Nil	Nil	Nil	Nil
2005[16]	Pancreatic	Yes (IHC, H&E)	Nil	Nil	Yes (laser scanning cytometry analysis)	Nil
2005[17]	Pancreatic	Yes (IHC)	Nil	Nil	Yes (Western blotting)	Nil
2005[18]	Brain	Yes (IHC)	Nil	Yes (RT-PCR, FISH, Northern blotting)	Yes (Western blotting)	Nil
2006[19]	Ovarian	Yes (IHC, ICC, H&E)	Yes (MLPA genomic profiling)	Yes (high-performance liquid chromatography, genotyping, RT-PCR)	Nil	Nil
2006[20]	Lung	Yes (histopathology)	Nil	Yes (SKY, CGH, and FISH)	Nil	Nil

Continued

TABLE 1.1 A Review of PDX Papers in the Years pre-2005, 2005–10, 2010–15, and Currently Describing Their Molecular Characterization—cont'd

Year	Tumor Subtype	Microscopy-Based Analysis	Next Generation Sequencing	Gene Expression Analysis	Protein Expression Analysis	Epigenomics
2006[21]	Human	Yes (IHC)	Nil	Yes (RT-PCR)	Yes (Western blotting, ELISA)	Nil
2006[22]	Brain	Yes (IHC)	Nil	Yes (RT-PCR/PCR, FISH)	Yes (Western blotting)	Nil
2007[23]	Colorectal	Yes (IHC, H&E)	Nil	Yes (qRT-PCR)	Nil	Nil
2007[24]	Breast	Yes (IHC)	Nil	Yes (RT-PCR)	Yes (Western blotting)	Nil
2007[25]	Pancreatic	Yes (IHC)	Nil	Yes (RT-PCR, eTAG)	Yes (Western blotting)	Nil
2007[26]	Breast	Yes (histology and IHC)	Nil	Yes (CGH, RT-PCR)	Yes (Western blotting)	Nil
2008[27]	Ovarian	Yes (IHC)	Nil	Yes (RNAseq, Affymetricx GeneChip SNP)	Nil	Nil
2008[28]	Lung cancer	Yes (IHC)	Yes (whole genomic sequencing)	Yes (RT-PCR, PCR)	Yes (Western blotting, immunoblotting)	Nil
2009[29]	Pancreatic	Yes (IHC)	Nil	Nil	Yes (Western blotting)	Nil
2011[30]	Breast	Yes (IHC)	Nil	Yes (whole genome microarray)	Yes (Western blotting)	Nil

2012[31]	Renal cell	Nil	Yes (whole exome sequencing)	Yes (copy number array, human genome microarray)	Nil	Nil
2012[32]	Colorectal	Yes (IHC)	Yes (targeted panel genome sequencing)	Yes (CGH)	Nil	Nil
2012[33]	Lung	Nil	Nil	Yes (ARMS, PCR, and FISH)	Nil	Nil
2012[34]	Breast	Yes (IHC)	Nil	Nil	Yes (Western blotting)	Nil
2012[35]	Breast	Yes (IHC)	Nil	Yes (whole genome microarray)	Yes (Western blotting)	Nil
2013[36]	Pancreatic	Yes (IHC)	Nil	Nil	Yes (ELISA)	Nil
2013[37]	Lung	Yes (IHC)	Nil	Yes (qRT-PCR, FISH)	Yes (Western blotting)	Nil
2013[38]	Breast	Yes (IHC)	Nil	Nil	Yes (Western blotting)	Nil
2013[39]	Melanoma	Yes (IHC)	Nil	Yes (qRT-PCR, genotyping)	Yes (Western blotting)	Nil
2014[40]	Sarcoma	Yes (IHC)	Nil	Yes (microarray, qRT-PCR)	Nil	Nil
2014[41]	Pancreatic	Yes (IHC)	Nil	Yes (FISH)	Nil	Nil
2014[42]	Renal cell	Yes (IHC)	Nil	Yes (qRT-PCR)	Yes (Western blotting, ELISA)	Nil

ARMS, amplification refractory mutation system; *CGH*, comparative genomic hybridization; *ELISA*, enzyme-linked immunosorbent assay; *eTAG*, expressed sequence tag; *FISH*, fluorescence in situ hybridization; *H&E*, hematoxylin and eosin stain; *IHC*, immunohistochemistry; *MLPA*, multiplex ligation-dependent probe amplification; *qRT-PCR*, quantitative real time-polymerase chain reaction; *RT-PCR*, real-time polymerase chain reaction; *SKY*, spectral karyotyping; *SNP*, single nucleotide polymorphism.

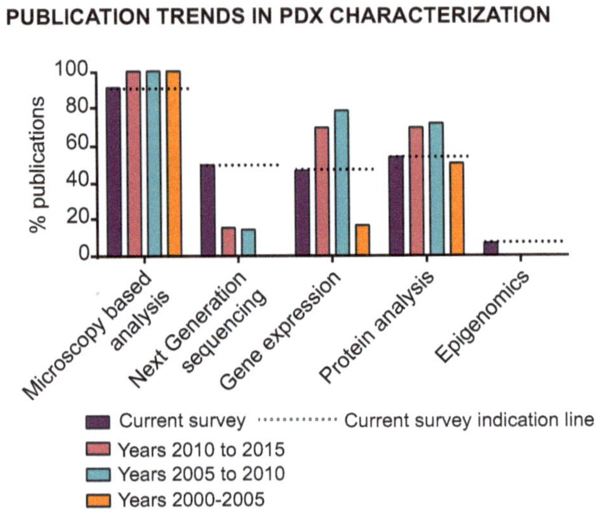

FIGURE 1.4 Trends in types of molecular characterization performed in the years pre-2005, 2005–10, 2010–15, and currently. $N=33$ publications.

PDX Program Expenditure

The cost of running a PDX program varies among different institutes. These costs include animal procurement, animal husbandry, bioservices, lease of animal space, PDX generation, maintenance, and staff salaries. A major portion of PDX program expenditure is also required for the optional application of molecular characterization including next generation sequencing, advance protein expression assays, and epigenetic analysis, all of which will improve the utility of PDX cohorts and the quality of the program. The hallmark of a successful PDX program is that it is able to control costs in areas of PDX development and maintenance. It also includes establishing secure funding to ensure continued development of the resource, enabling critical preclinical analysis of tumor biology and drug response and resistance. Two-thirds of all academic PDX programs obtain funding from national research government grants and philanthropic support. Only a third of the respondents reported receiving some form of financial support from their collaboration with industry.

In terms of the expenditure, the majority of the respondents' PDX program (53.7%, 34/64 respondents) operated on a budget of US$300,000 or less annually. Taking into count the requirements of a whole PDX program, this is a small annual working budget for a PDX program, highlighting the need for improvement of funding to enable a PDX program to increase its throughput and efficiency.

On average, the global annual cost of running a PDX program is US$380,681 based on information provided by all respondents. Regionally,

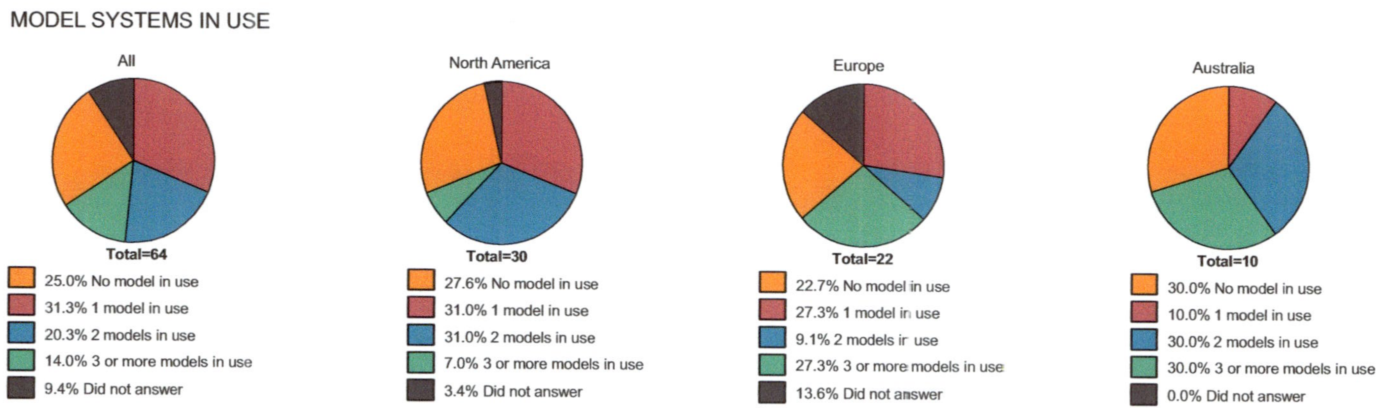

FIGURE 1.5 PDX model development by region The models include systems to develop PDX-derived cell lines, PDX-derived organoids, patient tumor–derived organoids, new generation culture media, and recombination techniques (such as inductive mesenchyme or cancer-associated fibroblasts). The number of respondents are underneath each graph and the percentages shown in the legend key.

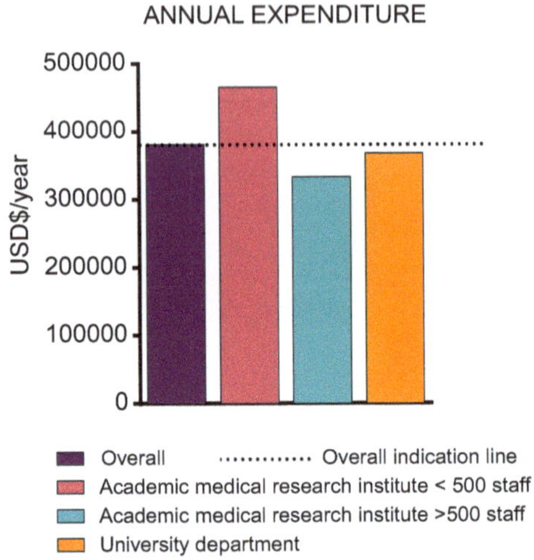

FIGURE 1.6 Average capital expenditure for PDX programs in different countries. The average annual cost of a PDX program is US$380,681 annually, US$385,958 in Europe, US$332,352 in North America, US$303,125 in Australia. A total of 44/64 respondents answered this question, 10 respondents did not know their annual budget, and 10 respondents skipped this question.

European PDX programs are the costliest with an annual expenditure of US$385,958, when compared with North American programs (US$332,352) and Australia (US$303,125) (Fig. 1.6). Regional cost variables may contribute to the differences in the annual expenditure. However, it is interesting to note that PDX program expenditure in larger research institutes is smaller when compared with that in smaller institutes. This is relevant given that most PDX programs in North America are run within large research institutes. Shared facilities and scientific technology platforms can drive down the cost of PDX program allowing a more competitive environment. The smaller research institutes that predominate in Europe may not share the same privileges or access to centralized facilities. Although spending less annually, the programs in North America did not characterize their PDX as robustly as did their European counterparts in next generation sequencing, protein analysis, and epigenetic analysis. In contrast, PDX programs situated within universities as opposed to medical research institutes appeared to have lower expenditure, and universities make less use of molecular characterization of their PDX models. Of the three common cancer types, the average expenditure for breast, colorectal, and lung cancer programs (excluding respondents who did not know their annual budgets) were $352,000, $361,905, and $419,048, respectively. There is a positive correlation between the extent of PDX model development and annual expenditure (described in Section 3.4). For example, lung cancer PDX programs report the most development of extending their PDX and report higher average annual expenditure.

Governance and Occupational Health and Safety

Proper governance guidelines for each PDX program should be designed with the inclusions of good policy and practice and consideration of appropriate OHS measures. Good governance practice for an academic PDX program includes:

- Obtaining appropriate consent from patients for the use of study material;
- Securing patient data storage with reliable systems to enable return of results of clinical significance to patients;
- Developing secure PDX tracking data systems to track PDX mouse lineages;
- In-built animal welfare monitoring system including availability of trained veterinarians;
- Occupational safety measures in handling biohazard materials, such as patient tumor materials and extended derivatives, with auditable reporting systems available.

The outcome of this survey confirmed that most PDX programs can improve on governance practices. All respondents reported that appropriate consent had been obtained from patients, except in one case where consent was obtained as part of a larger clinical trial. About 55% (30/55 respondents) of PDX programs have a secure study database with data coded by an ID which can be reliably reidentified if required. Thirty-five percent (19/55 respondents) implement restricted access only to study-related personnel and store clinical and study data on separate databases and separate servers. Of note, only 18% (10/55 respondents) of PDX programs return results of potential clinical significance back to the patient. Although the majority of PDX programs perform at least one method of ensuring patient data confidentiality, this could be an area that could be improved. Only 55% (29/53 respondents) have database management systems to track their PDX mice and PDX treatments. However, randomizing and assigning mice to particular treatments is usually performed manually without the use of computer software and over half (54%, 29/54 respondents) of PDX programs reported not double-blinding assessors to the treatment arm of the PDX model during scoring of tumor kinetics.

All PDX mice are immunocompromised. Screening PDX recipient mice for murine and human viruses should ensure that the PDX animals are healthy and prevent spread of transmissible disease. In most cases, good animal handling practice involving using personal protective equipment, such as gloves and safety glasses should suffice. There is an expectation where mouse facilities/bioservices should routinely perform animal screening for viruses or retroviruses. Fifty-one percent (29/57 responders) of PDX programs report routine murine virology tests and only 16% (9/57 responders) screen for murine retroviruses. Notably, the screening for human viruses, such as HIV and hepatitis B viral screen was performed by only 26% of PDX programs (15/57 responders). Of these, five responders obtained tissue from the biobank, meaning only 38% (5/13 responders) of biobanks perform human virology tests, or that the awareness of this type of testing was not high among responders. Twenty-one percent (12/57 responders) indicated routine screening for human viruses and retroviruses, with adequate reporting systems in place for returning human viral results to patients. No Australian PDX programs report screening human viruses/retroviruses. The survey did not capture whether institutes have different reporting systems for viral pathogens. For example, institutions may choose to test the tumor sample before implantation, test the patient directly, or place all PDX animals in animal biosafety level 2 facilities which automatically cover the safety risk of the typical viral pathogens so that testing may not be necessary. It should be noted that institutions may decide to use one or a combination of these reporting systems.

Clinical Relevance of PDX Program

The clinical relevance of a PDX program is establishing that each PDX tumor maintains a range of characteristics consistent with the original biological behavior of the patient's tumor from which it was derived. This should include careful correlation of patient clinical outcomes with the response of the PDX to standard therapies and any relevant other therapies in vivo. The process includes validation of the original histopathology of the patient's tumor and collection of long-term patient clinical outcome data, which may take a considerable time to obtain depending on the patient's prognosis.

The findings of this survey revealed that the majority of academic PDX programs routinely reviewed the histopathology results of the patient's tumor (79%, 48/60 respondents) and collect patient's clinical data following their cancer treatment (77%, 46/60 respondents) (data not shown). Despite this, only 40% (24/60 respondents) of these programs reported routinely documenting correlation of their PDX model outcomes with the patients' clinical outcomes. This could merely reflect the current stages of each PDX program, whether they are at the early phase of generating and validating the PDX models or at the later stages where clinical outcome data is available and preclinical assessment of response to standard therapy has been completed. This is reflected by the leading type of research publication from each PDX program being one that focuses on the design and characterization of PDX models from that particular PDX program (41%, 26/64 respondents), the analysis of drug interactions (30%, 19/64 respondents), and investigation of biomarkers (20%, 13/64 respondents).

FROM ACADEMIA TO COMMERCIALIZATION

An important goal of a PDX program is the generation of robust preclinical data to support the development of novel therapeutics, especially in their transition to early-phase human clinical trials.[2] Streamlined collaborations increase the availability and sharing of valuable, well-validated and annotated PDX models that can in turn speed preclinical discovery. The licensing of PDX models in return for fee can aid academic PDX programs in maintaining, generating, and developing additional PDX models to ensure long-term viability of the resource.

Globally, 30% (19 of 64 respondents) reported licensing one or more of their PDX models to industry in return for a fee (Fig. 1.7A). Programs that do

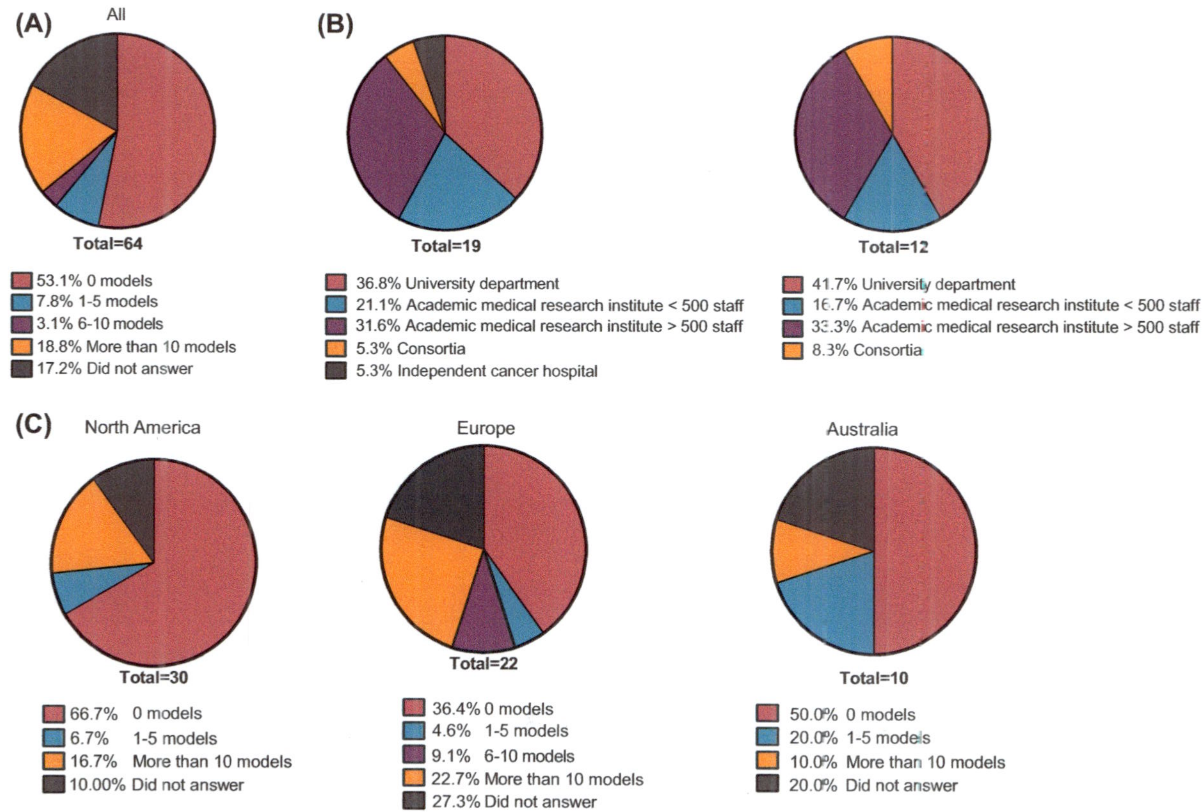

FIGURE 1.7 Licensing of PDX models by (A) overall number of models licensed, (B) type of institution or institutions that license more than 10 models and (C) by region.

license appear to be able to easily generate additional PDX models for licensing, with 12 of 19 respondents licensing more than 10 PDX models, 2 of 19 having licensed between 6 and 10 PDX models, and 5 of 19 respondents having licensed between one to five PDX models. All these respondents disclosed receiving financial return for their PDX models.

In terms of the types of institution that had licensed their PDX models, we found similar numbers of PDX programs from universities (37%, 7/19 respondents) and medical research institutes (53%, 10/19 respondents) involved in this process (Fig. 1.7B). There were also a similar number of PDX programs from universities (42%, 5/12 respondents) and medical research institutes (50%, 6/12 respondents) that had licensed more than 10 PDX models (Fig. 1.7B). Regionally, Europe had the highest percentage of PDX programs licensed (36%, 8/22 respondents) and programs that had licensed more than 10 models (23%, 5/22 respondents) (Fig. 1.7C). This was followed by North America (27%, 8/30 respondents; and 20%, 6/30 respondents, respectively) and Australia (30%, 3/10; and 0%, 0/10 respondents, respectively). It is worth noting that two of the European PDX programs involved in licensing a high number of PDX models were consortia. Of all programs that had licensed (19 respondents), the majority (79%, 15/19 respondents) licensed from a collaboration with a public hospital, followed by private collections (32%, 6/19 respondents) biobanks (26%, 5/19 respondents), and research consortia (11%, 2/19 respondents).

The tumor subtypes of PDX that have been successfully licensed include nine breast cancer PDX models, five colorectal cancer PDX models, five lung cancer PDX models, and six ovarian cancer PDX models. This leaves 64% (34/53 respondents) of the PDX models within the academic programs as unlicensed. It is unclear if these PDX models are still undergoing development and validation, or, whether there is a lack of understanding or estimation of the value of PDX models to their own research programs. There is a large potential in the area of licensing PDX models between institutes and industries. In the future, it will be useful to understand whether licensing from academia to industry involves simple service contracts or whether there are ongoing financial returns that would benefit the longevity of the academic PDX program.

A SUCCESSFUL PDX PROGRAM

Core Metrics

Thus far this chapter has described current PDX program practice. To aid in ranking all PDX programs surveyed according to their degree of success, four core metrics were selected. The top five ranked PDX programs were then analyzed together. The four main core metrics chosen were:

1. Extensive use of routine molecular- and cellular-based characterization of their PDX models;
2. Substantial annual expenditure on the PDX programs with reliable multiple sources of financial funding;

3. Advancement in PDX model development, particularly those programs utilizing or developing three or more PDX model derivatives. The mode derivatives described included PDX-derived cell lines, PDX-derived organoids, parallel patient-derived organoids, the use of new generation culture media, and recombination technology (such as inductive mesenchyme and use of cancer-associated fibroblasts);
4. Successful commercialization of PDX models as an indicator of robustly characterized and annotated PDX models and commercial value of the PDX models.

Consortia were omitted from this ranking.

To provide a more holistic review of the top ranked PDX programs a further four metrics were also included in the analysis and ranking of PDX programs. These included:

5. Correlation of patient clinical outcome with PDX outcome, to validate the clinical relevance of the PDX model;
6. Publications produced from the PDX model, which include the impact factors and strengths of the publications not only spanning the PDX model techniques but also demonstrating the context of PDX outcome data by the analysis of five or more models in one publication;
7. Governance in relation to established governance processes in place within the institute for handling and storing confidential patient data and appropriate OHS practices;
8. Number of efforts to widen the program's collaborative base, such as creating standardized approaches to collecting PDX patient outcome data, standardized approaches to collecting PDX treatment efficacy data, standardized approaches to collecting PDX genomic/other molecular data, and collaborative agreements between academic laboratories with or without financial terms.

We assessed respondents in all eight key areas as key performance indicators (KPIs) for a successful PDX program (Table 1.2).

Characteristics of the Top Five PDX Programs Ranked

All of the top five ranked PDX programs were located in North America (3) or Europe (2). The two PDX programs from Europe were led by basic scientists and two of the three PDX programs from North America were led by clinician-scientists. No university-based PDX programs were listed in the top five ranked programs, and most (four of five) PDX programs were from large medical research institutes except for one European respondent. The average expenditure of the top five was higher (US$820,000/year) than that of the average PDX program (US$380,681/year) (Fig. 1.8A). The top five responders performed better routine molecular characterization in next generation sequencing, gene expression analysis and protein analysis (Fig. 1.8B), as well as development of PDX model derivatives than the average of all academic PDX programs (Fig. 1.8C).

TABLE 1.2 Key Performance Indicators of the Top Five Ranked PDX Programs

Country	Type of Laboratory	Lead Principle Investigator	Tumor Subtypes (0–23)	Routine Characteri-zation (0–13)	PDX Model Development (0–4)	Correlating Clinical Outcome to PDX Data (Y/N)	Publication Types (0–4)	Licensed >10 PDX models?	Governance and OHS (0–3)	Annual Budget/ No. of Sources	Collaboration (0–5)
North America	MRI >500 staff	Basic scientist	4	13	1	N	4	Y	3	$750,000–1,000,000/ 4 sources	5
North America	MRI >500 staff	Clinician scientist	19	11	1	Y	0	Y	3	150,000–300,000/ 1 source	NA
North America	MRI >500 staff	Clinician scientist	2	7	0[b]	Y	0	Y	3	1,000,000–2,000,000/ 3 sources	1
Europe	MRI >500 staff	Basic scientist	7	7	3	Y	NA	Y	2	750,000–1,000,000/ 4 sources	NA
Europe	MRI <500 staff	Basic scientist	3	2	4	Y[a]	NA	Y	0	750,000–1,000,000/ 2 sources	4

MRI, medical research institute; *N*, no; *NA*, not applicable; *Y*, yes.
[a]*In special circumstances when results are available from the hospital.*
[b]*Intend to test all.*

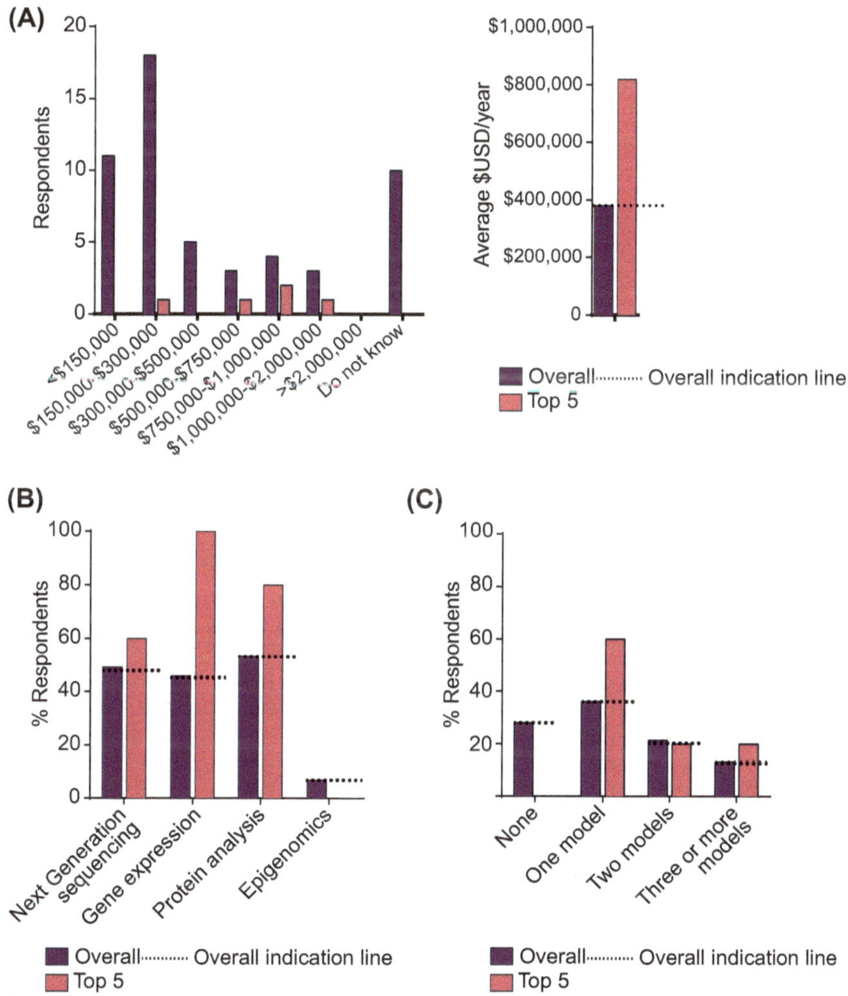

FIGURE 1.8 The top five PDX programs categorized by (A) annual expenditure, (B) extent of molecular characterization, and (C) models in use to develop their own PDX models.

Based on the metrics used for ranking the PDX program, none of the PDX programs excelled in all the KPIs. The top ranked responder from North America performed well in seven of eight KPIs, with the exception that no correlation with patient outcome data was reported and only one type of PDX model derivative had been developed (Table 1.2). Similarly, the second ranked PDX program, which was also from North America, included a large range of tumor subtypes with excellent molecular characterization, but reported no intention to develop PDX model derivatives, other than developing PDX-derived cell lines.

The third ranked PDX program extensively characterized its models but had no PDX model derivatives in use, although it had the intention to develop them.

All three PDX programs from North America described good governance and OHS indices, indicating that standardized, streamlined governance systems are in place. In relation to other PDX programs, two of these five programs had low annual budgets of US$150,000–300,000 despite achieving highly on other KPIs (Fig. 1.8A). One possible reason for this lies in potential offset of costs by being in a large medical research institute. These programs would be linked to a core platform facility with preexisting infrastructure and research capacity for in-house molecular testing. Other preexisting collaborations that satisfy various needs within the PDX program may also exist, making the total cost of the program difficult to determine.

The fourth and fifth ranked PDX programs were located in Europe. Both European PDX programs were well established in developing PDX models and reported wide collaboration. One of the PDX program scored low in the OHS performance index, and both declined to comment on their publication achievements.

The outcome of this analysis suggests that even within the highly ranked PDX programs by described KPI's, no single PDX program performed highly across all eight KPIs and that there were areas for recommendation for improvement.

RECOMMENDATIONS FOR IMPROVING CURRENT PDX PRACTICES

The standards of academic PDX programs vary according to funding constraints, opportunities for collaboration, links with local medical health institutes, and availability of specific specialty expertise (for example, a particular tumor subtype). Despite this there is a desirable gold standard which each institute should aspire to attain to maintain a successful PDX program. We identify three main areas for improvement and make future recommendations.

Molecular Characterization

Informative, high-quality PDX models require fairly extensive molecular characterization, including newer genomic sequencing technologies. This should complement other routine PDX characterization, such as histopathology, immunohistochemistry, tumor volume/kinetics analysis, and response to the standard treatment for that type of PDX. Newer and more informative molecular analysis involving next generation sequencing, such as candidate panel testing, RNA-Seq, and low-coverage whole genome sequencing should be performed when possible. Protein expression analysis, such as reverse-phase protein arrays and epigenomic analysis should be explored and would greatly increase the value of existing PDX models. It was notable that epigenomic analysis was only used under special circumstances and not reported as routine by any respondent. The relative novelty, lack of access, or cost associated with these epigenomic techniques highlights a future area of improvement. To remain competitive with other PDX programs, each PDX program should aim to access a facility platform to ensure that robust characterization is feasible.

Future recommendations: Each PDX program should aim to expand beyond gene sequencing technologies and start embracing other analyses, such as protein analysis and epigenomics. The rapid analysis of sequencing and other analyses, to achieve the aim of "personalized medicine" will depend on the active involvement of bioinformaticists and genomicists.

Governance

All PDX programs should have in place standardized processes to obtain appropriate consent of all patients, secure storage facility for sensitive patient data, a reliable capacity to return results of clinical significance to the individual patient, a centralized system for experimental design and tracking of experimental animals, and the implementation of health reporting systems to protect both the experimental mice and laboratory staff working with human cancer tissues. Incorporating the role of facility managers has the potential of reducing the governance procedures for lead investigators in PDX programs.

Future recommendations: Increasingly, ethics committees, industry, and regulators are accepting preclinical PDX drug response analyses as relevant data. These results are used to shape the design of early-phase clinical trials of novel cancer therapeutics. To ensure the success of such trials, standardized and universally accepted governance processes need to be in place. Robust governance will speed the transition of animal-derived preclinical data into the generation of human trials. Dedicated and well-trained facility core managers may enable scientists to focus on their research program. It is therefore recommended that all PDX programs be aware or have platforms in place for best practice governance obligations, which may vary from country to country.

Collaboration

It would be rare for one PDX program alone to be able to absorb all the financial strain and extensive characterization of its models on its own. In contrast, there are clear benefits to fostering strong collaboration and networking opportunities with other PDX and non-PDX research programs, both within academic and industry settings. The majority of PDX programs report that the strength of their programs was the capacity to collaborate widely and in doing so, to be able to secure a wide source of intellectual, technical, and financial support.

Future recommendations: There is a huge potential and opportunity for both academic and industry laboratories to partner through consortia. Consortia can provide a firm platform for laboratories to harmonize and streamline existing PDX models. This can include instituting transparent and well-governed mechanisms to ensure academic fairness, as well as protection of patients' liberty and confidentiality. It may also provide opportunities to train clinician scientists in academic programs, such as Europe, where most programs are led by basic scientists. Collaborations within consortia can also increase the quality of preclinical data produced to further engage with industry partners. There is a need for better education on the benefits of partnerships with industry and academia. These partnerships should not be limited to simple service agreements. We recommend a move toward ongoing funding agreements between industry and academic laboratories. Money received from industry should be rolled back into the academic scientific PDX infrastructure, ensuring ongoing characterization and viability of the PDX resource.

SUMMARY AND CONCLUDING COMMENTS

The majority of PDX programs publish validation of the quality of their PDX models, methods for improving take rates, and establishing correlations between clinical and PDX outcome data. A range of PDX programs have reported on tumor context–specific efficacy of novel therapeutics (reviewed in Lodhia et al.[2]). However, the majority of PDX programs do not have sufficiently well-characterized models to generate reliable drug response data to be shaping clinical trial design consistently. To broaden the potential preclinical benefits of PDX it will be imperative to focus on building the necessary platforms, including governance and engagement with industry, to enable this to become a reality.

ACKNOWLEDGMENTS

Supported by grants from the National Health and Medical Research Council Australia (Project Grants 1057831, 1062702, 1081178) and the Stafford Fox Medical Research Foundation; by the Cancer Council Victoria (Sir Edward Dunlop Fellowship in Cancer Research to CLS), Victorian Cancer Agency (Fellowship to CLS), the Clinical Australian Postgraduate Award scholarship (to GYH), the Clinician Researcher Top Up PhD Cancer Therapeutic scholarship (to GYH), by the Australian Cancer Research Foundation, and by an Operational Infrastructure Support Grant from the Victorian State Government.

REFERENCES

1. Hidalgo M, Amant F, Biankin AV, Budinska E, Byrne AT, Caldas C, et al. Patient-derived xenograft models: an emerging platform for translational cancer research. *Cancer Discov* 2014;**4**(9):998–1013.
2. Lodhia KA, Hadley AM, Haluska P, Scott CL. Prioritizing therapeutic targets using patient-derived xenograft models. *Biochim Biophys Acta* 2015;**1855**(2):223–34.
3. Hudson WA, Li Q, Le C, Kersey JH. Xenotransplantation of human lymphoid malignancies is optimized in mice with multiple immunologic defects. *Leukemia* 1998;**12**(12):2029–33.
4. Firestone B. The challenge of selecting the 'right' in vivo oncology pharmacology model. *Curr Opin Pharmacol* 2010;**10**(4):391–6.

5. Shultz LD, Brehm MA, Garcia-Martinez JV, Greiner DL. Humanized mice for immune system investigation: progress, promise and challenges. *Nat Rev Immunol* 2012;**12**(11):786–98.
6. Puig I, Chicote I, Tenbaum SP, Arques O, Herance JR, Gispert JD, et al. A personalized preclinical model to evaluate the metastatic potential of patient-derived colon cancer initiating cells. *Clin Cancer Res* 2013;**19**(24):6787–801.
7. Whiteford CC, Bilke S, Greer BT, Chen Q, Braunschweig TA, Cenacchi N, et al. Credentialing preclinical pediatric xenograft models using gene expression and tissue microarray analysis. *Cancer Res* 2007;**67**(1):32–40.
8. Siolas D, Hannon GJ. Patient-derived tumor xenografts: transforming clinical samples into mouse models. *Cancer Res* 2013;**73**(17):5315–9.
9. Ocana A, Pandiella A, Siu LL, Tannock IF. Preclinical development of molecular-targeted agents for cancer. *Nat Rev Clin Oncol* 2011;**8**(4):200–9.
10. Presnell SC, Werdin ES, Maygarden S, Mohler JL, Smith GJ. Establishment of short-term primary human prostate xenografts for the study of prostate biology and cancer. *Am J Pathol* 2001;**159**(3):855–60.
11. Krasagakis K, Almond-Roesler B, Geilen C, Fimmel S, Krengel S, Chatzaki E, et al. Growth and characterization of a cell line from a human primary neuroendocrine carcinoma of the skin (Merkel cell carcinoma) in culture and as xenograft. *J Cell Physiol* 2001;**187**(3):386–91.
12. Ribatti D, Raffaghello L, Pastorino F, Nico B, Brignole C, Vacca A, et al. In vivo angiogenic activity of neuroblastoma correlates with MYCN oncogene overexpression. *Int J Cancer* 2002;**102**(4):351–4.
13. Ray S, Almasan A. Apoptosis induction in prostate cancer cells and xenografts by combined treatment with Apo2 ligand/tumor necrosis factor-related apoptosis-inducing ligand and CPT-11. *Cancer Res* 2003;**63**(15):4713–23.
14. Verschraegen CF, Hu W, Du Y, Mendoza J, Early J, Deavers M, et al. Establishment and characterization of cancer cell cultures and xenografts derived from primary or metastatic Mullerian cancers. *Clin Cancer Res* 2003;**9**(2):845–52.
15. Li ZY, Ni S, Yang X, Kiviat N, Lieber A. Xenograft models for liver metastasis: relationship between tumor morphology and adenovirus vector transduction. *Mol Ther* 2004;**9**(5):650–7.
16. Davis DW, Takamori R, Raut CP, Xiong HQ, Herbst RS, Stadler WM, et al. Pharmacodynamic analysis of target inhibition and endothelial cell death in tumors treated with the vascular endothelial growth factor receptor antagonists SU5416 or SU6668. *Clin Cancer Res* 2005;**11**(2 Pt 1):678–89.
17. Hylander BL, Pitoniak R, Penetrante RB, Gibbs JF, Oktay D, Cheng J, et al. The anti-tumor effect of Apo2L/TRAIL on patient pancreatic adenocarcinomas grown as xenografts in SCID mice. *J Transl Med* 2005;**3**(1):22.
18. Giannini C, Sarkaria JN, Saito A, Uhm JH, Galanis E, Carlson BL, et al. Patient tumor EGFR and PDGFRA gene amplifications retained in an invasive intracranial xenograft model of glioblastoma multiforme. *Neuro-Oncology* 2005;**7**(2):164–76.
19. Indraccolo S, Tisato V, Agata S, Moserle L, Ferrari S, Callegaro M, et al. Establishment and characterization of xenografts and cancer cell cultures derived from BRCA1$^{-/-}$ epithelial ovarian cancers. *Eur J Cancer* 2006;**42**(10):1475–83.
20. Cutz JC, Guan J, Bayani J, Yoshimoto M, Xue H, Sutcliffe M, et al. Establishment in severe combined immunodeficiency mice of subrenal capsule xenografts and transplantable tumor lines from a variety of primary human lung cancers: potential models for studying tumor progression-related changes. *Clin Cancer Res* 2006;**12**(13):4043–54.
21. Elaraj DM, Weinreich DM, Varghese S, Puhlmann M, Hewitt SM, Carroll NM, et al. The role of interleukin 1 in growth and metastasis of human cancer xenografts. *Clin Cancer Res* 2006;**12**(4):1088–96.

22. Sarkaria JN, Carlson BL, Schroeder MA, Grogan P, Brown PD, Giannini C, et al. Use of an orthotopic xenograft model for assessing the effect of epidermal growth factor receptor amplification on glioblastoma radiation response. *Clin Cancer Res* 2006;**12**(7 Pt 1):2264–71.
23. Dangles-Marie V, Pocard M, Richon S, Weiswald LB, Assayag F, Saulnier P, et al. Establishment of human colon cancer cell lines from fresh tumors versus xenografts: comparison of success rate and cell line features. *Cancer Res* 2007;**67**(1):398–407.
24. Ghadersohi A, Pan D, Fayazi Z, Hicks DG, Winston JS, Li F. Prostate-derived Ets transcription factor (PDEF) downregulates survivin expression and inhibits breast cancer cell growth in vitro and xenograft tumor formation in vivo. *Breast Cancer Res Treat* 2007;**102**(1):19–30.
25. Rubio-Viqueira B, Jimeno A, Cusatis G, Zhang X, Iacobuzio-Donahue C, Karikari C, et al. An in vivo platform for translational drug development in pancreatic cancer. *Clin Cancer Res* 2006;**12**(15):4652–61.
26. Marangoni E, Vincent-Salomon A, Auger N, Degeorges A, Assayag F, de Cremoux P, et al. A new model of patient tumor-derived breast cancer xenografts for preclinical assays. *Clin Cancer Res* 2007;**13**(13):3989–98.
27. Kortmann U, McAlpine JN, Xue H, Guan J, Ha G, Tully S, et al. Tumor growth inhibition by olaparib in BRCA2 germline-mutated patient-derived ovarian cancer tissue xenografts. *Clin Cancer Res* 2011;**17**(4):783–91.
28. Fichtner I, Rolff J, Soong R, Hoffmann J, Hammer S, Sommer A, et al. Establishment of patient-derived non-small cell lung cancer xenografts as models for the identification of predictive biomarkers. *Clin Cancer Res* 2008;**14**(20):6456–68.
29. Cao P, Maira SM, Garcia-Echeverria C, Hedley DW. Activity of a novel, dual PI3-kinase/mTor inhibitor NVP-BEZ235 against primary human pancreatic cancers grown as orthotopic xenografts. *Br J Cancer* 2009;**100**(8):1267–76.
30. Oakes SR, Vaillant F, Lim E, Lee L, Breslin K, Feleppa F, et al. Sensitization of BCL-2-expressing breast tumors to chemotherapy by the BH3 mimetic ABT-737. *Proc Natl Acad Sci USA* 2012;**109**(8):2766–71.
31. Sivanand S, Pena-Llopis S, Zhao H, Kucejova B, Spence P, Pavia-Jimenez A, et al. A validated tumorgraft model reveals activity of dovitinib against renal cell carcinoma. *Sci Transl Med* 2012;**4**(137):137ra175.
32. Julien S, Merino-Trigo A, Lacroix L, Pocard M, Goere D, Mariani P, et al. Characterization of a large panel of patient-derived tumor xenografts representing the clinical heterogeneity of human colorectal cancer. *Clin Cancer Res* 2012;**18**(19):5314–28.
33. Zhang J, Zhang L, Su X, Li M, Xie L, Malchers F, et al. Translating the therapeutic potential of AZD4547 in FGFR1-amplified non-small cell lung cancer through the use of patient-derived tumor xenograft models. *Clin Cancer Res* 2012;**18**(24):6658–67.
34. Dave B, Landis MD, Tweardy DJ, Chang JC, Dobrolecki LE, Wu MF, et al. Selective small molecule Stat3 inhibitor reduces breast cancer tumor-initiating cells and improves recurrence free survival in a human-xenograft model. *PloS One* 2012;**7**(8):e30207.
35. Ma CX, Cai S, Li S, Ryan CE, Guo Z, Schaiff WT, et al. Targeting Chk1 in p53-deficient triple-negative breast cancer is therapeutically beneficial in human-in-mouse tumor models. *J Clin Invest* 2012;**122**(4):1541–52.
36. Pawaskar DK, Straubinger RM, Fetterly GJ, Hylander BH, Repasky EA, Ma WW, et al. Synergistic interactions between sorafenib and everolimus in pancreatic cancer xenografts in mice. *Cancer Chemother Pharmacol* 2013;**71**(5):1231–40.
37. Zhang XC, Zhang J, Li M, Huang XS, Yang XN, Zhong WZ, et al. Establishment of patient-derived non-small cell lung cancer xenograft models with genetic aberrations within EGFR, KRAS and FGFR1: useful tools for preclinical studies of targeted therapies. *J Transl Med* 2013;**11**:168.

38. Vaillant F, Merino D, Lee L, Breslin K, Pal B, Ritchie ME, et al. Targeting BCL-2 with the BH3 mimetic ABT-199 in estrogen receptor-positive breast cancer. *Cancer Cell* 2013;**24**(1):120–9.
39. Das Thakur M, Salangsang F, Landman AS, Sellers WR, Pryer NK, Levesque MP, et al. Modelling vemurafenib resistance in melanoma reveals a strategy to forestall drug resistance. *Nature* 2013;**494**(7436):251–5.
40. Stewart E, Goshorn R, Bradley C, Griffiths LM, Benavente C, Twarog NR, et al. Targeting the DNA repair pathway in Ewing sarcoma. *Cell Rep* 2014;**9**(3):829–41.
41. Al-Ejeh F, Pajic M, Shi W, Kalimutho M, Miranda M, Nagrial AM, et al. Gemcitabine and CHK1 inhibition potentiate EGFR-directed radioimmunotherapy against pancreatic ductal adenocarcinoma. *Clin Cancer Res* 2014;**20**(12):3187–97.
42. Su B, Zhao W, Shi B, Zhang Z, Yu X, Xie F, et al. Let-7d suppresses growth, metastasis, and tumor macrophage infiltration in renal cell carcinoma by targeting COL3A1 and CCL7. *Mol Cancer* 2014;**13**:206.

Chapter 2

Role of Companies and Corporations in the Development and Utilization of PDX Models

J. Snyder[1], O. Duchamp[2], K. Paz[3], P. Sathyan[4]

[1]*University of Washington School of Medicine, Seattle, WA, United States;* [2]*Oncodesign, Dijon Cedex, France;* [3]*Champions Oncology, Hackensack, NJ, United States;* [4]*KEW Group Inc, Cambridge, MA, United States*

INTRODUCTION

Although much of the early work related to patient-derived tumor xenograft (PDX) research was initiated by academic centers, commercial entities have subsequently taken on a critical role in supporting the development, improvement, and assessment of the PDX technology. According to a 2014 *Cancer Letters* manuscript on PDX models, at the time of publication, there were at least eight commercial providers (companies/institutions/organizations) of PDX services within North America, five within Europe, and three within Asia,[1] and the market is constantly growing, emphasizing the importance of this technology as an oncology research tool. In addition, several pharmaceutical companies that do not have an in-house PDX program, or have only limited number of models, have entered into partnership with academic centers or companies to support model development, optimization, and testing. Collaborative efforts linking academia, industry, and pharmaceutical partners have been established in different geographic regions to maximize the potential of this technology in revolutionizing oncology drug discovery and patient care. Several companies have also expanded their PDX banks and service repertoire by acquiring other entities. Examples include the acquisition of PRECOS Ltd, a UK-based contract research organization, and Molecular Response by Crown Bioscience Inc. (CrownBio), and Oncotest GmbH by Charles River.

This chapter discusses the role of the industry in advancing development and utility of PDX models, primarily based on a survey of major providers of PDX

Patient Derived Tumor Xenograft Models. http://dx.doi.org/10.1016/B978-0-12-804010-2.00026-6

services. A web-based search and data from previous publications were used to identify 16 commercial providers of PDX services worldwide (Table 2.1), and a detailed survey was conducted and distributed electronically to representatives in these organizations. The survey attempted to give a comprehensive overview

TABLE 2.1 Commercial Providers of PDX Services Worldwide

Provider	Website Address
Champions Oncology, Hackensack, NJ, USA	http://www.championsoncology.com
Charles River Laboratories, Wilmington, MA, USA	http://www.criver.com
Crownbio, Santa Clara, CA, USA	http://www.crownbio.com
Deshpande Laboratories, Bhopal, Madhya Pradesh, India	http://deshpandelab.com
Experimental Pharmacology and Oncology, Berlin-Buch, Germany	http://www.epo-berlin.com
GenScript, Piscataway, NJ, USA	http://www.genscript.com
Horizon/SAGE Laboratories Cambridge, UK, England, and St. Louis, MO, USA	https://www.horizondiscovery.com/in-vivo-models/pdx
The Jackson Laboratory, Sacramento, CA, USA	https://www.jax.org/jax-mice-and-services/in-vivo-pharmacology/oncology-services/pdx-tumors#
Living Tumor Laboratory, Vancouver, British Columbia, Canada	http://www.livingtumorcentre.com
Oncodesign, Dijon Cedex, France	http://www.oncodesign.com
Pharmaron, Beijing, China	http://www.pharmaron.com/
Shanghai LIDE Biotech Co, Ltd, Shanghai, China	http://www.lidebiotech.com
Urolead, Strasbourg, France	http://www.urolead.com/ips/products-and-services
WuXi AppTec, Shanghai, China	http://www.wuxiapptec.com
Xenopat, L'Hospitalet de Llobregat, Barcelona, Spain	http://www.xenopat.com
XenTech, Paris, France	http://www.xentech.eu/

of the field and included technical questions regarding tissue selection, transport, mouse strain, implantation procedure, and storage of samples. It also incorporated platform-related questions regarding inventory, cancer type selection, services offered, challenges associated with the procedures, and future directions anticipated within the PDX space aiming at improving and advancing the platform. Complete (seven) or partial (one) responses were obtained from three commercial providers primarily serving the United States and North America, three primarily serving Europe, one primarily serving Asia, and one providing worldwide services. Results were analyzed together and, when relevant, according to geographical regions. Importantly, due to the limited number of participants, survey results must be interpreted with caution. The limited number of overall complete responses also precluded statistical analyses. Company representatives, websites, and publications were also used to obtain some information regarding specific services. A similar survey was distributed to academic centers with PDX programs, and the results of this survey are presented in Section IV, Chapter 1.

PDX INVENTORY AND TUMOR SAMPLES

Number and Type of Models in PDX Bank

Tumor types specified in the survey questionnaire included hematological, bladder, brain, breast, lung, kidney, pancreatic, ovarian, cervical, prostate, colorectal, gastroesophageal, head and neck, as well as bone tumors; melanoma; skin cancer (nonmelanoma); liver and biliary tumors; and sarcoma. Most companies responding to the survey reported having >200 models in their PDX tumor bank while adding 6–10 models to their inventory each quarter. One respondent reported adding 21–30 models and two reported adding >31 models to their inventory each quarter. While there are companies that specialize in one tumor type (eg, breast cancer) or a narrow range of tumor types (eg, kidney, prostate, bladder), most survey respondents reported that their inventory is composed of a wide variety of tumor types (≥10). The most common tumor type in the inventory of all respondents was breast cancer (subtype unspecified), with most respondents reporting >11 models in their inventory (Fig. 2.1A). Most respondents also reported having >11 models of lung, pancreatic, and colorectal neoplasms (Fig. 2.1A). The least common tumor type was skin cancer (nonmelanoma), followed by bone, prostate, cervical, and hematological neoplasms (Fig. 2.1A). Respondents with the aforementioned tumor types reported having less than 11 models for these indications (Fig. 2.1A). This may be attributed to technical difficulties in collecting ample amount of these patient tumors and/or to low tumor engraftment rates of these PDX models. "Other" tumor types in inventories added by survey respondents included mesothelioma. Other tumor types not included in the survey but present in inventories include testicular, small intestine, duodenal, and thymic tumors, and chordoma. Responses did not

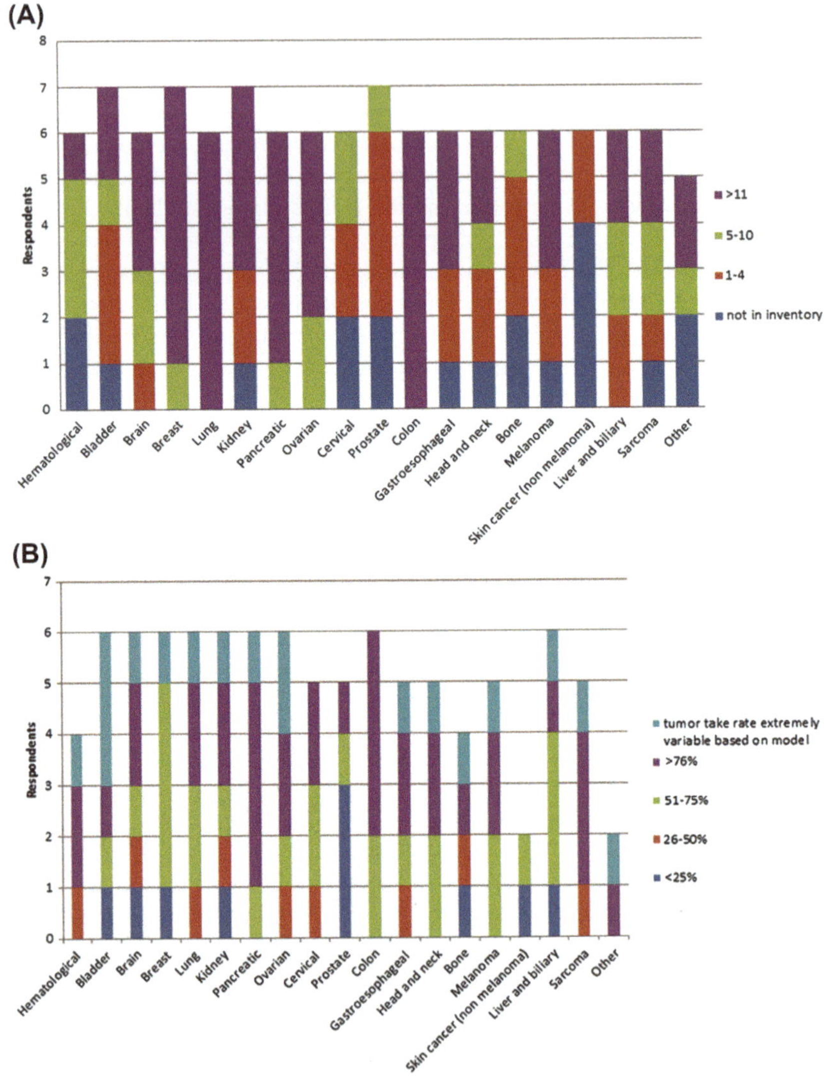

FIGURE 2.1 **(A) PDX tumor inventory.** A PDX tumor inventory of survey participants is presented with number of models present within each tumor type. Legend: *blue* indicates that the tumor type is not present in the PDX bank; *red* indicates that one to four models are present; *green* indicates that 5–10 models are present; *purple* indicates that >11 models are present. In this survey, the threshold for number of models is low and therefore does not distinguish between PDX tumor inventories having highly abundant tumor types with >40 models and medium inventories of 11–39 models. **(B) Engraftment rate by tumor type.** Estimated engraftment rate by number of survey respondents. *Royal blue* indicates estimated engraftment rate of <25%, *red* indicates rate of 26–50%, *green* indicates rate of 51–75%, and purple indicates rate of >76%. The *light blue bars* indicate respondents who declined to give an engraftment rate due to variability within the tumor type based on model.

appear to vary dramatically by geographic area served. In general, results on the frequency of PDX models by cancer subtype were similar for the academic and industry surveys. However, the threshold in the survey was quite low and failed to highlight inventory differences between highly abundant tumor types with >40 models and medium inventories of >11 models.

Success Rate of PDX Model Establishment

PDX take rate may refer to the engraftment of the primary human tumor in the mice or to the engraftment rate of a model between two mouse generations (including recovery from cryopreservation).[2] In the context of approximate tumor take rate in their inventory, most respondents listed their tumor take rate at >51% for the majority of tumor types, although the specific tumor engraftment rate per cancer indication varies greatly (Fig. 2.1B). A higher tumor take rate (>76%) was reported by most respondents for pancreatic, colorectal, and sarcoma models (Fig. 2.1B). Some respondents (three of five) felt that the engraftment rate for prostate samples was lower (<25%) (Fig. 2.1B). The engraftment rates for bladder, brain, kidney, and bone neoplasms were reported to be extremely variable based on tumor model by several respondents (Fig. 2.1B), probably due to the low abundance of these cancer indications in some or many inventories. These results are in alignment with those gathered from the academic survey with the exception of lung and pancreatic cancer models that appeared to have a higher engraftment rate in the industry survey.

Tumor and Disease Status

Different factors affect the engraftment rate, the quality of the tumor bank, and its clinical and translational relevance. Treatment-naive or pretreatment tumors may have different applications when subjected to drug sensitivity tests. Some tumors are harvested from the primary cancer site, whereas others are derived from metastatic lesions. Survey respondents reported that the majority of their patient tumors were treatment naive (four of seven). Similarly, most survey respondents reported that the majority of their patient tumors were primary (four of six), although two respondents reported that the majority of their patient tumors were metastatic. One survey respondent commented that approximately 15% of their models are established with patient metastases, whereas some models are established with the primary and metastatic tumors from the same patient.

PRACTICE AND PROTOCOLS

Type of Tumor Tissue Used in PDX Model Development and the Origin and Source of Samples

Tissue used in PDX model development may be collected during surgery or biopsy and may be subjected to various processing methods, such as mechanical or chemical digestion of tumor fragments.[3,4] All survey respondents (seven of seven) implanted fresh tumor fragments in the attempt to create a PDX model, and many (four of seven) listed this as the preferred sample which yields very good results in PDX model generation. Two respondents reported using fresh tumor minced and three respondents reported using dimethyl sulfoxide (DMSO) cryopreserved tumor in the generation of PDX tumors. Only one respondent reported using freshly digested tumor. The majority of respondents (seven of eight) reported that their PDX tumor samples were obtained during surgery. Some respondents (four of eight) reported that tumor samples were obtained via a biopsy and less often (three of eight) via fine-needle aspirate. Recent publications have described successful tumor engraftment for small cell lung cancer and prostate cancer following needle biopsy[5,6]; obtaining samples for implantation via this technique may become more common.

Shipping of Patient Tumors

Given the requirement for obtaining patient tumor samples from hospitals or research facilities distant from the implantation centers, a mechanism for efficient transport of tumor samples is essential. Many survey respondents (four of seven) reported seeing a difference in tumor take rate based on method of transportation. Most survey respondents (six of seven) reported transporting samples chilled, with two respondents reporting that samples were transported following a slow freezing process using DMSO. Survey respondents reported occasionally shipping samples overnight (all seven respondents) and using a specialized transport medium (six of seven), with all respondents reporting an average transport time of less than 24 h between tumor collection and implantation (all seven respondents). During storage and transport, temperature was checked by an automatic system or by the transporter.

Storage

Banked tumors in repositories may include DMSO-cryopreserved samples, snap frozen samples, optimal cutting temperature samples, formalin-fixed paraffin-embedded (FFPE) samples, FFPE tissue microarray, and extracted DNA and RNA samples. Survey respondents reported storing banked tumors using cryopreservation (six of seven) with >75% success in engrafting most PDX models from cryopreservation, regardless of the tumor type. For breast and liver and biliary neoplasms, two of six respondents estimated 51–75% success in bringing tumors back from cryopreservation (Fig. 2.2).

Mouse Models

Mouse strain is an important factor in PDX model development. Although nude and SCID mice were traditionally used, more immunodeficient mouse strains, such as NSG mice have been reported to be more receptive to human

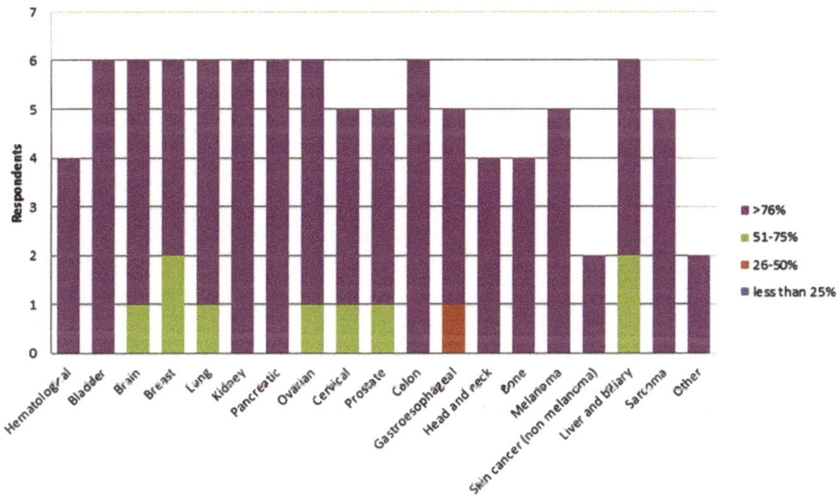

FIGURE 2.2 Approximate engraftment rate by tumor type following cryopreservation. *Blue* indicates <25% successful engraftment, *red* indicates 26–50% success, *green* indicates 51–75% success, and *purple* indicates >76% success in successfully growing the tumor type in the mouse following cryopreservation.

tumor engraftment, particularly for some hematological neoplasms.[7] The most common mouse strain used by survey respondents was the athymic nude (nu/nu) mouse (six of seven), although nude, NOD/SCID (*Prkdc*^{scid}; five of seven respondents), NOG, and NSG (both are NOD/SCID/IL2Rγ^{null}; five of seven respondents) are all commonly used. These results differ from those of the survey of academic institutions, in which the NSG mouse strain was most commonly used (45 respondents), followed by SCID mice (15 respondents) and nude mice (14 respondents). It could not be discerned from the present survey whether different mice strains were used for particular tumor models; however, most respondents reported using multiple strains within the same institution, suggesting that this is the case in some instances. Consideration of mouse strain in the development of PDX models is discussed further in Section I, Chapter 5.

Tumor Implantation

The choice of implantation site may affect tumor engraftment rates as well as ease of patient tumor placement and monitoring of xenograft growth.[3,4] Possibilities include subcutaneous implantation in the mouse flank, orthotopic implantation, which although more technically challenging and time consuming may more accurately mimic the tumor in the patient, and heterotopic sites, such as the subrenal capsule, which may increase engraftment rate over the subcutaneous method because of higher tissue perfusion and which may also shorten time to engraftment.[3,4,8] The most common implantation site reported in our survey was subcutaneous flank (all seven), although heterotopic (four of seven) and orthotopic [including intraperitoneal (four of seven), mammary fat pad (five of seven), and intracerebral (three of seven)] implantation sites were all commonly reported.

Tumor Monitoring

The method used to monitor tumor growth is related to the implantation site as subcutaneous flank and fat pad tumors are often more amenable to physical measurement; however, orthotopic techniques will require advanced imaging, such as ultrasound, magnetic resonance imaging (MRI) and computed tomography (CT). All survey respondents reported using physical measurement (calipers) to monitor tumor volume and growth, with three of seven reporting using ultrasound imaging, one reporting using MRI/CT, and four reporting using other imaging techniques to monitor tumor growth. Other imaging modalities include micro–positron emission tomography used in combination with MRI and CT for internal tumor growth monitoring.

Tumor Growth in the Mouse

Low-passage PDX models (<10) in the mouse may have an advantage in terms of preserving the molecular and genetic integrity of the patient's tumor.[4] Six of seven survey respondents required up to five mouse generations on an average to establish a model stock, with one survey respondent reporting an average of 6–10 generations to establish a stock. Responses to the question, "What is the maximal mouse generation you would go up to?" were variable and ranged from 1 to 20 generations. In general, respondents indicated that the number of generations to establish a stock and the maximal mouse generation used does not vary based on the tumor model. The length of time that first-generation tumors grow in the mouse also varied among survey respondents and ranged from 1–2 months to 3–12 months. Time to grow for second-generation (P2 and beyond) tumors was shorter compared with first-generation (P1) tumors. Responses for length of time to grow for tumors brought back from cryopreservation ranged from 1–2 to 4–6 months.

Tumor Characterization

Comparison of the PDX model with the original patient tumor is crucial to assess whether tumor characteristics, such as histology, grade, genetics, epigenetics, gene and protein expression, and post-translational modification, have been retained.[3] Five of seven survey respondents reported checking clonal variability and six of seven reported monitoring changes in the stromal content of tumors. In all cases (seven of seven), histology was used in PDX model validation and immunohistochemistry was used by most respondents (six of seven) for specific protein expression monitoring (Fig. 2.3). Gene expression analysis using gene

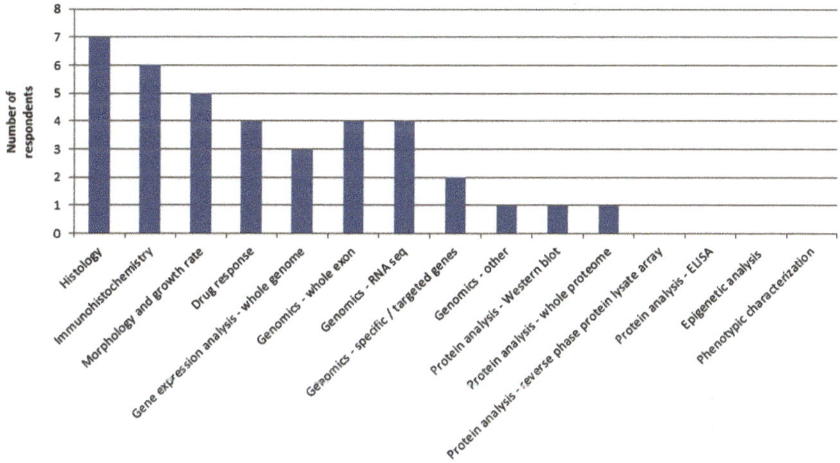

FIGURE 2.3 **Methods used to verify tumor integrity.** Various techniques performed in the characterization of PDX models are presented by frequency of use by survey respondents. *ELISA*, enzyme-linked immunosorbent assay.

array or RNA sequencing, as well as targeted or whole exome sequencing, were used to characterize PDX models by four of seven respondents. Protein analysis using Western blot and proteomics was used infrequently (one respondent each) to characterize models. The most common methods to monitor changes in tumor characteristics were growth rate (five of seven) and histology (five of seven), followed by genomics in two cases, and proteomics in one case. No survey respondent reported using epigenomics in molecular characterization as a routine test but one respondent is testing methylation status occasionally. Results of PDX model validation and molecular characterization were similar to the academic survey, although Western blotting was used more frequently (51%) by academic respondents. In general, industry survey respondents felt that their models were stable throughout the different passages in the mice and reported limited drift in models characteristics.

Patient Data

The use of patient tumors and medical information requires strict practices to protect privacy and to inform patients of their rights and the benefits and risks associated with the program. All survey respondents used patient informed consent to allow research and commercial use. Most survey respondents reported collecting patient data and sharing these data with PDX clients. In addition to patient medical information obtained during the time of tumor implantation, most respondents (six of seven) collected additional patient data, such as response to treatment and disease progression. Four of seven respondents reported that occasionally additional tumor samples from the same individual were collected and implanted upon disease progression to generate another PDX model to look for genetic changes and to compare drug sensitivity.

Among survey respondents, all reported that patient data relating to demographics, molecular profile, and response to therapy were collected. Five of six respondents made an effort to obtain the pathology report. Three of six respondents reported collecting laboratory results, although the survey did not specify what type of laboratory reports were collected. Imaging results were collected in one case. Occasionally, circulating tumor cells, circulating tumor DNA, and other samples, such as peripheral blood mononuclear cell (PBMC) and serum were also collected for some patients.

MODEL DEVELOPMENT, CHALLENGES, AND FUTURE DIRECTIONS

PDX Model Development and Services Offered

Companies create PDX models and expand their tumor banks or individual tumors to offer services for patients and care givers (two of seven respondents), academic centers (four of seven), or pharmaceutical companies (all seven respondents), which each present a set of unique requirements and challenges. In addition to PDX model generation, services provided by these companies include mechanism-of-action studies and biomarker discovery and validation (five of seven). Five of seven respondents reported offering additional services outside of PDX models including generation of primary human cancer cell lines (four of seven) and PDX-derived organoids (four of seven).

Other services identified included pharmacokinetic/pharmacodynamic testing, drug response testing, Avatar services, coclinical trials, and humanized mice.

Appendix 1 lists additional information provided by some companies who responded to an email query sent out separately from the survey.

Avatar Services

Avatar models are "personalized mouse models"[1] created from a patient's tumor developed to guide therapeutic decisions for that individual in the clinic.[7] Avatar models aid interpretation of genomic data and direct empirical therapy, as a strong correlation has been reported between drug activity in the Avatar and clinical outcome in the patients.[9,10] For the purpose of this chapter, we define Avatar models as used in personalized medicine in conjunction with the patient's oncologist for predicting drug response for an individual patient. Avatar services are further discussed in Section V.

Coclinical Trials

Coclinical trials involve the generation of PDX from clinical trial patients during the clinical trial.[1,3,11] The goal is to study questions that cannot be studied in the actual patient to maximize the information gathered in this trial. Coclinical trials are further discussed in Section V.

Development and Use of Humanized Mice

Humanized mice offer the advantage of a more human immune response in the PDX model, as the lack of a human immune response has been a criticism of PDX models, although challenges exist in implanting aspects of a human immune system which still is tolerant of the tumor graft growth.[7,12] Humanized mice, harboring human immune system, were commonly used by survey respondents (five of seven). This differs from the academic survey, in which only three respondents were using a humanized hematopoietic system in mouse model. Examples of proprietary humanized mouse models offered or in development by some commercial providers include PDX-bearing humanized -NSG and PDX-bearing humanized-NSG-SGM3 mice available from Jackson Laboratories for immuno-oncology research; human hematopoietic stem cell engrafted CIEA NOG mouse from Taconic Laboratories suitable for combined immune system and tumor xenograft studies; X-mice from Oncodesign which combines PDX models and liver or immune system humanized mice; and ImmunoGrafts from Champions Oncology which combines the TumorGraft (a type of patient-derived xenograft) and humanized mice (NSG mice reconstituted with human hematopoietic cells).

Program Costs

Many survey respondents (four of seven) estimated the average annual cost to run their PDX program (including salaries, caging and equipment for mouse maintenance, laboratory and surgical equipment, molecular analyses, transportation, and data storage) at >$2,000,000. One survey respondent each indicated the annual cost of their program at <$499,000 and $500–749,000. Two survey respondents preferred not to answer or did not respond to this question. Annual costs for industry providers of PDX services, as expected, was in general much higher than those of academic PDX programs.

Challenges in the Field

The majority (four of seven) of survey respondents felt that most challenges with PDX models are related to the human samples as opposed to the mouse models (one of seven). Five of seven respondents also reported challenges regarding international shipping of samples. We identified three particular areas of challenges: challenges in model creation and tumor bank maintenance and growth, challenges in personalized medicine and serving the patient, and challenges in serving biotech and pharmaceutical companies.

The Role of Collaboration

Survey respondents viewed collaboration with other companies and academic institutions favorably, commenting that consortium efforts and collaborations would be likely to enhance the efficacy of PDX development pipelines, increase the rate of innovation and identification of cancer therapies and biomarkers, and help focus international efforts on the development of rare models for specific, less represented subpopulation of cancers.

Examples include the formation of several local and international PDX consortia, such as Center of Resource for Experimental Models of Cancer and Innovative MODels Initiative (IMODI),[4] two French initiatives discussed further in Section V. Other examples of collaborations include the participation by Champions Oncology Inc. in multiple coclinical drug trials with various academic and pharmaceutical partners and the Primary Human Tumor Consortium formed between Jackson Laboratories and more than 20 cancer centers to create a library of PDX tumors for the global research community.[7]

INTERVIEW WITH COMPANY REPRESENTATIVES REGARDING CHALLENGES AND FUTURE DIRECTIONS IN PDX DEVELOPMENT

Given the limited number of survey respondents and to obtain a more in-depth view regarding challenges and future directions in the PDX industry space, we interviewed two scientists who represent companies that offer a broad range of PDX services for their opinions. This interview was conducted separately from the survey and represents only the opinions of the individuals interviewed. Keren Paz is the former Chief Scientific Officer for Champions Oncology, Inc., in New Jersey, USA. Olivier Duchamp is the Director of Scientific Partnership and Technology Transfer for Oncodesign in Dijon Cedex, France.

Q: What do you see as the major obstacles and challenges in the PDX field in regard to model and tumorbank generation, Avatar service to patients and oncologists, drug development service to biopharma partners, and coclinical trials?

Are there any new directions to overcome these challenges?

Challenges and Future Directions in Model Creation and Tumor Bank

K. Paz: Indeed, while the PDX technology is, undoubtedly, the most reliable preclinical tool available nowadays for oncology research, it doesn't come without challenges.

Building a strong, translationally relevant tumor bank relies on two major factors—well thought-after patient selection and high engraftment rate. Although the most relevant patient population is often a moving target, due, in large, to the evolution and progress in drug discovery, the general notion is that PDX models generated from samples obtained from patients with profiles similar to those enrolled in clinical trials present the greatest value to the oncology research community. Often, therefore, tumors from metastatic lesions of heavily pretreated patients are advantageous compared to those obtained from the primary mass of a treatment-naive patient. These tumor samples, however, are difficult to acquire since patients at this advanced stage are no longer candidates for surgical resection.

The engraftment rate is a result of the quality and quantity of the tissue, the time from surgery to implantation, the aggressiveness of the disease, and the treatment history of the patient. Oftentimes, the most desirable tumors are difficult to collect and engraft. At Champions, an effort is made to strategize tumor selection according to the most up-to-date research requirements. Moreover, in order to minimize technical hurdles, such as time to implantation, a decision was made to employ several implantation centers around the world, with highly trained teams, working around the clock and performing implantations not only from surgeries but also from a small amount of biopsy tissue.

O. Duchamp: PDX are only tools that may help cancer understanding, drug development, and patient treatment. There have been a lot of models that have been developed by the companies with a huge investment during these last 10 years. All companies now have medium to large collections of models, but they all have approximately the same types of models. In term of novel developments, we now have to focus our efforts on the development of underrepresented cancers or subtypes of cancers in PDX collections worldwide. Underrepresentation may be due to technical issues (low tumor take rate or clonal selection in mice, ie, prostate, breast, myeloma), rarity, or tumor sample accessibility. Even though PDX are now considered as "better" at mimicking the human cancer pathologies than the cell line–derived models, there are still many stromal components that are missing in our models to completely mimic the human situation. We need to consider the entirety of the cancer pathology and not only the tumor epithelial cells. Moreover, the diversity of models, the costs of model development, PDX collection maintenance, and quality control of all these collections seems also to be a big challenge in the near future.

To circumvent these disadvantages of PDX models, we at Oncodesign and many other research groups are working on the humanization of the tumor microenvironment including the immune system or the chronic inflammation in specific organs associated with some cancers (liver, colon, lung…) and the development of metastatic models. Metastases are highly frequent in syngeneic models even in ectopic situations, but PDX models are rarely metastatic, suggesting that the tumor microenvironment is an essential actor in the tumor dissemination process. Probably, the stroma humanization will help understanding of tumor dissemination mechanisms and the development of new therapeutic agents.

K. Paz: I agree that an important barrier in PDX development is the immune system. Despite a great advancement in the field of immune oncology, immune compromised mice cannot be used to assess response to these drugs. The development of humanized mouse models represents a tremendous breakthrough in the field. These models encompass both human immune system and human cancer and, therefore, can be used to test immune therapy drugs as single agents and in combination.

Challenges in Personalized Medicine and Serving Patients

K. Paz: The most significant challenge of the Avatar service, whereby a personalized PDX model is generated on behalf of an individual patient, followed by a panel of drug sensitivity tests, to help guide patient care, is the turnaround time. The interval between tumor implantation and reporting of test results can be as short as three months, in some rare cases, but more frequently between six and nine months.

While an effort is made to shorten the process without compromising the integrity and fidelity of the tumor, it is imperative to engage in an open and honest communication with oncologists, patients, and families to evaluate, in advance, the potential utility and benefit of the service given the specific disease status and time restrictions.

Challenges in Serving Pharmaceutical Companies

O. Duchamp: The usefulness of PDX models for better selecting efficacious new drugs is still not clearly demonstrated. It's a complex question. Today, PDX models are not the best models for the pharmacological evaluation of drugs targeting the tumor environment. For immune oncology drugs, we use syngeneic mice models, but we have known for several decades that the murine immune system is not identical to the human one. In the same way, metastatic PDX models are very rare, and consequently, it is difficult to evaluate the effectiveness of a drug on the tumor metastatic dissemination.

For pharmaceutical companies, it is like a nightmare to find the right PDX models that could answer their questions: does the model exist? Where? In which conditions? The only way to address this challenge is the initiation of an international database that may be linked to an international biobank.

Moreover, PDX models are valuable for in vivo proof of concept with lead compounds, but not really useful for drug screening and hit selection. To address this limitation, we may develop in vitro/ex vivo assays (primoculture, tumorspheres, organoids) based on biological samples coming from PDX models in order to increase the chance of selecting compounds that will be rapidly active in in vivo PDX models.

K. Paz: The spectrum of PDX testing for biopharmaceutical companies is enormous and includes efficacy assessment, mechanism of action studies, pharmacokinetics evaluation, and biomarker discovery. These experiments can be conducted using PDX models derived from a tumor bank or as part of coclinical program, whereby PDX models are generated on behalf of pharma partners, using their clinical trial patient samples.

Aside for the obvious challenges of engraftment rate and model availability, a major debate in the field is around precision and reproducibility. Due to the in vivo nature of the PDX technology, the unique cross talk between the different components of the tumor and its simulation of human cancer, heterogeneity, clonal variation, microenvironment shift, and minor molecular drifts may exist. These phenomena are, in fact, the essence of the platform that maintains and underlines the biological properties of the disease in the most authentic manner.

Challenges in Coclinical Trials

O. Duchamp: Coclinical trial is a new paradigm that has been introduced recently. For me it's not entirely clear how they are to be uniformly successfully implemented given the technical limitations we are facing. For example, while coclinical trials should be of value for tumor types with known in vivo take rates >80%, how can we decide to adapt or optimize the treatment strategy in patients based on PDX model outcomes knowing that for some cancers we will have a tumor engraftment rate <25% or patients for whom the tumor does not grow in mice? In addition, for many clinical trials, surgery or biopsies are not planned or not possible in the targeted patient populations, or tumor material not available for in vivo xenograft. Further, the pharmacokinetics and the metabolism of drugs should be different in mice and in patients. In this case, liver-humanized mice bearing PDX may represent a solution. Finally, there are questions about how to manage the drug combinations in PDX models and which doses of each drug to use.

Q: What do you foresee for the future of PDX services as regards collaboration between academia and industry?

K. Paz: Multiple collaborations with companies, hospitals, and academic centers allow the collection of the most relevant tumor samples in order to build a robust bank.

O. Duchamp: As PDX models are now considered common tools for both academic and industrial research, cooperation with all the end users seems the only way to correctly orient, create, characterize, and qualify the PDX models. Some national or international consortia have been initiated during these past 4 years in this way. At Oncodesign, we have initiated the IMODI program. This national consortium offers an opportunity to increase the rate of innovation and identification of cancer therapies and biomarkers, with the creation of an organized structure designed for the development of personalized medicine which directly benefits patients. From an industrial point of view, the main advantages of integrating the IMODI consortium are: the selection and anticipation of cancer pathologies of interest based upon clinical and pharmaceutical industry needs; standardization of ethical, quality control, and technical processes in regard to industrial requirements; a centralized biobank and database; the freedom of use of all the results for internal research by each partner; an organized IP management; payment of royalties based on the commercialization of models and results by all the small and medium enterprises; and the reduction of individual costs annually dedicated to the development and characterization of models.

SUMMARY AND CONCLUDING COMMENTS

In contrast to academic programs, most commercial providers of PDX services have large annual budgets allocated to their PDX programs and maintain a large and varied inventory of tumor models. Some commercial providers are performing only PDXs, whereas others offer a range of services. In general, results did not appear to differ dramatically by the predominant geographic area served. Industry providers of PDX services have identified several challenges in the field, but through areas, such as humanized mouse development, refinements in avatar services and coclinical trials, and the development of consortia and collaborative efforts are seeking to address these challenges and advance the field.

APPENDIX 1. ADDITIONAL INFORMATION ON SOME COMPANIES PROVIDING AND SUPPORTING PDX MODEL DEVELOPMENT

Information for this table was obtained from commercial providers who responded to an email query, distinct from the survey, which requested a brief description of current services offered. This table is not comprehensive, as not all companies responded to the query, and information is presented as provided by the company. For more information on services offered by commercial providers of PDX services, a list of company contact information including website addresses is included in Section IV, Chapter 1, Table 2.1.

Company	Services
Champions Oncology, Hackensack, NJ, and Baltimore, MD, USA	• Over 500 established PDX models (Champions TumorGraft) and ~1000 models under development; subcutaneous and orthotopic engraftments • Extensive clinical, molecular, and growth profiling • Avatar services to guide patients' care • Efficacy drug sensitivity, mechanism of action, pharmacokinetics, dose finding, and safety studies • Immunotherapy studies with humanized mice (ImmunoGraft) • Coclinical studies with pharmaceutical partners and academic cancer centers
Horizon/SAGE Laboratories, Cambridge, UK, England, and St. Louis, MO, USA	• Comprehensive collection of published breast cancer PDX models (Li et al., 2013), including 8 ER+, 2 HER2+, and 12 triple-negative breast cancer models • Highly characterized PDX models with genetic fidelity confirmed by WGS of originating tumor, early and late passages • Comprehensive patient history, WGS, RNA Seq, and estradiol responsiveness available • In vivo efficacy studies available at our St. Louis facility; models also available to license in your own facility

Company	Services
The Jackson Laboratory, Sacramento, CA, USA	• Therapeutic development, drug response evaluation of multiple drugs alone or in combination • Preclinical efficacy testing of immuno-oncology compounds using platforms humanized with both PDX and human immune systems • Access to over 400 early-passage PDX models with a spectrum of relevant mutations and detailed characterization data including genomics (RNA Seq, gene expression, and SNPs), SOC, tumor growth data, histological data, and pathology images • PDX live tumor engrafted NSG mice ready for preclinical enrollment
Oncodesign, Dijon Cedex, France	• PDX products and services • Pharmacological drug evaluation (PK/PD, efficacy, combination, resistance, mechanism of action) • Preclinical phase 2 studies • Drug and biomarker discovery
Shanghai LIDE Biotech Co, Ltd, Shanghai, China	• PDX and CDX model establishment • In vivo efficacy study with PDX models and CDX models • Tumor sensitivity assay • Human immuno-oncology model establishment • Biomarker analysis • Circulating tumor cell detecting
Taconic, Hudson, NY, USA	• Human hematopoietic stem cell-engrafted CIEA NOG mouse suitable for combined immune system and tumor xenograft studies • Human PBMC-engrafted CIEA NOG mouse models for immuno-oncology research • Human GM-CSF and IL-3 transgenic NOG mice for AML engraftment and extended lineage reconstitution upon hematopoietic stem cell engraftment
Urolead, Strasbourg, France	• Collection of 60 PDX models in the oncourological sphere: kidney, bladder, and prostate cancers • Histological, molecular, and genetic characterizations • Access to clinical and pathological status of patient • Preclinical platform for drug efficacy studies • Repository of tumors, protein lysates, DNA/RNA extracts
Xenopat, L'Hospitalet de Llobregat, Barcelona, Spain	• Patient-derived orthotopic xenograft models (orthoxenografts) characterized by a high degree of histologic, genetic, epigenetic, and drug response correlation with the original (primary or metastatic) tumor • Orthoxenobank including ovarian, colorectal, testicular, lung, endometrial, breast, pancreatic, pediatric, and rare tumors, among others, for drug development • Personalized oncologic treatment guidance in real time. Generation of PDOX from primary and metastatic tumors including biopsy-obtained samples
XenTech, Paris, France	• Large collection of over 40 breast cancer PDX models • More than 140 PDX models of adult and pediatric solid tumors • In vivo drug efficacy testing and biomarker discovery services • Comprehensive molecular and drug response database

AML, acute myeloid leukemia; *CDX*, cell line-derived xenograft models; *GM-CSF*, granulocyte macrophage colony stimulating factor; *IL-3*, interleukin 3; *PD*, pharmacodynamic; *PDX*, patient-derived tumor xenograft; *PDOX*, patient-derived orthotopic xenografts; *PK*, pharmacokinetic; *SOC*, standard of care; *SNP*, single nucleotide polymorphism; *WGS*, whole genome sequencing.

REFERENCES

1. Malaney P, Nicosia SV, Dave V. One mouse, one patient paradigm: new avatars of personalized cancer therapy. *Cancer Lett* 2014;**344**(1):1–12.
2. Zhang X, Claerhout S, Prat A, Dobrolecki LE, Petrovic I, Lai Q, et al. A renewable tissue resource of phenotypically stable, biologically and ethnically diverse, patient-derived human breast cancer xenograft models. *Cancer Res* 2013;**73**(15):4885–97.
3. Hidalgo M, Amant F, Biankin AV, Budinska E, Byrne AT, Caldas C, et al. Patient-derived xenograft models: an emerging platform for translational cancer research. *Cancer Discov* 2014;**4**(9):998–1013.
4. Siolas D, Hannon GJ. Patient-derived tumor xenografts: transforming clinical samples into mouse models. *Cancer Res* 2013;**73**(17):5315–9.
5. Anderson WC, Boyd MB, Aguilar J, Pickell B, Laysang A, Pysz MA, et al. Initiation and characterization of small cell lung cancer patient-derived xenografts from ultrasound-guided transbronchial needle aspirates. *PLoS One* 2015;**10**(5):e0125255.
6. Lin D, Wyatt AW, Xue H, Wang Y, Dong X, Haegert A, et al. High fidelity patient-derived xenografts for accelerating prostate cancer discovery and drug development. *Cancer Res* 2014;**74**(4):1272–83.
7. Shultz LD, Goodwin N, Ishikawa F, Hosur V, Lyons BL, Greiner DL. Human cancer growth and therapy in immunodeficient mouse models. *Cold Spring Harb Protoc* 2014;**7**:694–708.
8. Dong X, Guan J, English JC, Flint J, Yee J, Evans K, et al. Patient-derived first generation xenografts of non-small cell lung cancers: promising tools for predicting drug responses for personalized chemotherapy. *Clin Cancer Res* 2010;**16**(5):1442–51.
9. Garralda E, Paz K, Lopez-Casas PP, Jones S, Katz A, Kann LM, et al. Integrated next-generation sequencing and avatar mouse models for personalized cancer treatment. *Clin Cancer Res* 2014;**20**(9):2476–84.
10. Hidalgo M, Bruckheimer E, Rajeshkumar NV, Garrido-Laguna I, De Oliveira E, Rubio-Viqueira B, et al. A pilot clinical study of treatment guided by personalized tumorgrafts in patients with advanced cancer. *Mol Cancer Ther* 2011;**10**(8):1311–6.
11. Nardella C, Lunardi A, Patnaik A, Cantley LC, Pandolfi PP. The APL paradigm and the "co-clinical trial" project. *Cancer Discov* 2011;**1**(2):108–16.
12. Cassidy JW, Caldas C, Bruna A. Maintaining tumor heterogeneity in patient-derived tumor xenografts. *Cancer Res* 2015;**75**(15):2963–8.

Section V

Challenges & Future of PDX Models

Chapter 1

Patient-Derived Tumor Xenograft: Present and Future Challenges and Applications

G. Inghirami[1,2,3], P.T. Tinkey[4], E. de Stanchina[5], R.K. Uthamanthil[6]
[1]Weill Cornell Medical College, New York, NY, United States; [2]University of Torino, Torino, Italy; [3]New York University School of Medicine, New York, NY, United States; [4]The University of Texas MD Anderson Cancer Center, Houston, TX, United States; [5]Memorial Sloan Kettering Cancer Center, New York, NY, United States; [6]Fred Hutchinson Cancer Research Center, Seattle, WA, United States

INTRODUCTION

In the February 2016 issue of *Nature* magazine, Heidi Ledford discussed the decision of the National Cancer Institute (NCI) to launch a rejuvenated repository of clinically annotated cancer models, derived from primary patient samples.[1] Once this program reaches full maturity, patient-derived xenograft (PDX) models will replace the NCI-60 human cancer cell line panel from NCI drug screening programs. It is anticipated that the NCI will distribute cells or PDXs with genomic and clinical data, corresponding to defined human cancers and selected subsets. The program includes the generation of PDX-derived cell lines that can be used for biochemical studies and drug screening experiments as well as companion intratumoral fibroblast cell lines. These are expected to be instrumental in understanding how the host contributes to tumor development and growth and mechanisms involved in sustaining resistant phenotypes. The NCI estimates that ultimately a total of 1000 models will be generated.

This decision was reached as a response to widespread demand for better cancer models which more reproducibly and accurately recapitulate human cancers. In the past 25 years, industries and academic centers have screened more than 100,000 compounds. However, only 1 in 10,000 reaches the clinical arena and is ultimately commercialized. There is a general agreement that, although many issues contribute to the current inefficient drug discovery pipelines, deficiencies in in vivo models add substantially to the low rate of success. As James Doroshow, Director of the Division of Cancer Treatment and Diagnosis at the

Patient Derived Tumor Xenograft Models. http://dx.doi.org/10.1016/B978-0-12-804010-2.00027-8

NCI in Bethesda, Maryland states, "thirty years ago, the idea was that if you found a drug that worked on six breast cancer cell lines, then you could use it to treat breast cancer; well, it doesn't work that way."

The NCI's initiative is in line with the objectives of many other analogous programs. In Europe, 17 institutions have created a multiinstitutional network, known as EurOPDX, a consortium that currently holds over 1500 PDXs. Similarly, academic centers in the United States, Canada, and China and private laboratories including the Jackson Laboratory, Champions Oncology, and others have developed a very large array of PDXs. Finally, pharmaceutical companies have stepped into the arena with Novartis, a Swiss pharma giant, leading the way with the generation of 1000 PDXs.

Although PDX models are expected to substantially broaden the way in vivo studies are designed and executed and they are anticipated to reshape drug discovery programs, many issues are emerging and new hurdles need to be solved. In this chapter, we will briefly discuss some of them and discuss future avenues, new applications, and possible solutions to the most pressing questions.

TECHNICAL IMPROVEMENTS

Tumor Type Representation

It is well established that the rate of successful implantation is linked to multifactorial events, and to the unique properties of individual specimens. The nature of tumor cells is one factor that has been proven to influence PDX engraftment rates. For instance, fully transformed lesions and metastatic processes can readily engraft,[2–4] whereas low-grade lesions have a limited rate of success and/or require special conditions.[5] Among primary lesions, colon,[2] head and neck,[6] squamous lung cancers,[7] and hepatocellular[8] carcinomas are easily implantable. By contrast, primary and even metastatic prostate cancers are difficult to establish even in highly immunocompromised mice,[9–11] although some success has been obtained recently using circulating tumor cells.[12] This has led to an imbalanced portfolio of PDX models worldwide. While many models have been developed, the repertoires of most organizations include the same types of tumors and are instead lacking in rare and harder to engraft cancers. A worldwide coordinated effort is required to identify and prioritize development of PDX biobanks so that a complete bank of rare and underrepresented tumors can be established. For tumor models that do exist, often only one stage of the tumor is represented. A further refinement will be to continue to build well-annotated banks that include PDX models from all stages of cancer progression, from early, treatment-naive stages to metastatic and relapsed and/or chemorefractory cancers.

Sample Collection and Processing Methods

One of the major limitations in PDX development is connected to the source, collection, and processing of the neoplastic samples. With rare exception[13] the currently available PDXs were generated using surgically resected samples, cell suspensions from pleural and peritoneal fluid, and, in the case of hematopoeitic disorders, from blood and/or bone marrow aspirates. However, it is desirable to extend the PDX preparations to scenarios that utilize less invasive surgical approaches, such as fine-needle aspirates and core biopsies.[13–15] The use of these minimally invasive procedures would allow for collections of multiple samples from the same patient along disease progression. This way, well-annotated PDX models, representing different stages of disease progression, could be established from the same patient (ie, from naive, resistant, and metastatic tumor sites). Finally, successful implants have recently been established using circulating tumor cells, a strategy that also allows the generation of models at different time points.[16]

Timely tissue transfer and processing also represents a major technical challenge, as it has been demonstrated that prolonged tissue ischemia time impairs engraftment.[7] These hurdles can be overcome to an extent by establishing a multiprofessional team devoted to specific tasks within the program, and by implementing standard operating procedures for all steps. However, many limitations still remain: for example, collection of postmortem samples through rapid autopsy programs, which can be a valuable source of tumor material, are often performed several hours after the patient's death, despite the best team efforts to coordinate prompt sample collection.

Biobanking

The process of cryopreservation of PDX samples could also be refined, to improve their long-term viability. In fact, it is known that different types of tissues react differently to cooling, and both the cryoprotectant and cooling rate required for proper preservation vary widely depending on the origin of the tissue.[17] In addition, it has been observed that, depending upon the technique used for cryopreservation, the antigenicity of the preserved tissue varies significantly.[18,19] This can potentially have implications in tumor immunotherapy studies using cryopreserved PDX samples. In addition, cryopreservation techniques lead to reduced viability of cells[20] and the potential for selection of tumor cells based on cold tolerance is possible. Many large PDX programs use standard tissue-freezing techniques that can lead to intracellular ice crystal formation and cell death. While the use of dimethylsulfoxide (DMSO) and other cryoprotectants reduces this damage, the use of programmed/controlled rate freezing techniques might further improve preservation of tumor characteristics. As discussed in the Global Surveys presented in Section IV, better utilization of existing biobanks [and use of commonly accepted standard operating procedures (SOPs)] will be beneficial.

Sample Implantation

Implantation techniques also play a major role in establishing and standardizing the use of PDX models. Although preservation of tumor heterogeneity in

PDX models is a big advantage, it can also be a hindrance in conducting studies using early-passage PDX models. Various tumor chunks from the same tumor/patient can show different growth rate characteristics[21] and sometime lead to the expansion of different populations (personal communications) in mice. In addition to the difficulties in getting enough numbers of homogeneous tumors for experiments, this also opens up the possibility of different tumors forming from spatially separated genetically different subclones. It is possible that mincing the tumor tissue and injecting a mixture (or a cell suspension) might better represent tumor heterogeneity across all mice instead of implanting chunks from various areas of the tumor. This, however, will lead to the disruption of the tumorigenic niches and thus more investigation needs to be done in this area to determine what process may be preferable for different tumor types.

In fact, different implantation techniques may be employed to increase the take rate in different tumor types. For example, implanting breast cancer samples in the mammary fat pad provides a more faithful microenvironment.[22–24] Moreover, implantation into the inguinal fat pads seems to be correlated to higher take rates than implantation into the thoracic pads, implying the relevance of local tissue microenvironment.[25] More recently, intraductal (into the milk ducts) injection of breast cancer tissue has been shown to yield invasive carcinomas.[26] Implantation of tumor samples under the kidney capsule and/or within the kidneys, although technically more challenging, seems also to provide some advantages, potentially owing to the highly vascular nature of the kidney tissue.[27] Development of better implantation techniques that are unique to specific tumor types may further advance the utility of these models. While progress is being made on different fronts, it is important that appropriate implantation routes and conditional settings (ie, hormonal therapies, lymphokine administration, coimplant of protumorigenic factors) be defined for each individual type of cancer.

It must also be noted that, due to differences in basic husbandry programs between institutions, a multitude of environmental variables can have different impacts on tumor implantation. Variations in the content of diet, water quality, microbial flora, environment temperatures, and enrichment programs may cause differences in tumor take and growth rate between institutions. This highlights the need to develop rigorous, consistent standards for use in global PDX programs.

Variable success in establishing PDXs may be explained with the emerging notion that the relationship between tumors, and the host is highly dynamic, requires the presence of multifunctional elements, and changes over time. The end product is a unique liaison, in which both compartments have bilaterally educated each others and they are ultimately dependent on one another.[28] Thus the inappropriate mix of elements, and/or of cells not properly preconditioned, even when orthotropic routes of implantations are used, may result in failures. Overall, these considerations justify more rigorous studies in which the features of both tumor and host elements are precisely defined.

Clinical Application

Prolonged intervals for the generation and propagation of PDX is a major limitation of these models. Typically, long periods are required for tumors to grow, frequently exceeding 6–7 months,[29] whereas only a minority grows within a few weeks of implantation. Thus, PDX can seldom be used to guide the therapeutic decision of the donor patients, and even when information from the model becomes available, patients will have meanwhile undergone multiple rounds of therapies and/or have developed chemorefractory diseases. In these settings, the patient-specific relevance of information that can be drawn by the PDX generated from the original lesions remains questionable. Exceptions do exist; for example, very informative models established from bladder cancers can effectively guide therapeutic decision in patients with a recurrence after many months after surgery.[30] In addition, the development of in vitro or ex vivo systems derived from PDX models could supplement the need for faster feedback to the patient. At the same time we believe that efforts should be made to accelerate the mouse model development.

It is now evident that we need to establish very large libraries of cancer-specific PDXs, with the broadest cancer representation within individual cancer types. These libraries must include detailed clinical and molecular annotation and the construction of molecular classifiers capable of stratifying individual entities in multiple and parceled subsets. In parallel, these cohorts should be challenged with a variety of drugs to define the most successful combination for each individual subset.[31] This may be achieved by using innovative trial strategies currently being tested to improve cancer drug discovery and treatment (http://www.cancer.gov/about-cancer/treatment/clinical-trials/nci-supported/nci-match). If these all-inclusive objectives are reached, it will be possible to match any naive cancer patient to a specific group of PDXs and thus predict the best and most likely to succeed treatment option for any specific case. This is a monumental task, which requires the coordinated efforts of all available PDX networks as well as dedicated support of the pharmaceutical industry and an enormous financial patronage.

PDX MOLECULAR CHARACTERIZATION

Sample Annotation

It is reasonable to speculate that more than 5000 different PDXs have been established so far; however, the usefulness of these models varies according to their level of characterization. As gathered from the surveys in this book (Section IV), there is no universal standard for the minimum annotation that should be performed for PDX models. While a majority of programs both in academia and industry perform histology and immunohistochemistry to confirm that their PDX models correlate with the corresponding patient tumor, in many cases annotations are limited to those analyses. Less commonly, gene expression and copy number variation analyses have been executed. Limited information is generally available on whole exon and/or genomic profiling. Data on epigenetic fingerprints have been rarely described. Although difficult, we strongly believe that comprehensive molecular characterization (ie, next generation sequencing (NGS), whole exome sequencing (WES), total RNA, methylation and proteomic/metabolomics profile) for each PDX should become mandatory. This information is essential for the comparison of the patient tumor to the matched PDX and to appropriately interpret the biological features and responses of the PDX to drugs. This will require an enormous financial effort, a meticulous and highly efficient organization, and the creation of dedicated databases capable of integrating the findings from the PDX with the corresponding clinical patient information. This emphasizes the need to develop centralized, collaborative working groups that can set standards, enforce protocols, pool resources, and streamline the sharing of data and models between contributing members.

Clonal Selection

Although there is a general consensus that the majority of PDXs closely mimic their corresponding donor samples and shows responses similar to those seen in patients, the data regarding the precise genomic and epigenetic correspondence of primary tumors and PDX are largely lacking. In fact, it is not a common practice to collect and then analyze the germline DNA with the DNA of the tumor and the first derived PDX. It is even more rare that genomic data is derived from serial passages or on multiple PDXs obtained from the same donor implanted in multiple mice. Without these data, it is virtually impossible to define the real correspondence between the PDX and patient tumor. In the case of acute lymphoblastic leukemias, it has been shown that selected clones have the highest probability of engraftment success. These frequently correspond to minor populations that can eventually emerge after chemotherapy in humans.[32] This is a phenomenon seen in several other contexts, where more aggressive clones emerge during serial passages.[33] This is an interesting occurrence that suggests that PDXs may predict the clonal evolution and tumor progression that naturally occurs in humans, but in a shorter period. Eirew and colleagues[34] have shown that by using deep-genome and single-cell sequencing methods in breast cancer models, clonal selection after engraftment can be observed in both primary and metastatic breast tumors. In their study, they observed that there was a considerable range varying from extreme selective engraftment of minor clones (<5%) to moderate polyclonal expansions. Of note, ongoing clonal dynamics along multiple passages was observed in tumors which had displayed an initial modest selection. The authors were also able to demonstrate that major mutation clusters related predictably to the most abundant clonal genotypes and that similar clonal expansion patterns emerged in independent grafts derived from the same starting lesion. Collectively, these data suggest that, in a constant mouse environment, selected clones bearing distinct genomic aberrations can determine the tumor evolutionary trajectories, consistent with a clonal selection process. This and other studies clearly demonstrate that more precise molecular fingerprints are required to evaluate PDX and that there is need not only to determine their spontaneous evolution but also to assess the changes that occur after treatment. This will provide a new avenue for the utilization of these models, which could allow us to foresee and/or anticipate in coclinical trials the evolution that can occur in humans.

Protumorigenic Signatures

Genomic analysis can provide relevant data on the protumorigenic signals provided by the host[35,36] allowing the stratification of primary neoplasms among histologically indistinguishable primary patient samples with similar genetic alterations.[37] Indeed, recent data have demonstrated that the bioinformatic deconvolution of mouse host and human cancers permits the generation of signatures, which are highly informative of the operational circuitries in the cancer environments, that then can robustly predict disease relapses.[35,36] It must now be established whether the mouse compartment of PDX models can faithfully recapitulate the microenvironment properties of different types of tumors and early-stage lesions. In fact, several studies have demonstrated that the profiles of PDXs closely resemble those seen in metastatic settings and relapsed patients.[22,23,38–40] These phenotypes are shared by tumors implanted orthotopically or subcutaneously and maintained over multiple passages.[22] At this point, it is unclear whether this correspondence is due to the fact that many PDXs were generated from end-stage diseases or whether the mouse can only support and provide a unique protumorigenic environment. Thus, these questions will only be answered by studying PDXs derived from many different types of cancers (solid vs liquid) and from early or premalignant lesions [myelodysplastic syndromes (MDS) vs acute myeloid leukemia (AML), Barrett esophagus vs carcinomas, hepatomas vs hepatocarcinomas, etc.].

INNOVATIVE PDX DERIVATIVE MODELS

Since the global signatures of primary tumor and PDX is largely influenced by the contribution of the host elements, it may be feasible to establish transcription classifiers, derived from the tumor and the host cells,[35,36] capable of predicting clinical responses.[40] This is epitomized by the study of Daniel et al.[41] who compared the profiles of small cell lung cancer PDXs with their derived cell lines. In this investigation, the authors demonstrated that the cell lines derived from the PDXs substantially diverged from the donor samples and their transcriptomic signatures could not be reestablished once they were regrown in vivo. This result suggests that "never in culture" PDX more closely recapitulate cancer patients, potentially because of less clonal evolution and maintenance of the tumor microenvironment.[41]

Nonetheless, there is still a great demand to establish in vitro models from PDX, with the hope to use them for drug and genomic discovery programs. These programs are currently ongoing in many academic institutions and are sponsored by the NCI, which is actively working to establish pairs of PDX and correspondent cell lines. As a result of these efforts, we have learned that there are major limitations in the generation of stable lines from many PDXs. However, the use of special media and/or coculture with stromal, endothelial, and other types of supporting cells has provided new and successful avenues.[42] Conditionally reprogrammed cell culture (CRC) strategies can be used to selectively expand epidermal cells and cultures containing irradiated feeder cells and Rho-associated protein kinase inhibitors favoring the preferential proliferation of tumor epithelial elements.[43] In 2014, Crystal et al. established multiple lines from primary samples and used them to identify novel combinatorial therapeutic panels for resistant non–small cell lung cancers.[44] Thus, it is conceivable that analogous modalities may be used to take advantage of established PDXs. This is a very active line of investigation with private companies establishing PDX-derived 2D and three-dimensional (3D) models (http://www.oncotest.com/oncotest-cell-lines.html). In parallel, academic institutions have established cell line "factories" to create public collections of genomically characterized disease models of every major cancer type. The objective is to determine best practices to ensure open, unfettered access to the new models for the scientific community (http://www.broadinstitute.org/cellfactory). Initial attempts were mainly performed using fresh primary cancer samples, but the same strategy has now been adopted using PDX-derived material (Weinstock D., Personal communication).

Although these new strategies are very promising, it remains unclear whether these PDX-derived lines are subject to the same selection that occurred in the generation of currently available cell lines. Indeed, it is unclear whether clones than can emerge in CRCs, leading to expansion of highly homogeneous lines, do not represent the richer heterogeneity of the PDX tumors. Several lines of investigation now suggest that these concerns can be lessened by establishing 3D organoid cultures, in which PDX cells are grown in matrixes supplemented with feeder/nursing cells. Highly annotated and characterized human organoids provide a new and powerful tool to overcome some of the insurmountable obstacles faced with handling of primary lesions.[45] Organoids more closely mimic the biological characteristics of tumors[46,47] and allow for the utilization of toxicological and pharmacological programs and genomic remodeling.[48] The ability to use organoids might be critical in the case of rare and underrepresented neoplasms, for which there are no available models.

Alternative methods include the in vitro growth of mechanically dissociated PDX tumors. These tumor spheres can remain alive for many days/weeks and can be propagated in culture after gentle mechanical manipulation or short enzymatic digestion.[49] Tumor spheres are easily generated using advanced cancers and can re-create well-differentiated neoplasms.[50] In the case of prostate-derived lesions, they faithfully maintain the phenotype of the original tumor (endocrine) and can be propagated in NSG mice (Puca L., personal communication).

Mechanical and or fluorescent-based approaches have been used to select unique populations to favor implantation of cancer cells or can help show distant colonization. Liu and colleagues have demonstrated that the selection of CD44-enriched breast cancer stem cells facilitates the orthotopic engraftment of breast cancer cells and the spontaneous development of metastases.[51] Tumor growth and distant colonization can be determined using reporter markers, ie, luciferase, introduced into the tumor cells using retro,[52] lenti,[53,54] or adenoviral[55] preparations. Nevertheless, the percentage of efficient transduction varies considerably from <1% to 99%,[56] depending on the reported cassette (luciferase, NGFR, cherry, etc.), tumor type, proliferative tumor rates, etc. To improve transduction and to select the desired cell population, Picco et al. have recently used a system that takes advantage of the different sensitivities of mouse and tumor cells to diphtheria toxin (DT). Direct injecting of a green fluorescent protein-diphtheria toxin receptor (GFP-DTR) lentiviral vector into patient-derived tumorgrafts followed by systemic DT administration allowed efficient selection of human cells transduced with microRNA sequences engineered to downregulate the ubiquitous DPH2 gene, a key enzyme for the biosynthesis of the DT target diphthamide.[57] Luciferase-based modalities are quite inexpensive, easily applicable, and high throughput; however, they remain relatively insensitive and do not provide information on dynamic tumor growth patterns, rapid drug responses, and metabolic activity.

Finally, a detailed characterization of dynamic tumor growth patterns, rapid drug responses, and metabolic activity are as important as the molecular characterization of the tumor. To this end, small animal imaging techniques, including computed tomography, magnetic resonance imaging (MRI), and positron emission tomography, may need to be employed for a more detailed characterization of PDX models.[58,59] These modalities can be instrumental to define new and rapid biomarkers of clinical responses.[60] In addition, in search of sensitive biomarkers, we and others have recently tested sensitive protocols using small amounts of plasma, taking advantage of deep sequencing platforms using liquid biopsy protocols. These strategies precisely define tumor burden and give relevant data on response to therapies, having demonstrated that they are more sensitive compared with conventional MRI and luciferase-based tests and can be used to promptly guide therapeutic interventions and to rapidly define clonal selection and the possible occurrence of resistant phenotypes. As for human clinical trials, this approach will eventually allow the implementation of personalized programs in oncology.[61]

THE HOST (MOUSE) ASPECT OF PDX MODELS

There are multiple pressing questions related to the role of the host (mouse) in the establishment of PDX models, for example, what are the host limitations that lead to different take rates between various neoplasms? How can we accelerate the growth of tumors in the mouse (growth rate) so that patients are directly benefited by the use of PDX models in coclinical trials? While humanized mice models provide a platform to study tumor–immune interactions, how can we avoid graft-versus-host disease (GVHD) and related complications, therefore enabling longer studies? How does the host environment affect the tumor characteristics while growing in the mouse? What are the other confounding variables that can be introduced by the mouse model?

Many laboratories are currently addressing these questions and a few answers have recently emerged. More importantly, it is now recognized that these issues are highly relevant and that only through a real collaborative effort we will be eventually able to successfully solve them.

Engraftment Efficiency

It is well known that tumor take rates may differ depending upon the strain used for implantation (nude/SCID/NSG). Can the current limitations in establishing some type of tumors result from the limitations of the available mouse strains? Even the most successful groups have difficulty establishing PDXs from some cancer types, for example, some breast cancers or lymphomas (~30% engraftment rate), when compared with melanoma and squamous epithelial cancers (50–75% engraftment rate). Even then, it is unclear why only a fraction of these highly implantable cases can be propagated. In 2015, Stewart and colleagues showed that only 6 of 33 lung adenocarcinoma–bearing epidermal growth factor receptor (EGFR) mutations could be implanted. They further demonstrated that engrafting and nonengrafting patients had a differentially expressed gene set, which could be used to identify patients harboring EGFR-mutant tumor with significantly different prognoses. Finally, the PDXs established from these patients included models with variable sensitivity to first- and second-generation EGFR tyrosine kinase inhibitors (TKIs) and the monoclonal antibody cetuximab.[40] These data suggest that it may be possible to construct gene expression classifiers, which can predict implantation efficiency of specific tumor types, clearly underlying that certain neoplasms require well-defined conditions for in vivo growth, which are not provided by the current mouse strains.

Engineered Mouse Strains

To overcome some of the technical limitations, encouraging results have been obtained using engineered mouse strains, as in PDX of acute myeloid leukemias,[62] or the use of NOD/SCID-B2 or NSG mice in the case of the myelodysplastic syndrome,β[63,64] suggesting that improved host–tumor interactions and the profound impairment of the natural immunity play a critical role, at least in some models.[65] In line with this hypothesis, orthotropic implantation (also called patient-derived orthotopic tumor xenograft[66]) along with coimplantation of human immune cells[67] or stromal components[68,69] has been proved to facilitate tumor engraftments and to maintain stable phenotypes,[70] although exceptions have been described.[65] All these functionally diversified mouse elements can interact with human cells via pair ligand/receptor interactions and by secreting lymphokines and growth factors that can influence tumor cell behavior in a paracrine or juxtacrine fashion.

The Role of the Immune System

One of the major limitations of current PDX models is the absence of a competent immune system, which can be paired with the native stromal elements. Fully humanized mice may represent a viable solution and they should increase our chance of success. These models have a relatively robust lymphoid representation as well as partial reconstitution of human mesenchymal elements. Types of humanized mice available for PDX research, their advantages, and their limitations are described in detail in Section I, Chapter 6. As indicated above, the stromal microenvironment appears to play a critical role; but clear understanding of those protumorigenic properties is still largely elusive. Nevertheless, the relationship between stromal and cancer cells is now documented and has been proved to be remarkably stable. This has been recognized using transgenic nude mice expressing fluorescent proteins, which have shown that stromal cells can be expanded and propagated for several passages prior to their replacement by an incoming population of new colonizing cells.[71] We recently demonstrated using WES and RNAseq that in PDX lymphomas the ratio of mouse host elements to neoplastic cells is not random, but unique to each individual line and remains stable along serial passages. These data strongly suggest that the tumor cells of each individual PDX requires a unique support and this favors the emergence of selected phenotypes.

Novel methods are being developed to circumvent the limitations of humanized mice. GVHD is a significant limitation of humanized mouse models, substantially limiting prolonged observations; use of major histocompatibility complex (MHC) I and II or B2 knockout recipient mice may improve the application of peripheral blood mononuclear cell-reconstituted cancer models. Improved T-cell responses have been recently seen in human leukocyte antigen transgenic mice[72] and decreased GVHD reaction in B2-/MHC I-deficient NSG mice.[73] More recently, the concept of "immuno-avatars"—where a patient's immune system is reconstituted in the mouse with tumor from the same patient—are being developed. Toward this end, Morton and colleagues have taken advantage of reconstituted mice and studied the growth of patient-matched PDX of head and neck cancers.[74] They first demonstrated that human mesenchymal cells and B and T cells could home within the tumors and proved that XActMice display a transcriptome more closely resembling that of primary lesions compared with nonreconstituted NSG mice. Interestingly, XActMice also displayed increased intratumoral lymphatic vessel density, suggesting a partial but complex reconstitution of not only the lymphoid compartment but also the different elements of mesenchymal origin.[74] Thus, these chimera models represent a powerful tool for more precise studying the relationship between the tumor and host, which will allow testing of new immunomodulators (ie, anti-PD1, anti–CTLA-4) and biologicals (bifunctional antibodies). Moreover, they are powerful tools to study the effects of radiation and chemotherapy and can be employed to define how low doses of chemotherapy in combination with checkpoint inhibitors can induce robust immune responses (therapy-mediated vaccination). Thus it is not surprising that scientists as well as private organizations are currently exploring these strategies (https://www.jax.org/news-and-insights/jax-blog/2015/april/the-next-big-thing-in-cancer-modeling-patient-derived-xenografts-in-humaniz).

Although highly sophisticated and extremely useful, humanized models require high levels of technical skills and dedicated personnel and they remain very expensive, which limits the wide distribution and utilization of these PDX tumor models.

Development of Unrelated Malignancies

In mice xenograft models, multiple factors, infectious and noninfectious, have been linked to the development of tumors that are different from the implanted tumor xenografts. Some of these tumors are of murine origin, whereas others originate from nontumor cells from the implanted tissue. Development of these unrelated tumors can either cause failure of engraftment of the intended tumor or interfere with tumor development, tumor characteristics, and response to therapy.

Epstein-Barr Virus

One of the major viral agents identified is the Epstein-Barr Virus (EBV), which resides in human lymphoblastoid populations. For both solid and hematological disorders, the expansion of contaminating EBV+ lymphocytes in NSG mice, even from minute tissue samples, represents a common and serious limitation. The EBV-mediated lymphoma is being recognized as more common than previously thought.

Efficacious approaches to eliminate EBV contamination are largely impractical or financially prohibitive. In the case of solid tumors, the possibility of using anti-B-cell agents, ie, rituximab, in complement-efficient mice may represent a valuable solution. This approach, however, cannot be used in the generation of PDX of patients with B-cell lymphoproliferative disorders. In this latter scenario, the implementation of autologous anti-EBV T cells or engineered T cells may be a promising avenue but is technically challenging.[75,76] There are anecdotal reports that passaging the tumor through nude mice, if possible, may eliminate the EBV-related lymphoma.

Mouse Viruses

Mouse viruses that are endogenous or those contaminating biologicals can also lead to tumors that interfere with the primary PDX. In SCID (and NSG) mice, the NOD genome contains multiple copies of a unique endogenous ecotropic murine leukemia provirus locus (Emv-30, mapped to the proximal region of chromosome 11), typified by the family of murine leukemia virus (MuLV). This provirus was indicated in thymomagenesis in SCIDs.[77] In 2014 a report indicated that human tumor-mediated paracrine stimulation can induce AML of mouse origin, and that Emv-30 provirus can cause the origination of neoplasia without a recombination event.[78] MuLV is also known to contaminate human tumor cell lines that are passaged in mice, including three cell lines from the NCI-60 cell line collection at NCI-Frederick.[79,80] Similarly, Matrigel contaminations of lactate dehydrogenase–elevating virus are undesirable and difficult to eliminate.[51,81] Mouse parvovirus is another agent that can reside in tumor tissue and interfere with the tumor growth and pathology. While biological contaminants can be avoided by stringent quality control of tissues and biologicals, as well as high-quality rodent health monitoring programs, detection of activation of endogenous viruses may need frequent tumor characterization as well as testing mice for contamination.

Horizontal Oncogenesis

A third way of contamination of PDX tumors by tumors of murine origin is by recruitment and transformation of mouse cells by human tumors. This phenomenon was reported in 1982 as "horizontal oncogenesis"[82] in nude mice carrying human xenografts. Although its incidence is relatively low, it has been reported sporadically.[83] There could be multiple ways of horizontal oncogenesis. It was reported that non-cell-of-origin-derived cells within the glioma environment in the mouse can be corrupted to become bona fide tumor, which deviates from the generally established view of gliomagenesis.[84] Jacobsen et al. reported direct evidence using an experimental model system for the malignant transformation of normal host stroma induced by fusion with malignant epithelium.[85] The hybrid cells thus generated were capable of forming highly aggressive tumors, demonstrating significant role of stroma in the growth of the tumor that has contribution from the mouse host.

Therefore, continuous improvement of mouse models through use of transgenic techniques and immunomodulation as well as better understanding the tumor microenvironment is critical. More efficient data-gathering techniques, including advanced imaging techniques are critical in using mouse models for the best outcome. Equally important is guarding against pathogens and tumorigenic processes that can take advantage of the limitations of the host and have the potential of significantly altering/influencing the PDX experiment.

CLINICAL TRIALS AND DATA REPORTING

With the development of personalized programs for the treatment of cancer patients, the molecular stratification of patients (ie, single nucleotide polymorphism profile) and their tumors are a prerequisite for the delivery of the most appropriate therapies and the right dosage. In the arena of drug development and clinical trials the old paradigm of delivering a single combination of compounds to patients with similar histological disorders has become obsolete. The design of umbrella, basket, and matched trails has brought new hopes and unlocked innovative applications. A similar approach is now being performed using either genetically engineered mouse models (GEMM) or PDX mice, within the general framework of the mouse hospital.[86,87] Thus, coclinical mouse trials can be concurrently executed in parallel with human trials, providing the unique opportunity to predict responses, anticipate toxicity, and facilitate real-time patients' adjustments.[86,88] This design enables the delivery of identical treatments to both the human patients and the corresponding PDXs and rapid translation of the data into the clinic arena.

So far, several pre- or coclinical trials have tested the efficacy of drugs specifically targeting drivers of aberrant genetic defects of human cancers,[86,88,89] either in GEMM or PDX models. Pitter and colleagues evaluated a combination of AKT and mTOR inhibitors in human glioblastoma,[90] and Bertotti et al. proved that overexpressing HER cetuximab-resistant colon cancer PDXs are effectively treated by inhibiting the HER2 signaling pathway.[2] Of note, both mouse studies fostered the design of human trials currently underway at the Memorial Sloan Kettering Cancer Center (NCT01051557) and in Italy under the guidelines of the Institute for Cancer Research and Treatment at Candiolo, respectively. In line with these investigations, Von Hoff[91] and Frese[92] have demonstrated that the combination of gemcitabine plus nab-paclitaxel in mice was an active regimen in patients with advanced pancreatic cancer. This led to a phase 3 clinical trial, which confirmed the original phase 1 and 2 data, and further established that nab-paclitaxel plus gemcitabine improved overall survival, progression-free survival, and response rate of pancreatic cancer patients.[93]

In 2011, Hidalgo's group explored an alternative usage of PDXs.[94] In their study, they tested 63 drugs, resulting in 232 treatment regimens, in PDX models derived from chemorefractory tumor cells. Although this approach was highly demanding and very costly, it demonstrated the power of PDX in searching for personalized treatment in a selected cohort of patients. We envision that this strategy can now be used to test small libraries of compounds targeting well-defined lesions in relatively limited libraries of PDX bearing identical mutations, or from PDX derived from naive or chemoresistant individuals. Finally, cell lines or short in vitro culture of PDX cells may be used to select drug candidates from large chemical libraries. Positive hits can be then cross-validated in the same PDX from which the lines were derived or alternatively in other PDXs, bearing lesions with same phenotypes or genetic defects. It is likely that the most efficient use of PDX models will result from a combination of innovative in vitro and in vivo models used simultaneously to support drug discovery, high-throughput screening, and coclinical trials data and predict patient response. Moreover, the best combination of models may vary by the cancer and tumor type. Thus, the development of a comprehensive, universally accessible database will be a critical part of the required infrastructure to guide best practices and use of resources.

Although these objectives are highly desirable, mouse clinical trials are still surrounded with many technical and scientific uncertainties that need to be solved before their usage will be collectively embraced. Indeed, the establishment of mouse hospitals entails the construction of dedicated facilities (imaging, surgical suits, etc.) and integrated programs which bridge clinical, experimental, translational, and research units and dedicated pharmacy suites.[87] These requirements are currently impairing a broader utilization of PDX models, whose comprehensive usage remains limited to big pharma[31] and to selected institutions. Moreover, the cost of generating and maintaining PDX models is at present prohibitive and thus we anticipate that combined mouse and human trials will only flourish after lower costs are reached and larger collections of PDX are readily available. In parallel, the efficacy of PDX models in guiding the therapy for individual cancer patients and improving the success of human clinical trials must be proven. If this is achieved, clinical oncologists will be more likely to perform concurrent mouse and human trials, a practice that has not yet been accepted into the experimental oncology arena.

Many studies have already proved that PDX are highly informative and more predictive than conventional in vitro models for the selection of novel and/or effective drugs.[27,31,40,95–98] Thus we anticipate that PDX will become the preferred tool in future preclinical drug programs.

Nevertheless, PDX trials still require standardized protocols and more universal data analyses. Actually, many studies have been using individualized protocols and the global community is still missing a uniform approach to the design and execution of preclinical studies. This is critical to address issues like human cancer heterogeneity, to dissect the complex genomic landscape of cancers, and to discover the great variety of mechanisms leading to cancer resistance. Dose and time schedules and ultimately different results (tumor regression, biomarkers, progression-free survival and overall survival, tumor recurrence) remain quite variable among different studies and unified protocols will be mandatory to address these problems.

Finally, we need to apply the same biostatistical rules and strategies that are in place in human trials for the analysis of the PDX-derived data.[99–101] These will ultimately dictate the appropriate number of mice and the selection of drugs for further clinical development. Since the number of mice that can be tested needs to be relatively small, innovative biochemical/molecular readouts and statistical analyses should be developed. Toward this end the identification of biomarkers may improve clinical prediction in selected subgroups of cancer patients.[102] Moreover, the discovery of biomarkers will facilitate the transition from unselected randomized controlled clinical trials to biomarker-driven clinical trials; this, however, requires new discovery modalities and improved preclinical models of cancer.[103] Integration of PDX from naive and chemoresistant tumors and genomic platforms is expected to decipher mechanisms of acquired drug resistance that emerge over time and support the discovery of clinical biomarkers of chemoresistance.[104]

CURRENT AND FUTURE ACCESSIBILITY OF PDX MODELS

It is now accepted that the global success of PDX models will depend on the creation of large and well-annotated libraries and on their collective distribution and usage worldwide by the academic communities and the private sectors. In many smaller, academic programs, resources are focused on the creation and use of models for the laboratory's specific research purpose; resources for collaboration, documentation, and distribution of the models are not prioritized or available. Based on recent surveys, PDX centers have been established in North America, Europe, and Australia, and a few exist in China and Japan, with much fewer locations in South America and Middle Eastern countries. These initiatives have led to the creation of large pools of PDX libraries for most common human cancers in industrialized countries, with some clear deficiencies (ie, lymphoma PDX). Although highly ambitious, it is critical that similar initiatives are embraced in underrepresented countries and in specific geographic regions. Indeed, only when a universal PDX program is in place will it be possible to study models of rare cancers seen in unique populations, selected regions, or from different ethnicities. The universal PDX libraries will thus become an invaluable tool to define the oncogenic role of driver mutations and their association with different codrivers as well as a platform to dissect the role of infective agents in different races and genomic landscapes.

Of note, surveys showed that biobanks are infrequently used as a source of tumor for PDX studies. The use of biobanks should be promoted and supported as a worldwide resource.

Although the current PDX programs are mainly present in industrialized countries, the new initiatives sponsored by national institutes and foundations constitute a valuable asset from which an integrated network can be constructed. Relevant initiatives are currently supported by the France Center of Resource for Experimental Models of Cancer consortium, by dedicated European programs, and by the NCI in the United States. The next step will be to somehow integrate these separate programs to create larger consortia. This is only possible via a close and productive international cooperation, dedicated infrastructures, and adequate financial support from national/international programs, private foundations, and pharmaceutical industries. Toward this end, we hope that such a universal program will be embraced by international organizations like the World Health Organization.

Nevertheless, several hurdles still need to be unraveled. Effective and sophisticated PDX units require professional teams and dedicated infrastructures that are very expensive, which limits the development and broad utilization of PDX. Costs can be decreased by expanding the number of established PDX lines, improving SOPs, and streamlining mouse clinical trials. We also predict that educational courses and dedicated programs will create a new generation of professional operators and that closer relationships between basic scientists, translational scientists, and oncologists will be encouraged. As part of this, expert clinical-scientists in PDX models will become critical. The complexities of transfer regulations, intellectual property rights, and commercialization represent additional obstacles that have greatly constrained the general expansion of the PDX methodology. Thus, new attention should be focused on biobanking[105] and streamlining processes to support the academic and industrial usage of PDXs.[106–108] Finally, dedicated laboratory information management systems should be constructed and adopted among units within a PDX network.[109]

Finally, we are convinced that the most successful application of PDX will only be reached by rigorous, complete, and consistent clinical and molecular annotation of PDX models. Indeed, the current lack of a comprehensive genomic characterization of engrafted tumors is a clear limitation. It is very important that scientists and private organizations recognize the critical value of fully annotated models and of genomic fingerprints of matched normal controls, primary lesions, and patient-matched PDXs. These requirements are essential to avoid expansive and time-consuming research activities on poorly annotated and scantly informative models. In this context, dedicated support is necessary to create public repositories for the upload and storage of clinical, genomic, and functional data. This in turn will encourage an open and widespread use of PDX models. Annotated libraries are also anticipated to improve patients' stratification and anticancer treatments, as molecular/biological fingerprints will drive therapeutic decisions. Moreover, it will be possible to identify unique functional subsets of tumors that will foster the development of up front "ad hoc" therapies in cancer patients.

In conclusion, PDXs represent an extremely promising model for the study and characterization of human cancers. Although there are several problems that must be resolved, PDXs will indeed provide invaluable information on the tumor biology and the host–tumor interactions, and they will eventually contribute to improving the daily management of many cancer patients.

REFERENCES

1. Ledford H. US Cancer Institute to overhaul tumour cell lines. Veteran cells to be retired in favour of fresh tumour samples grown in mice. *Nature* 2016;**530**(391).
2. Bertotti A, Migliardi G, Galimi F, et al. A molecularly annotated platform of patient-derived xenografts ("xenopatients") identifies HER2 as an effective therapeutic target in cetuximab-resistant colorectal cancer. *Cancer Discov* 2011;**1**(6):508–23.
3. Garrido-Laguna I, Uson M, Rajeshkumar NV, et al. Tumor engraftment in nude mice and enrichment in stroma- related gene pathways predict poor survival and resistance to gemcitabine in patients with pancreatic cancer. *Clin Cancer Res* 2011;**17**(17):5793–800.
4. Nemati F, Sastre-Garau X, Laurent C, et al. Establishment and characterization of a panel of human uveal melanoma xenografts derived from primary and/or metastatic tumors. *Clin Cancer Res* 2010;**16**(8):2352–62.
5. Bagnara D, Kaufman MS, Calissano C, et al. A novel adoptive transfer model of chronic lymphocytic leukemia suggests a key role for T lymphocytes in the disease. *Blood* 2011;**117**(20):5463–72.

6. Sun S, Zhang Z. Patient-derived xenograft platform of OSCC: a renewable human bio-bank for preclinical cancer research and a new co-clinical model for treatment optimization. *Front Med* 2016;**10**(1).
7. Guerrera F, Tabbo F, Bessone L, et al. The influence of tissue ischemia time on RNA integrity and patient-derived xenografts (PDX) engraftment rate in a non-small cell lung cancer (NSCLC) biobank. *PLoS One* 2016;**11**(1):e0145100.
8. Gu Q, Zhang B, Sun H, et al. Genomic characterization of a large panel of patient-derived hepatocellular carcinoma xenograft tumor models for preclinical development. *Oncotarget* 2015;**6**(24):20160–76.
9. Lawrence MG, Pook DW, Wang H, et al. Establishment of primary patient-derived xenografts of palliative TURP specimens to study castrate-resistant prostate cancer. *Prostate* 2015;**75**(13):1475–83.
10. Russell PJ, Russell P, Rudduck C, Tse BW, Williams ED, Raghavan D. Establishing prostate cancer patient derived xenografts: lessons learned from older studies. *Prostate* 2015;**75**(6):628–36.
11. Godebu E, Muldong M, Strasner A, et al. PCSD1, a new patient-derived model of bone metastatic prostate cancer, is castrate-resistant in the bone-niche. *J Transl Med* 2014;**12**:275.
12. Williams ES, Rodriquez-Bravo V, Chippada-Venkata U, et al. Generation of prostate cancer patient derived xenograft models from circulating tumor cells. *J Vis Exp* 2015;**105**:53182.
13. Anderson WC, Boyd MB, Aguilar J, et al. Initiation and characterization of small cell lung cancer patient-derived xenografts from ultrasound-guided transbronchial needle aspirates. *PLoS One* 2015;**10**(5):e0125255.
14. Allaway RJ, Fischer DA, de Abreu FB, et al. Genomic characterization of patient-derived xenograft models established from fine needle aspirate biopsies of a primary pancreatic ductal adenocarcinoma and from patient-matched metastatic sites. *Oncotarget* 2016;**7**(13).
15. Gandara DR, Mack PC, Bult C, et al. Bridging tumor genomics to patient outcomes through an integrated patient-derived xenograft platform. *Clin Lung Cancer* 2015;**16**(3):165–72.
16. Hodgkinson CL, Morrow CJ, Li Y, et al. Tumorigenicity and genetic profiling of circulating tumor cells in small-cell lung cancer. *Nat Med* 2014;**20**(8):897–903.
17. Bakhach J. The cryopreservation of composite tissues: principles and recent advancement on cryopreservation of different type of tissues. *Organogenesis* 2009;**5**(3):119–26.
18. Ketheesan N, Kearney JN, Ingham E. The effect of cryopreservation on the immunogenicity of allogeneic cardiac valves. *Cryobiology* 1996;**33**(1):41–53.
19. Ingham E, Matthews JB, Kearney JN, Gowland G. The effects of variation of cryopreservation protocols on the immunogenicity of allogeneic skin grafts. *Cryobiology* 1993;**30**(5):443–58.
20. Baust JM, Van B, Baust JG. Cell viability improves following inhibition of cryopreservation-induced apoptosis. *In Vitro Cell Dev Biol Anim* 2000;**36**(4):262–70.
21. Maekawa H, Tadanori Y, Kawada K, Yoshiharu S. Summary of 50 cases of patient derived colorectal cancer xenografts: problems and tips to obtain appropriate results in translational researches. In: *AACR special conference on patient derived cancer models: present and future applications from basic science to the clinic New Orleans*. 2016.
22. Mattie M, Christensen A, Chang MS, et al. Molecular characterization of patient-derived human pancreatic tumor xenograft models for preclinical and translational development of cancer therapeutics. *Neoplasia* 2013;**15**(10):1124–36.
23. Sivanand S, Pena-Llopis S, Zhao H, et al. A validated tumorgraft model reveals activity of dovitinib against renal cell carcinoma. *Sci Transl Med* 2012;**4**(137).
24. Visonneau S, Cesano A, Torosian MH, Miller EJ, Santoli D. Growth characteristics and metastatic properties of human breast cancer xenografts in immunodeficient mice. *Am J Pathol* 1998;**152**(5):1299–311.

25. Fleming JM, Miller TC, Meyer MJ, Ginsburg E, Vonderhaar BK. Local regulation of human breast xenograft models. *J Cell Physiol* 2010;**224**(3):795–806.
26. Vockentanz L, Nopora A. Development of next generation breast cancer PDX models by applying intramammary fat pad and intra ductal tumor transfer. In: *AACR special conference on patient derived cancer models: present and future applications from basic science to the clinic New Orleans*. 2016.
27. Hidalgo M, Amant F, Biankin AV, et al. Patient-derived xenograft models: an emerging platform for translational cancer research. *Cancer Discov* 2014;**4**(9):998–1013.
28. Rafii S, Butler JM, Ding BS. Angiocrine functions of organ-specific endothelial cells. *Nature* 2016;**529**(7586):316–25.
29. Morton CL, Houghton PJ. Establishment of human tumor xenografts in immunodeficient mice. *Nat Protoc* 2007;**2**(2):247–50.
30. Pan CX, Zhang H, Tepper CG, et al. Development and characterization of bladder cancer patient-derived xenografts for molecularly guided targeted therapy. *PLoS One* 2015;**10**(8):e0134346.
31. Gao H, Korn JM, Ferretti S, et al. High-throughput screening using patient-derived tumor xenografts to predict clinical trial drug response. *Nat Med* 2015;**21**(11):1318–25.
32. Clappier E, Gerby B, Sigaux F, et al. Clonal selection in xenografted human T cell acute lymphoblastic leukemia recapitulates gain of malignancy at relapse. *J Exp Med* 2011;**208**(4): 653–61.
33. Petrillo LA, Wolf DM, Kapoun AM, et al. Xenografts faithfully recapitulate breast cancer-specific gene expression patterns of parent primary breast tumors. *Breast Cancer Res Treat* 2012;**135**(3):913–22.
34. Eirew P, Steif A, Khattra J, et al. Dynamics of genomic clones in breast cancer patient xenografts at single-cell resolution. *Nature* 2015;**518**(7539):422–6.
35. Isella C, Terrasi A, Bellomo SE, et al. Stromal contribution to the colorectal cancer transcriptome. *Nat Genet* 2015;**47**(4):312–9.
36. Calon A, Lonardo E, Berenguer-Llergo A, et al. Stromal gene expression defines poor-prognosis subtypes in colorectal cancer. *Nat Genet* 2015;**47**(4):320–U362.
37. Poirier JT, Gardner EE, Connis N, et al. DNA methylation in small cell lung cancer defines distinct disease subtypes and correlates with high expression of EZH2. *Oncogene* 2015;**34**(48):5869–78.
38. Ding L, Ellis MJ, Li SQ, et al. Genome remodelling in a basal-like breast cancer metastasis and xenograft. *Nature* 2010;**464**(7291):999–1005.
39. Garrido-Laguna I, Uson M, Rajeshkumar NV, et al. Tumor engraftment in nude mice and enrichment in stroma-related gene pathways predict poor survival and resistance to gemcitabine in patients with pancreatic cancer. *Clin Cancer Res* 2011;**17**(17):5793–800.
40. Stewart EL, Mascaux C, Pham NA, et al. Clinical utility of patient-derived xenografts to determine biomarkers of prognosis and map resistance pathways in EGFR-mutant lung adenocarcinoma. *J Clin Oncol* 2015;**33**(22):2472–U2494.
41. Daniel VC, Marchionni L, Hierman JS, et al. A primary xenograft model of small-cell lung cancer reveals irreversible changes in gene expression imposed by culture in vitro. *Cancer Res* 2009;**69**(8):3364–73.
42. Dangles-Marie V, Pocard M, Richon S, et al. Establishment of human colon cancer cell lines from fresh tumors versus xenografts: comparison of success rate and cell line features. *Cancer Res* 2007;**67**(1):398–407.
43. Liu XF, Ory V, Chapman S, et al. Rock inhibitor and feeder cells induce the conditional reprogramming of epithelial cells. *Am J Pathol* 2012;**180**(2):599–607.
44. Crystal AS, Shaw AT, Sequist LV, et al. Patient-derived models of acquired resistance can identify effective drug combinations for cancer. *Science* 2014;**346**(6216):1480–6.

45. Gao D, Vela I, Sboner A, et al. Organoid cultures derived from patients with advanced prostate cancer. *Cell* 2014;**159**(1):176–87.
46. Sato T, Vries RG, Snippert HJ, et al. Single Lgr5 stem cells build crypt-villus structures in vitro without a mesenchymal niche. *Nature* 2009;**459**(7244):262–5.
47. Boj SF, Hwang CI, Baker LA, et al. Organoid models of human and mouse ductal pancreatic cancer. *Cell* 2015;**160**(1–2):324–38.
48. Matano M, Date S, Shimokawa M, et al. Modeling colorectal cancer using CRISPR-Cas9-mediated engineering of human intestinal organoids. *Nat Med* 2015;**21**(3):256–62.
49. Pauli C, Puca L, Robinson BD, et al. An emerging role for cytopathology in precision oncology. *Lab Investig* 2016;**96**:113A.
50. Weiswald LB, Richon S, Validire P, et al. Newly characterised ex vivo colospheres as a three-dimensional colon cancer cell model of tumour aggressiveness. *Br J Cancer* 2009;**101**(3):473–82.
51. Liu HP, Patel MR, Prescher JA, et al. Cancer stem cells from human breast tumors are involved in spontaneous metastases in orthotopic mouse models. *Proc Natl Acad Sci USA* 2010;**107**(42):18115–20.
52. Jaffee EM, Dranoff G, Cohen LK, et al. High-efficiency gene-transfer into primary human tumor explants without cell selection. *Cancer Res* 1993;**53**(10):2221–6.
53. Vick B, Rothenberg M, Sandhofer N, et al. An advanced preclinical mouse model for acute myeloid leukemia using patients' cells of various genetic subgroups and in vivo bioluminescence imaging. *PLoS One* 2015;**10**(3):e0120925.
54. Terziyska N, Alves CC, Groiss V, et al. In vivo imaging enables high resolution preclinical trials on patients' leukemia cells growing in mice. *PLoS One* 2012;**7**(12).
55. Song LJ, Kauss MA, Kopin E, et al. Optimizing the transduction efficiency of capsid-modified AAV6 serotype vectors in primary human hematopoietic stem cells in vitro and in a xenograft mouse model in vivo. *Cytotherapy* 2013;**15**(8):986–98.
56. Vick B, Rothenberg M, Sandhofer N, et al. An advanced preclinical mouse model for acute myeloid leukemia using patients' cells of various genetic subgroups and in vivo bioluminescence imaging. *PLoS One* 2015;**10**(3).
57. Picco G, Petti C, Trusolino L, Bertotti A, Medico E. A diphtheria toxin resistance marker for in vitro and in vivo selection of stably transduced human cells. *Sci Rep* 2015;**5**.
58. Braekeveldt N, Wigerup C, Gisselsson D, et al. Neuroblastoma patient-derived orthotopic xenografts retain metastatic patterns and geno- and phenotypes of patient tumours. *Int J Cancer* 2015;**136**(5):E252–61.
59. Blattmann C, Thiemann M, Stenzinger A, et al. Establishment of a patient-derived orthotopic osteosarcoma mouse model. *J Transl Med* 2015;**13**:136.
60. Ellis L, Shah P, Hammers H, et al. Vascular disruption in combination with mTOR inhibition in renal cell carcinoma. *Mol Cancer Ther* 2012;**11**(2):383–92.
61. Girotti MR, Gremel G, Lee R, et al. Application of sequencing, liquid biopsies and patient-derived xenografts for personalized medicine in melanoma. *Cancer Discov* 2015;**6**(3).
62. Saito Y, Yuki H, Kuratani M, et al. A pyrrolo-pyrimidine derivative targets human primary AML stem cells in vivo. *Sci Transl Med* 2013;**5**(181). 181ra152.
63. Thanopoulou E, Cashman J, Kakagianne T, Eaves A, Zoumbos N, Eaves C. Engraftment of NOD/SCID-beta2 microglobulin null mice with multilineage neoplastic cells from patients with myelodysplastic syndrome. *Blood* 2004;**103**(11):4285–93.
64. Muguruma Y, Matsushita H, Yahata T, et al. Establishment of a xenograft model of human myelodysplastic syndromes. *Haematologica* 2011;**96**(4):543–51.

65. Zhang X, Claerhout S, Prat A, et al. A renewable tissue resource of phenotypically stable, biologically and ethnically diverse, patient-derived human breast cancer xenograft models. *Cancer Res* 2013;**73**(15):4885–97.
66. Hoffman RM. Patient-derived orthotopic xenografts: better mimic of metastasis than subcutaneous xenografts. *Nat Rev Cancer* 2015;**15**(8):451–2.
67. Vudattu NK, Waldron-Lynch F, Truman LA, et al. Humanized mice as a model for aberrant responses in human T cell immunotherapy. *J Immunol* 2014;**193**(2):587–96.
68. Proia DA, Kuperwasser C. Reconstruction of human mammary tissues in a mouse model. *Nat Protoc* 2006;**1**(1):206–14.
69. Ginestier C, Hur MH, Charafe-Jauffret E, et al. ALDH1 is a marker of normal and malignant human mammary stem cells and a predictor of poor clinical outcome. *Cell Stem Cell* 2007;**1**(5):555–67.
70. Zhang XM, Claerhout S, Prat A, et al. A renewable tissue resource of phenotypically stable, biologically and ethnically diverse, patient-derived human breast cancer xenograft models. *Cancer Res* 2013;**73**(15):4885–97.
71. Suetsugu A, Katz M, Fleming J, et al. Multi-color palette of fluorescent proteins for imaging the tumor microenvironment of orthotopic tumorgraft mouse models of clinical pancreatic cancer specimens. *J Cell Biochem* 2012;**113**(7):2290–5.
72. Shultz LD, Saito Y, Najima Y, et al. Generation of functional human T-cell subsets with HLA-restricted immune responses in HLA class I expressing NOD/SCID/IL2r gamma(null) humanized mice. *Proc Natl Acad Sci USA* 2010;**107**(29):13022–7.
73. Pino S, Brehm MA, Covassin-Barberis L, et al. Development of novel major histocompatibility complex class I and class II-deficient NOD-SCID IL2R gamma chain knockout mice for modeling human xenogeneic graft-versus-host disease. *Mouse Models Drug Discov Methods Protoc* 2010;**602**:105–17.
74. Morton JJ, Bird G, Keysar SB, et al. XactMice: humanizing mouse bone marrow enables microenvironment reconstitution in a patient-derived xenograft model of head and neck cancer. *Oncogene* 2016;**35**(3):290–300.
75. Hanley PJ, Cruz CR, Savoldo B, et al. Functionally active virus-specific T cells that target CMV, adenovirus, and EBV can be expanded from naive T-cell populations in cord blood and will target a range of viral epitopes. *Blood* 2009;**114**(9):1958–67.
76. De Angelis B, Dotti G, Quintarelli C, et al. Generation of Epstein-Barr virus-specific cytotoxic T lymphocytes resistant to the immunosuppressive drug tacrolimus (FK506). *Blood* 2009;**114**(23):4784–91.
77. Prochazka M, Gaskins HR, Shultz LD, Leiter EH. The nonobese diabetic scid mouse: model for spontaneous thymomagenesis associated with immunodeficiency. *Proc Natl Acad Sci USA* 1992;**89**(8):3290–4.
78. Triviai I, Ziegler M, Bergholz U, et al. Endogenous retrovirus induces leukemia in a xenograft mouse model for primary myelofibrosis. *Proc Natl Acad Sci USA* 2014;**111**(23):8595–600.
79. Sfanos KS, Aloia AL, Hicks JL, et al. Identification of replication competent murine gammaretroviruses in commonly used prostate cancer cell lines. *PLoS One* 2011;**6**(6):e20874.
80. Zhang YA, Maitra A, Hsieh JT, et al. Frequent detection of infectious xenotropic murine leukemia virus (XMLV) in human cultures established from mouse xenografts. *Cancer Biol Ther* 2011;**12**(7):617–28.
81. Whittle JR, Lewis MT, Lindeman GJ, Visvader JE. Patient-derived xenograft models of breast cancer and their predictive power. *Breast Cancer Res* 2015;**17**.

82. Goldenberg DM, Pavia RA. In vivo horizontal oncogenesis by a human tumor in nude mice. *Proc Natl Acad Sci USA* 1982;**79**(7):2389–92.
83. Menendez C, Salvador B, Munoz M, Banos N, Sarno F, Lopez-Cases PP. When murine tumors are thought to be human: a draw back of patient derived xenografts. In: *AACR special conference on patient derived cancer models: present and future applications from basic science to the clinic. New Orleans*. 2016.
84. Fomchenko EI, Dougherty JD, Helmy KY, et al. Recruited cells can become transformed and overtake PDGF-induced murine gliomas in vivo during tumor progression. *PLoS One* 2011;**6**(7):e20605.
85. Jacobsen BM, Harrell JC, Jedlicka P, Borges VF, Varella-Garcia M, Horwitz KB. Spontaneous fusion with, and transformation of mouse stroma by, malignant human breast cancer epithelium. *Cancer Res* 2006;**66**(16):8274–9.
86. Nardella C, Lunardi A, Patnaik A, Cantley LC, Pandolfi PP. The APL paradigm and the "co-clinical trial" project. *Cancer Discov* 2011;**1**(2):108–16.
87. Clohessy JG, Pandolfi PP. Mouse hospital and co-clinical trial project–from bench to bedside. *Nat Rev Clin Oncol* 2015;**12**(8):491–8.
88. Chen Z, Cheng K, Walton Z, et al. A murine lung cancer co-clinical trial identifies genetic modifiers of therapeutic response. *Nature* 2012;**483**(7391):613–7.
89. Stebbing J, Paz K, Schwartz GK, et al. Patient-derived xenografts for individualized care in advanced sarcoma. *Cancer* 2014;**120**(13):2006–15.
90. Pitter KL, Galban CJ, Galban S, et al. Perifosine and CCI 779 co-operate to induce cell death and decrease proliferation in PTEN-intact and PTEN-deficient PDGF-driven murine glioblastoma. *PLoS One* 2011;**6**(1):e14545.
91. Von Hoff DD, Ramanathan RK, Borad MJ, et al. Gemcitabine plus nab-paclitaxel is an active regimen in patients with advanced pancreatic cancer: a phase I/II trial. *J Clin Oncol* 2011;**29**(34):4548–54.
92. Frese KK, Neesse A, Cook N, et al. nab-Paclitaxel potentiates gemcitabine activity by reducing cytidine deaminase levels in a mouse model of pancreatic cancer. *Cancer Discov* 2012;**2**(3):260–9.
93. Von Hoff DD, Ervin T, Arena FP, et al. Increased survival in pancreatic cancer with nab-paclitaxel plus gemcitabine. *N Engl J Med* 2013;**369**(18):1691–703.
94. Hidalgo M, Bruckheimer E, Rajeshkumar NV, et al. A pilot clinical study of treatment guided by personalized tumorgrafts in patients with advanced cancer. *Mol Cancer Ther* 2011;**10**(8):1311–6.
95. Marangoni E, Poupon MF. Patient-derived tumour xenografts as models for breast cancer drug development. *Curr Opin Oncol* 2014;**26**(6):556–61.
96. Fichtner I, Slisow W, Gill J, et al. Anticancer drug response and expression of molecular markers in early-passage xenotransplanted colon carcinomas. *Eur J Cancer* 2004;**40**(2):298–307.
97. Weroha SJ, Becker MA, Enderica-Gonzalez S, et al. Tumorgrafts as in vivo surrogates for women with ovarian cancer. *Clin Cancer Res* 2014;**20**(5):1288–97.
98. Migliardi G, Sassi F, Torti D, et al. Inhibition of MEK and PI3K/mTOR suppresses tumor growth but does not cause tumor regression in patient-derived xenografts of RAS-mutant colorectal carcinomas. *Clin Cancer Res* 2012;**18**(9):2515–25.
99. Ma J, Hobbs BP, Stingo FC. Statistical methods for establishing personalized treatment rules in oncology. *Biomed Res Int* 2015;**2015**:670691.
100. Chen Y, Chen Z, Mori M. A new statistical decision rule for single-arm phase II oncology trials. *Stat Methods Med Res* 2016;**25**(1):118–32.
101. Jeong JH. Statistical analysis in cancer clinical trials. *Anticancer Drugs* 2008;**19**(Suppl. 1):S9–10.

102. Jimeno A, Tan AC, Coffa J, et al. Coordinated epidermal growth factor receptor pathway gene overexpression predicts epidermal growth factor receptor inhibitor sensitivity in pancreatic cancer. *Cancer Res* 2008;**68**(8):2841–9.
103. Gandara DR, Li T, Lara Jr PN, et al. Algorithm for codevelopment of new drug-predictive biomarker combinations: accounting for inter- and intrapatient tumor heterogeneity. *Clin Lung Cancer* 2012;**13**(5):321–5.
104. Gandara DR, Van Dyke T, Z W-O, et al. Enhancing EGFR-directed therapies through a novel research platform integrating data from genetically engineered mice, patient derived xenografts and clinical trials (IGXT). *J Thor Oncol* 2011;**6**.
105. Macilotti M, Penasa S, Tomasi M. Consent, privacy and property in the Italian biobanks regulation: a hybrid model within EU? *Ethics Law Gov Biobanking Natl Eur Int Approaches* 2015;**14**:53–77.
106. Anderson M. Xenotransplantation: a bioethical evaluation. *J Med Ethics* 2006;**32**(4):205–8.
107. Kelland LR. Of mice and men: values and liabilities of the athymic nude mouse model in anticancer drug development. *Eur J Cancer* 2004;**40**(6):827–36.
108. Bertotti A, Trusolino L. From bench to bedside: does preclinical practice in translational oncology need some rebuilding? *JNCI Journal Natl Cancer Inst* 2013;**105**(19):1426–7.
109. Baralis E, Bertotti A, Fiori A, Grand ALAS. A software platform to support oncological data management. *J Med Syst* 2012;**36**(1):S81–90.

Index

'*Note:* Page numbers followed by "f" indicate figures and "t" indicate tables.'

H

I

O

P

R

U

V

W

X

Kolibri 360 GmbH
Ferdinand-Jühlke-Straße 7
99095 Erfurt, Deutschland
produktsicherheit@kolibri360.de